DRUGS AND THE FUTURE:

BRAIN SCIENCE, ADDICTION AND SOCIETY

Drugs and the Future: Brain Science, Addiction and Society

Scientific Coordinators

DAVID NUTT
Psychopharmacology Unit, University of Bristol, UK

TREVOR W. ROBBINS
Department of Experimental Psychology and MRC
Centre for Behavioural and Clinical Neuroscience, University of Cambridge, UK

GERALD V. STIMSON
International Harm Reduction Association, Melbourne, Australia

MARTIN INCE
Science Writer, London, UK

and

ANDREW JACKSON
Department of Trade and Industry, UK

ELSEVIER

AMSTERDAM • BOSTON • HEIDELBERG • LONDON
NEW YORK • OXFORD • PARIS • SAN DIEGO
SAN FRANCISCO • SINGAPORE • SYDNEY • TOKYO

Academic Press is an imprint of Elsevier

While the Office of Science and Innovation commissioned a portion of these reviews, the views are those of the authors, are independent of Government and do not constitute government policy.

Academic Press is an imprint of Elsevier
30 Corporate Drive, Suite 400, Burlington, MA 01803, USA
525 B Street, Suite 1900, San Diego, California 92101-4495, USA
84 Theobald's Road, London WC1X 8RR, UK

This book is printed on acid-free paper. ∞

Library of Congress Cataloging-in-Publication Data
Application submitted

British Library Cataloguing-in-Publication Data
A catalogue record for this book is available from the British Library.

ISBN 13: 978-0-12-370624-9
ISBN 10: 0-12-370624-6

For information on all Academic Press publications
visit our Web site at www.books.elsevier.com

Printed in the United States of America
06 07 08 09 10   9 8 7 6 5 4 3 2 1

Contents

Contributors

Richard Ashcroft
Imperial College, London, UK

David Ball
King's College, University of London, UK

Virginia Berridge
London School of Hygiene and Tropical
Medicine
London, UK

Alastair V Campbell
Centre for Ethics in Medicine
University of Bristol, UK

Ben Capps
University of Bristol, UK

Rudolf N Cardinal
Department of Experimental Psychology
and MRC Centre for Behavioural and
Clinical Neuroscience
University of Cambridge, UK

Jonathan Cave
University of Warwick, UK

David Cowan
University of London, UK

Val Curran
University College, London, UK

Patricia DiCiano
Department of Experimental Psychology
and MRC Centre for Behavioural and
Clinical Neuroscience
University of Cambridge, UK

Colin Drummond
St George's Hospital Medical School,
London, UK

Theodora Duka
University of Sussex, UK

Barry J Everitt
Department of Experimental Psychology
and MRC Centre for Behavioural and
Clinical Neuroscience
University of Cambridge, UK

Hugh Garavan
Trinity College, Dublin, Eire

Christine Godfrey
University of York, UK

Peter W Halligan
School of Psychology
Cardiff University, UK

Gordon Hay
Centre for Drug Misuse Research
University of Glasgow, UK

Kim GC Hellemans
Department of Experimental Psychology
and MRC Centre for Behavioural and
Clinical Neuroscience
University of Cambridge, UK

Tim Hickman
University of Lancaster, UK

Brian Hurwitz
King's College, University of London, UK

Leslie Iversen
University of Oxford, UK

Andrew Jackson
Office of Science and Innovation,
Department of Trade and Industry, UK

Roy Jones
The Research Institute for the
Care of the Elderly, Bath, UK

Terry Jones
University of Manchester, UK

Jonathan LC Lee
Department of Experimental Psychology
and MRC Centre for Behavioural and
Clinical Neuroscience
University of Cambridge, UK

Anne Lingford-Hughes
University of Bristol, UK

Charlie Lloyd
York, UK

Neil McKeganey
Centre for Drug Misuse Research
University of Glasgow, UK

Kelly Morris
University of Bristol, UK

Peter Morris
University of Nottingham, UK

Joanne Neale
School of Health and Social Care
Oxford Brookes University, UK

David Nutt
University of Bristol, UK

Jim Orford
Alcohol, Drugs, Gambling and Addiction
Research Group, School of Psychology,
University of Birmingham, UK

David Osselton
Forensic Science Service, UK

Marcus Pembrey
University of Bristol, UK

Ian Ragan
CIR Consulting Ltd,
London, UK

Trevor W. Robbins
Department of Experimental Psychology
and MRC Centre for Behavioural and
Clinical Neuroscience
University of Cambridge, UK

Steven Robinson
Forensic Science Service, UK

Robin Room
School of Population Health, Melbourne
University, and AER Alcohol Policy
Research Centre, Turning Point
Alcohol & Drug Centre, Melbourne,
Australia

John Rothwell
University College, London, UK

Barbara Sahakian
University of Cambridge, UK

David N. Stephens
University of Sussex, UK

Gerald V. Stimson
International Harm Reduction Association,
Australia

Caroline Tapping
King's College, University of London, UK

Danielle Turner
University of Cambridge, UK

Neil Vickers
King's College, University of London, UK

Steve Williams
Institute of Psychiatry, UK

Foreword
Drugs and the Future

Charles R. Schuster, PhD

Distinguished Professor of Psychiatry and Behavioral Neurosciences
Wayne State University School of Medicine

The use of psychotropic drugs to modify sensation, perception, mood, and behaviour has been ubiquitous in human societies since time immemorial. Alcohol, caffeine, coca, nicotine, opium, peyote, marijuana, mescaline and many other substances have been used in a variety of cultures in the world for religious ceremonies, healing by shamans, or as a brief escape from the rigours of a difficult existence. The scientific development of safe and effective psychotropic drugs for the treatment of psychiatric and neurological disorders is, however, a relatively recent phenomenon. Only in the past 50 years have we developed highly specific and effective drugs for the treatment of neurological and psychiatric disorders. Progress is being made in our understanding of the pathophysiology of neurodegenerative and psychiatric disorders including substance abuse and dependence. Coincident with these significant therapeutic gains, we are learning more about the fundamental neural mechanisms underlying cognition, motor function, perception, motivation, and mood states. Unquestionably, we will see continued progress in our understanding of the etiology of neurological and psychiatric disease states and, hopefully, in the development of ways to prevent and more effectively treat these problems. In so doing we will inexorably discover new means to alter our mood, perceptions and cognition.

We have in the past generally discounted the possibility that psychotropic agents might be useful for improving normal performance. Extensive research has demonstrated that certain medications can enhance cognitive and motor task performance that has been degraded by fatigue or boredom. The United Sates Department of Defense, for example, sanctions the use of such drugs for pilots who must remain on duty for extended periods of time. Now, however, we are faced with the likelihood of discovering new psychotropic agents that will augment the optimal performance of non-disordered individuals, allowing them to work not only longer, but also more efficiently and productively. It is also likely that we will develop – through rational design or serendipity – psychotropic agents that can enhance such human qualities as empathy, sympathy, spirituality, and compassion. Psychotropic drugs have been used by many to enhance creativity, with mixed results. Undoubtedly, as we continue mainstream development of psychotherapeutic agents, new 'psychedelic' agents will also be discovered. This will force us to give serious reconsideration to the manner in which we view the use of currently available 'psychedelic' agents that in most countries are banned as illegal drugs. Could these compounds and ones yet to be discovered lead to more creative thinking in the arts and sciences? Could they increase spirituality and feelings of compassion for the less fortunate? If they do, how will or should these agents be sanctioned and regulated?

What will all of this mean to future generations? Great promise, but the potential for unintended adverse consequences as well. I believe that the following ethical and procedural issues must be considered in sanctioning the development and distribution of psychotropic agents that enhance normal performance and other desirable human qualities. First, I am concerned about access to such psychotropic agents. Will they be prescribed by physicians? How will physicians decide for whom they will prescribe such psychotropic agents? How will they be paid for? If only individuals who can afford to pay for these agents can access them, are we further separating individuals by socioeconomic level? Are we in danger of creating a modern-day equivalent to a behavioural eugenics movement or a caste system? Further, will ambitious young workers escalate their use of such agents in an attempt to better compete with their peers? The current furore over the use of performance-enhancing anabolic steroids by athletes in the United States portends some of the problems we will have with 'steroids for the mind.' Finally, what will happen to one's sense of satisfaction for a job well done if the successful performance is at least partly attributable to a pill? If increased compassion or empathy can be achieved by ingesting a psychotropic agent, will this alter our veneration for these human attributes?

I do not mean to diminish the possible benefits that might accrue from new psychotropic agents for enhancing normal performance and other desirable human qualities. It seems conceivable that, if an entire population received a psychotropic agent that boosts memory function, we would not equalise individual differences but rather increase the population mean for memory function. This could be true for all of the human mental functions that psychotropic agents might enhance. This is, of course, a utopian view, but conceivable. Unfortunately, the reality is that such agents would be disproportionately available for the wealthier nations' populations potentially further widening the socioeconomic gap between nations of the world.

As is true with all medications, fashioning rational policies requires that we balance the risks and benefits of these agents for the individual and society in general. We must also seriously consider alternatives to psychotropic agents for enhancing normal performance. Much can be achieved using educational and other behavioral approaches to enhance our mental performances. Clearly, we can also do a better job of nurturing the human qualities of empathy, compassion and spirituality by means other than psychotropic agents, probably at lower cost and with reduced likelihood of adverse side effects. Nevertheless, we should not prejudge the potential benefits of psychotropic agents for purposes other than treatment of disease. Whether or not we oppose this application of psychotropic drugs based on ethical principles, they will be developed. Once developed, it will be difficult to contain their distribution and use. It is far better that we begin our public discourse now on policies to productively use these agents rather than wait until they are here.

Introduction

Sir David King, ScD FRS
Chief Scientific Adviser to HM Government;
Head of the Office of Science and Innovation

From the day we are born to the day we die, drugs help to keep us healthy, happy and strong. Over the next 20 years, drugs for mental health treatments are likely to be important to a growing proportion of the population, and legal and illegal so-called 'recreational' drugs will continue to have a significant impact on society at every level.

Though the changes we saw in the second half of the twentieth century were dominated by developments in computers and telecommunications, biology and medicine also made huge strides. The greatest changes we will see in the twenty-first century may be brought to us through developments in our understanding of the brain. These advances may offer revolutionary treatments for the brain, and could see the end of neurodegenerative disorders such as Alzheimer's and Parkinson's diseases. We should also see much improved treatments for addictions and other mental health disorders, and the development of new 'recreational' drugs some of which might lead to fewer harms and lower risks of addiction than the substances in use today.

Such changes are to be welcomed, but it is possible that we will also see fundamental advances of a new kind which will revolutionise the way we think. We are on the verge of developments which could possibly move us into a world where we could take a drug to help us learn, think faster, relax, sleep more efficiently or even subtly alter our mood to match that of our friends. This would have implications for individuals, and could lead to a fundamental change in the way we behave as a society.

But the brain is delicate. Anything we take can have unexpected and unwanted effects. Just as we may see new advances in the treatment of addiction, we could also see continuing use of existing and novel 'recreational' drugs. These drugs bring with them the potential for considerable harm with significant potential negative impact on individuals, families and communities. This is not a future we want to fall into unprepared.

This Foresight project provides us with the evidence for what future science may allow us to do in this area, and highlights the key opportunities and challenges of the next 20 years. It is essential that we use this information to decide the course we want to take as a nation, and take action to get us there.

Acknowledgements

This project would not have been possible without the commitment of many collaborators. We would especially like to thank members of the OSI Foresight directorate including Dr Claire Craig, Dr Andrew Jackson, Joanne Marsden, manager of the project, her colleagues Mary Lawrence, Gerard Rand, James Withers, Samuel Danqah and Jane Jackson, and members of the stakeholder group including its successive chairs, Lord Warner and Jane Kennedy MP of the Department of Health, our advisory group, all the science review authors and referees, and for their work on the scenarios, Andrew Curry and Rachel Kelnar of the Henley Centre and Alister Wilson of Waverley Management Consultants. The enthusiastic support of Sir David King, head of the Office of Science and Innovation and chief scientific adviser to the UK government, was vital to our success.

Drugs Futures 2025? was an independent analysis based on a thorough review of the evidence. It was commissioned by the OSI, part of the UK government, but its findings are not government policy.

1

Drugs Futures 2025

Professor David Nutt, Professor Trevor Robbins and Professor Gerry Stimson

Over the past 10 years there have been significant advances in our understanding of areas such as neuroscience, genetics, pharmacology, psychology and social policy. This new knowledge has moved us to a new level in our understanding of how brains work, how chemicals affect the brain's performance and, in turn, how this affects our behaviour.

The Foresight project whose work has given rise to this book, and to which the editors were science advisors, was set up to consider how we can manage the use of psychoactive substances in the future to the best advantage of the individual, the community and society.

The project was set up by the UK Government's Office of Science and Innovation because of its awareness that current scientific advances in this area may have wide-reaching implications for society over the next 20 years. They are likely to be applied to provide a better understanding of mental health, and of treatments to enhance it, of the varying effects of legal and illegal drugs on different individuals, and of the nature of addiction itself as well as treatments for it. We are also finding out about mental processes themselves. This development brings with it the potential for cognition enhancers, substances that can enhance the performance of our brain in specific ways, such as improving short-term memory or increasing our speed of thought.

In the developed world, we live in an age where the majority find themselves in physical health and prosperity. As our material situation has improved, attention has turned increasingly to our mental state. We do not expect merely to be well fed and housed. We also pursue happiness for ourselves and others.

At the same time, we expect more from our brains. Our knowledge of the way human brains and behaviour work has been growing apace. This knowledge has brought significant gains through better treatments for many mental health disorders and the diagnosis of new conditions such as attention-deficit hyperactivity disorder (ADHD).

At the same time, our growing knowledge has contributed to the increased use of chemicals to affect the brain. We term these psychoactive substances. Despite the decline in the use of tobacco, one of the principal recreational drugs, the volume and range of recreational substance use in the UK is growing, and there has been an increase in the use of medicines such as cognition enhancers intended to improve mental performance.

We are on the verge of a revolution in the specificity and function of the psychoactive substances available to us. In particular, we expect to know far more in the near future about their effects on individual users, a development driven by our knowledge of the human genome and its expression in individuals.

There has been significant investment in research on drugs and the brain, and it is starting to bear fruit. Many of the advances have been unexpected and are still not understood. But they suggest that we are on the verge of major change. In particular, new approaches are being developed for medicines for mental health. Preventative treatments are being trialled for Alzheimer's disease and we may be able to develop them for schizophrenia. At the same time, pharmacogenetics is allowing us to identify people at higher risk of adverse – or in some cases even beneficial – drug side-effects.

We are learning more about how the brain regenerates itself. This may play a key role in helping us to treat mental health disorders and reduce natural mental decline with age, an acute social and medical problem in the developed and developing worlds.

There have been significant advances in our understanding of addiction and of the treatments available for it. Our knowledge of the harms of recreational drugs is increasing and we may be able to use this growing body of evidence to help us to make better decisions about their use. For example, it is clear that children and adolescents are much more vulnerable than adults to harm and addiction. Drugs are being developed which help people to forget experiences. In the future it might be possible to 'unlearn' an addiction. Vaccines are being trialled that might allow us to stop the action of nicotine, cocaine and perhaps in future other drugs on the brain. Genomics is helping us to identify why certain groups of people are at greater or lesser risk of harm from recreational drugs, or of becoming addicted to them, than others. This could allow education, drug counselling and medical treatments for addiction to be targeted more precisely. Experimental work suggests that it may be possible in some cases to separate the effect of a psychoactive substance from its addictive properties. This could pave the way to non-addictive recreational drugs. But as with any new substance the risks will need to be assessed. It may also be possible to produce a recreational substance with similar effects to alcohol but

fewer harms. Such new drugs raise social and ethical issues, as do new psychoactive substances intended to improve the performance of the healthy brain.

These advances will be set against a backdrop of new expectations and social views. There is a large unmet need for medicines for mental health. It is set to increase as the population ages and with improvements in diagnosis. This increasing need, and the rise of the 'consumer patient', will keep pressure on Government to find treatments for mental health disorders and for the natural decline of mental capabilities with age. There is an increase in self-treatment as people buy medicines online and use alternatives such as natural health foods and 'healthy options' food lines, and a blurring of the distinction between medicines for mental health and foods.

These advances raise the hope that harms from recreational drug use and from mental disorder can be reduced. But they bring with them the risk that behaviour once regarded as normal can become unacceptable and be regarded as needing treatment. This 'medicalisation' of normal life may grow as we increase our understanding of behaviour and recognise certain behaviours as medical conditions. It is not clear how far this trend will go, and to some extent it goes against the desire for more 'natural' approaches to diet and medicine. We have already seen excessively active children diagnosed as having ADHD, and excessively shy people being diagnosed as having social anxiety disorder. Effective treatments have been made available for both conditions.

We can see a trend for the use of medicines in areas such as the control of mood to become more acceptable. But there is also increasing concern about the risks of new medicines and the climate for new drug development is less positive than in the past. We accept far less risk with new drugs than with some drugs already available over the counter. Despite an increasing expectation that there is a pill to solve every problem, pharmaceutical companies are under increasing pressure to reduce prices, while the discovery and development costs for new drugs are soaring. It costs in the order of $1 billion and takes 10 years to develop and approve a drug. There is a danger that pharmaceutical companies could withdraw from the development of new medicines for mental health.

It is undisputed that substance misuse can lead to significant harm to individuals, families and communities. The current economic and social costs of illicit drug use to the UK are in the order of £13 billion a year. Crime accounts for most of this cost. Health harms are also significant, with an estimated 350 000 problem drug users in the UK. Many of these are injecting users and are at risk of transmitting hepatitis C and HIV infections. There are estimated to be more than 100 000 children in England, Scotland and Wales with a mother who is a problem drug user.

Apart from caffeine, which is the most-used psychoactive substance but is rarely associated with serious harm, alcohol and tobacco are the main legal drugs. In the UK, alcohol is associated with 22 000 premature deaths a year, 30 000 hospital admissions and 50% of violent crime. Harm associated with alcohol costs the UK economy about £20 billion per year. Smoking is in decline in the UK but is associated with a fifth of all deaths, 106 000 per year, and a third of all cancers. Because people from lower socioeconomic categories are more likely to smoke, tobacco is a contributor to health inequalities.

There are also about 300 000 problem gamblers in the UK, and significant numbers of sufferers from other damaging non-drug behaviour, such as eating disorders, that may be regarded as addictive.

We can anticipate both continued use of recreational psychoactive substances and greater sophistication in the way people use them. Better information is allowing users of such drugs to create the experience they want by combining existing and novel substances in new ways. Despite the sophistication of some drug users, this could lead to significant increased risks because certain combinations can increase harms significantly.

The market for treatments for addiction is small and there is a potential for stigma to be attached to any business that might develop treatments for illicit drugs. So, although the impact of addiction on society is significant, pharmaceutical companies have little incentive to develop treatments for addiction.

In the future there could be an increasing expectation that the regulatory structure for recreational psychoactive substances should match our understanding of their harms. Decisions on the regulatory approach to recreational drugs must take into account the harms to the individual and others, the benefits, society's view (including the ethical perspective) of the acceptability of the substance, and people's rights to use a substance that is currently legal.

We are now starting to see the use of cognition enhancers by the healthy. They are developed for health treatments and then found and used by healthy people. For example, methylphenidate (known as Ritalin), a treatment for ADHD, and modafinil, a treatment for narcolepsy, are being used to improve alertness and performance by groups including students. Both of these drugs are licensed for use on prescription only. Also under investigation are a group of chemicals called ampakines that enhance the actions of the neurotransmitter glutamate in the brain, and have been shown to enhance verbal recall in healthy elderly volunteers.

Though the effects of these developments are uncertain and some may be far in the future, we need to take action now if we are to manage the risks. Continuing too long with current frameworks could create a risk that the pharmaceutical industry pulls out of the market for the development of new medicines for mental health. We may see an increase in self-treatment, with individuals using approaches that are outside the normal regulatory safeguards. We may also see new conditions diagnosed and treated, shaping the acceptability of new patterns of behaviour in society, without a full dialogue about the consequences.

There is currently no regulatory framework for the development of drugs for the healthy in the UK. The use of animals in drug testing is envisaged in British law only for preventing or curing disease, not for developing compounds to make life better for people who are well.

Our research on attitudes within the pharmaceutical industry suggests that the companies involved see many problems in becoming involved in developing these drugs and few incentives to do so.

In the same way, future approaches to the management of recreational drugs require solid information, and time to engage in a dialogue with the public before change. One strong message from our analysis is that any change to the legal status of a recreational drug could lead to unexpected negative effects if society is not ready for it. Reducing harm from the use of recreational drugs is as much about having the right culture for their use as it is about the policy for their management. Encouraging the responsible use of alcohol rather than binge drinking is a case in point. This is important whether we are increasing or decreasing the level of control. If control is increased over a particular substance, users may try to find a way around the change, possibly leading to other forms of harm. But if controls are lessened without a culture that supports sensible use of the substance, more harm can also result.

Cognition enhancers involve a specific and interesting set of issues. If they become practical, 'mental cosmetics' could become accepted and create new expectations about the performance and behaviour of individuals and groups. Policies in such a situation should seek to minimise harm and to consider the social and ethical issues. We would need to understand the risks of the cognition enhancers that were in use to regulate them effectively, and to consider what role the UK pharmaceutical industry might play in this market.

What strategic choices do we face about drugs and the brain in the coming 20 years?

In the field of medicines for mental health we may have to:

- accept a new system for developing medicines for mental health, or maintain the status quo and risk the withdrawal of pharmaceutical companies from this market;
- allow definitions of 'normal' behaviour to alter and allow more treatment of everyday variation in mental capacity, at the risk of an overmedicated society, or encourage non-drug approaches;
- regulate drugs and foods with medical uses consistently, at the risk of excessive control, or accept different levels of regulation;
- accept self-treatment for mental health conditions, or attempt to control and monitor it.

For recreational drugs, some choices that face society are:

- consider a public sector role in developing treatments for addiction, or accept that they are likely to emerge only slowly as spin-offs from other pharmaceutical developments;
- allow individuals to have and use information on their possible susceptibility to drugs, or have such knowledge mediated by professionals such as doctors and counsellors;
- explore less harmful alternatives to today's recreational drugs, or seek to reduce their use;
- use present methods to watch for drug harms in individuals, or support the development of new methods which might make drug use less available for individuals at the risk of compromising their rights;
- undertake a long-term social investigation of what drives recreational drug use, or deal with it via current patterns of regulation based mainly on the criminal justice system;
- use a consistent, harms-based approach to regulating drug use, or see each drug in its wider ethical or social context.

Key choices on cognition enhancers include:

- accept their spread and the possible development of 'haves' and 'have-nots' and of a significant percentage of the population being dependent on them, or have a debate in society on their use and base management approaches on the results;
- support UK business as a producer of enhancers in the hope of getting an early lead in a significant market, or accept that other countries will get the commercial benefits.

We recognise that these are not all simple binary choices. It may be possible, for example, to tolerate increased drug use while encouraging education to make its risks more apparent to potential users. Nor is society a single entity. It will probably continue to contain some groups which accept drug use, some which reject it strongly, and others in between.

In common with other Foresight projects, this one was designed to produce insights into possible developments, but it has not generated any forecasts. Instead, it has pointed to potential changes which we believe government, industry, medical professionals, the voluntary sector responsible for caring for drug abusers, and others including the general public may wish to consider.

Although all Foresight projects consider complex topics, we feel that this one had a particularly difficult set of issues to cope with. It is only five years since the unveiling of the human genome and we are only now finding out how influential its discovery will prove to be. Many effects concerned with drugs and the brain doubtless have a genetic component. But the way genetic makeup turns into human physiology and behaviour is far from simple. It may well turn out that our new knowledge only allows us to predict general susceptibility to addiction rather than forecasting it absolutely.

We have not tried to predict how society's attitude to psychoactive substances will change. The decline in smoking – in both incidence and social acceptability – is a startling example of a rapid change in drug use. But many drug markets are very conservative and innovation in them can be very slow, as the decades between the development of Ecstasy and its entry into widespread use suggest. The spread of the web as an information source and of small-scale chemical synthesis as a practical technology implies that new, smaller and more informal drug suppliers could emerge as a challenge to today's patterns of both legal and illicit trade.

It is possible that drug use will become more widely accepted in society, but there are substantial minorities in the UK, such as the Muslim community, which reject it.

It is also possible that in 20 years, drug regulation and control will have been realigned so that drugs are controlled according to the harm for which they are responsible, and are regarded more as a concern of the health system than for criminal justice. However, such reform would have to match society's expectations. Alcohol, for example, is responsible for many serious harms. But it is also enjoyed by millions of people, is legal despite restrictions on its sale, creates large tax revenues, and most importantly, is part of the social fabric of the UK.

The Drugs Futures 2025? project enlisted the support of academic experts ranging from neuroscientists to economists. We are sure that the expert reviews of the science that they produced, which make up the remaining chapters of this book, are the most thorough analyses ever written of the issues faced by the UK and other countries in the sphere of legal and illegal drug use and their interaction with brain science.

2

Foresight

Andrew Jackson

1 INTRODUCTION

In times gone by, kings and queens looked to prophets and signs in the sky as they decided what to do for the good of their nation. Today, presidents and prime ministers still have to take decisions of vital importance, but the prophets are gone. The question could be whether to go to war, or how to invest money to support the health of their people. Should we build more hospitals to treat disease, or more sports centres in the hope of reducing the incidence of chronic disease?

Recent events such as the tsunami which hit Indonesia on Boxing Day 2004, and the 11 September 2001 attacks on the US, have once again raised the question of how can we find out about future risks and opportunities in the minds of people and governments alike.

In the UK, the government's chief scientist directs a programme to advise on exactly this question. Unlike its ancient predecessors, it uses scientific evidence rather than auguries as the basis for its advice.

2 WHAT IS FORESIGHT?

Technology Foresight is used by governments across the world to explore how technology might play out in the future. The aim is usually to look for opportunities which could be exploited and threats which could be avoided, or at least prepared for.

The UK Government introduced its Foresight programme in 1992. The underlying thought was to provide an environment in which business and the science community could work together to decide how the UK could make the most of the UK's strength in science. The challenge from the beginning was the breadth of the programme, which meant that its outputs varied in quality.

In 2002 steps were taken to address this weakness when the programme was relaunched in a new form by Professor Sir David King, the UK Government's Chief Scientific Adviser. The new programme was changed in several key ways that were important to its eventual success.

- It focuses on only three or four areas at any one time. This means that its projects have the resources to look in depth at the issue they are addressing, engaging key stakeholders in the process and producing a firm science evidence base to inform the visions of the future that it develops.

- Issues are carefully chosen to be ones where the programme can add value. Projects either look at how science and technology can be used to help the UK respond to important strategic issues, or at how science and technology might develop, considering potential future uses of that science and its wider social implications. The Brain Science, Addiction and Drugs (BSAD) project that has given rise to this book is a case in point. Four other projects have been completed under the new programme, two looking from the perspective of a strategic issue and two exploring the development of a new area of science (see Box).

Flood Futures 2080 considered how flood risks could change over the next 80 years and what we could do to manage this risk.

Cyber Trust and Crime Prevention looked at how information technology might develop in the future, and the possible consequences for trust and crime.

Cognitive Systems considered developments in our understanding of how living systems think and how they might help us develop intelligence in computers.

Exploiting the Electromagnetic Spectrum looked at how developments in areas such as optics, near infrared and magnetic resonance imaging could support technology in the future. The possibilities it included ranged from hand-held personal health scanners such as the tricorder seen in *Star Trek* to CCTV-type technology for security that could see whether someone is carrying a weapon, explosives or drugs.

- Experts from science work as part of the team, so that the quality of the science is assured. We have succeeded in attracting leading scientists to the projects, adding both to the authority of the projects and to the quality of their findings. Trevor Robbins, David Nutt and Gerry Stimson were the project experts on the BSAD project. They were critical to the project's success and we worked very closely with them throughout the project

- All projects start by commissioning 'state of the art' reviews, such as those that make up most of the chapters of this book. These set out our current understanding of the science and look forward to consider future capabilities

- The futures process we follow is designed to match the needs of the project. We do not think that there is a single right approach to futures work. We first decide the issues we want to look at and then design the approach which will best help us to answer the questions we have raised.

- Each project is led by a minister from a department of the UK Government. Winning their support assures us that we are looking at an area where we can make a contribution to policy at the highest level.

3 WHAT APPROACH DID WE USE TO EXPLORE THE FUTURE OF DRUG USE?

We decided to look at the future of brain science and drugs because of rapid advances in neuroscience, and concern about the impact that drugs were having on society. We started with a series of workshops and one-to-one interviews with experts in the field to help decide the scope of the project. The future is a big place, and agreeing the field of study is critical to the success of the project. Too narrow, and it will miss important potential changes; too wide, and it will be too shallow to raise issues worth investigating.

We were soon faced with several dilemmas. As we spoke to more experts it became clear that there was no clear distinction between the various types of drugs.

For example, drugs for mental health were sometimes used for recreational purposes. So we decided to look at all chemicals which had an effect on the brain's performance – so-called psychoactive substances. In our initial work we discussed how to minimise any harm but time and time again it was pointed out to us that there were also benefits. In fact, it would distort the issue if we did not consider the benefits of mental health treatments.

So, we finally came down to our project question: how can we manage the use of psychoactive substances in the future to best advantage for the individual, community and society?

The risk with any exercise of this type is that we will end up collecting only a small part of the evidence necessary to answer the question in a thorough way. So having decided the project question, we consider what subsidiary questions we would need to answer in order to answer our main question. This approach is generally called issues tree analysis. The aim is to produce a set of questions which are mutually exclusive and completely exhaustive. This led us to three further questions. What will be the psychoactive substances of the future? What interventions in addiction will be available in future? What will the future impacts of psychoactive substances be?

We then sought input from 15 different areas of science in the form of state-of-science reviews to answer these questions. This evidence became the basis of the future visions we created.

We used two futures techniques, horizon scanning and scenarios. The aim of the horizon scan is to look across all the evidence we have and to consider which developments are likely to have the greatest impact, whether good or bad, as we walk towards 2025. There is no way to weigh each of the suggested advances against each other. Instead the small group of experts and the central futures team each picked out what they thought, from their areas of expertise, might have greatest impact. We then spent a day together discussing what

we each thought, testing and developing our ideas.

The horizon scan of course picked up many potential advances, for example the development of vaccines for illicit drugs and the use of cognition-enhancing drugs by the healthy. The case was strong for each of the possible advances we identified. In the case of new drugs, there was scientific evidence of their feasibility. New behaviours were ones which either a small group was already following, or which society had followed in the past.

Even with this evidence it was unclear how the potential advances in science would play out in society. For example, would society embrace cognition enhancers for the healthy, or decide that in the longer term it is better to live with the brains we were born with?

So we decided to produce some scenarios which would play out how society might respond to these advances. The first step in the development of our scenarios was to think about the things we know could change over the next 20 years and which would set the context. We developed a list of more than 60 factors. To give an example of their range, four were:

- the ageing of the population,
- changing views of the rights of individuals to choose what is best for them,
- advances in our capability to use genetic information,
- pressure on pharmaceutical companies to reduce the risk of their products, increasing the regulatory cost of new treatments.

Rather than produce thousands of scenarios, each playing out different permutations of the way these factors could interact, we decided to pick just four scenarios which we thought were at the four corners of the map of the possible futures. None of these would be the preferred future, but they would each help us to understand a good percentage of the risks and opportunities in a manageable way. They would also provide a framework which we could use to test policy for robustness against future changes.

To ensure that we were seeing the extremes of possible future developments, we decided to picture two uncertainties which had great variability and were important in understanding the answer to our project's question. Six different sets of uncertainties were considered before we picked the two we used as the basis for the scenarios. These were:

- whether decisions in the future would be based on the latest scientific evidence or the latest social view,
- whether the focus for our use of drugs in society would be for enhancement of our performance or for treatment of disease.

This was one of the richest parts of the exercise, as we wrestled intellectually to decide which drivers of change would matter most to the question we were considering. This was an important process to go through. It is via conflict that futures work delivers its greatest insights.

We then spent six months discussing and developing with a wide range of experts and practitioners what would happen in each of the four scenarios. Again there was much disagreement, as we chipped away at each other's ideas until we had honed four scenarios, each of which were internally consistent.

It soon became clear that the project was raising issues which would be significant for society. So we decided that before we published our findings, we should have a public engagement exercise to expose members of the public to a range of the possible developments. The public quickly alighted on three areas which they were most concerned about:

- the possibility of vaccines against recreational drugs. They were concerned that they could be used to restrict an individual's freedom if given without consent,

- greater understanding of the causes of mental capabilities and moods. They were concerned that if there is a medical reason for a wider range of behaviours, society might decide to define what 'normal' is and impose medication so that all are 'normal',
- individual choice versus society's right to protect itself. They thought that individuals should be free to choose what they did, though they accepted the current rules on what was and was not illegal. It might be concluded that what they did not want was change that would restrict their freedom any further.

4 WHAT HAPPENS NEXT?

One of the greatest challenges for any piece of futures work is to make things happen. If it presents a future which is too challenging, it is difficult to get anyone to take it seriously. If it is too close to what we already know, people say that it tells them nothing new and they will not change their behaviour on the basis of reading it. Whichever is the problem, the consequence is the same. The destiny of most futures work is to collect dust on a shelf.

Although some copies of our final report, *Drugs Futures 2025?*, may stay on the shelf, it has also led to clear action. The UK Government recognised the importance of the issues raised by the report. Ministers from four departments have supported an independent review of the issues raised by the project. The Government has asked the UK's Academy of Medical Sciences to consider the issues and make recommendations for action. Action on the part of government and others has followed all of the Foresight reports. So perhaps in the UK, Foresight is starting to fill the role of the prophet for the future!

CHAPTER

3

Neuroscience of Drugs and Addiction

Trevor Robbins, Rudolf Cardinal, Patricia DiCiano, Peter Halligan, Kim Hellemans, Jonathan Lee and Barry Everitt

1   EXECUTIVE SUMMARY

Brain science is at the core of our future understanding of how drugs affect behaviour, and their consequent impact on society. Extraordinary advances in the last three decades have meant that we now understand much about the connectivity of the brain and how its functionality depends on chemical messages passing between nerve cells, or neurons, in the form of neurotransmitters they release which bind to receptors. Psychoactive substances exert their effects by affecting the regulation of neurotransmitters or simulating their actions at their receptors, and subsequently within the nerve cell itself, often in highly specific ways. We understand how many drugs work in molecular terms and where they may work, at least initially, in the brain. Moreover, we now understand in broad terms how different parts of the brain work at a systems level to produce behavioural and cognitive output.

Major advances have been made on two fronts. First, our understanding of the major neural components of the 'reward' or reinforcement system in the brain in animals has improved. This mediates the influence both of events such as food and sex on learning, and of drugs of abuse. Second, understanding has improved in cognitive neuroscience, elucidating how the human brain processes information, particularly within the cerebral cortex. Convergence between these areas is beginning to enable us to understand the neurobiological underpinnings of the effects of psychoactive substances in humans, even within a societal context.

For example, the emerging theme of neuroeconomics promises to reveal how the cognitive apparatus of the brain constrains the assumptions of rational decision-making in traditional economic theory. A complementary advance has been the application of some aspects of neural decision-making theory to the explanation of the behaviour of individual substance abusers.

Our burgeoning understanding of how psychoactive substances affect brain function includes a growing realisation of their long-term effects, both neural and behavioural. Vulnerability or susceptibility to some actions of psychoactive substances, including both cognitive enhancement and dependence, appear to depend on individual differences based on genetic or environmental, including developmental, factors. It is becoming clear that the future impact of neuroscience will be realised through interactions with diverse disciplines including cognitive and social psychology, physics, molecular biology and genomics. This expansion of knowledge is influencing our attitudes to such important areas as the treatment of mental illness, the potential for augmenting cognitive function through psychoactive substances, and the study of drug use and abuse. Thus, the concept of addiction itself is undergoing radical change. Although many in society still view drug abuse as a social or moral problem best handled through the criminal justice system, the growing scientific evidence suggests instead that addiction is a chronic, relapsing and treatable brain disorder that can result from prolonged effects of drugs on the brain.

2 INTRODUCTION

Communication within the brain depends on the release of neurotransmitter substances. Many agents, including drugs, but also nutrients and transcranial magnetic or deep brain stimulation, exert their effects through chemical neurotransmission. Many psychoactive drugs work on chemical systems that not only control behaviour, but also respond to behavioural change. Many forms of behaviour, ranging from transcendental meditation to compulsive eating or gambling, may regulate the functioning of the chemical systems of the brain.

In the last 50 years or so, the list of chemical neurotransmitter substances in the brain has lengthened from two to over 60 (Feldman *et al.*, 1997; Cooper *et al.*, 2002). The neurotransmitters include amino-acids and monoamines and structurally more complex neuropeptides. The list is likely to be extended, leading to further drug development. The discovery of new neurotransmitters goes hand in hand with the mapping of the neurons that contain them in the brain. These substances are not distributed homogeneously in the central nervous system, but are contained within defined tracts and clusters of cells, which may be organised in a complex arrangement to form functional, interconnected brain systems. Moreover, at the synapses between neurons, these substances interact as ligands with complex protein molecules called receptors on the neuronal membranes, to which they bind and thus transduce their chemical signals. There are often several distinct receptor subtypes for a given neurotransmitter, and these are also widely distributed within the brain, generally but not always matching the mapping of the neurotransmitter systems themselves. Further complexity is conferred by variations in protein subunits making up the receptors. The many functional effects of drugs such as nicotine and benzodiazepines such as diazepam can be attributed in part to different receptor subtypes operating preferentially in different brain regions. The discovery of 'orphan' receptors without obvious neurotransmitter ligands in different brain regions indicates the possibility of further discoveries of new psychoactive substances (Civelli *et al.*, 1999; Preskorn, 2001). In the past, the discovery of psychoactive drugs has often predated the discovery of the endogenous neurotransmitter ligand (e.g. endorphin and enkephalins in the case of opiates such as morphine and heroin, and β-carbolines in the case of the benzodiazepines), as well as the brain receptors upon which they act (Cooper *et al.*, 2002).

The biophysical actions of neurotransmitters at specific receptors range from short-lived electrochemical effects at ion channels to slower cellular signalling via receptors linked to biochemical cascades (e.g. 'second messengers') and gene transcription. The old adage of one neurotransmitter per neuron has long been disproved by discoveries that many of the actions of the 'classical' neurotransmitters, such as acetylcholine (ACh), noradrenaline (NA), serotonin (5-HT) and dopamine (DA), are augmented by coreleased peptides (Cooper *et al.*, 2002). The chemical neurotransmitters affect the functioning of dense, but generally highly organised, sets of connections, conveniently referred to as neuronal networks. They do this either by affecting fast signalling, whether excitatory or inhibitory, within the network, or by slower and spatially more diffuse modulations across the nodes of the network. An individual neuron is subject to many different influences from distinct neurotransmitter systems. The activity of a particular cell and thus of entire networks can be adjusted by variations in the syntax of chemical messages impinging on the cell.

Several neurological and neuropsychiatric disorders have chemical pathologies for which a strategy of pharmacological replacement of deficient systems has been adopted. L-DOPA medication in Parkinson's disease is the classic example, where the loss of DA-containing cells of the substantia nigra leads to the characteristic motor symptoms. L-DOPA remediates some of the cognitive deficits associated with Parkinson's disease (Cools *et al.*, 2001), but also produces some undesirable cognitive and emotional side-effects, including for some patients a drive to abuse the drug (Lawrence *et al.*, 2003). L-DOPA's therapeutic effects also tend to diminish with long-term treatment, leading to a gamut of other attempts to treat the disorder which includes other dopaminergic drugs, deep-brain stimulation, neurosurgery and the neural transplantation of embryonic nigral cells (Walter and Vitek, 2004). Especially in view of the ethical problems posed by the last-named, a future approach will almost certainly involve the use of stem cells engineered to produce DA. A similar approach to the treatment of Alzheimer's disease with cholinergic drug treatments (including nicotine) has proved less successful, although such treatment does improve some functions, notably attention (Levin, 2002). The future strategy (as with the treatment of stroke) is likely to hinge on neuroprotection, preventing through drug treatment the neuronal loss occurring as a consequence of the initial pathology (Citron, 2002).

Many other disorders that result in cognitive or mood-related deficits are now treated with drugs. These include depression, treated with monoamine reuptake inhibitors such as the selective 5-HT reuptake inhibitors (SSRIs), schizophrenia, treated by DA receptor blockers, and attention-deficit hyperactivity disorder (ADHD), which is treated effectively with amphetamine-like stimulant drugs such as methylphenidate (Ritalin; Solanto *et al.*, 2001). A number of cognitive disorders arising from brain dysfunction have been treated on an experimental basis: these include Korsakoff's syndrome (arising from alcoholism), which has been treated with drugs affecting noradrenergic transmission, acute brain injury (treated with DA receptor agonists), and stroke (treated with amphetamine). Whilst the molecular bases of these drugs' actions at the cellular level are well defined, the mechanistic basis of any of these therapeutic effects is less clear. The most effective anti-psychotic drug,

clozapine, is also one of the least specific in pharmacological terms. Anti-depressants such as the SSRIs may work via effects on neurogenesis in the hippocampus (Duman, 2004). Nevertheless, given the therapeutic efficacy of most of these drugs, and strong evidence from animal models of cognitive function, there is optimism that cognitive and mood-related disorders will continue to respond to interventions based on psychoactive substances.

One of the most promising developments from experimental neuroscience has arisen from a neuronal model of learning called long-term potentiation (LTP). It can occur in subtly different forms in many forebrain regions, but has been investigated most intensively in the hippocampus (Thomas and Malenka, 2003). LTP crucially depends on the excitatory amino-acid neurotransmitter glutamate, and its actions at the AMPA- and N-methyl-*d*-aspartate (NMDA) receptor subtypes. Several agents affecting glutamate transmission have been developed, including some (such as the AMPA-kines) that have been shown to have positive effects on learning in the laboratory for both normal animals and humans, and have been subject to preliminary clinical trials (Lynch, 2002). Some NMDA receptor antagonists, such as ketamine, have recently been shown to have significant abuse potential (Curran and Morgan, 2000). In a more speculative vein, drugs enhancing the transcription factor CREB (cAMP response element binding protein) could also emerge from advances in the application of basic neuroscience (Tully *et al.*, 2003).

The phenomenon of beneficial effects in normal subjects lacking discernible brain dysfunction is not restricted to drugs affecting glutamate receptors. In specific situations, which may include the infusion of drugs locally to specific brain regions in experimental animals and the engagement of particular cognitive functions, many positive drug effects have been reported for compounds acting on the classical cholinergic, noradrenergic, serotoninergic or dopaminergic systems (Arnsten and Robbins, 2002).

Only some of these systems have also been associated with drug dependence. Thus the positive effects of cholinergic drugs on attention and aspects of mnemonic function are not accompanied by mood-altering effects of potential recreational use.

The prediction of psychopharmacological efficacy is often confounded by the surprising emergence of new substances which may have initially appeared to be innocuous or which were initially established in some other functional context. The effective anti-narcoleptic modafinil (Mignot *et al.*, 2002) has stimulant-like actions, but does not appear primarily to affect the brain neurotransmitters implicated in the effects of stimulant drugs such as amphetamine and methylphenidate. This drug has mild beneficial effects on tests of short-term memory and planning, as well as an anti-impulsive action, both in normal adults and in patients with ADHD (Turner *et al.*, 2004). Its beneficial effects on vigilance and other aspects of human performance have led to its well-publicised use by the military.

These effects indicate again the possibility of cognitive enhancement in intact individuals. Increasing evidence of individual variability in intellectual function in normal subjects that occurs as a function of genotypical variation (Mattay *et al.*, 2003) and in association with factors such as fatigue or under-arousal in the work-place, may promote self-medication. But although modafinil emerged from a scientific programme of drug development, we do not know how it works. The fact that modafinil is not widely abused indicates that it is feasible to dissociate stimulant from reinforcing actions of drugs of abuse. Whether this dissociation arises from the pharmacokinetic actions of the drug, which is relatively slow-acting, or its distinct neurochemical actions, is a theoretically, as well as practically, important issue.

Self-medication prompted by a perceived need to elevate the activation of particular brain neurochemical systems might also affect other domains of forebrain functioning. The need to enhance activation of the dopaminergic reinforcement ('reward') system might explain why individuals use cocaine and other psychomotor stimulants that operate primarily through this system. Such a view is consistent with evidence that euphoria produced by drugs such as cocaine and methylphenidate may depend on initially low levels of striatal DA (D2) receptors, as revealed by positron emission tomography, which may be indicative of low basal mood states (Volkow *et al.*, 1999a; Figure 3.1). It may also be relevant to the identification of individuals who indulge in certain behavioural addictions such as gambling (Reuter *et al.*, 2005). Whether these individual differences arise from genetic or environmental influences is still to be determined.

3 NEUROPSYCHOLOGY OF REINFORCEMENT LEARNING AND ADDICTION

Motivated action can be examined by studying instrumental conditioning, the process by which animals alter their behaviour when there is a contingency between their behaviour and a reinforcing outcome (Thorndike, 1911). Reinforcement learning (Minsky, 1961; Russell and Norvig, 1995; Haykin, 1999) has been studied for a long time (Thorndike, 1905; Thorndike, 1911; Grindley, 1932; Guthrie, 1935; Skinner, 1938; Hull, 1943). At its most basic level, it is the ability to learn to act on the basis of important outcomes such as reward and punishment. Events that strengthen preceding responses are called positive reinforcers, while events whose removal strengthens preceding responses are called negative reinforcers (Skinner, 1953). If reinforcers are defined by their effect on behaviour, then, to avoid a circular argument, behaviour cannot be said to have altered as a consequence of reinforcement (Skinner, 1953). However, to explain behaviour rather than merely describe it, internal processes such as motivation must also be accounted for. Central motivational states, such as hunger

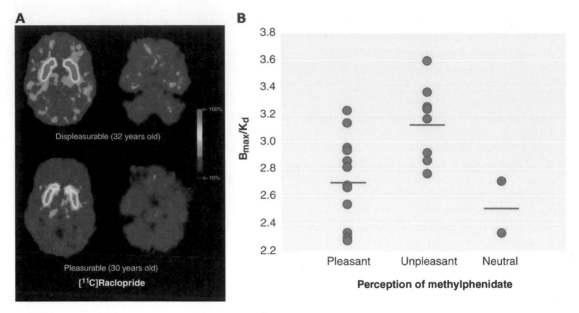

FIGURE 3.1 **(A)** Distribution volume images of $[^{11}C]$raclopride at the levels of the striatum (left) and cerebellum (right) in a healthy male subject who reported the effects of methylphenidate as pleasant and in a healthy male subject who reported them as unpleasant. $100\% = 25$ ml/mg; $10\% = 0.4$ ml/mg. **(B)** D2 receptor levels (B_{max}/K_d) in 23 healthy male subjects who reported the effects of methylphenidate as pleasant, unpleasant, or neutral. B_{max}/K_d values were lower in subjects who reported the effects of methylphenidate as pleasant than in those who reported them as unpleasant. The horizontal lines represent the means for the B_{max}/K_d estimates for the different groups. (From Volkow *et al.*, 1999c). Reprinted, with permission, from *American Journal of Psychiatry*. Copyright (1999) American Psychiatric Association. (This figure appears in the colour plate section.)

and thirst, account parsimoniously for a great deal of behavioural variability (Erwin and Ferguson, 1979; Toates, 1986; Ferguson, 2000). For example, water deprivation, eating dry food, hypertonic saline injection, and the hormone angiotensin II all induce a common state – thirst – that has multiple effects. Thirsty animals drink more water, drink water faster, perform more of an arbitrary response to gain water, and so on. The ideas of motivational state entered early theories of reinforcement. For example, it was suggested that events that reduce 'drive' states such as thirst are positively reinforcing (Hull, 1943). However, on its own, this simple model cannot account for many instrumental conditioning phenomena, let alone 'unnatural' reinforcement such as drug addiction.

Modern neuropsychological theories recognise that many processes contribute to a simple act such as pressing a lever to receive food or a drug (Dickinson, 1994). Rats and humans exhibit goal-directed action, which is based on knowledge of the contingency between one's actions and their outcomes, and knowledge of the value of those outcomes. These two representations interact so that we work for that which we value (Dickinson, 1994; Dickinson and Balleine, 1994). Environmental stimuli provide information about what contingencies may be in force in a given environment (Colwill and Rescorla, 1990; Rescorla, 1990a,b). Remarkably, the value system governing goal-directed action is not the brain's only one. This 'cognitive' value system exists alongside (Balleine and Dickinson, 1991) the valuation process that determines our reactions when we actually experience a goal such as food, termed 'liking', 'hedonic reactions', or simply 'pleasure' (Garcia, 1989). Under many normal circumstances the two values reflect one another and change together. However, the fact that they are different means that animals must learn which outcomes are valuable in a given motivational state, a process referred to as incentive learning. For example, rats do not know that to eat a particular food while sated is not as valuable as to eat the same food while hungry until they have actually eaten the food while sated (Balleine, 1992).

Just as there is more than one value system, there is more than one route to action, and not all action is goal-directed. With time and training, actions can become habitual (Adams, 1982), that is, elicited by direct stimulus–response (S–R) associations. S–R habits are less flexible than goal-directed action, because their representation contains no information about what the final outcome will be, and cannot alter quickly if the desirability of a particular outcome changes. But they may help reduce the demands on the cognitive, goal-directed system in familiar settings.

Stimuli that predict reward may become conditioned stimuli (CS), associated with the reward (unconditioned stimulus, US) through pavlovian associative learning. Pavlovian CS can influence instrumental behaviour directly (pavlovian–instrumental transfer, PIT) and can serve as the goals of behaviour, termed conditioned reinforcement (Estes, 1948; Lovibond, 1983; Dickinson, 1994; Dickinson and Balleine, 1994; Cardinal et al., 2002).

Seen in this context, the major neuropsychological theories of drug addiction – none of them mutually exclusive – can be summarised:

3.1 Direct Positive Effects of Drugs; Self-medication; Tolerance

Drugs are taken for their positive effects. These may include euphoria, enhanced social experiences, enhanced intellectual or attentional performance, and an enhanced effect of other reinforcers such as food or sex (Wikler, 1965, 1973; Altman et al., 1996;

Feldman et al., 1997), as indicated in Chapter 6, Pharmacology and Treatments.

An aspect of this may be that people 'self-medicate' to achieve a desired level of mood, social performance, and so on (Khantzian, 1985; Weiss and Mirin, 1986; Altman et al., 1996; Markou et al., 1998; Newhouse et al., 2004), although the extent to which this occurs is debated (e.g. Castaneda et al., 1994; Newhouse et al., 2004). Furthermore, the effect of the drug depends upon the user's expectations (Mitchell et al., 1996) and prior mood, and varies between people (Uhlenhuth et al., 1981; de Wit et al., 1986).

Tolerance to pleasant drug effects may build up, requiring the user to take more drugs to achieve the same effect. Tolerance can be due to a decrease in drug bioavailability ('metabolic tolerance'), a reduction in the number or responsiveness of receptors or intracellular mechanisms ('pharmacodynamic tolerance'), or a compensatory mechanism ('behavioural tolerance') (Feldman et al., 1997). Tolerance may develop with chronic use, but in the case of cocaine, can develop in a single session (Fischman, 1989), perhaps explaining cocaine 'bingeing'. Metabolic tolerance is seen to barbiturates, ethanol and opiates (Feldman et al., 1997). Pharmacodynamic tolerance is seen to a wide range of drugs including barbiturates, ethanol, opiates, amphetamine, cocaine, nicotine and caffeine (Feldman et al., 1997). Behavioural or conditioned tolerance has been observed to opiates, ethanol, nicotine, benzodiazepines and other drugs (Siegel, 1975, 1976; Krasnegor, 1978; Dafters and Anderson, 1982; Siegel, 1999). Since conditioned tolerance may be situation-specific (Siegel, 1999) and the lethality of drugs may be increased if the environment changes, the opponent process model of addiction (Solomon and Corbit, 1974; Koob et al., 1989) suggests that a key component of addiction is the development of behavioural (Epping-Jordan et al., 1998) and neuroanatomical (Weiss et al., 1992; Maisonneuve and Kreek, 1994) tolerance, which can counteract the effects of the drug (Siegel et al., 1982).

3.2 Conditioning and Sensitisation

Conditioned stimuli associated with the pleasant aspects of drug-taking may act to promote drug-taking. Drug-associated cues including mood states, people, locations, and abuse paraphernalia may induce some of the primary effects of drugs (Kenny et al., 2003), but can also induce craving in addicts, and trigger relapse (Siegel, 1988; Tiffany and Drobes, 1990; Gawin, 1991; O'Brien et al., 1998). Addicts may also work directly for drug-associated stimuli (conditioned reinforcement), leading them in turn to the drug itself.

Sensitisation ('inverse' or 'reverse' tolerance) occurs when repeated doses of a drug enhance one or more of its effects. Prototypically, moderate, spaced doses of amphetamine enhance the subsequent locomotor response to it (Robinson and Berridge, 1993; Altman et al., 1996; Kalivas et al., 1998). Sensitisation can exhibit environmentally-specific conditioned properties (Post and Weiss, 1988), and changes in drug pharmacodynamics (Pettit et al., 1990). It has been suggested that the ability of drug-associated CSs to promote drug-seeking or craving also sensitises as a consequence of repeated drug-taking (Robinson and Berridge, 1993; Wyvell and Berridge, 2001).

3.3 Withdrawal and Conditioned Withdrawal

Some drugs, notably the opiates and alcohol, produce powerful physical withdrawal syndromes. Thus, it is possible to consider addiction within the framework of both rewarding and aversive consequences (Bechara et al., 1998). Withdrawal symptoms are improved by the drug, so the drug is taken to escape from withdrawal (Wikler, 1965, 1973). However, demonstrations that the neural substrates mediating physical signs of dependence are separate from those of reward (Bozarth and Wise, 1984) support earlier behavioural evidence that physical dependence is not a necessary correlate of opiate addiction. In withdrawal,

incentive learning operates for drugs of abuse just as for natural reinforcers. Just as hunger increases the hedonic impact of food (Berridge, 1991), which teaches the animal that it is more worth working for food when it is hungry (Dickinson and Balleine, 1994), rats learn that heroin has a high value in the state of opiate withdrawal (Hutcheson et al., 2001a). Hedonic impact may be a 'common currency' for determining the value of widely varying reinforcers (Cabanac, 1992). Environmental stimuli may become associated with withdrawal (Goldberg and Schuster, 1967; O'Brien et al., 1975, 1976, 1977) and CSs for withdrawal may then provoke drug-taking just as withdrawal itself does (Wikler, 1965, 1973).

Drugs such as cocaine that do not produce obvious physical withdrawal syndromes may nonetheless have unpleasant after-effects on mood (Koob and Bloom, 1988; Gawin, 1991; Markou and Koob, 1991; Koob et al., 1997; Knackstedt et al., 2002), which may promote drug-taking in the same way that physical withdrawal does. 'Opponent process' theories (Solomon and Corbit, 1973, 1974; Solomon, 1980a,b; Koob et al., 2004) use the idea that a long-lasting unpleasant process opposes the euphoric effects of drugs, and that with chronic use, the euphoric effects diminish while the dysphoric process comes to dominate, leading to drug-taking via negative reinforcement.

3.4 Habit Learning

Drugs may activate habit-learning systems so that actions that led to the drug are reinforced directly, creating powerful stimulus-resonse habits or 'involuntary' responses (O'Brien and McLellan, 1996; Tiffany and Carter, 1998; Robbins and Everitt, 1999; Everitt et al., 2001; Everitt and Wolf, 2002). A hallmark of habitual responding directly is that it persists stimulus–response habits even if the reinforcer's value is reduced (Dickinson, 1994). Habits are sometimes thought of as 'compulsive' responding when they occur at an abnormally high level, since they do not depend on the current value of the goal. Alcohol seeking may primarily reflect habitual responding (Dickinson *et al.*, 2002), and while cocaine-seeking can be goal-directed (Olmstead *et al.*, 2001), under some circumstances responding for cocaine can be more habitual than responding for natural reinforcers (Miles *et al.*, 2003). Similarly, soon after acquisition, cocaine-seeking is readily suppressed by an aversive CS, but this suppression is lost after prolonged experience of cocaine (Vanderschuren and Everitt, 2004). Craving and habits both capture something of the casual definition of addiction as 'compulsive' behaviour (e.g. APA, 1994; Leshner, 1997; Koob *et al.*, 1998).

3.5 Individual Vulnerability

People who become drug addicts may be more vulnerable than other people to one or more of these neuropsychological effects, as well as being more predisposed to try drugs of abuse in the first place. Vulnerability to drug effects is discussed in greater detail in Section 7.

3.6 Comparison of Drug-taking to Alternative Activities

From a behavioural-economic perspective, addicts weigh up the benefits and costs of drug-taking. They may do so rationally (Stigler and Becker, 1977; Becker and Murphy, 1988), or may exhibit decision-making flaws characteristic of humans, such as focusing inappropriately on short-term rather than long-term goals and being inconsistent in their choices (Ainslie, 1975, 1992; Herrnstein and Prelec, 1992; Heyman, 1996; Rachlin, 1997, 2000; Ainslie, 2001); see Section 11.

Drug addicts may be predisposed to act even more for short-term benefit than other people, or drugs may induce decision-making deficits (Petry *et al.*, 1998; Bickel *et al.*, 1999; Madden *et al.*, 1999; Rogers *et al.*, 1999a; Volkow *et al.*, 1999a; Ainslie and Monterosso, 2003; Bickel and Johnson, 2003; Mitchell, 2003; Vuchinich and Heather, 2003). There

is some evidence that self-control deficits may be a reversible consequence of cigarette dependence (Bickel *et al.*, 1999; Bickel and Johnson, 2003).

None of these theories, or indeed levels of explanation, is adequate on its own (Heather, 1998). For example, although heroin may be taken to alleviate withdrawal, heroin self-administration can persist in the absence of withdrawal (Bozarth and Wise, 1981, 1984), and although heroin has euphoric effects, humans will work for doses that they cannot subjectively distinguish from a placebo (Lamb *et al.*, 1991). To seek a single theory of drug addiction is to miss the point that drugs of abuse have many effects, people take drugs for many reasons, and those reasons vary between people.

4 THE NEURAL SYSTEM BASIS OF REINFORCEMENT LEARNING: RELEVANCE TO NATURAL MOTIVATION AND DRUG ADDICTION

Considerable progress has been made in establishing some of the mechanisms by which neural structures respond to appetitive and aversive events. To some extent these structures can be compared directly to the psychological processes known to influence animals' responding for rewards.

A number of limbic cortical and subcortical structures in the brain play a role in assessing the value of reinforcers and of the stimuli that predict them, and in actions directed at obtaining those reinforcers or stimuli (Cardinal *et al.*, 2002; Figure 3.2). Their relevance to addiction has been considered many times before (e.g. Altman *et al.*, 1996; Volkow and Li, 2004), and influential theories of addiction have postulated that drugs of abuse 'short-circuit' or 'hijack' the neural mechanisms underlying reward or motivation (Tiffany, 1990; Grace, 1995; White, 1996; Bechara *et al.*, 1998; Phillips *et al.*, 2003).

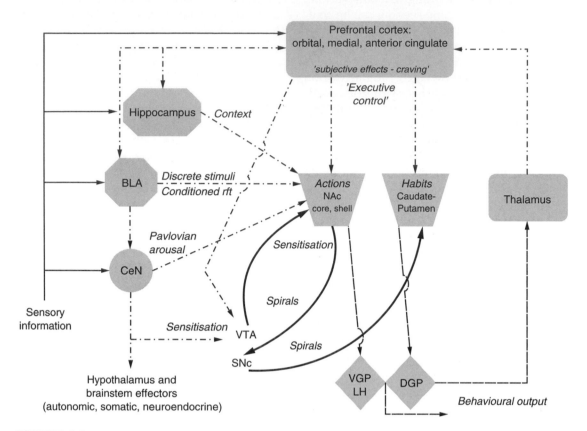

FIGURE 3.2 Schematic representation of limbic circuitry including cortex, ventral striatum, and pallidum, that tentatively localises functions involved in addiction discussed in the text including: (i) processing of discrete and contextual drug-associated conditioned stimuli – basolateral amygdala and hippocampal formation, respectively, with a special role of the basolateral amygdala in mediating conditioned reinforcement and the central amygdala in pavlovian (or conditioned) arousal; (ii) goal-directed actions ('action–outcome' associations) – involving the interaction of prefrontal cortex with other structures, perhaps including the nucleus accumbens; (iii) 'habits' (stimulus–response learning) – dorsal striatum. Both (ii) and (iii) involve interactions between cortical projections to striatal domains, modulated by DA. (iv) 'Executive control' – prefrontal cortical areas; (v) subjective processes, such as craving, activate areas such as orbital and anterior cingulate cortex, as well as temporal lobe structures including the amygdala, in functional imaging studies; (vi) 'behavioural output' is intended to subsume ventral and dorsal striatopallidal outflow via both brainstem structures and re-entrant thalamo-cortical loop circuitry; (vii) 'spirals' refers to the serial, spiralling interactions between the striatum and midbrain DA neurons that are organised in a ventral-to-dorsal progression (Haber *et al.*, 2000); (viii) sensitisation refers to the enhancement of drug and conditioned responses that is a consequence of earlier drug exposure and is at the heart of theories of addiction and relapse. The neural basis of stress-induced relapse, which involves the bed nucleus of the stria terminalis, central amygdala and their noradrenergic innervation is not illustrated. Dot-dashed arrows: glutamatergic pathways; Dashed arrows: GABAergic pathways; bold arrows: dopaminergic pathways. The transmitter used by central amygdala neurons is less certain, but is probably glutamate and also a neuropeptide(s). Abbreviations: BLA: basolateral amygdala; CeN: central nucleus of the amygdala; VTA: ventral tegmental area; SNc: substantia nigra pars compacta; DGP, dorsal globus pallidus; LH, lateral hypothalamus; NAc, nucleus accumbens; rft, reinforcement; VGP, ventral globus pallidus. This diagram is modified from Altman *et al.*, 1996 and Everitt and Wolf, 2002.

4.1 The Role of DA in the Nucleus Accumbens in Motivation and Learning

The discovery that rats would work hard to stimulate regions of their brain electrically (intracranial self-stimulation, or ICSS; Olds and Milner, 1954) was historically important. Many sites that support ICSS lie on the path of dopaminergic neurons from the substantia nigra pars compacta (SNc) and ventral tegmental area (VTA) to limbic sites including the ventral striatum (nucleus accumbens, Acb), and ICSS is substantially reduced after Acb DA depletion (Fibiger et al., 1987). The rate at which rats learn to respond for ICSS is correlated with the degree of potentiation of synapses made by cortical afferents onto striatal neurons, a potentiation that requires DA receptors (Reynolds et al., 2001). The discovery that deep brain stimulation and transcranial magnetic stimulation can influence cognition, affect and motor performance in humans means that we cannot discount this means of altering brain function. Deep brain stimulation of the subthalamic nucleus has been successful with severe Parkinson's disease, and may have applications in obsessive compulsive disease and clinical depression (George, 2003) but care is needed as the stimulation can be self-administered, and in the case of Parkinson's disease, dramatic emotional sequelae have been reported (Schneider et al., 2003).

4.2 DA: Motivation, Reward and Pleasure

An early suggestion was that Acb DA mediated the pleasurable aspects of reward (Wise, 1981, 1982; Wise and Bozarth, 1985). There is now strong evidence against this simple idea. Certainly, DA is released in response to appetitive reinforcers (e.g. Fiorino et al., 1993; Wilson et al., 1995; Schultz et al., 1997; Berridge and Robinson, 1998; Schultz, 1998; Schultz et al., 1998; Schultz and Dickinson, 2000; Datla et al., 2002, Ito et al., 2002; Carelli and Wightman, 2004;

Young, 2004), intra-Acb DA agonists are reinforcing (Phillips et al., 1994a), animals may adjust their drug-taking to maintain high Acb DA levels (Pettit and Justice, 1989), and some aspects of naturally- and drug-reinforced responding depend on Acb DA (e.g. Pettit et al., 1984; Caine and Koob, 1994; Baker et al., 1998; Ikemoto and Panksepp, 1999; Dickinson et al., 2000; Parkinson et al., 2002; Salamone and Correa, 2002; Salamone et al., 2003). However, Acb DA does not mediate 'pleasure' (Fibiger and Phillips, 1988; Robbins and Everitt, 1992; Berridge and Robinson, 1998; Volkow et al., 1999a), though its release may correlate with activity in other systems that do, and reinforcement operates in its absence (Ettenberg et al., 1982; Pettit et al., 1984). Measured by microdialysis techniques, DA is also released in response to aversive stimuli, CSs that predict them, and other salient stimuli (see e.g. Salamone, 1994; Horvitz, 2000; Young, 2004), which would be consistent with a more general motivational role. CSs that have been paired with reward also elicit approach (Brown and Jenkins, 1968); this effect also depends on the Acb (Parkinson et al., 1999a,b, 2000c) and its DA innervation. DA may also be involved in learning this approach response, again perhaps under the control of the central nucleus of the amygdala (CeA; Parkinson et al., 2000a,b,c; Hall et al., 2001; Cardinal et al., 2002a; Parkinson et al., 2002; Phillips et al., 2003; see Figure 3.2). Acb DA also contributes directly to subjects' motivation to work hard (Ikemoto and Panksepp, 1999; Salamone and Correa, 2002; Salamone et al., 2003).

Hedonic assessment of rewards themselves, or 'liking', does not depend on dopaminergic processes (Pecina et al., 1997; Berridge and Robinson, 1998; Dickinson et al., 2000; Pecina et al., 2003). Instead, it involves opioid mechanisms in the nucleus accumbens shell (AcbSh) and other systems in the pallidum and brainstem (Berridge, 2000; Kelley and Berridge, 2002). Intra-Acb μ opioid agonists also affect food preference, increasing the intake of highly palatable foodstuffs including fat, sweet foods, salt, and ethanol (Zhang *et al.*, 1998; Zhang and Kelley, 2000; Kelley *et al.*, 2002a; Zhang and Kelley, 2002; Will *et al.*, 2003), while chronic ingestion of chocolate induces adaptations in endogenous Acb opioid systems (Kelley *et al.*, 2003). However, the notion that 'pleasure' can be mediated by receptors in a sub-cortical nucleus is perhaps too simple. Activity in this circuitry is probably subject to further processing in cortical (particularly prefrontal cortical) circuits, before attribution and accompanying subjective commentary (Altman *et al.*, 1996).

4.3 DA and Learning

The notion that DA 'stamps in' the learning of stimulus–response connections has considerable support. It has acute effects that modulate corticostriatal transmission, and also lasting effects. The combination of presynaptic and postsynaptic activity normally induces long-term depression of corticostriatal synapses, but if the same pattern of activity is paired with a pulse of DA, then the active synapses are strengthened (Reynolds and Wickens, 2002). Natural reinforcers, drugs of abuse, and CSs that predict either, trigger increases in DA release in the Acb (Berridge and Robinson, 1998; Datla *et al.*, 2002; Ito *et al.*, 2002; Carelli and Wightman, 2004; Young, 2004). DA neurons fire to unexpected rewards, or to unexpected stimuli that predict reward (Schultz *et al.*, 1997, 1998; Schultz, 1998; Schultz and Dickinson, 2000). DA neuron firing may be a teaching signal used for learning about actions that lead to reward (Schultz *et al.*, 1997). The Acb similarly responds to anticipated rewards (Schultz *et al.*, 1992; Miyazaki *et al.*, 1998; Martin and Ono, 2000; Schultz *et al.*, 2000; Breiter *et al.*, 2001; Knutson *et al.*, 2001; de la Fuente-Fernandez *et al.*, 2002; Cromwell and Schultz, 2003; Elliott *et al.*, 2003; McClure *et al.*, 2003; Bjork *et al.*, 2004; Zink *et al.*, 2004). Other parameters of tonic DA neuronal firing may signal reward uncertainty, possibly relevant to the understanding of

gambling behaviour (Fiorillo *et al.*, 2003; Schultz, 2004).

Targets of DA neurons certainly influence instrumental behaviour. Structures that learn from the DA 'teaching signal' probably include the dorsal striatum and prefrontal cortex (PFC) (see Figure 3.2), but much attention has focused on the Acb. Blockade of *N*-methyl-D-aspartate (NMDA) glutamate receptors in the nucleus accumbens core (AcbC) has been shown to retard instrumental learning for food (Kelley *et al.*, 1997), as has inhibition or over-stimulation of protein kinase A (PKA) within the Acb (Baldwin *et al.*, 2002a). Concurrent blockade of NMDA and DA D1 receptors in the AcbC synergistically prevents learning (Smith-Roe and Kelley, 2000). Once the response has been learned, subsequent performance is not impaired by NMDA receptor blockade within the AcbC (Kelley *et al.*, 1997). Furthermore, infusion of a PKA inhibitor (Baldwin *et al.*, 2002a) or a protein synthesis inhibitor (Hernandez *et al.*, 2002) into the AcbC after instrumental training sessions impairs subsequent performance, implying that PKA activity and protein synthesis in the AcbC contribute to the consolidation in memory of instrumental behaviour.

However, it is clear that the Acb is not required for simple instrumental conditioning but rather is implicated in providing extra motivation for behaviour, especially when such motivation is triggered by pavlovian CSs, or when reinforcers are delayed or require substantial effort to obtain. Rats with Acb or AcbC lesions acquire lever-press responses on sequences of random ratio schedules at normal or slightly reduced levels (Corbit *et al.*, 2001; de Borchgrave *et al.*, 2002) and are fully sensitive to changes in the action–outcome contingency (Balleine and Killcross, 1994; Corbit *et al.*, 2001; de Borchgrave *et al.*, 2002). Thus, the Acb is not critical for goal-directed action (see Cardinal *et al.*, 2002b). Rather, it appears to be critical for some aspects of motivation that promote responding for rewards in real-life situations. For example, the Acb plays a role in promoting responding for delayed rewards (Cardinal *et al.*, 2001; Cardinal and Cheung, 2005) and is required for pavlovian CSs to provide a motivational boost to responding (Hall *et al.*, 2001a; de Borchgrave *et al.*, 2002), i.e. for PIT. PIT has sometimes been termed 'wanting' (Wyvell and Berridge, 2000, 2001), although 'wanting' could equally refer to the instrumental incentive value underpinning true goal-directed action or pavlovian arousal itself. PIT can be further enhanced by injection of amphetamine into the Acb (Wyvell and Berridge, 2000) and depends on DA (Dickinson *et al.*, 2000), possibly under the control of the CeA (Hall *et al.*, 2001a). Other motivational effects of pavlovian CSs also depend on the Acb, for example, the capacity of CSs to act as conditioned reinforcers of instrumental behaviour.

The neural basis of conditioned reinforcement has been investigated using the 'acquisition of a new response' procedure, in which subjects work only for a conditioned stimulus that has previously been associated with a natural reinforcer such as food or water. From these studies, it is clear that the basolateral amygdala (BLA) and AcbC are important in the ability to respond normally for conditioned reinforcement (Cador *et al.*, 1989; Burns *et al.*, 1994; Parkinson *et al.*, 1999a; Everitt and Robbins, 2000). In naturalistic situations, rewards are frequently available only after a delay, require considerable effort to achieve, and are signalled by environmental stimuli. Thus, the Acb is central to a number of processes that require motivation (Mogenson *et al.*, 1980). Functional neuroimaging evidence supports this conclusion in humans (Knutson *et al.*, 1999; Breiter *et al.*, 2001).

4.4 Action–outcome Contingency Knowledge, Planning and Value: the Prefrontal Cortex and Amygdala

The prefrontal cortex (specifically, prelimbic cortex) is required for rats to represent the contingencies between actions and their outcomes (Balleine and Dickinson, 1998; Corbit and Balleine, 2003), and acquisition of instrumental responses on a simple schedule is disrupted by blocking NMDA and DA D1 receptors in the PFC (Baldwin *et al.*, 2002b). This is relevant to evidence from cognitive neuroscience that sectors of the human PFC are important for volitional processes (see Section 9.13 and Figure 3.2).

The PFC is also involved in extinction (Myers and Davis, 2002), the cessation of responding when a CS or response is no longer paired with reinforcement. Extinction is not 'unlearning' but involves the learning of new, inhibitory associations (see Mackintosh, 1974; Delamater, 2004). Lesions of the ventral medial PFC interfere with the extinction of pavlovian conditioned freezing in the rat (Morgan *et al.*, 1993; Morgan and LeDoux, 1995, 1999). The PFC interacts with the amygdala, an important site of CS–US association in this task (see Davis, 2000; LeDoux, 2000a), and may suppress conditioned freezing when it is no longer appropriate (Garcia *et al.*, 1999; Myers and Davis, 2002; Quirk *et al.*, 2003; Rosenkranz *et al.*, 2003).

The orbitofrontal cortex (OFC) is part of the PFC with a particular role in the assessment of reinforcer value. It has bidirectional connections to the amygdala, and both are heavily implicated in the retrieval of the value of primary reinforcers based on information from CSs (Cardinal *et al.*, 2002b; Balleine *et al.*, 2003; Lindgren *et al.*, 2003; Pickens *et al.*, 2003; O'Doherty, 2004). In humans, the OFC and amygdala are also activated during extinction of pavlovian conditioning (Gottfried and Dolan, 2004). The amygdala regulates the DA signal to the Acb (Everitt *et al.*, 2000; Parkinson *et al.*, 2000a; Hall *et al.*, 2001a; Cardinal *et al.*, 2002b; Phillips *et al.*, 2003). Goal-directed action requires that action–outcome contingencies interact with the incentive value of goals (Dickinson, 1994; Dickinson and Balleine, 1994) and the connection between the amygdala and the PFC (Pitkänen, 2000) may provide this functional link (Coutureau *et al.*, 2000; Arana *et al.*, 2003; Gottfried *et al.*, 2003; Holland and Gallagher, 2004).

4.5 Relevance to Drug Addiction

It has been suggested that these motivational and learning processes are particularly significant in some addictions, and their modification may have therapeutic potential. The existence of dissociable parallel brain systems mediating the associative control over addiction sits comfortably within the classic dichotomy of behavior into pavlovian (Pavlov, 1927) or instrumental learning (Thorndike, 1905). A number of influential theories of addiction have postulated the existence of multiple parallel processes, each with its own independent, but interacting, neural system (Tiffany, 1990; Grace, 1995; White, 1996; Bechara *et al.*, 1998; Phillips *et al.*, 2003).

DA systems are affected by virtually all of the major classes of drugs of abuse, ranging from the psychomotor stimulants to opioids, alcohol and nicotine, as well as by natural reinforcers such as food. Some abused drugs are particularly potent in this regard. Both food and drugs of abuse increase Acb DA, but the DA response to drugs of abuse may not habituate to the same extent as that to food (Di Chiara, 1998, 2002). Sensitisation occurs following psychostimulant administration directly into the VTA, which induces hypersensitivity to DA in the Acb (Cador *et al.*, 1995) and enhances the response to pavlovian CSs associated with reward (Harmer and Phillips, 1999; Taylor and Horger, 1999; Wyvell and Berridge, 2001). In animal models of drug-seeking behaviour controlled by drug-associated stimuli (Everitt and Robbins, 2000), lesions of the AcbC or disruption of its glutamatergic neurotransmission reduce drug-seeking (Di Ciano and Everitt, 2001; Hutcheson *et al.*, 2001a), probably by reducing the motivational impact of the CSs. DA D3 receptors are particularly concentrated in the Acb and amygdala (Sokoloff *et al.*, 1990), and D3 receptor antagonists (Vorel *et al.*, 2002;

Di Ciano *et al.*, 2003) and partial agonists (Pilla *et al.*, 1999; Cervo *et al.*, 2003) reduce cue-controlled cocaine-seeking or relapse to cocaine-taking in animal models. Some manipulations that reduce drug-seeking or reinstatement of drug-taking in animal models, such as DA D3 receptor antagonists, do not reduce food-seeking in a similar manner (Vorel *et al.*, 2002; Di Ciano *et al.*, 2003). It is not yet clear to what extent sensitisation contributes to human addiction (Sax and Strakowski, 2001), but it has been suggested that a sensitised response to drug-associated cues contributes to drug craving – that this 'incentive motivational' system becomes sensitized (Robinson and Berridge, 1993). In current animal models, drug sensitization enhances responding for food, or responding to CSs for food (Taylor and Horger, 1999; Wyvell and Berridge, 2001; Olausson *et al.*, 2003), but in human addiction, responding for non-drug reinforcement declines relative to that for drug reinforcement (APA, 2000). However, pre-treatment with psychomotor stimulants results in animals being willing to work harder for cocaine and this may reflect an effect of sensitization on the motivation to seek drugs (Vezina, 2004).

The well-known ability of psychomotor stimulants to potentiate conditioned reinforcement (Taylor and Robbins, 1984), depends upon the integrity of the dopaminergic innervation of the Acb, especially the AcbSh (Parkinson *et al.*, 1999a). This might be one possible basis for understanding why psychomotor stimulant drugs are themselves reinforcing; they enhance the reinforcing effects of environmental stimuli. The importance of conditioned reinforcers is that they allow the mediation and maintenance of long chains of behaviour, including drug-seeking behaviour, over delays to primary reinforcement.

Although potent as conditioned reinforcers when presented contingently, CSs paired with drug infusions do not increase drug-seeking when presented noncontingently to animals (Kruzich *et al.*, 2001; Deroche-Gamonet *et al.*, 2002; Di Ciano and Everitt, 2003). Thus, conditioned reinforcement appears to be reliant on the contingency between the response and the CS, irrespective of the motivational value of the US (Parkinson *et al.*, 2005). Indeed, the reliance of drug-seeking and taking on drug-associated conditioned reinforcers is underscored by further findings that cocaine self-administration is lower in the absence of any contingent CS (Semenova and Markou, 2003). Indeed, nicotine self-administration in animals is difficult to acquire in the absence of conditioned reinforcers (Caggiula *et al.*, 2002), suggesting that conditioned reinforcers may form part of a powerful stimulus complex, along with the drug, in maintaining drug use. Similarly, conditioned reinforcement maintained by CSs previously paired with oral alcohol can be persistent (Shahan, 2002) and the ability to maintain responding is independent of the drug (Shahan *et al.*, 2003), suggesting that this type of drug-seeking has a habitual quality. The impact of conditioned reinforcement on drug-seeking is persistent and relatively impervious to extinction. It can maintain responding independently from the drug with which it was paired, suggesting that it may depend upon a separate neural system from that which mediates the effects of the drug itself (Shahan, 2002; Di Ciano and Everitt, 2004a).

In experimental models of addictive behaviour in which drug-associated conditioned reinforcers support and maintain prolonged bouts of seeking behaviour (Everitt and Robbins, 2000), the functional integrity of a neural system involving the BLA and AcbC is of major importance (see Figure 3.2). Thus, lesions of the BLA or AcbC, but not the AcbSh, greatly impair the acquisition of cocaine-seeking behaviour (Whitelaw *et al.*, 1996; Ito *et al.*, 2004). There is also neurochemical specificity in these BLA and Acb mechanisms. DA receptor blockade, but not AMPA receptor blockade in the BLA, reduces established cue-controlled cocaine seeking. The reverse is true in the AcbC, where AMPA, but not DA receptor blockade, has this effect (Di Ciano and Everitt, 2004b). It has additionally been established that disconnection of the BLA and AcbC by blocking DA receptors in the BLA on one side of the brain and AMPA receptors in the AcbC on the other has the same effect of dramatically reducing cocaine seeking (Di Ciano and Everitt, 2004b). These data provide the strongest evidence that the BLA and AcbC function serially as components of a neural system that mediates these conditioned influences on drug-seeking (see Figure 3.2).

In functional imaging studies of human drug addicts, the amygdala is consistently activated by exposure to cocaine-, heroin-, food- and sex-associated stimuli in a way that is correlated with drug craving (e.g. Grant *et al.*, 1996; Gottfried *et al.*, 2003). Other regions commonly activated by drug-associated stimuli include the anterior cingulate cortex, OFC and occasionally the Acb (Grant *et al.*, 1996; Childress *et al.*, 1999; Sell *et al.*, 1999; Garavan *et al.*, 2000). These data show that in both animals and humans, limbic cortical-ventral striatopallidal circuitry is associated with emotional learning and in processes related to drug craving, addiction and relapse.

4.6 Habits and the Dorsal Striatum

The development of stimulus–response habits may depend on dorsal striatal plasticity (Packard and McGaugh, 1996), which may in turn depend on DA receptors (Reynolds *et al.*, 2001; Reynolds and Wickens, 2002). The balance between habits and goal-directed behaviour may also be regulated by the prelimbic and infralimbic cortex (Killcross and Coutureau, 2003), subdivisions of the rat PFC. Recent functional neuroimaging data in humans supports the hypothesis that the ventral and dorsal striatum are also involved differentially in pavlovian and instrumental learning (O'Doherty *et al.*, 2004).

Dorsal striatal DA release to CSs is a correlate of well-established cocaine-seeking (Ito *et al.*, 2002). By contrast, such DA release is not seen in the AcbC region (Ito *et al.*, 2000). Consistent with the electrophysiological data (Schultz *et al.*, 1998), DA release is only observed there when the CS is presented in a surprising context. Comprehensive studies of chronic cocaine self-administration in monkeys indicate a progressive involvement of limbic, association and sensorimotor striatal domains, with autoradiographic changes evident first in the ventral, and then in the dorsal striatum (Nader *et al.*, 2002; Porrino *et al.*, 2004). These data support the notion that there may be a stage of stimulus–reward or action–outcome learning that precedes stimulus–response habit learning. These phases may be mediated respectively by the ventral and dorsal striatum, either successively, or more probably in a temporally overlapping manner, possibly via the recently characterised 'cascading' neural connectivity that links these different corticostriatal loops (Haber *et al.*, 2000; see Figure 3.2). Thus, drug addiction is conceived in terms of a switch between these modes of learning, operating across the corticostriatal circuitry, from ventral striatal (i.e. Acb) to dorsal striatal domains.

5 NEUROBIOLOGY OF RELAPSE

A key feature of drug addiction is the high propensity to relapse, even after protracted periods of abstinence. The prevalent animal model of relapse utilises the so-called extinction-reinstatement procedure recently reviewed by Shaham and colleagues (Shaham *et al.*, 2003) in a double issue of *Psychopharmacology* (volume 168, issues 1–2) devoted to this subject. The usual form of this procedure is to train rats to press a lever to self-administer a drug and then to extinguish the instrumental act of lever pressing by omitting drug infusions. Following extinction, three manipulations generally accepted to be of importance in precipitating relapse in abstinent human drug addicts can 'reinstate' drug-seeking responses by increasing lever pressing although the drug remains unavailable. They are exposure to drug-associated stimuli, experimenter-administered drug, or 'stress,' usually an electric shock to the feet. However, extinction of the instrumental act of drug self-administration is not generally a means by which human addicts achieve abstinence. Abstinence is more likely to arise through an active decision to abstain or through abstinence imposed by the law or by treatment. Moreover, since the extinguished response is so readily reinstated, it is unlikely that extinction training will provide an effective clinical approach to treatment. Extinction of the acquired properties of drug-associated stimuli through their non-reinforced exposure has been attempted as a therapeutic strategy, but with limited success (O'Brien *et al.*, 1990; O'Brien *et al.*, 1992), most likely because cue exposure in the clinic is unlikely to reduce the properties of drug cues in the original drug-associated environment.

Neurobiologically, these ways of inducing relapse in the extinction-reinstatement model depend upon both common and discrete elements of limbic cortical-ventral striatopallidal circuitry. Most studies have involved the reinstatement of cocaine-seeking behaviour, but there are also studies with heroin and nicotine.

5.1 Drug-cue-induced Reinstatement

The neural basis of cue-induced reinstatement has been reviewed extensively (Kalivas and McFarland, 2003; Shaham *et al.*, 2003). It is prevented by reversible or permanent inactivation of the BLA and reversible inactivation of the dorsal mPFC (Meil and See, 1997; Kalivas and McFarland, 2003; Kalivas *et al.*, 2003). Inactivation of the OFC also attenuates cue-induced reinstatement of drug seeking (Fuchs *et al.*, 2004). Systemically injected D1 and D3 DA receptor antagonists block cued reinstatement (Ciccocioppo *et al.*, 2001; Di Ciano and Everitt, 2003), as do intra-BLA, but not intra-Acb, infusions of D1 DA receptor antagonists (See *et al.*, 2001) – consistent with the effects of D1 and D3 DA receptor antagonism in the BLA on cocaine-seeking measured under a second-order schedule (Di Ciano and Everitt, 2004b). Perhaps surprisingly, inactivation of the Acb does not attenuate cue-induced reinstatement (Kalivas and McFarland, 2003), yet this structure is important for conditioned reinforcement and other pavlovian influences on instrumental behaviour, while AMPA receptor blockade attenuates cocaine-seeking under a second-order schedule (Di Ciano and Everitt, 2001). Although limbic cortical-ventral striatopallidal systems are implicated in the conditioned control of drug-seeking and reinstatement after extinction, much remains to be established in terms of the processes occurring in cortical and subcortical structures and the ways in which different subsystems interact. While the BLA mediates reinstatement following exposure to discrete, cocaine-associated stimuli, the hippocampus may underlie the motivational impact of contextual stimuli (see Figure 3.2). Theta-burst stimulation of the hippocampus, a form of experimental deep brain stimulation, has been shown to reinstate extinguished cocaine-seeking in a manner that depended on glutamate transmission in the VTA. It was suggested that this might mimic the process by which reinstatement occurs when animals are placed in a context associated with drug-taking, rather than in response to discrete cocaine cues (Vorel *et al.*, 2001). Indeed, dorsal hippocampal inactivation attenuates context-induced reinstatement of drug seeking, as does inactivation of the dorsal mPFC (Fuchs *et al.*, 2005). These data are in accord with the suggestion of a differential involvement of the amygdala in conditioning to discrete, and the hippocampal formation in conditioning to contextual, stimuli (Selden *et al.*, 1991; McDonald and White, 1993). Moreover, electrophysiological and *in vivo* neurochemical studies have demonstrated that hippocampal, amygdala and PFC projections interact in the Acb in a way that is modulated by mesolimbic DA and that, in turn, can modulate the release of DA (O'Donnell and Grace, 1995; Blaha *et al.*, 1997; Di Ciano *et al.*, 1998; Pennartz *et al.*, 2000; Floresco *et al.*, 2001). Thus, hippocampal, amygdala and PFC mechanisms may influence drug-seeking through their convergent projections to the Acb, perhaps competing for access to response strategies subserved by different cortical-striato-pallido-thalamo cortical re-entrant loops (see Figure 3.2). The mPFC is clearly important in reinstatement – whether

induced by cues, contexts, drugs or stress – following extinction of the instrumental seeking response (McFarland and Kalivas, 2001; Fuchs *et al.*, 2005). Determining the psychological process that the mPFC subserves in these settings is an important goal.

The vigour of conditioned reinstatement of cocaine seeking increases with the duration of withdrawal (Grimm *et al.*, 2001), suggesting that neuroadaptations to chronic cocaine self-administration and withdrawal interact with the motivation to seek cocaine when cocaine cues are present in the environment. These findings may provide insight into the possible mechanisms that underlie the persistence or 'incubation' of cocaine-seeking reported to occur over time in abstinent cocaine addicts. The mechanisms underlying this incubation effect have been shown to depend upon the upregulation of the extracellular signal-regulated kinase (ERK) signalling pathway specifically within the CeA (Lu *et al.*, 2005). Thus, exposure to cocaine-associated stimuli increased cocaine-seeking and also ERK phosphorylation in the CeA, but not BLA, substantially more after 30 days than after one day of cocaine withdrawal, so the incubation effect was correlated with ERK upregulation in the CeA. Inhibition of ERK phosphorylation in the CeA, but not BLA, after 30 days of withdrawal greatly decreased cocaine-seeking, whereas stimulation of ERK phosphorylation in the CeA, but not BLA, increased cocaine-seeking after one day of withdrawal. Thus the mechanisms mediating drug-cue-induced relapse and its enhancement during protracted withdrawal appear to depend upon two dissociable mechanisms in the BLA and CeA, respectively.

5.2 Drug-induced Reinstatement

Drug-induced reinstatement by 'priming' (i.e. non-contingent or experimenter administered cocaine or heroin – often given intraperitoneally and not intravenously) can be attenuated by D1-like dopamine receptor antagonists (Shaham and Stewart, 1996). In neuroanatomical studies it has been shown that drug-induced reinstatement can be blocked by inactivation of the VTA, dorsal mPFC, AcbC and ventral pallidum, called the 'motor subcircuit' by Kalivas and colleagues (McFarland and Kalivas, 2001; Kalivas and McFarland, 2003; Kalivas *et al.*, 2003; see Figure 3.2). Moreover, DA receptor antagonists infused into the mPFC or AcbSh also attenuate drug-induced reinstatement (see Shaham *et al.*, 2003). Antagonists at AMPA, but not NMDA receptors in the ACb, block reinstatement induced by systemic or intra-mPFC cocaine and, by contrast, AMPA receptor agonists infused into the Acb reinstate cocaine seeking (Cornish *et al.*, 1999; Cornish and Kalivas, 2000). The effects of cocaine or heroin to reinstate extinguished responding are mimicked by systemic injections of D2, but not D1, receptor agonists (Self and Nestler, 1998) and by infusions of cocaine, amphetamine or DA itself directly into either the Acb or mPFC (Stewart and Vezina, 1988; Cornish and Kalivas, 2000; McFarland and Kalivas, 2001). Antagonists at μ opiate receptors prevent the effects of heroin and alcohol, but not cocaine, on reinstatement (Shaham and Stewart, 1996; Le *et al.*, 1999) and a CB1 receptor antagonist has also been shown to prevent the reinstatement effects of cocaine (De Vries *et al.*, 2001).

5.3 Stress-induced Reinstatement

Reinstatement can be induced by several stressors, including footshock, food deprivation and also CNS administration of corticotrophin releasing factor CRF (see Shaham *et al.*, 2003). Inactivation of the dorsal mPFC prevents footshock-induced reinstatement; this area of the PFC is commonly involved in cued-, drug- and stress-induced reinstatement (McFarland *et al.*, 2004). Additional and unique neural circuitry appears to be critical for the effects of stress, including the CeA, bed nucleus of the stria terminalis (BNST) and the noradrenergic medullary tegmentum which innervates these structures (Aston-Jones *et al.*, 1999; Shaham *et al.*, 2000a,b). Thus, the following manipulations all block stress-induced reinstatement:

intra-BNST, but not intra-amygdala, infusions of a CRF antagonist; systemic and intracerebroventricular, but not intra-locus coeruleus, injections of an alpha-2 noradrenergic receptor agonist; intra-BNST and intra-amygdala alpha-2 noradrenergic receptor antagonists; and destruction of the ventral noradrenergic bundle originating in the medullary noradrenergic cell groups (see Shaham *et al.*, 2003 for review). The CRF-containing projections between the CeA and BNST have also been shown to be a critical link between these structures in mediating stress-induced relapse (Shaham *et al.*, 2003). Thus, two neural systems implicated in stress responses in general – one utilising NA and the other CRF – are implicated along with the mPFC in mediating relapse induced by footshock stress in the extinction-reinstatement procedure. The generally accepted mechanism is that stress activates the medullary noradrenergic neurons and leads to activation of the CRF system within the BNST and possibly the CeA (see Kalivas and McFarland, 2003; Shaham *et al.*, 2003, for reviews). How this subcortical, neuroendocrine mechanism interfaces with the mPFC is not altogether clear, nor is how this impinges on limbic cortical ventral striatopallidal circuitry.

One of the reasons for developing and studying the neural basis of relapse in experimental animals is to develop treatments that will promote abstinence. Intensive experimental investigation of this area has yielded detailed information on the neural systems and neurochemical mechanisms underlying cue-, stress- and drug-induced relapse. An important issue for resolution is the extent to which the effects on reinstatement of cues, drug or stress actually depend upon the prior process of instrumental extinction. If they do, their utility in human addiction, where this extinction process does not occur, may be slight. D3 DA receptor antagonists appear to have efficacy in both the cued-reinstatement procedure and ongoing, cue-controlled cocaine-seeking suggesting that this dopaminergic target might affect the conditioned process common to both.

In addition, the GABA-B receptor agonist baclofen both attenuates drug seeking that depends upon drug-associated conditioned reinforcers in rats (Di Ciano and Everitt, 2003) and also attenuates cue-induced activation of limbic cortical areas in cocaine-addicted humans (Brebner *et al.*, 2002). New pharmacological treatments to prevent relapse may emerge from this rich preclinical data on experimental models of reinstatement in animals.

6 NEUROADAPTATIONS – INTRACELLULAR CASCADES

The chronic administration of drugs of abuse results in the induction of intracellular cascades within the limbic corticostriatal circuitry. Although different drugs act at different receptor targets on the cell surface, there is a degree of convergence in their downstream signalling pathways. Interaction between the drug and its target results in either the opening of a ligand-gated channel, or the activation of a receptor-linked G-protein (Koob and Nestler, 1997), both of which induce intracellular cascades. One common action of drugs is the activation of the transcription factor CREB and components of the cAMP signalling pathway, such as adenylyl cyclase (AC) and protein kinase A (PKA) (Duman *et al.*, 1988; Terwilliger *et al.*, 1991; Guitart *et al.*, 1992a; Unterwald *et al.*, 1993; Konradi *et al.*, 1994; Cole *et al.*, 1995; Ortiz *et al.*, 1995; Turgeon *et al.*, 1997; Carlezon *et al.*, 1998; Rubino *et al.*, 2000; Asher *et al.*, 2002; Shaw-Lutchman *et al.*, 2003). CREB regulates the transcription of genes whose promoters contain the CRE element, and is thought to be a site of convergence of intracellular cascades as it can be activated through phosphorylation at serine 133 by several different protein kinases (Shaywitz and Greenberg, 1999; De Cesare and Sassone-Corsi, 2000). Therefore alterations in CREB and the cAMP signalling pathway may represent common neuroadaptations of different drugs of abuse.

Opiates and cannabinoids acutely inhibit adenylyl cyclase and the cAMP signalling pathway (Dill and Howlett, 1988; Duman *et al.*, 1988; Childers, 1991), resulting in a decrease in phosphorylated CREB (Guitart *et al.*, 1992a). In contrast, acute administration of ethanol and stimulants increases the activity of the cAMP signalling pathway (Yang *et al.*, 1996; Shaw-Lutchman *et al.*, 2003). However, in all cases, there is a common chronic upregulation of the cAMP signalling pathway that is accompanied by tolerance to the acute intracellular response to drugs of abuse (Dill and Howlett, 1988; Guitart *et al.*, 1992a; Carlezon *et al.*, 1998; Self *et al.*, 1998; Pliakas *et al.*, 2001). The switch from acute inhibition to chronic upregulation of the cAMP pathway with repeated opioid administration is poorly understood, though it is known to involve adaptations in G-protein properties resulting from their persistent stimulation (Watts, 2002), and neuroadaptive changes in protein kinase systems (Liu and Anand, 2001). Furthermore, few downstream targets have been identified that mediate the functional effects of cAMP and CREB upregulation. Among the proteins whose levels are increased by chronic drug administration in a CREB dependent manner are AC, tyrosine hydroxylase (TH), the rate-limiting enzyme in DA synthesis, and the opioid peptide dynorphin (Daunais and McGinty, 1994; Cole *et al.*, 1995; Lane-Ladd *et al.*, 1997; Carlezon *et al.*, 1998; Chao *et al.*, 2002). Dynorphin stimulates κ-opioid receptors, resulting in an inhibition of DA release (Shippenberg and Rea, 1997), and the effects of CREB upregulation on drug reward are blocked by κ-opioid antagonists (Carlezon *et al.*, 1998; Pliakas *et al.*, 2001). Dynorphin mRNA levels are increased in the striatum of cocaine abusers *post-mortem* (Hurd and Herkenham, 1993). Therefore neuroadaptations in cAMP signalling, resulting in dynorphin upregulation, may partially underlie tolerance to the effects of drugs of abuse.

Repeated intermittent administration of addictive drugs results in sensitisation of, rather than tolerance to, some of the behavioural and rewarding effects of drugs.

The VTA is required for the initiation of behavioural sensitisation (Vanderschuren and Kalivas, 2000), and long-lasting adaptations in the Acb are correlated with the expression of sensitisation (Henry and White, 1995; Churchill *et al.*, 1999; Thomas *et al.*, 2001). Transient increases of GluR1 subunits in the VTA are important for the triggering of sensitisation (Carlezon and Nestler, 2002). The resultant persistent increase in calcium signalling and calcium/calmodulin-stimulated (CaM) kinase activation have also been implicated in behavioural sensitisation (Licata and Pierce, 2003). CaM kinase II stimulates the mitogen-activated protein (MAP) kinase signalling pathway (Seger and Krebs, 1995), which is known to be involved in sensitisation (Pierce *et al.*, 1999). Sensitisation may also be mediated by a chronic drug-induced downregulation of the *Homer* gene family. Developmental genetic knockout of *Homer1* or *Homer2* in drug-naïve rats mimics the sensitised response to acute drug administration observed in rats experiencing withdrawal (Szumlinski *et al.*, 2004). Specifically, *Homer* downregulation is critically important in the Acb, as localised antisense-mediated knockdown of *Homer1* expression in the Acb similarly induces sensitisation (Ghasemzadeh *et al.*, 2003), and virally-mediated rescue of *Homer2* in the Acb of *Homer2* knockout mice reverses the drug-sensitised phenotype (Szumlinski *et al.*, 2004).

One neuroadaptation that has attracted particular interest is the upregulation of the chronic Fos-related antigen ΔFosB. Levels of ΔFosB are increased in the Acb for up to four weeks following drug administration (Hope *et al.*, 1994; Moratalla *et al.*, 1996; Nye and Nestler, 1996), and ΔFosB is also progressively upregulated with repeated drug administration (Nestler, 2001). This suggests that it is involved in behavioural sensitisation, a hypothesis that is strongly indicated by the demonstration that ΔFosB overexpression in the Acb sensitises behavioural and rewarding responses to cocaine and morphine (Kelz *et al.*, 1999), whereas a reduction inhibits responses to cocaine (Peakman *et al.*, 2003) and *fosB* knockout mice do not develop behavioural sensitisation (Hiroi *et al.*, 1997). Therefore, ΔFosB may be a 'molecular switch' (Kelz and Nestler, 2000), that enables the sensitisation of responses to drugs of abuse and long-term adaptations underlying addiction that persist through withdrawal. Again, the current challenge is to identify downstream targets of ΔFosB signalling, one of which may be cyclin-dependent kinase 5 (cdk5) (Chen *et al.*, 2000; Bibb *et al.*, 2001).

Upon withdrawal from drugs, which may be precipitated experimentally by the administration of an antagonist, there is a further increase in the activity of the cAMP signalling pathway beyond the level observed during tolerance (Duman *et al.*, 1988; Guitart *et al.*, 1992a). This reflects a state of dependence upon drugs of abuse, whereby when in withdrawal, the molecular cascades underlying reward are altered, resulting in an amotivational state (Carlezon *et al.*, 1998; Self *et al.*, 1998; Pliakas *et al.*, 2001; Walters and Blendy, 2001; Newton *et al.*, 2002; Nestler and Malenka, 2004). Mice deficient in CREB display reduced opiate dependence (Maldonado *et al.*, 1996; Lane-Ladd *et al.*, 1997; Valverde *et al.*, 2004) showing that cAMP signalling is important for both tolerance and dependence. A focus for current and future research is the characterisation of the downstream targets of CREB, such as dynorphin, that are required for the development of tolerance and dependence.

Neuroadaptations implicated in drug-induced reinstatement (Section 5) include the expression of *AGS3* (*activator of G protein signalling 3*), the blockade of which prevents cocaine-induced relapse to cocaine seeking (Bowers *et al.*, 2004), and a lowering of extracellular glutamate through reduction of cystine-glutamate exchange, the restoration of which also prevents cocaine-primed relapse (Baker *et al.*, 2003). Drug-cue-induced reinstatement exhibits a time-dependent increase through withdrawal, with cue-induced cocaine, methamphetamine, heroin and sucrose seeking behaviours incubating over time (Grimm *et al.*, 2001, 2002;

Shalev *et al.*, 2001; Shepard *et al.*, 2004). Molecular changes that correlate with this incubation effect may be important for cue-induced relapse to drug seeking. With short periods of withdrawal, transient increases are observed in tyrosine hydroxylase activity and cdk5 protein levels in the VTA (Berhow *et al.*, 1995; Lu and Wehner, 1997), and more persistent increases in PKA activity occur in the Acb (Terwilliger *et al.*, 1991; Berhow *et al.*, 1995; Lu and Wehner, 1997). However, the closest correlate of incubation appears to be the progressive upregulation of BDNF protein in the VTA (Grimm *et al.*, 2003; Lu *et al.*, 2003). BDNF appears to be involved in the persistence of the incubation effect rather than being critical for incubation itself, evidenced by the demonstration that intra-VTA infusion of BDNF protein increases cocaine seeking over and above the incubation-related elevation (Lu *et al.*, 2004).

BDNF has a well-established role in hippocampal LTP and learning and memory (Lu and Chow, 1999; Schinder and Poo, 2000; Yamada *et al.*, 2002). Therefore there is a similarity between the molecular mechanisms of drug addiction and learning and memory that also applies to the other intracellular cascades described, particularly the involvement of CREB (Nestler, 2002). Furthermore, drugs of abuse induce changes in the VTA and Acb that are reminiscent of the influential cellular models of learning and memory LTP and long-term depression (LTD) (Thomas and Malenka, 2003). One important issue that concerns research into both drug addiction and learning and memory is the longevity of both processes. All the molecular neuroadaptations described thus far are impermanent, and though some are indeed long-lasting, none can account for the compulsion and relapse that are observed months or even years after withdrawal. It is increasingly thought that morphological changes in synaptic structure are the only process by which the plasticity underlying both drug addiction and learning and memory can become near-permanent (Nestler and Malenka, 2004). BDNF is necessary for the neuronal growth and synaptic remodelling associated with learning and memory (McAllister *et al.*, 1999; Schinder and Poo, 2000; Tyler *et al.*, 2002; Yamada *et al.*, 2002), and its putative role in incubation, as well as sensitisation (Horger *et al.*, 1999; Pierce *et al.*, 1999), suggests that morphological plasticity may be critically involved in drug addiction.

Many genes have been implicated in synaptic plasticity (Abraham *et al.*, 1991; Nestler, 2001; Crombag *et al.*, 2002; Dudai, 2002), and recently the involvement of *cdk5* in addiction-related permanent plasticity has attracted great attention. *Cdk5* is regulated by ΔFosB (Chen *et al.*, 2000; Bibb *et al.*, 2001), providing a link between the longest-lasting molecular adaptation and permanent plasticity (Chao and Nestler, 2004), while cdk5 mediates the proliferation of striatal dendritic spines in response to chronic administration of cocaine (Bibb *et al.*, 2001; Norrholm *et al.*, 2003). Such structural changes are likely to involve neurofilaments, which are elements of the cytoskeletal architecture of neurons (Lee and Cleveland, 1996; Toni *et al.*, 1999). There is evidence for hyperphosphorylation of neurofilament proteins both in rodents and in human opiate addicts *postmortem* (Beitner-Johnson *et al.*, 1992; Ferrer-Alcon *et al.*, 2000; Jaquet *et al.*, 2001). The mechanisms underlying neuroadaptations in synaptic morphology will be a focus of future research investigating the mechanisms of the long-lasting plasticity mediating drug addiction.

Synaptic morphology can also be altered by the production of new neurons. This neurogenesis is increasingly believed to play a role in drug-induced neuroadaptation. The few studies that have been conducted suggest that chronic exposure to drugs of abuse decreases neurogenesis in the hippocampus (Abrous *et al.*, 2002; Nixon and Crews, 2002; Crews and Nixon, 2003; Eisch and Mandyam, 2004; Yamaguchi *et al.*, 2004). A parallel is found in studies of depression, in which decreased hippocampal neurogenesis is observed (Kempermann and Kronenberg, 2003; Malberg and Duman, 2003; Duman, 2004). In contrast, learning and memory are associated with an increase in hippocampal neurogenesis (Gould and Gross, 2002; Shors *et al.*, 2002), and one action of antidepressant drugs is to increase hippocampal neurogenesis and neuronal growth (Blows, 2000; Malberg and Duman, 2003; Castren, 2004). This may suggest a potential avenue for the treatment of addiction. Some antidepressants may work partly by increasing neurogenesis. Antidepressants are sometimes, but not always, effective medications for drug dependence (Hughes *et al.*, 2004; Szerman *et al.*, 2005).

Though further delineation of the molecular pathways involved in drug addiction will be a focus of future research, an important challenge will be to integrate the resulting information, as the same molecular candidates are implicated in several aspects of drug addiction. BDNF is associated with incubation, relapse, sensitisation and permanent plasticity. Furthermore, neuroadaptations occur throughout the limbic corticostriatal circuitry. Although molecular changes have been localised to particular brain areas, their relevance to behaviour is only beginning to be determined in a spatially localised manner. Array technology has recently been used both *in vitro* and *in vivo* to produce large sets of information on the upregulation of genes following the administration of drugs of abuse (Thibault *et al.*, 2000; Gonzalez-Nicolini and McGinty, 2002; Li *et al.*, 2002; Pollock, 2002; Toda *et al.*, 2002), but it will be several years before it can be established whether such neuroadaptations are merely correlative, or critical for the development of addiction.

The similarity between the molecular processes implicated in drug addiction and those firmly established in learning and memory will guide future research. One exciting prospect is the possible manipulation of drug-associated memories long after they have been acquired. Studies of fear conditioning have demonstrated that previously learned memories for stimulus-aversive outcome associations can be disrupted in a retrieval-dependent manner, so that they are not expressed subsequently in retrieval tests (Nader *et al.*, 2000). This impairment of the reconsolidation of memories has also been observed in several other learning and memory paradigms (Przybyslawski and Sara, 1997; Przybyslawski *et al.*, 1999; Bozon *et al.*, 2003; Eisenberg *et al.*, 2003; Suzuki *et al.*, 2004), including a study of appetitive incentive learning (Wang *et al.*, 2005), and also in humans (Walker *et al.*, 2003), and may be extended to drug addiction. Drug-associated environmental stimuli elicit strong craving and increase the chance of relapse in abstinent individuals. The potential to reduce the impact of these cues through disrupting the reconsolidation of their association with addictive drugs may be a future avenue of research. Stimulus–addictive drug associations are supported by the same neuroanatomical substrates as both appetitive and aversive associations (Everitt *et al.*, 2000; LeDoux, 2000), further underlining the similarity between addiction and learning, and the upregulation of *Zif268* in the amygdala is strongly correlated with the reconsolidation of both stimulus–drug and stimulus–footshock associations (Hall *et al.*, 2001b; Thomas *et al.*, 2003), providing a prospective target for functional studies. *Zif268* has recently been shown to be a specific marker of the reconsolidation of hippocampal-dependent contextual fear memories (Lee *et al.*, 2004). Moreover, it appears that the molecular mechanisms of consolidation and reconsolidation are doubly dissociable, at least in the hippocampus (Lee *et al.*, 2004; Figure 3.3). It may be possible to target the reconsolidation of previously-learned maladaptive memories that are important in drug addiction (Nader, 2003).

7 VULNERABILITY TO ADDICTION

A significant proportion of the population take drugs of abuse at least once in their lifetime. Many individuals are capable of maintaining prolonged recreational use.

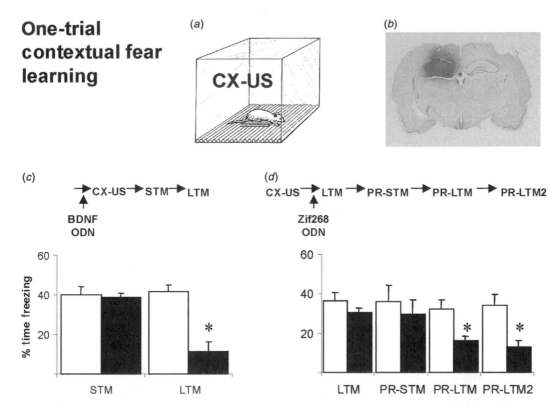

FIGURE 3.3 The consolidation and reconsolidation of contextual fear memories are mediated by independent cellular processes. Rats are fear-conditioned to a novel context (*a*), and infused into the dorsal hippocampus with antisense oligodeoxynucleotides (ODN) 90 minutes before conditioning or memory reactivation (*b*). Subsequently, tests for long-term memory show that BDNF is required specifically for consolidation (*c*), whereas Zif268 is necessary only for reconsolidation (*d*). Based on data reported in Lee *et al.*, 2004.

Only a few develop a true addiction (O'Brien *et al.*, 1986). In the last few decades, the identification of the factors that determine these individual differences in propensity for addiction has become one of the major targets of drug abuse research. Emerging data from both clinical and animal experiments suggest that there exist 'vulnerable' phenotypes and genotypes that are more predisposed to drug abuse (Piazza *et al.*, 2000). Elucidating the nature of these vulnerabilities could help prevent addiction in the predisposed population.

7.1 Individual Differences in Humans

Enormous differences between the subjective and reinforcing effects of drugs in humans are well-documented (de Wit *et al.*, 1986; Abi-Dargham *et al.*, 2003; Fergusson *et al.*, 2003). Individuals who prefer the effects of amphetamine to placebo show increased ratings of euphoria and positive mood, compared to anxiety and depression in subjects that choose placebo over amphetamine (de Wit *et al.*, 1986). Recent advances in imaging technology have yielded exciting information about the neural correlates of these subjective differences. In one recent report, the intensity of the high induced by methylphenidate was significantly correlated with levels of released DA. Subjects who had the greatest increase perceived the most intense high (Volkow *et al.*, 1999b). Further, the magnitude of decrease in D2 receptor availability

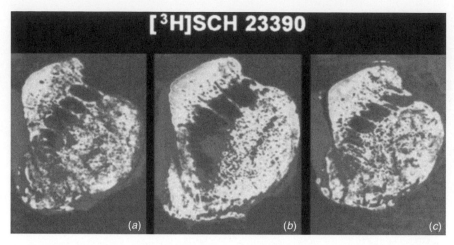

FIGURE 3.4 Representative colour-coded autoradiograms depicting specific D1 binding using [³H]SCH-23390 at the level of the posterior ventral precommissural striatum of a control rhesus monkey (panel *a*) and from a representative monkey in the chronic 0.03 mg/kg cocaine per injection (panel *b*) and 0.3 mg/kg cocaine per injection (panel *c*) groups. The autoradiogram is scaled in fmol/mg wet-weight tissue. (From Nader *et al.*, 2002.) Reprinted, with permission, from *Neuropsychopharmacology* 27: 35-46 (http://www.nature.com/npp/index.html). Copyright (2002) Macmillan Publishers Ltd.

is significantly associated with the positive reinforcing effects of the psychomotor stimulant methylphenidate (Volkow *et al.*, 1999b; Figure 3.1), and release of DA in response to *d*-amphetamine correlates with self-reports of 'drug wanting' and the personality trait of novelty-seeking (Leyton *et al.*, 2002). In support of these findings, rhesus monkeys with extensive cocaine self-administration history show significant decreases in D_2 receptor densities throughout the striatum compared to monkeys with a history of food reinforcement (Nader *et al.*, 2002; Figure 3.4). These data suggest that pre-existing differences between subjects in the rate of DA release and/or D_2 receptor distribution may play a role in the predisposition to drug abuse. The cause and exact nature of these functional differences is not known.

7.2 Animal Models in the Study of Individual Differences

Individual differences in conditioned and unconditioned responses to drugs of abuse have been reliably demonstrated in animals (Piazza *et al.*, 1998). In particular, the propensity to acquire intravenous self-administration (IVSA) in rats can be predicted by the behavioural reactivity of an individual rat to a stressful situation, such as exposure to a novel environment (e.g. Altman and Das, 1966; Piazza *et al.*, 1990, 1991a). In this model, the propensity to develop drug SA can be represented by dividing animals into subgroups based on their locomotor response to a novel environment. Animals with an activity score above the mean for the entire group, so-called 'high responders' (HRs), show enhanced acquisition of psychostimulant IVSA (Altman and Das, 1966; Piazza *et al.*, 1990, 1991a; Marinelli and White, 2000) compared to animals with an activity score below the median of the group, the 'low responders' (LRs).

Further studies show that individual differences in drug intake originate from vertical shifts in the dose–response curve for intravenous cocaine- self-administration, and these vertical shifts can be predicted by reactivity to novelty (Piazza *et al.*, 2000). HR/LR groups also show differences in drug-mediated behaviours, such as increased locomotor response to systemic administration of cocaine, amphetamine, and morphine (Hooks *et al.*, 1991a,b, 1992a; Kalinichev *et al.*, 2004), enhanced psychostimulant-induced behavioural sensitisation (Jodogne *et al.*, 1994; Chefer *et al.*, 2003; Hooks *et al.*, 2004), and stronger contextual conditioning to drugs (Jodogne *et al.*, 1994).

Behavioural differences between HRs and LRs appear to be mediated by differences in dopaminergic neuronal structure and function. For example, HRs show increased cocaine- (Chefer *et al.*, 2003), amphetamine- (Hooks *et al.*, 1992b), and stress- (Rouge-Pont *et al.*, 1993) induced DA levels in the Acb, as well as a higher 3,4-dihydroxyphenylacetic acid (DOPAC)/DA ratio in this region (Piazza *et al.*, 1991b). Data from electrophysiological studies demonstrate higher basal firing rates and bursting activity of DA neurons in the ventral tegmental area and, to a lesser extent, the SNc in HRs (Jodogne *et al.*, 1994). Structurally, HRs have increased DAT numbers (Chefer *et al.*, 2003) and greater B_{max} for D1 binding sites (Hooks *et al.*, 1994) in the Acb. Regulatory mechanisms of the mesolimbic DA system also differ between HRs and LRs. Recent data indicate that HRs express lower levels of tyrosine hydroxylase levels and CCK-mRNA, part of the intrinsic inhibitory input to dopaminergic VTA neurons, but higher levels of PPE-mRNA, part of the extrinsic facilitating input to these neurons (Lucas *et al.*, 1998).

These behavioural and neurochemical differences are accompanied by differences in activity of the hypothalamic–pituitary–adrenal axis (HPA), the system primarily activated under stressful situations. Animals designated as HR have higher novelty-induced corticosterone secretion compared to LR rats (Piazza *et al.*, 1991b), and self-administration of amphetamine is positively correlated with corticosterone levels after two hours of exposure to stress (Piazza *et al.*, 1991b). The work of Piazza and his colleagues suggests that individual differences in vulnerability to addiction can be modelled in animals, and that these differences are related to altered structure and function of the DAergic and HPA systems.

Nonetheless, the developmental cause of these behavioural and neural differences is not known.

7.3 Environmental Influences on the Developing Brain

Environmental experience may contribute to individual differences in vulnerability to drug addiction. Early adverse experience, such as childhood sexual or physical abuse, is one of the most important biological and environmental factors that are associated with vulnerability to substance abuse (Gordon, 2002). The prevailing view is that these stressors influence the development of neural systems that underlie the expression of behavioural and endocrine responses to stress and reward. Although clinical data confirm a relationship between early adverse experience and substance abuse, it is not known whether this relationship is direct or indirect. Recent developments using animal models of early adverse environmental experience have been important in elucidating the causal nature of this relationship.

7.4 Effects of Disrupted Maternal Care

One animal model of early adverse experience takes the form of disrupted maternal care, whereby infant rats experience repeated episodes of prolonged maternal separation (MS) during the first two weeks after birth. This consistently gives rise to profound behavioural, neural, and endocrine differences in adult animals. It leads to increased behavioural reactivity in response to stressors (Meaney *et al.*, 1988; Ogawa *et al.*, 1994; Wigger and Neumann, 1999), and these behaviours are accompanied by altered structure and function of neural regions involved in HPA activation (Plotsky and Meaney, 1993; Noonan *et al.*, 1994; Avishai-Eliner *et al.*, 1999; Huot *et al.*, 2002).

Recent work using these models has attempted to form a causal relationship between disrupted maternal care, reactivity to stressors, and individual differences rat strains (Ranaldi *et al.*, 2001). Another important question is whether prenatal exposure to drugs of abuse facilitates the development of drug dependence in general. In one study, prenatal exposure to morphine enhanced rates of heroin and of cocaine self-administration (Ramsey *et al.*, 1993).

Adolescence is another period during which the brain undergoes many complex changes that can have a prolonged impact on decision-making and cognitive processes (Giedd *et al.*, 1999; Spear, 2000). In addition, adolescents are more likely to experiment with illicit drugs, which may be due in whole or in part to the increase in sensation- and novelty-seeking that is characteristic of adolescence (Stansfield *et al.*, 2004). Recent clinical data suggest that adolescent exposure to drugs of abuse is associated with increased risk of addiction in adulthood (Estroff *et al.*, 1989; Kelley *et al.*, 2004). Not unlike the data from prenatal exposure research, studies using animal models suggest that rodents with adolescent exposure to drugs such as methylphenidate (Achat-Mendes *et al.*, 2003; Brandon *et al.*, 2003), nicotine (Abreu-Villiça *et al.*, 2004a; Collins *et al.*, 2004; Kelley and Rowan, 2004; Schochet *et al.*, 2004), cannabinoids (Pistis *et al.*, 2004), MDMA (Ecstasy) (Morley-Fletcher *et al.*, 2002; Achat-Mendes *et al.*, 2003), and alcohol (Philpot and Kirstein, 2004; White and Swartzwelder, 2004) also show behavioural and neural changes indicative of tolerance to these and other drugs, which persist into adulthood. Adolescent-exposed animals tested as adults show a behavioural and neural profile that is different from adult animals administered a similar drug regime (e.g. Pistis *et al.*, 2004; Schochet *et al.*, 2004). This suggests differential long-term neuroadaptive responses to drugs, possibly related to immature or still-developing plasticity mechanisms in the PFC. One potential confound for these studies is that the majority of them look at effects of non-contingent drug administration during the periadolescent period on later adult behaviour and neurochemistry. Future studies should aim at exploring how self-administration

drug experience during adolescence influences drug-mediated behaviours and neural changes when tested in adulthood.

7.8 Genetic Factors Involved in Vulnerability to Addiction

Individual differences in genetic make-up critically influence susceptibility to addiction. Although some aspects of vulnerability may be unique for specific substances, most known genetic influences are common to all drugs of abuse. Recent estimates suggest that genetic components explain 40-60 per cent of overall vulnerability to addiction (Tsuang *et al.*, 1999; Uhl, 1999, 2004). These data do not support single-gene models for the inheritance of addiction vulnerability. Contributions from allelic variations in several genes are likely to be involved. Genetic components do not necessarily impact upon the initiation of drug use, but instead influence progression from regular use to dependence (Tsuang *et al.*, 1999; Uhl, 2004). Recent data are yielding information on which chromosomal regions, genes, haplotypes, and allelic variants provide exactly what genetic influence on vulnerability to drug abuse.

Although there are numerous candidate genes influencing addiction and addictive behaviours, human studies have generally focused on identifying genes associated with dopaminergic function. A number of studies report a significant association between substance dependence and polymorphisms of dopaminergic receptor genes (DRD1, DRD2, DRD3, DRD4). Subjects with a history of drug use show increased frequency of homozygosity for the restriction polymorphism Dde 1 of the DRD2 gene (Comings *et al.*, 1997), and several studies have demonstrated a link between the presence of the A1 allele of the DRD2 Taq 1 polymorphism and drug dependence (Smith *et al.*, 1992; O'Hara *et al.*, 1993; Comings *et al.*, 1994). Polymorphisms of the DRD3 gene have recently been identified in 96 rat strains and substrains (Smits *et al.*, 2004), although there is good evidence that this gene does not play a major role in the genetic vulnerability to alcoholism (Gorwood et al., 1995; de Jong and de Kloet, 2004). Novelty-seeking, a personality trait often observed in addicts, is significantly associated with the 7-repeat allele of the DRD4 exonic polymorphism (Ebstein et al., 1996).

Individual differences in genetic polymorphisms have functional outcomes. Individuals homozygous or heterozygous for the 7- (or longer) repeat allele (DRD4 L) report significantly higher craving after consumption of alcohol compared to individuals classified as DRD4 S (Hutchison et al., 2002). Further, although olanzapine reduces craving for alcohol in both DRD4 S and DRD4 L individuals, it only reduces cue- and alcohol priming-induced craving in DRD4 L individuals (Hutchison et al., 2003).

7.9 Animal Models used in the Study of Genetic Neurovulnerability to Addiction

The role of genetic factors in contributing to drug-related behaviours can be examined using inbred rodent strains, which, in contrast to outbred strains, provide a stable genotype. Two inbred rat strains that differ in responses to drugs of abuse are Lewis (LEW) and Fischer 344 (F344) rats. In comparison to F344 rats, LEW rats show greater behavioural responses to several drugs, including oral self-administration (Suzuki et al., 1988, 1992, 1998), intravenous acquisition of self-administration of morphine (Ambrosio et al., 1995) and cocaine (Kosten et al., 1997), place conditioning (Guitart et al., 1992b; Kosten et al., 1994), and locomotor sensitisation (Camp et al., 1994; Kosten et al., 1994).

These strains also differ in properties of their mesolimbic DA systems. LEW rats have lower basal extracellular DA metabolite levels in the Acb (Camp et al., 1994; Strecker et al., 2004) and lower numbers of spontaneously active DA neurons in the VTA (Minabe et al., 1995). They also show a more prolonged elevation of DA levels in

the ventral striatum following acute cocaine administration (Camp et al., 1994; Strecker et al., 2004). At a biochemical level, LEW rats express higher levels of tyrosine hydroxylase in the VTA, but lower levels in the Acb, than F344 rats (Haile et al., 2001). Finally, strain differences are also observed in HPA function. Although F334 have higher basal and stress-induced levels of glucocorticoids, LEW rats show a more prolonged elevation of corticosterone following exposure to a stressor (Dhabhar et al., 1993).

Differences in susceptibility to the reinforcing properties of cocaine, amphetamine, morphine and ethanol have been described among inbred strains of mice (Cunningham et al., 1992; Henricks et al., 1997; Cabib et al., 2000; Conversi et al., 2004). A number of studies have demonstrated that mice belonging to the inbred strains C57BL/6 (C57) and DBA/2 (DBA) differ in their behavioural and neural responses to drugs of abuse (Zocchi et al., 1998; He and Shippenberg, 2000; Kuzmin and Johansson, 2000; Murphy et al., 2001; Conversi et al., 2004; Orsini et al., 2004; Ventura et al., 2004). The data suggest that the C57 genotype can be characterised as 'drug-preferring' and the DBA genotype as 'drug-resistant'. Sensitivity to the unconditioned locomotor effects of amphetamine (Cabib et al., 2000) and level of locomotor activity in a novel environment (Orsini et al., 2004) are both susceptible to the influence of environmental manipulations such as food restriction when measured in these strains. These data provide information on genetic–experience interactions, and suggest a possible homology between these phenotypes and psychostimulant-induced place preference (Orsini et al., 2004).

7.10 The Influence of Gender on Vulnerability

Epidemiological data suggest a greater prevalence of substance use disorders among men, but recent surveys show increased rates of substance dependence in women (Brady and Randall, 1999; Samhsa, 2000). These that exposure to alcohol in developing rats led to severe reductions of glutamate receptors of the AMPA subtype in the neocortex (Bellinger *et al.*, 2002) (see also section 7.7). These adverse actions on the brain and intellect, as well as the social burden of domestic violence arising from the heightened aggression produced by abuse, and overall greater morbidity and mortality, place alcohol among the most behaviourally toxic of all psychoactive substances. However, not all alcohol consumption has adverse effects. There is consistent evidence of significant beneficial health effects of drinking alcohol (and associated substances such as the polyphenols of red wine) in small amounts, which reduces the incidence of strokes and dementia (Pinder and Sandler, 2004).

By contrast with alcohol, the evidence for deleterious cognitive effects of cannabis intoxication is controversial. Any significant effects may depend on chronic use over many years in that small sub-population of users who become addicted (Rogers and Robbins, 2001). However, accumulating evidence suggests that cannabis can act as a triggering factor for schizophrenia (Arseneault *et al.*, 2004).

9 DRUG ADDICTION: A SOCIAL COGNITIVE NEUROSCIENCE PERSPECTIVE

Until recently, the gap between social cognition and molecular and cellular neuroscience has seemed unbridgeable, given the complexities of linking social constructs such as theory of mind with simple causal neural networks (Adolphs, 2003). However, the emergence of cognitive neuropsychology in the 1970s illustrated the potential of a productive synthesis of cognitive psychology and clinical neuroscience in addressing common questions of how the mind/brain works. Cognitive neuroscience will continue to prove important in the objective evaluation of cognitive effects of drugs and the intellectual sequelae of chronic drug use.

A similar initiative in 'social cognitive neuroscience', embracing developments in 'affective neuroscience' and 'neuroeconomics' promises to be of considerable importance for understanding the nature of addiction in its social context.

Social cognitive neuroscience (SCN) is a systematic and theoretically-driven approach designed to understand social and emotional phenomena in terms of the interaction between motivations and social factors that influence behaviour, information-processing mechanisms that underlie social-level phenomena, and the brain mechanisms that instantiate cognitive-level processes (Cacioppo and Berntson, 2002; Adolphs, 2003; Blakemore *et al.*, 2004; Ochsner, 2004). The concern with neural substrates underlying normal social cognitive mechanisms links social neuroscience to the basic neurosciences and has been facilitated by the increasing availability of methodologies for investigating neural function in non-brain-damaged adults. SCN bridges the gap between social cognition and neuroscience by exploring how the brain influences social process as well as how social processes influence the brain (Harmon-Jones and Devine, 2003). Of particular interest is the issue of whether the processes that give rise to social cognition are a subset of more general cognitive operations, or whether instead there are unique processes governing social cognition (Adolphs, 2003; Blakemore *et al.*, 2004).

Although still in its infancy, the social cognitive neuroscience approach has already been applied successfully to a broad range of topics in the social sciences (Adolphs, 2003) and neuropsychiatric conditions, which potentially include addiction (Grady and Keightley, 2002). It is proving possible to elucidate the neural and cognitive mechanisms underlying more complex social constructs such as volition (Spence and Frith, 1999); attribution theory (Klein and Kihlstrom, 1998; Ochsner and Lieberman, 2001; Adolphs, 2003); self-regulation (Levesque *et al.*, 2004); cognitive reappraisal (Ochsner *et al.*, 2002); attitudes (Ochsner and Lieberman, 2001); mental representation of self (Kelley *et al.*, 2002a; Klein *et al.*, 2002); reward (O'Doherty *et al.*, 2003a); beliefs (Samson *et al.*, 2004); emotions (Ochsner and Feldman, 2001; Dolan, 2002), deception (Spence *et al.*, 2004); empathy (Decety and Jackson, 2004); theory of mind (Stuss *et al.*, 2001); cognitive control MacDonald *et al.*, 2000); intuition (Lieberman, 2000); moral emotions (Kroll and Egan, 2004) and complex social and economic judgements such as decision-making (Lieberman *et al.*, 2003; Glimcher and Rustichini, 2004).

9.1 Addiction as a Disorder of Social Cognition

Viewing it as a complex brain disorder, it is possible to consider the main behavioural characteristics of drug addiction in terms of at least four impairments of social cognition:

9.1.1 *Impairment in the Processing and Representation of Saliency or Rewards*

Many modern theories of drug use and dependence assign central prominence to the role of compulsive craving in drug use and relapse. Until recently it was believed that addiction was predominantly driven by reward processes mediated by limbic circuits (Blum *et al.*, 2000). However, results from recent neuroimaging studies implicate a highly interconnected network of brain areas including orbital and medial PFC, amygdala, striatum and dopaminergic midbrain in reward processing (see sections 4 and 5). Distinct reward-related functions can be attributed to different components of this network. The OFC is involved in coding stimulus reward value and in concert with the amygdala and ventral striatum is implicated in representing predicted future reward. These frontal areas are frequently activated in addicted subjects during intoxication, craving, and bingeing, but deactivated during withdrawal (Volkow *et al.*, 2003a,b). The same regions are also involved in higher-order cognitive and motivational

functions, such as the ability to track, update, and modulate the salience of a reinforcer as a function of context and expectation and the ability to control and inhibit prepotent responses. Cognitive theories have been influential by embedding craving within a network based on social learning theory (Niaura, 2000; Drummond, 2001). According to Goldstein and Volkow (2002) these results imply that addiction involves brain areas involved in several cortically regulated cognitive and emotional processes including the overvaluing of drug reinforcers, the undervaluing of alternative reinforcers, and deficits in inhibitory control for drug responses.

9.1.2 *Impairment of Social Reasoning and Decision Making*

The PFC has been implicated in guiding social cognition (decision making and inhibitory control) by eliciting emotional states that serve to bias cognition, a role that is further supported by investigations of normal decision making and social reasoning studies (Adolphs, 2003). The effects of damage to medial and orbital PFC are consistent with a role for these regions in guiding the strategic adoption of someone else's point of view (Stuss *et al.*, 2001) and impaired performance in reasoning about social exchange (Stone *et al.*, 2002). Compromised decision making could contribute to the development of addiction and undermine attempts at abstinence. The behaviour of those addicted to drugs could be viewed as demonstrating faulty decision making given their inability to discontinue self-destructive drug-seeking behaviours. A go/no-go response inhibition task in which working memory demands were varied (Kaufman *et al.*, 2003; Hester and Garavan, 2004) demonstrates that the compromised abilities of cocaine users to exert control over strong prepotent urges were associated with reduced activity in both anterior cingulate and right prefrontal cortices. The results suggest a neuroanatomical basis for this dysexecutive component in addiction, supporting the importance of cognitive functions in prolonging abuse or predisposing users towards relapse. Abnormalities in the PFC are found consistently in most drug-addicted subjects using imaging studies (Goldstein and Volkow, 2002; Bolla *et al.*, 2003; Ersche *et al.*, 2005). Thus, one might expect that the disruptions of self-monitoring and decision-making processes observed in drug-addicted subjects (Rogers *et al.*, 1999a; Bechara and Damasio, 2002) might possibly arise from drug dependent disruption of these prefrontal functions. However, as described in section 8, an alternative possibility is that the deficits are not a consequence of drug-taking, but that both arise from premorbid changes in the PFC. Furthermore, it is even possible that the drug-taking behaviour might arise from a propensity to self-medication.

9.1.3 Impairment of Voluntary Control

The issue of volition is central to social cognition since most consider willed action as essential to social democracy and to social constructs such as guilt, responsibility, accountability, law and sanctioning deviant behaviour. Drug addiction is typically portrayed as a compulsive drive to take drugs despite awareness of serious adverse consequences. The self-perceived 'loss of control' where the addict seems unable or unwilling to control their drug use is traditionally viewed as 'voluntary' despite studies showing long-lasting changes in the brain that could compromise crucial elements of the volitional system (Peoples, 2002; Morse, 2004; Volkow and Li, 2004). Campbell (2003) has argued that addiction should be considered a disease of volition caused by a cognitive impairment involving an inability to recall the negative effects of the addictive behaviour.

Historically however, the construct of 'will' has been generally defined as the capacity to choose what action to perform or withhold (Frith *et al.*, 1991) and in a recent review Zhu (2004) distinguishes three

stages of volition: the mental act of decision making; the mental act of initiating voluntary action; and the mental activity of executive control. According to Zhu (2004) the essential engagement of the ACC in all three types of volition suggests a pivotal role in sustaining the volitional function. Other imaging studies implicate PFC, SMA and lateral PFC (Frith *et al.*, 1991; Spence *et al.*, 1998).

Dysfunction in these regions has been associated with neuropsychiatric disorders of action including hysterical weakness, alien hand and schizophrenia (Marshall *et al.*, 1997; Spence *et al.*, 1998), and have also been found in relation to issues of deception and malingering (Ward *et al.*, 2003; Spence *et al.*, 2004). Spence and Frith (1999) suggest that 'the dorsolateral PFC and the brain regions with which it is connected are essential to performing willed action, and that diseases or dysfunction of these circuits may be associated with a variety of disorders of volition, such as Parkinson's disease, 'utilisation' behaviour, 'alien' and 'phantom' limbs, delusions of 'alien control', and the passivity phenomena of schizophrenia.

The issue of impaired volition raises possible ethical issues about the capacity of addicted persons to give 'free and informed' consent to participate in studies that involve detecting neural abnormalities in addiction and treatments designed to reduce their addiction. Research involving persons who are cognitively or physically impaired in their decision making or volitional control would require special ethical consideration (Brody, 1998) because they may not be capable of providing informed consent. The view among addiction researchers has been that drug-dependent people are able to give free and informed consent to participate in research studies and clinical trials so long as they are not intoxicated or suffering acute withdrawal symptoms at the time that they give consent (Adler, 1995; Gorelick *et al.*, 1999; Hall *et al.*, 2004). However Cohen (2002) controversially argues that 'the nature and pathology of untreated substance dependence make the condition inherently incompatible with a rational, internally uncoerced and informed consent on the part of those volunteering to receive addictive drugs in a non-therapeutic research setting'.

9.1.4 Impairment of Awareness of the Serious Adverse Consequences

Drug-addicted individuals use drugs despite apparently knowing the long-term physical and psychological consequences. Rinn *et al.* (2002) tested the hypothesis of this lack of apparent awareness by suggesting that it was a product of cognitive failure rather than an emotion-driven rejection of the truth. In their study they found persistent denial to be significantly correlated with greater impairment of executive function, verbal memory, visual inference, and mental speed. Self-awareness deficits are common after traumatic brain injury (McGlynn and Schacter, 1989) and reflect a person's 'inability to recognise deficits or problem circumstances caused by neurological injury' (Barco *et al.*, 1991). Such awareness disorders are believed to reflect a complex interaction between neurological, psychological and social factors depending on lesion location and cognitive dysfunction (McGlynn and Schacter, 1989).

10 THE MIND/BRAIN INTERFACE: NEUROBEHAVIOURAL ECONOMICS OF ADDICTION

10.1 Basic Principles of Behavioural Economics

Behavioural economics, a merging of traditional economic theory with psychological studies of choice (Rachlin *et al.*, 1976; Allison, 1979), offers different perspectives on addiction. Much of economics is based on utility theory (von Neumann and Morgenstern, 1947; Russell and Norvig, 1995), which assumes that agents are rational and exhibit certain reasonable attributes of preference. For example, one assumption is transitivity of preference: if an agent prefers A to B and B to C, then it must prefer A to C or it would easily be exploited by more rational agents. Given these assumptions, there must exist a utility function that assigns unidimensional values to real-world multidimensional events or outcomes, such that the agent prefers outcomes with higher utility. Psychologically and neurally, a similar process must also happen (Shizgal, 1997) if only to decide access to motor output. Agents can then use their knowledge about the world, and about the consequences of their actions (which may be uncertain), to act so as to maximise their expected utility (Arnauld and Nicole, 1662). Rational behaviour need not require complex, explicit thought. Conversely, if people are logical, then we can infer their value system by observing their behaviour (Friedman, 1990; Williams, 1994).

A direct application of traditional economics to addiction is the calculation of elasticity of demand for goods, such as drugs. In a barter economy, and therefore in animal experiments, the 'price' of a commodity has no absolute meaning. We can speak of price only in terms of what other commodities an animal will give up to obtain the good, and that may depend on the specific commodities being traded (Friedman, 1990; Rachlin, 2003; Vuchinich and Heather, 2003). In humans, elasticity has a more general meaning, since humans use a monetary economy. Money is a single commodity that is substitutable for almost all others (fungible), so we can calculate elasticity as the change in consumption as money price changes. Elasticity is defined as the proportional change in consumption divided by the proportional change in price. Elasticity is usually negative (we consume less as price goes up), so elasticities between −1 and 0 represent relatively 'inelastic' demand (consumption is not reduced much by price increases) and elasticities below −1 represent relatively 'elastic' demand (consumption is strongly affected by price).

10.2 Addiction in Behavioural Economic Terms

An obvious way to think about addiction is that demand for drugs is inelastic compared to demand for other things. The more someone is addicted, the more inelastic their demand is – they will therefore sacrifice other commodities (work, money, social interaction) rather than sacrifice the drug. Alcohol demand in rats can be more inelastic than demand for food (Heyman *et al.*, 1999; Heyman, 2000). Yet drug demand is not completely inelastic, and addiction is not an all-or-nothing phenomenon. Most users of heroin, cocaine, and alcohol do not use extremely large amounts, as the stereotype of an addict would suggest. Instead, most use infrequently, or 'chip' (NHSDA, 2001; MacCoun, 2003a). Furthermore, over 75 per cent of those dependent on an illicit drug recover (Warner *et al.*, 1995; Heyman, 2003). In fact, the elasticity of demand for cigarettes is typically about −0.4 (Gruber *et al.*, 2002; Chaloupka *et al.*, 2003); that is, if the price goes up by 10%, consumption goes down by 4%. When the price goes up, some people quit altogether and others smoke less. As for most commodities, elasticity varies with price: smokers working for cigarette puffs in the laboratory are fairly inelastic when the price is low ($\varepsilon = -0.56$), but become more elastic when the price goes up ($\varepsilon = -1.58$) (Bickel *et al.*, 1995a; DeGrandpre and Bickel, 1995). Probably for this reason, elasticity is greater for poorer smokers, for whom cigarettes are proportionally more expensive (Gruber *et al.*, 2002). In the UK, elasticity of demand for alcohol varies from −1.69 for wine through −0.86 for spirits to −0.76 for beer (Smith, 1999). Participation price elasticities (the effect of price on the number of people using a drug) are about −0.90 to −0.80 for heroin and −0.55 to −0.36 for cocaine. Overall elasticities (the effect of price on the total amount consumed) are about −1.80 to −1.60 for heroin and −1.10 to −0.72 for cocaine (Saffer and Chaloupka, 1995).

Elasticity also varies with motivational state and other factors. Animals' demand for food is more inelastic when they are hungry and if there are no alternative ways of obtaining food (Hursh, 1978). Similarly, demand for cigarettes is more inelastic when smokers have been abstinent (Madden and Bickel, 1999). From a policy perspective, it is also important to consider cross-price elasticity. If a policy reduces consumption of drug A, will the benefits be mitigated by increased consumption of drug B? In the case of alcohol and cigarettes, the two are either complements ($\varepsilon < 0$) or independent, so reducing consumption of one tends to reduce (or not affect) consumption of the other (Gruber *et al.*, 2002). Similar analyses have been conducted for other drugs and non-drug reinforcers (Bickel *et al.*, 1995b).

10.3 Irrationality and its Consequences for Addiction

Some economists have described addiction as rational (Becker and Murphy, 1988), in that addicts take the future consequences of their behaviour into account and have stable preferences. In rational addiction theory, addiction arises because the quantities of the addictive good consumed at different time periods are complements, which can lead to unstable states. This accounts for binges of consumption. Assuming rationality allows us to predict behaviour much better than not assuming it unless we can predict the specific way in which people will be irrational (Friedman, 1990). A contribution of rational addiction theory (Stigler and Becker, 1977; Becker and Murphy, 1988) was therefore to consider price as a major influence on the consumption of addictive drugs (MacCoun, 2003b). However, the premise that drug addicts choose rationally, maximising their total happiness, has been criticised (Winston, 1980; Ainslie and Monterosso, 2003; MacCoun, 2003b). Certainly, humans do not always choose according to rational norms. They deviate from the optimum when making decisions (Kahneman *et al.*, 1982; Heckerman *et al.*, 1992; Chase *et al.*, 1998; Mullainathan, 2002) because human cognitive abilities are limited ('bounded rationality') and because people frequently make choices that are not in their long-term interest ('bounded willpower').

In particular, humans and animals do not discount the future in a consistent way (Ainslie, 1975, 2001). It is rational to value future rewards somewhat less than immediate rewards (Figure 3.5(a)). Steep temporal discounting (temporal 'myopia' or short-sightedness) leads to short-termism and impulsive choice (Figure 3.5(b)). The shape of the temporal discounting function is also very important (Figure 3.5(c)). Simple economic models assume exponential temporal discounting, which leads to preferences that are temporally consistent (what is preferred at time x is also preferred at

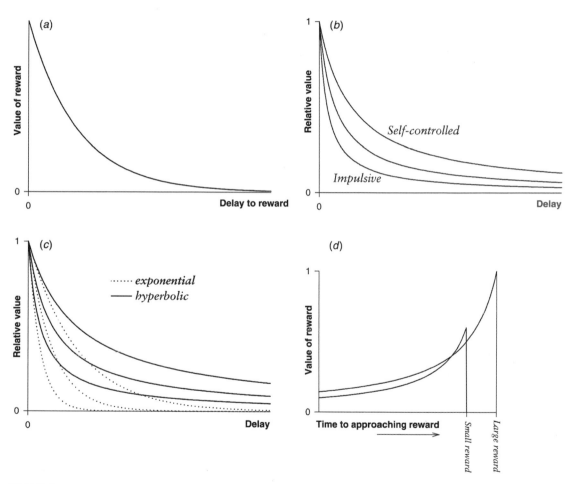

FIGURE 3.5 Temporal discounting. (*a*) The value of a reward declines the more it is delayed. (*b*) Some individuals do not value future rewards very much (they discount steeply) and are impulsive. Others value future rewards more, and are self-controlled. (*c*) Animals and people tend to discount the future in a hyperbolic, not exponential, way. (*d*) This leads to preference reversal. If a subject chooses between a big reward and a small reward when both are a long way in the future, he'll choose the big one. But as time passes and he gets closer in time to both, there may come a point at which preference reverses, he values the small reward more highly, and he chooses the smaller reward – he acts impulsively.

time y). But animals and people actually exhibit hyperbolic temporal discounting (Ainslie, 1975; Mazur, 1987; Mazur *et al.*, 1987; Grace, 1996; Richards *et al.*, 1997). This leads to preferences (Ainslie, 1975, 1992, 2001; Bradshaw and Szabadi, 1992) that depend on when a choice is made (preference reversal; Figure 3.5(d)). Therefore, many major behavioural economic theories of addiction (Ainslie, 1975, 1992, 2001; Herrnstein and Prelec, 1992; Heyman, 1996; Rachlin, 1997, 2000a) emphasise that addiction results from the maximisation

of short-term rather than long-term utility (MacCoun, 2003b; Vuchinich and Heather, 2003), with preferences that are inconsistent over time thanks to hyperbolic discounting, and that drug addictions (Rachlin, 2003) are bad because short-term selection of drugs leads to lower long-term overall utility. Consumption of drugs reduces the value of future activities – the 'primrose path' to addiction (Figure 3.6). Knowing that one is predisposed to be temporally inconsistent allows the use of self-control strategies (Ainslie, 2001; Ainslie

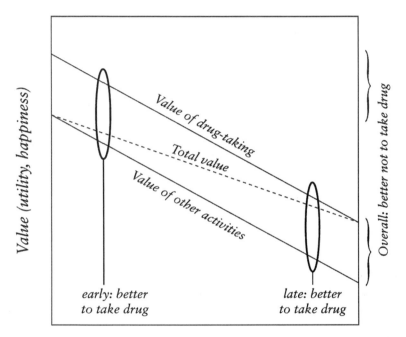

Proportion of behaviour allocated to drug use
[drug consumption ÷ (drug consumption + other activities)]

FIGURE 3.6 Good now, bad in the long run – the 'primrose path' to addiction (Herrnstein and Prelec, 1992; Rachlin, 1997, 2003; Vuchinich and Heather, 2003). At any point, drug-taking has a higher value than other activities, so you take the drug. But drug-taking lowers both the value of future drug-taking (e.g. alcohol consumption causes tolerance, meaning that future alcohol isn't worth as much) and the value of other activities (e.g. the more alcohol you consume, the less you socialise and the worse you are at socialising; the more heroin you take, the worse you are at your job). So as you drink more, your total happiness goes down – you'd be better off not being an alcoholic. But even when you are an alcoholic, drinking now is worth more than not drinking now – for you are sensitive to local, not global, utility. As Rachlin (2000b) puts it: 'The alcoholic does not choose to be an alcoholic. Instead he chooses to drink now, and now, and now, and now. The pattern of alcoholism emerges in his behaviour ... without ever having been chosen'.

and Monterosso, 2003; Homer, ~800 BC), such as precommitment to a particular course of action, which improve long-term utility.

Economic theories of addiction are also relevant when considering the extent to which drug use is voluntary. The diagnostic criteria for drug dependence (APA, 2000) include a compulsion to take a drug, yet drug use can be voluntary. Drug use certainly has utility to the user; this may be in the form of euphoria, enhanced social experiences, or enhanced intellectual performance (Feldman *et al.*, 1997). It is debatable whether even addicts take drugs involuntarily. Just because someone says they don't want to smoke and then later smokes doesn't mean they're smoking involuntarily – it might simply be that they're inconsistent (Schaler, 2000; Skog, 2003). Furthermore, not everyone who smokes wants to give up. Appreciating these differences leads to a broader classification of addiction (Figure 3.7).

The fact that people do not act to maximise their total long-term expected

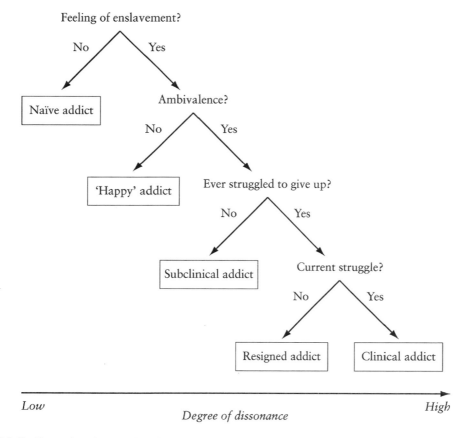

FIGURE 3.7 Skog's (2003) view of addiction. A person may be unaware that it is difficult for him or her to live without a drug. Such a person is enslaved, but unaware; Skog calls them 'naïve' addicts. He offers the example of a heavy drinker in Paris in World War II, who had never realised that he was dependent on alcohol until rationing came along and he was limited to one litre of wine per week. Then there are those who know that life would be harder without, but are happy with this situation: 'happy' addicts, such as the typical 1950s smoker who thought that smoking was good for you (or at least, not bad). Those who are aware smoking is bad for you but feel no particular motivation to cut back are called 'subclinical' addicts by Skog. Finally, there are those who have tried and failed but are not trying at the moment, and those in an active struggle to quit.

Altman, J. and Das, G.D. (1966) Behavioral manipulations and protein metabolism of the brain: effects of motor exercise on the utilization of leucine-H 3. *Physiology and Behavior* 1: 105.

Altman, J., Everitt, B.J., Glautier, S., Markou, A., Nutt, D., Oretti, R., Phillips, G.D., and Robbins, T.W. (1996) The biological, social and clinical bases of drug addiction: commentary and debate. *Psychopharmacology* 125: 285–345.

Ambrosio, E., Goldberg, S.R., and Elmer, G.I. (1995) Behavior genetic investigation of the relationship between spontaneous locomotor activity and the acquisition of morphine self-administration behavior. *Behavioural Pharmacology* 6: 229.

Anderson, I.M., Richell, R.A., and Bradshaw, C.M. (2003) The effect of acute tryptophan depletion on probabilistic choice. *J Psychopharmacol* 17: Mar 3–7.

Anglin, M.D., Hser, Y.I., and McGlothlin, W.H. (1987) Sex differences in addict careers. 2. Becoming addicted. *Drug and Alcohol Dependence* 13: 59.

APA (1994) *Diagnostic and statistical manual of mental disorders, version IV (DSM-IV).* Washington DC: American Psychiatric Association.

APA (2000) *Diagnostic and Statistical Manual of Mental Disorders*, 4th edition, text revision (DSM-IV-TR). Washington DC: American Psychiatric Association.

Arana, F.S., Parkinson, J.A., Hinton, E., Holland, A.J., Owen, A.M., and Roberts, A.C. (2003) Dissociable contributions of the human amygdala and orbitofrontal cortex to incentive motivation and goal selection. *J Neurosci* 23: 22 Oct, 9632–9638.

Arnauld, A. and Nicole, P. (1662) *La logique, ou l'art de penser [Logic, or the Art of Thinking; the Port-Royal Logic].*

Arnsten, A.F. and Robbins, T.W. (2002) Neurochemical modulation of prefrontal cortical function in humans and animals. In: D. T. Stuss and R. T. Knight (eds), *Principles of frontal lobe function.* New York: Oxford University Press: 51–84.

Arseneault, L., Cannon, M., Witton, J., and Murray, R.M. (2004) Causal association between cannabis and psychosis: examination of the evidence. *Br J Psychiatry* 184: Feb 110–117.

Asher, O., Cunningham, T.D., Yao, L., Gordon, A.S., and Diamond, I. (2002) Ethanol stimulates cAMP-responsive element (CRE)-mediated transcription via CRE-binding protein and cAMP-dependent protein kinase. *J Pharmacol Exp Ther* 301: Apr 66–70.

Aston-Jones, G., Delfs, J.M., Druhan, J., and Zhu, Y. (1999) The bed nucleus of the stria terminalis. A target site for noradrenergic actions in opiate withdrawal. *Ann N Y Acad Sci* 877: 29 Jun 486–498.

Avishai-Eliner, S., Hatalski, C.G., Tabachnik, E., Eghbal-Ahmadi, M., and Baram, T.Z. (1999) Differential regulation of glucocorticoid receptor messenger RNA (GR-mRNA) by maternal deprivation in immature rat hypothalamus and limbic regions. *Brain Res Dev Brain Res* 114: 14 May 265–268.

Baer, J.S., Sampson, P.D., Barr, H.M., Connor, P.D., and Streissguth, A.P. (2003) A 21-year longitudinal analysis of the effects of prenatal alcohol exposure on young adult drinking. *Arch Gen Psychiatry* 60: Apr 377–385.

Baker, D.A., Fuchs, R.A., Specio, S.E., Khroyan, T.V., and Neisewander, J.L. (1998) Effects of intraaccumbens administration of SCH-23390 on cocaine-induced locomotion and conditioned place preference. *Synapse* 30: Oct 181–193.

Baker, D.A., McFarland, K., Lake, R.W., Shen, H., Tang, X.C., Toda, S., and Kalivas, P. W. (2003) Neuroadaptations in cystine-glutamate exchange underlie cocaine relapse. *Nat Neurosci* 6: Jul 743–749.

Baldwin, A.E., Sadeghian, K., Holahan, M.R., and Kelley, A.E. (2002a) Appetitive instrumental learning is impaired by inhibition of cAMP-dependent protein kinase within the nucleus accumbens. *Neurobiol Learn Mem* 77: Jan 44–62.

Baldwin, A.E., Sadeghian, K., and Kelley, A.E. (2002b) Appetitive instrumental learning requires coincident activation of NMDA and dopamine D1 receptors within the medial prefrontal cortex. *J Neurosci* 22: 1 Feb 1063–1071.

Balleine, B. (1992) Instrumental performance following a shift in primary motivation depends on incentive learning. *Journal of Experimental Psychology: Animal Behavior Processes* 18: 236–250.

Balleine, B. and Dickinson, A. (1991) Instrumental performance following reinforcer devaluation depends upon incentive learning. *Quarterly Journal of Experimental Psychology, Section B – Comparative and Physiological Psychology* 43: 279–296.

Balleine, B.W. and Dickinson, A. (1998) Goal-directed instrumental action: contingency and incentive learning and their cortical substrates. *Neuropharmacology* 37: 407–419.

Balleine, B.W. and Dickinson, A. (2000) The effect of lesions of the insular cortex on instrumental conditioning: evidence for a role in incentive memory. *Journal of Neuroscience* 20: 8954–8964.

Balleine, B. and Killcross, S. (1994) Effects of ibotenic acid lesions of the nucleus accumbens on instrumental action. *Behavioural Brain Research* 65: 181–193.

Balleine, B.W., Killcross, A.S., and Dickinson, A. (2003) The effect of lesions of the basolateral amygdala on instrumental conditioning. *J Neurosci* 23: 15 Jan 666–675.

Barco, P.P., Crosson, B., Bolesta, M.M., Werts, D., and Stout, R. (1991) Levels of awareness and compensation in cognitive rehabilitation. In: J.S. Kreutzer and P. H. Wehman (eds), *Cognitive rehabilitation for persons with traumatic brain injury: a functional approach.* Baltimore: P.H. Brookes: 129–146.

Bardo, M.T., Bowling, S.L., Rowlett, J.K., Manderscheid, P., Buxton, S.T., and Dwoskin, L.P. (1995) Environmental enrichment attenuates locomotor sensitization, but not in vitro dopamine release, induced by amphetamine. *Pharmacol Biochem Behav* 51: Jun–Jul 397–405.

Bardo, M.T., Klebaur, J.E., Valone, J.M., and Deaton, C. (2001) Environmental enrichment decreases intravenous self-administration of amphetamine in female and male rats. *Psychopharmacology (Berl)* 155: May 278–284.

Barr, C.S., Newman, T.K., Schwandt, M., Shannon, C., Dvoskin, R.L., Lindell, S.G., Taubman, J., Thompson, B., Champoux, M., Lesch, K.P., Goldman, D., Suomi, S.J., and Higley, J.D. (2004a) Sexual dichotomy of an interaction between early adversity and the serotonin transporter gene promoter variant in rhesus macaques. *Proc Natl Acad Sci USA* 101: 12358–12363.

Barr, C.S., Newman, T.K., Lindell, S., Becker, M.L., Shannon, C., Champoux, M., Suomi, S.J., and Higley, J.D. (2004b) Early experience and sex interact to influence limbic-hypothalamic-pituitary-adrenal-axis function after acute alcohol administration in rhesus macaques (*Macaca mulatta*). *Alcohol Clin Exp Res* 28: 1114–1119.

Bechara, A. and Damasio, H. (2002) Decision-making and addiction (part I): impaired activation of somatic states in substance dependent individuals when pondering decisions with negative future consequences. *Neuropsychologia* 40: 1675–1689.

Bechara, A., Nader, K., and van der Kooy, D. (1998) A two-separate-motivational-systems hypothesis of opioid addiction. *Pharmacol Biochem Behav* 59: 1–17.

Becker, J.B. (1999) Gender differences in dopaminergic function in striatum and nucleus accumbens. *Pharmacol Biochem Behav* 64: Dec 803–812.

Becker, G.S. and Murphy, K.M. (1988) A theory of rational addiction. *Journal of Political Economy* 96: 675–700.

Beitner-Johnson, D., Guitart, X., and Nestler, E.J. (1992) Neurofilament proteins and the mesolimbic dopamine system: common regulation by chronic morphine and chronic cocaine in the rat ventral tegmental area. *J Neurosci* 12: Jun 2165–2176.

Bellinger, F.P., Davidson, M.S., Bedi, K.S., and Wilce, P.A. (2002) Neonatal ethanol exposure reduces AMPA but not NMDA receptor levels in the rat neocortex. *Brain Res Dev Brain Res* 136: 30 May 77–84.

Berhow, M.T., Russell, D.S., Terwilliger, R.Z., Beitner-Johnson, D., Self, D.W., Lindsay, R.M., and Nestler, E.J. (1995) Influence of neurotrophic factors on morphine- and cocaine-induced biochemical changes in the mesolimbic dopamine system. *Neuroscience* 68: Oct 969–979.

Berridge, K.C. (1991) Modulation of taste affect by hunger, caloric satiety, and sensory-specific satiety in the rat. *Appetite* 16: 103–120.

Berridge, K.C. (1996) Food reward: Brain substrates of wanting and liking. *Neuroscience and Biobehavioral Reviews* 20: 1–25.

Berridge, K.C. (2000) Measuring hedonic impact in animals and infants: microstructure of affective taste reactivity patterns. *Neuroscience and Biobehavioral Reviews* 24: 173–198.

Berridge, K.C. and Robinson, T.E. (1998) What is the role of dopamine in reward: hedonic impact, reward learning, or incentive salience? *Brain Research Reviews* 28: 309–369.

Bezard, E., Dovero, S., Belin, D., Duconger, S., Jackson-Lewis, V., Przedborski, S., Piazza, P.V., Gross, C.E., and Jaber, M. (2003) Enriched environment confers resistance to 1-methyl-4-phenyl-1,2,3,6-tetrahydropyridine and cocaine: Involvement of dopamine transporter and trophic factors. *Journal of Neuroscience* 23: 10999.

Bibb, J.A., Chen, J., Taylor, J.R., Svenningsson, P., Nishi, A., Snyder, G.L., Yan, Z., Sagawa, Z.K., Ouimet, C.C., Nairn, A.C., Nestler, E.J., and Greengard, P. (2001) Effects of chronic exposure to cocaine are regulated by the neuronal protein Cdk5. *Nature* 410: 15 Mar 376–380.

Bickel, W.K. and Johnson, M.W. (2003) Junk time: pathological behavior as the interaction of evolutionary and cultural forces. In: N. Heather and R. E. Vuchinich (eds), *Choice, behavioral economics and addiction*. Oxford: Elsevier: 249–271, 276–278.

Bickel, W.K., DeGrandPre, R.J., Higgins, S.T., Hughers, J.R., and Badger, G. (1995a) Effects of simulated employment and recreation on drug taking: a behavioral economic analysis. *Experimental and Clinical Psychopharmacology* 3: 467–476.

Bickel, W.K., DeGrandpre, R.J., and Higgins, S.T. (1995b) The behavioral economics of concurrent drug reinforcers: a review and reanalysis of drug self-administration research. *Psychopharmacology (Berl)* 118: Apr 250–259.

Bickel, W.K., Odum, A.L., and Madden, G.J. (1999) Impulsivity and cigarette smoking: delay discounting in current, never, and ex-smokers. *Psychopharmacology* 146: 447–454.

Bizot, J., Le Bihan, C., Puech, A.J., Hamon, M., and Thiébot, M. (1999) Serotonin and tolerance to delay of reward in rats. *Psychopharmacology* 146: 400–412.

Bjork, J.M., Knutson, B., Fong, G.W., Caggiano, D.M., Bennett, S.M., and Hommer, D.W. (2004) Incentive-elicited brain activation in adolescents: similarities and differences from young adults. *J Neurosci* 24: 25 Feb 1793–1802.

Bjornson, W., Rand, C., Connett, J.E., Lindgren, P., Nides, M., Pope, F., Buist, A.S., Hoppe-Ryan, C., and O'Hara, P. (1995) Gender differences in smoking cessation after 3 years in the Lung Health Study. *Am J Public Health* 85: Feb 223–230.

Blaha, C.D., Yang, C.R., Floresco, S.B., Barr, A.M., and Phillips, A.G. (1997) Stimulation of the ventral subiculum of the hippocampus evokes glutamate receptor-mediated changes in dopamine efflux in the rat nucleus accumbens. *Eur J Neurosci* 9: May 902–911.

Blakemore, S.J., Winston, J., and Frith, U. (2004) Social cognitive neuroscience: where are we heading? *Trends Cogn Sci* 8: May 216–222.

Blanc, G., Herve, D., Simon, H., Lisoprawski, A., Glowinski, J., and Tassin, J.P. (1980) Response to stress of mesocortico-frontal dopaminergic neurones in rats after long-term isolation. *Nature* 284: 265.

Blows, W.T. (2000) The neurobiology of antidepressants. *J Neurosci Nurs* 32: Jun 177–180.

Blum, K., Braverman, E.R., Holder, J.M., Lubar, J.F., Monastra, V.J., Miller, D., Lubar, J.O., Chen, T.J., and Comings, D.E. (2000) Reward deficiency syndrome: a biogenetic model for the diagnosis and treatment of impulsive, addictive, and compulsive behaviors. *J Psychoactive Drugs* 32 Suppl: Nov i–iv, 1–112.

Bolla, K.I., Eldreth, D.A., London, E.D., Kiehl, K.A., Mouratidis, M., Contoreggi, C., Matochik, J.A., Kurian, V., Cadet, J.L., Kimes, A.S., Funderburk, F.R., and Ernst, M. (2003) Orbitofrontal cortex dysfunction in abstinent cocaine abusers performing a decision-making task. *Neuroimage* 19: Jul 1085–1094.

Bowers, M.S., McFarland, K., Lake, R.W., Peterson, Y.K., Lapish, C.C., Gregory, M.L., Lanier, S.M., and Kalivas, P.W. (2004) Activator of G protein signaling 3: a gatekeeper of cocaine sensitization and drug seeking. *Neuron* 42: 22 Apr 269–281.

Bozarth, M.A. and Wise, R.A. (1981) Intracranial self-administration of morphine into the ventral tegmental area in rats. *Life Sci* 28: 2 Feb 551–555.

Bozarth, M.A. and Wise, R.A. (1984) Anatomically distinct opiate receptor fields mediate reward and physical dependence. *Science* 224: 4 May 516–517.

Bozon, B., Davis, S., and Laroche, S. (2003) A requirement for the immediate early gene zif268 in reconsolidation of recognition memory after retrieval. *Neuron* 40: 695–701.

Bradshaw, C.M. and Szabadi, E. (1992) Choice between delayed reinforcers in a discrete-trials schedule – the effect of deprivation level. *Quarterly Journal of Experimental Psychology, Section B – Comparative and Physiological Psychology* 44B: 1–16.

Brady, K.T. and Randall, C.L. (1999) Gender differences in substance use disorders. *Psychiatr Clin North Am* 22: Jun 241–252.

Brake, W.G., Zhang, T.Y., Diorio, J., Meaney, M.J., and Gratton, A. (2004) Influence of early postnatal rearing conditions on mesocorticolimbic dopamine and behavioural responses to psychostimulants and stressors in adult rats. *European Journal of Neuroscience* 19: 1863–1874.

Brandon, C.L., Marinelli, M., and White, F.J. (2003) Adolescent exposure to methylphenidate alters the activity of rat midbrain dopamine neurons. *Biological Psychiatry* 54: 1338–1344.

Brebner, K., Childress, A.R., and Roberts, D.C. (2002) A potential role for GABA(B) agonists in the treatment of psychostimulant addiction. *Alcohol Alcohol* 37: Sep–Oct 478–484.

Breiter, H.C., Aharon, I., Kahneman, D., Dale, A., and Shizgal, P. (2001) Functional imaging of neural responses to expectancy and experience of monetary gains and losses. *Neuron* 30: May 619–639.

British Heart Foundation (2004) *Give up before you clog up* [anti-smoking advertising campaign], UK.

Brody, H. (1998) Ethics in managed care. A matter of focus, a matter of integrity. *Mich Med* 97: Dec 28–32.

Brown, P.L. and Jenkins, H.M. (1968) Autoshaping of the pigeon's keypeck. *Journal of the Experimental Analysis of Behavior* 11: 1–8.

Buka, S.L., Shenessa, E.D., and Niaura, R. (2003) Elevated risk of tobacco dependence among offspring of mothers who smoked during pregnancy: a 30-year prospective study. *American Journal of Psychiatry* 160: 1978–1984.

Burns, L.H., Everitt, B.J., Kelley, A.E., and Robbins, T.W. (1994) Glutamate–dopamine interactions in the ventral striatum: role in locomotor activity and responding with conditioned reinforcement. *Psychopharmacology (Berl)* 115: 516–528.

Cabanac, M. (1992) Pleasure: the common currency. *J Theor Biol* 155: 21 Mar 173–200.

Cabib, S., Orsini, C., Le Moal, M., and Piazza, P.V. (2000) Abolition and reversal of strain differences in behavioral responses to drugs of abuse after a brief experience. *Science* 289: 463–465.

Cacioppo, J.T. and Berntson, G.G. (2002) Social neuroscience. In: J.T. Cacioppo, G.G. Berntson, R.M. Adolphs, C.S, Carter, R.J. Davidson, M. McClintock, B.S. McEwen, M.J. Meaney, D.L. Schacter, E.M. Sternberg, S.S. Suomi, and S.E. Taylor (eds), *Foundations in social neuroscience*. Cambridge, MA: MIT Press.

Cador, M., Robbins, T.W., and Everitt, B.J. (1989) Involvement of the amygdala in stimulus–reward associations: interaction with the ventral striatum. *Neuroscience* 30: 77–86.

Cador, M., Bjijou, Y., and Stinus, L. (1995) Evidence of a complete independence of the neurobiological substrates for the induction and expression of behavioral sensitization to amphetamine. *Neuroscience* 65: 385–395.

Caggiula, A.R., Donny, E.C., White, A.R., Chaudhri, N., Booth, S., Gharib, M.A., Hoffman, A., Perkins, K.A., and Sved, A.F. (2002) Environmental stimuli promote the acquisition of nicotine self-administration in rats. *Psychopharmacology (Berl)* 163: Sep 230–237.

Caine, S.B. and Koob, G.F. (1994) Effects of mesolimbic dopamine depletion on responding maintained by cocaine and food. *J Exp Anal Behav* 61: Mar 213–221.

Camp, D.M., Browman, K.E., and Robinson, T.E. (1994) The effects of methamphetamine and cocaine on motor behavior and extracellular dopamine in the ventral striatum of Lewis versus Fischer 344 rats. *Brain Research* 668: 180–193.

Campbell, W.G. (2003) Addiction: a disease of volition caused by a cognitive impairment. *Can J Psychiatry* 48: Nov 669–674.

Cardinal, R.N. and Cheung, T.H.C. (2005) Nucleus accumbens core lesions retard instrumental learning and performance with delayed reinforcement in the rat. *BMC Neuroscience* 6: 9.

Cardinal, R.N., Pennicott, D.R., Sugathapala, C.L., Robbins, T.W., and Everitt, B.J. (2001) Impulsive choice induced in rats by lesions of the nucleus accumbens core. *Science* 292: 2499–2501.

Cardinal, R.N., Parkinson, J.A., Lachenal, G., Halkerston, K.M., Rudarakanchana, N., Hall, J., Morrison, C.H., Howes, S.R., Robbins, T.W., and Everitt, B.J. (2002a) Effects of selective excitotoxic lesions of the nucleus accumbens core, anterior cingulate cortex, and central nucleus of the amygdala on autoshaping performance in rats. *Behav Neurosci* 116: Aug 553–567.

Cardinal, R.N., Parkinson, J.A., Hall, J., and Everitt, B.J. (2002b) Emotion and motivation: the role of the amygdala, ventral striatum, and prefrontal cortex. *Neuroscience and Biobehavioral Reviews* 26: 321–352.

Cardinal, R.N., Robbins, T.W., and Everitt, B.J. (2003) Choosing delayed rewards: perspectives from learning theory, neurochemistry, and neuroanatomy. In: N. Heather and R. E. Vuchinich (eds), *Choice, behavioral economics and addiction*. Oxford: Elsevier: 183–213, 217–218.

Carelli, R.M. and Wightman, R.M. (2004) Functional microcircuitry in the accumbens underlying drug addiction: insights from real-time signaling during behavior. *Curr Opin Neurobiol* 14: Dec 763–768.

Carlezon, W.A., Jr. and Nestler, E.J. (2002) Elevated levels of GluR1 in the midbrain: a trigger for sensitization to drugs of abuse? *Trends Neurosci* 25: Dec 610–615.

Carlezon, W.A., Jr., Thome, J., Olson, V.G., Lane-Ladd, S.B., Brodkin, E.S., Hiroi, N., Duman, R.S., Neve, R.L., and Nestler, E.J. (1998) Regulation of cocaine reward by CREB. *Science* 282: 18 Dec 2272–2275.

Carrol, M.E., Campbell, U.C., and Heideman, P. (2001) Ketoconazole suppresses food restriction-induced increases in heroin self-administration in rats: sex differences. *Experimental and Clinical Psychopharmacology* 9: 307.

Carroll, M.E., Morgan, A.D., Campbell, U.C., Lynch, W.D., and Dess, N.K. (2002) Cocaine and heroin i.v. self-administration in rats selectively bred for differential saccharin intake: phenotype and sex differences. *Psychopharmacology* 161: 304.

Carroll, M.E., Lynch, W.J., Roth, M.E., Morgan, A.D., and Cosgrove, K.P. (2004) Sex and estrogen influence drug abuse. *Trends Pharmacol Sci* 25: 273–279.

Castaneda, R., Lifshutz, H., Galanter, M., and Franco, H. (1994) Empirical assessment of the self-medication hypothesis among dually diagnosed inpatients. *Compr Psychiatry* 35: May–Jun 180–184.

Castren, E. (2004) Neurotrophic effects of antidepressant drugs. *Curr Opin Pharmacol* 4: Feb 58–64.

Cervo, L., Carnovali, F., Stark, J.A., and Mennini, T. (2003) Cocaine-seeking behavior in response to drug-associated stimuli in rats: involvement of D3 and D2 dopamine receptors. *Neuropsychopharmacology* 28: Jun 1150–1159.

Chaloupka, F.J., Emery, S., and Liang, L. (2003) Evolving models of addictive behavior: from neoclassical to behavioral economics. In: N. Heather and R. E. Vuchinich (eds), *Choice, behavioral economics and addiction*. Oxford: Elsevier: 71–89.

Chao, J. and Nestler, E.J. (2004) Molecular neurobiology of drug addiction. *Annu Rev Med* 55: 113–132.

Chao, J.R., Ni, Y.G., Bolanos, C.A., Rahman, Z., DiLeone, R.J., and Nestler, E.J. (2002) Characterization of the mouse adenylyl cyclase type VIII gene promoter: regulation by cAMP and CREB. *Eur J Neurosci* 16: Oct 1284–1294.

Charness, M.E., Simon, R.P., and Greenberg, D.A. (1989) Ethanol and the nervous system. *N Engl J Med* 321: 17 Aug 442–454.

Chase, V.M., Hertwig, R., and Gigerenzer, G. (1998) Visions of rationality. *Trends in Cognitive Sciences* 2: 206–214.

Chefer, V.I., Zakharova, I., and Shippenberg, T.S. (2003) Enhanced responsiveness to novelty and cocaine is associated with decreased basal dopamine uptake and release in the nucleus accumbens: quantitative microdialysis in rats under transient conditions. *The Journal of Neuroscience* 23: 3076–3084.

Chen, W.J., Maier, S.E., and West, J.R. (1997) Prenatal alcohol treatment attenuated postnatal cocaine-induced elevation of dopamine concentration in nucleus accumbens: a preliminary study. *Neurotoxicology and Teratology* 19: 39–46.

Chen, J., Zhang, Y., Kelz, M.B., Steffen, C., Ang, E.S., Zeng, L., and Nestler, E.J. (2000) Induction of cyclin-dependent kinase 5 in the hippocampus by chronic electroconvulsive seizures: role of [Delta]FosB. *J Neurosci* 20: 15 Dec 8965–8971.

Childers, S.R. (1991) Opioid receptor-coupled second messenger systems. *Life Sci* 48: 1991–2003.

Childress, A.R., Mozley, P.D., McElgin, W., Fitzgerald, J., Reivich, M., and O'Brien, C.P. (1999) Limbic activation during cue-induced cocaine craving. *American Journal of Psychiatry* 156: 11–18.

Choong, K. and Shen, R. (2004) Prenatal ethanol exposure alters the postnatal development of the spontaneous electrical activity of dopamine neurons in the ventral tegmental area. *Neuroscience* 126: 1083.

Churchill, L., Swanson, C.J., Urbina, M., and Kalivas, P.W. (1999) Repeated cocaine alters glutamate receptor subunit levels in the nucleus accumbens and ventral tegmental area of rats that develop behavioral sensitization. *J Neurochem* 72: Jun 2397–2403.

Ciccocioppo, R., Sanna, P.P., and Weiss, F. (2001) Cocaine-predictive stimulus induces drug-seeking behavior and neural activation in limbic brain regions after multiple months of abstinence: reversal by D(1) antagonists. *Proc Natl Acad Sci USA* 98: 1976–1981.

Citron, M. (2002) Alzheimer's disease: treatments in discovery and development. *Nat Neurosci* 5 Suppl: Nov 1055–1057.

Civelli, O., Reinscheid, R.K., and Nothacker, H.P. (1999) Orphan receptors, novel neuropeptides and reverse pharmaceutical research. *Brain Res* 848: 27 Nov 63–65.

Cohen, P.J. (2002) Untreated addiction imposes an ethical bar to recruiting addicts for non-therapeutic studies of addictive drugs. *J Law Med Ethics* 30: 73–81.

Cole, R.L., Konradi, C., Douglass, J., and Hyman, S.E.A. (1995) Neuronal adaptation to amphetamine and dopamine: molecular mechanisms of prodynorphin gene regulation in rat striatum. *Neuron* 14: 813–823.

Collins, S.L., Montano, R., and Izenwasser, S. (2004) Nicotine treatment produces persistent increases in amphetamine-stimulated locomotor activity in periadolescent male but not female or adult male rats. *Developmental Brain Research* 153: 175–187.

Colwill, R.M. and Rescorla, R.A. (1990) Evidence for the hierarchical structure of instrumental learning. *Animal Learning and Behavior* 18: 71–82.

Comings, D.E., Muhleman, D., Ahn, C., Gysin, R., and Flanagan, S. (1994) The dopamine D2 receptor gene: a genetic risk factor in substance abuse. *Drug and Alcohol Dependence* 34: 175–180.

Comings, D.E., Gade, R., Wu, S., Chiu, C., Dietz, G., and Muhleman, D. (1997) Studies of the potential role of the dopamine D1 receptor gene in addictive behaviors. *Molecular Psychiatry* 2: 44–56.

Conversi, D., Orsini, C., and Cabib, S. (2004) Distinct patterns of Fos expression induced by systemic amphetamine in the striatal complex of C57BL/6JICo and DBA/2JICo inbred strains of mice. *Brain Research* 1025: 59–66.

Cools, R., Barker, R., Sahakian, B.J., and Robbins, T.W. (2001) Enhanced or impaired cognitive function in Parkinson's disease as a function of dopaminergic medication and task demands. *Cerebral Cortex* 11: 1136–1143.

Cooper, J.R., Bloom, F.E., and Roth, R.H. (2002) *The biochemical basis of neuropharmacology.* 8th edition. New York: Oxford University Press.

Corbit, L.H. and Balleine, B.W.N. (2003) The role of prelimbic cortex in instrumental conditioning. *Behav Brain Res* 146: 145–157.

Corbit, L.H., Muir, J.L., and Balleine, B.W. (2001) The role of the nucleus accumbens in instrumental conditioning: evidence of a functional dissociation between accumbens core and shell. *Journal of Neuroscience* 21: 3251–3260.

Cornish, J.L. and Kalivas, P.W. (2000) Glutamate transmission in the nucleus accumbens mediates relapse in cocaine addiction. *The Journal of Neuroscience* 20: RC89 81–85.

Cornish, J.L., Duffy, P., and Kalivas, P.W. (1999) A role for nucleus accumbens glutamate transmission in the relapse to cocaine-seeking behavior. *Neuroscience* 93: 1359–1367.

Coutureau, E., Dix, S.L., and Killcross, A.S. (2000) Involvement of the medial prefrontal cortex-basolateral amygdala pathway in fear-related behaviour in rats. *European Journal of Neuroscience* 12 (Supplement 11): 156.

Crews, F.T. and Nixon, K. (2003) Alcohol, neural stem cells, and adult neurogenesis. *Alcohol Res Health* 27: 197–204.

Crombag, H.S., Jedynak, J.P., Redmond, K., Robinson, T.E., and Hope, B.T. (2002) Locomotor sensitization to cocaine is associated with increased Fos expression in the accumbens, but not in the caudate. *Behav Brain Res* 136: 455–462.

Cromwell, H.C. and Schultz, W.J. (2003) Effects of expectations for different reward magnitudes on neuronal activity in primate striatum. *J Neurophysiol* 89: 2823–2838.

Cunningham, C.L., Niehus, D.R., Malott, D.H., and Prather, L.K. (1992) Genetic differences in the rewarding and activating effects of morphine and ethanol. *Psychopharmacology* 107: 385–393.

Curran, H.V. and Morgan, C. (2000) Cognitive, dissociative and psychotogenic effects of ketamine in recreational users on the night of drug use and 3 days later. *Addiction* 95: 575–590.

Dafters, R. and Anderson, G. (1982) Conditioned tolerance to the tachycardia effect of ethanol in humans. *Psychopharmacology (Berl)* 78: 365–367.

Dalley, J.W., Theobald, D.E., Berry, D., Milstein, J.A., Laane, K., Everitt, B.J., and Robbins, T.W. (2004) Cognitive sequelae of intravenous amphetamine self-administration in rats: evidence for selective effects on attentional performance. *Neuropsychopharmacology* 30: 525–537.

Datla, K.P., Ahier, R.G., Young, A.M., Gray, J.A., and Joseph, M.H.N. (2002) Conditioned appetitive stimulus increases extracellular dopamine in the nucleus accumbens of the rat. *Eur J Neurosci* 16: 1987–1993.

Daunais, J.B. and McGinty, J.F. (1994) Acute and chronic cocaine administration differentially alters striatal opioid and nuclear transcription factor mRNAs. *Synapse* 18: 35–45.

Davis, M. (2000) The role of the amygdala in conditioned and unconditioned fear and anxiety. In: J. P. Aggleton (ed.), *The amygdala: a functional analysis.* 2nd edition. New York: Oxford University Press: 213–287.

de Borchgrave, R., Rawlins, J.N., Dickinson, A., and Balleine, B.W.M. (2002) Effects of cytotoxic nucleus accumbens lesions on instrumental conditioning in rats. *Exp Brain Res* 144: 50–68.

De Cesare, D. and Sassone-Corsi, P. (2000) Transcriptional regulation by cyclic AMP-responsive factors. *Prog Nucleic Acid Res Mol Biol* 64: 343–369.

De Jong, I.E.M. and de Kloet, E.R. (2004) Glucocorticoids and vulnerability to psychostimulant drugs: Toward substrate and mechanism. *Annals of the New York Academy of Sciences* 1018: 192.

de la Fuente-Fernandez, R., Phillips, A.G., Zamburlini, M., Sossi, V., Calne, D.B., Ruth, T.J., and Stoessl, A.J. N. (2002) Dopamine release in human ventral striatum and expectation of reward. *Behav Brain Res* 136: 359–363.

De Vries, T.J., Shaham, Y., Homberg, J.R., Crombag, H., Schuurman, K., Dieben, J., Vanderschuren, L.J., and Schoffelmeer, A.N.O. (2001) A cannabinoid mechanism in relapse to cocaine seeking. *Nat Med* 7: 1151–1154.

de Wit, H., Uhlenhuth, E.H., and Johanson, C.E. (1986) Individual differences in the reinforcing and subjective effects of amphetamine and diazepam. *Drug Alcohol Depend* 16: 341–360.

Deatherage, G. (1972) Effects of housing density on alcohol intake in the rat. *Physiology and Behavior* 9: 55–57.

Decety, J. and Jackson, P.L.J. (2004) The functional architecture of human empathy. *Behav Cogn Neurosci Rev* 3: 71–100.

DeGrandpre, R.J. and Bickel, W.K. (1995) Human drug self-administration in a

medium of exchange. *Experimental and Clinical Psychopharmacology* 3: 349–357.

Delamater, A.R.A. (2004) Experimental extinction in Pavlovian conditioning: behavioural and neuroscience perspectives. *Q J Exp Psychol B* 57: 97–132.

Deroche-Gamonet, V., Piat, F., Le Moal, M., and Piazza, P.V. (2002) Influence of cue-conditioning on acquisition, maintenance and relapse of cocaine intravenous self-administration. *Eur J Neurosci* 15: 1363–1370.

Dhabhar, F.S., McEwen, B.S., and Spencer, R.L. (1993) Stress response, adrenal steroid receptor levels and corticosteroid-binding globulin levels – a comparison between Sprague-Dawley, Fischer 344 and Lewis rats. *Brain Research* 616: 89–98.

Di Chiara, G. (1998) A motivational learning hypothesis of the role of mesolimbic dopamine in compulsive drug use. *Journal of Psychopharmacology* 12: 54–67.

Di Chiara, G. (2002) Nucleus accumbens shell and core dopamine: differential role in behavior and addiction. *Behav Brain Res* 137: 75–114.

Di Ciano, P. and Everitt, B.J. (2001) Dissociable effects of antagonism of NMDA and AMPA/KA receptors in the nucleus accumbens core and shell on cocaine-seeking behavior. *Neuropsychopharmacology* 25: 341–360.

Di Ciano, P. and Everitt, B.J. (2003) Differential control over drug-seeking behavior by drug-associated conditioned reinforcers and discriminative stimuli predictive of drug availability. *Behav Neurosci* 117: 952–960.

Di Ciano, P. and Everitt, B.J. (2004a) Conditioned reinforcing properties of stimuli paired with self-administered cocaine, heroin or sucrose. *Neuropharmacology* 47: 202–213.

Di Ciano, P. and Everitt, B.J. (2004b) Direct interactions between the basolateral amygdala and nucleus accumbens core underlie cocaine seeking behavior by rats. *The Journal of Neuroscience* 24: 7167–7173.

Di Ciano, P., Blaha, C.D., and Phillips, A.G. (1998) Conditioned changes in dopamine oxidation currents in the nucleus accumbens of rats by stimuli paired with self-administration or yoked-administration of d-amphetamine. *Eur J Neurosci* 10: 1121–1127.

Di Ciano, P., Underwood, R.J., Hagan, J.J., and Everitt, B.J. (2003) Attenuation of cue-controlled cocaine-seeking by a selective D3 dopamine receptor antagonist SB-277011-A. *Neuropsychopharmacology* 28: 329–338.

Di Paolo, T., Poyet, P., and Labrie, F. (1981) Effect of chronic estradiol and haloperidol treatment on striatal dopamine receptors. *European Journal of Pharmacology* 73: 105.

Dickinson, A. (1994) Instrumental conditioning. In: N.J. Mackintosh (ed.) *Animal learning and cognition*. San Diego: Academic Press: 45–79.

Dickinson, A. and Balleine, B. (1994) Motivational control of goal-directed action. *Animal Learning and Behavior* 22: 1–18.

Dickinson, A., Smith, J., and Mirenowicz, J. (2000) Dissociation of Pavlovian and instrumental incentive learning under dopamine antagonists. *Behavioral Neuroscience* 114: 468–483.

Dickinson, A., Wood, N., and Smith, J.W. (2002) Alcohol seeking by rats: action or habit? *Q J Exp Psychol B* 55: 331–348.

Dill, J.A. and Howlett, A.C. (1988) Regulation of adenylate cyclase by chronic exposure to cannabimimetic drugs. *J Pharmacol Exp Ther* 244: 1157–1163.

Dolan, R.J. (2002) Emotion, cognition, and behavior. *Science* 298: 1191–1194.

Donny, E.C., Caggiula, A.R., Rowell, P.P., Gharib, M.A., Maldovan, V., Booth, S., Mielke, M.M., Hoffman, A., and McCallum, S. (2000) Nicotine self-administration in rats: estrous cycle effects, sex differences and nicotinic receptor binding. *Psychopharmacology (Berl)* 151: 392–405.

Drummond, D.C. (2001) Theories of drug craving, ancient and modern. *Addiction* 96: 33–46.

Dudai, Y. (2002) Molecular bases of long-term memories: a question of persistence. *Curr Opin Neurobiol* 12: 211–216.

Duman, R.S. (2004) Depression: a case of neuronal life and death? *Biol Psychiatry* 56: 140–145.

Duman, R.S., Tallman, J.F., and Nestler, E.J. (1988) Acute and chronic opiate-regulation of adenylate cyclase in brain: specific effects in locus coeruleus. *J Pharmacol Exp Ther* 246: 1033–1039.

Ebstein, R.P., Novick, O., Umansky, R., Priel, B., Osher, Y., and Blaine, D. (1996) Dopamine D4 receptor exon III polymorphism associated with the human personality trait of novelty seeking. *Nature Genetics* 12: 78–80.

Einon, D.F. and Sahakian, B.J. (1979) Environmentally induced differences in susceptibility of rats to CNS stimulants and CNS depressants: evidence against a unitary explanation. *Psychopharmacology* 61: 299–307.

Eisch, A.J. and Mandyam, C.D. (2004) Drug dependence and addiction, II: Adult neurogenesis and drug abuse. *Am J Psychiatry* 161: 426.

Eisenberg, M., Kobilo, T., Berman, D.E., and Dudai, Y. (2003) Stability of retrieved memory: inverse correlation with trace dominance. *Science* 301: 1102–1104.

Elliott, R., Newman, J.L., Longe, O.A., and Deakin, J.F. (2003) Differential response patterns in the striatum and orbitofrontal cortex to financial reward in humans: a parametric functional magnetic resonance imaging study. *J Neurosci* 23: 303–307.

Epping-Jordan, M.P., Watkins, S.S., Koob, G.F., and Markou, A. (1998) Dramatic decreases in brain reward function during nicotine withdrawal. *Nature* 393: 76–79.

Ersche, K.D., Fletcher, P.C., Lewis, S.W.G., Clark, L., Stocks-Gee, G., London, M., Deakin, J.B., Robbins, T.W., and Sahakian, B. (2005) Abnormal frontal activations related to decision-making in current and former amphetamine and opiate dependent individuals. *Psychopharmacology (Berl)* 180: 612–623.

Erwin, R.J. and Ferguson, E.D. (1979) The effect of food and water deprivation and satiation on recognition. *American Journal of Psychology* 92: 611–626.

Estes, W.K. (1948) Discriminative conditioning. II. Effects of a Pavlovian conditioned stimulus upon a subsequently established operant response. *Journal of Experimental Psychology* 38: 173–177.

Estroff, T.W., Schwartz, R.H., and Hoffman, N.G. (1989) Adolescent cocaine abuse: addictive potential, behavioral and psychiatric effects. *Clinical Pediatrics* 28: 550–555.

Ettenberg, A., Pettit, H.O., Bloom, F.E., and Koob, G.F. (1982) Heroin and cocaine intravenous self-administration in rats: mediation by separate neural systems. *Psychopharmacology (Berl)* 78: 204–209.

Evans, S.M., Haney, M., Fischman, M.W., and Foltin, R.W. (1999) Limited sex differences in response to 'binge' smoked cocaine use in humans. *Neuropsychopharmacology* 21: 445–454.

Everitt, B.J. and Robbins, T.W. (2000) Second-order schedules of drug reinforcement in rats and monkeys: measurement of reinforcing efficacy and drug-seeking behaviour. *Psychopharmacology (Berl)* 153: 17–30.

Everitt, B.J. and Wolf, M.E. (2002) Psychomotor stimulant addiction: a neural systems perspective. *J Neurosci* 22: 3312–3320.

Everitt, B.J., Cardinal, R.N., Hall, J., Parkinson, J.A., and Robbins, T.W. (2000) Differential involvement of amygdala subsystems in appetitive conditioning and drug addiction. In: J.P. Aggleton (ed.), *The amygdala: a functional analysis*. 2nd edition. New York: Oxford University Press: 353–390.

Everitt, B.J., Dickinson, A., and Robbins, T.W. (2001) The neuropsychological basis of addictive behaviour. *Brain Research Reviews* 36: 129–138.

Fantegrossi, W.E., Woolverton, W.L., Kilbourn, M., Sherman, P., Yuan, J., Hatzidimitriou, G., Ricaurte, G.A., Woods, J.H., and Winger, G. (2004) Behavioral and neurochemical consequences of long-term intravenous self-administration of MDMA and its enantiomers by rhesus monkeys. *Neuropsychopharmacology* 29: 1270–1281.

Feldman, R.S., Meyer, J.S., and Quenzer, L.F. (1997) *Principles of neuropsychopharmacology*. Sunderland, Massachusetts: Sinauer.

Ferguson, E.D. (2000) *Motivation: a biosocial and cognitive integration of motivation and emotion*. Oxford: Oxford University Press.

Fergusson, D.M., Horwood, L.J., Lynskey, M.T., and Madden, P.A. (2003) Early reactions to cannabis predict later dependence. *Archives of General Psychiatry* 60: 1033–1039.

Ferrer-Alcon, M., Garcia-Sevilla, J.A., Jaquet, P.E., La Harpe, R., Riederer, B.M., Walzer, C., and Guimon, J. (2000) Regulation of non-phosphorylated and phosphorylated forms of neurofilament proteins in the prefrontal cortex of human opioid addicts. *J Neurosci Res* 61: 338–349.

Fibiger, H.C. and Phillips, A.G. (1988) Mesocorticolimbic dopamine systems and reward. *Ann N Y Acad Sci* 537: 206–215.

Fibiger, H.C., LePiane, F.G., Jakubovic, A., and Phillips, A.G. (1987) The role of dopamine in intracranial self-stimulation of the ventral tegmental area. *J Neurosci* 7: 3888–3896.

Fiorillo, C.D., Tobler, P.N., and Schultz, W. (2003) Discrete coding of reward probability and uncertainty by dopamine neurons. *Science* 299: 1898–1902.

Fiorino, D.F., Coury, A., Fibiger, H.C., and Phillips, A.G. (1993) Electrical stimulation of reward sites in the ventral tegmental area increases dopamine transmission in the nucleus accumbens of the rat. *Behav Brain Res* 55: 131–141.

Fischman, M.W. (1989) Relationship between self-reported drug effects and their reinforcing effects: studies with stimulant drugs. *NIDA Res Monogr* 92: 211–230.

Floresco, S.B., Todd, C.L., and Grace, A.A. (2001) Glutamatergic afferents from the hippocampus to the nucleus accumbens regulate activity of ventral tegmental area dopamine neurons. *J Neurosci* 21: 4915–4922.

Fone, K.C.F., Shalders, K., Fox, Z.D., Arthur, R., and Marsden, C.A. (1996) Increased 5-HT 2C receptor responsiveness occurs on rearing rats in social isolation. *Psychopharmacology* 123: 346–352.

Fowler, S.C., Johnson, J.S., Kallman, M.J., Liou, J.R., Wilson, M.C., and Hikal, A.H. (1993) In a drug discrimination procedure isolation-reared rats generalize to lower doses of cocaine and amphetamine than rats reared in an enriched environment. *Psychopharmacology* 110: 115–118.

Francis, D.D., Diorio, J., Plotsky, P.M., and Meaney, M.J. (2002) Environmental enrichment reverses the effects of maternal separation on stress reactivity. *The Journal of Neuroscience* 22: 7840–7843.

Friedman, D.D. (1990) *Price theory: an intermediate text*. South-Western.

Frith, C.D., Friston, K., Liddle, P.F., and Frackowiak, R.S. (1991) Willed action and the prefrontal cortex in man: a study with PET. *Proceedings of the Royal Society of London, Series B – Biological Sciences* 244: 241–246.

Fuchs, R.A., Evans, K.A., Parker, M.P., and See, R.E. (2004) Differential involvement of orbitofrontal cortex subregions in conditioned cue-induced and cocaine-primed reinstatement of cocaine seeking in rats. *J Neurosci* 24: 6600–6610.

Fuchs, R.A., Evans, K.A., Ledford, C.C., Parker, M.P., Case, J.M., Mehta, R.H., and See, R.E. (2005) The role of the dorsomedial prefrontal cortex, basolateral amygdala, and dorsal hippocampus in contextual reinstatement of cocaine seeking in rats. *Neuropsychopharmacology* 30: 296–309.

Fulford, A.J. and Marsden, C.A. (1998) Conditioned release of 5-hydroxytriptamine in vivo in the nucleus accumbens following isolation-rearing in the rat. *Neuroscience* 83: 481.

Garavan, H., Pankiewicz, J., Bloom, A., Cho, J.K., Sperry, L., Ross, T.J., Salmeron, B.J., Risinger, R., Kelley, D., and Stein, E.A. (2000) Cue-induced cocaine craving: Neuroanatomical specificity for drug users and drug stimuli. *American Journal of Psychiatry* 157: 1789–1798.

Garcia, J. (1989) Food for Tolman: Cognition and cathexis in concert. In: T. Archer and

L.-G. Nilsson (eds), *Aversion, avoidance and anxiety*. Hillsdale, New Jersey: Erlbaum: 45–85.

Garcia, R., Vouimba, R.M., Baudry, M., and Thompson, R.F. (1999) The amygdala modulates prefrontal cortex activity relative to conditioned fear. *Nature* 402: 294–296.

Gawin, F.H. (1991) Cocaine addiction: psychology and neurophysiology. *Science* 251: 1580–1586.

Gendle, M.H., Strawderman, M.S., Mactutus, C.F., Booze, R.M., Levistsky, D.A., and Strupp, B.J. (2003) Impaired sustained attention and altered reactivity to errors in an animal model of prenatal cocaine exposure. *Developmental Brain Research* 147: 85–96.

George, M.S. (2003) Stimulating the brain. *Sci Am* 289: 66–73.

Ghasemzadeh, M.B., Permenter, L.K., Lake, R.W., and Kalivas, P.W. (2003) Nucleus accumbens Homer proteins regulate behavioral sensitization to cocaine. *Ann NY Acad Sci* 1003: 395–397.

Giedd, J.N., Blumenthal, J., Jeffries, N.O., Castellanos, F.X., Liu, H., Zijdenbos, A., Paus, T., Evans, A.C., and Rapoport, J. (1999) Brain development during childhood and adolescence: a longitudinal MRI study. *Nature Neuroscience* 2: 861–863.

Gjelsvik, O. (2003) Reason and addiction. In: N. Heather and R.E. Vuchinich (eds), *Choice, behavioral economics and addiction*. Oxford: Elsevier: 219–238, 245–247.

Glatt, S.J., Trksak, G.H., Cohen, O.S., Simeone, B.P., and Jackson, D. (2004) Prenatal cocaine exposure decreases nigrostriatal dopamine release in vitro: effects of age and sex. *Synapse* 53: 74–89.

Glimcher, P.W. and Rustichini, A. (2004) Neuroeconomics: the consilience of brain and decision. *Science* 306: 447–452.

Goldberg, S.R. and Schuster, C.R. (1967) Conditioned suppression by a stimulus associated with nalorphine in morphine-dependent monkeys. *J Exp Anal Behav* 10: 235–242.

Goldstein, R.Z. and Volkow, N.D. (2002) Drug addiction and its underlying neurobiological basis: neuroimaging evidence for the involvement of the frontal cortex. *Am J Psychiatry* 159: 1642–1652.

Gonzalez-Nicolini, V. and McGinty, J.F. (2002) Gene expression profile from the striatum of amphetamine-treated rats: a cDNA array and in situ hybridization histochemical study. *Brain Res Gene Expr Patterns* 1: 193–198.

Gordon, H.W. (2002) Early environmental stress and biological vulnerability to drug abuse. *Psychoneuroendocrinology* 27: 115–126.

Gorelick, D.A., Pickens, R.W., and Benkovsky, F.O. (1999) Clinical research in substance abuse: human subjects issues. In: H.A. Pincus, J.A. Lieberman, and S. Ferris (eds), *Ethics in psychiatric research: a resource manual for human subjects protection*. Washington, DC: American Psychiatric Association.

Gorwood, P., Martres, M.P., Ades, J., Sokoloff, P.H., Noble, E.P., Geijer, T., Blum, K., Neiman, J., Jonsson, E., and Feingold, J. (1995) Lack of association between alcohol-dependence and D3 dopamine receptor gene in three independent samples. *American Journal of Medical Genetics* 60: 529–531.

Gottfried, J.A. and Dolan, R.J. (2004) Human orbitofrontal cortex mediates extinction learning while accessing conditioned representations of value. *Nat Neurosci* 7: 1144–1152.

Gottfried, J.A., O'Doherty, J., and Dolan, R.J. (2003) Encoding predictive reward value in human amygdala and orbitofrontal cortex. *Science* 301: 1104–1107.

Gould, E. and Gross, C.G. (2002) Neurogenesis in adult mammals: some progress and problems. *J Neurosci* 22: 619–623.

Grace, A.A. (1995) The tonic/phasic model of dopamine system regulation: its relevance for understanding how stimulant abuse can alter basal ganglia function. *Drug and Alcohol Dependence* 37: 111–129.

Grace, R.C. (1996) Choice between fixed and variable delays to reinforcement in the adjusting-delay procedure and concurrent chains. *Journal of Experimental Psychology: Animal Behavior Processes* 22: 362–383.

Grady, C.L. and Keightley, M.L. (2002) Studies of altered social cognition in neuropsychiatric disorders using functional neuroimaging. *Can J Psychiatry* 47: 327–336.

Grant, S., London, E.D., Newlin, D.B., Villemagne, V.L., Liu, X., Contoreggi, C., Phillips, R.L., Kimes, A.S., and Margolin, A. (1996) Activation of memory circuits during cue-elicited cocaine craving. *Proc Natl Acad Sci USA* 93: 12040–12045.

Green, L. and Fisher, E.B. (2000) Economic substitutability: some implications for health behavior. In: W. K. Bickel and R. E. Vuchinich (eds), *Reframing health behavior change with behavioral economics*. Mahwah, NJ: Erlbaum: 115–144.

Green, T.A., Gehrke, B.J., and Bardo, M.T. (2002) Environmental enrichment decreases intravenous amphetamine self-administration in rats: dose-response functions for fixed- and progressive-ratio schedules. *Psychopharmacology* 162: 373–378.

Grimm, J.W., Hope, B.T., Wise, R.A., and Shaham, Y. (2001) Neuroadaptation. Incubation of cocaine craving after withdrawal. *Nature* 412: 141–142.

Grimm, J.W., Shaham, Y., and Hope, B.T. (2002) Effect of cocaine and sucrose withdrawal period on extinction behavior, cue-induced reinstatement, and protein levels of the dopamine transporter and tyrosine hydroxylase in limbic and cortical areas in rats. *Behav Pharmacol* 13: 379–388.

Grimm, J.W., Lu, L., Hayashi, T., Hope, B.T., Su, T.P., and Shaham, Y. (2003) Time-dependent increases in brain-derived neurotrophic factor protein levels within the mesolimbic dopamine system after withdrawal from cocaine: implications for incubation of cocaine craving. *J Neurosci* 23: 742–747.

Grindley, G.C. (1932) The formation of a simple habit in guinea pigs. *British Journal of Psychology* 23: 127–147.

Gruber, J. and Mullainathan, S. (2002) Do cigarette taxes make smokers happier? [Working Paper 8872]. National Bureau of Economic Research.

Gruber, J., Sen, A., and Stabile, M. (2002) Estimating price elasticities when there is smuggling: the sensitivity of smoking to price in Canada [Working Paper 8962]. National Bureau of Economic Research.

Guisado, E., Fernandez-Tome, P., Garzon, J., and del Rio, J. (1980) Increased dopamine receptor binding in the striatum of rats after long-term isolation. *European Journal of Pharmacology* 65: 463–464.

Guitart, X., Thompson, M.A., Mirante, C.K., Greenberg, M.E., and Nestler, E.J. (1992a) Regulation of cyclic AMP response element-binding protein (CREB) phosphorylation by acute and chronic morphine in the rat locus coeruleus. *J Neurochem* 58: 1168–1171.

Guitart, X., Beitner-Johnson, D.B., Marby, D.W., Kosten, T.A., and Nestler, E.J. (1992b) Fischer and Lewis rat strains differ in basal levels of neurofilament proteins and their regulation by chronic morphine in the mesolimbic dopamine system. *Synapse* 12: 242.

Guthrie, E.R. (1935) *The psychology of learning.* New York: Harper.

Haas, A.L. and Peters, R.H. (2000) Development of substance abuse problems among drug-involved offenders. Evidence for the telescoping effect. *Journal of Substance Abuse* 12: 241.

Haber, S.N., Fudge, J.L., and McFarland, N.R. (2000) Striatonigrostriatal pathways in primates form an ascending spiral from the shell to the dorsolateral striatum. *Journal of Neuroscience* 20: 2369–2382.

Hadaway, P.F., Alexander, B.K., Coambs, R.B., and Beyerstein, B.L. (1979) The effect of housing and gender on preference for morphine-sucrose solutions in rats. *Psychopharmacology* 66: 87–91.

Haile, C.N., Hiroi, N., Nestler, E.J., and Kosten, T.A. (2001) Differential behavioral responses to cocaine are associated with dynamics of mesolimbic dopamine proteins in Lewis and Fischer 344 rats. *Synapse* 41: 179–190.

Hall, F.S. (1998) Social deprivation of neonatal, adolescent, and adult rats has distinct neurochemical and behavioural consequences. *Critical Reviews in Neurobiology* 12: 129–162.

Hall, F.S., Humby, T., Wilkinson, L.S., and Robbins, T.W. (1997a) The effects of isolation-rearing on preference by rats for a novel environment. *Physiology and Behavior* 62: 299.

Hall, F.S., Humby, T., Wilkinson, L.S., and Robbins, T.W. (1997b) The effects of isolation-rearing of rats on behavioural responses to food and environmental novelty. *Physiol Behav* 62: 281–290.

Hall, F.S., Wilkinson, L.S., Humby, T., Inglis, W., Kendall, D.A., Marsden, C.A., and Robbins, T.W. (1998) Isolation rearing in rats: pre- and postsynaptic changes in striatal dopaminergic systems. *Pharmacology, Biochemistry and Behavior* 59: 859–872.

Hall, J., Parkinson, J.A., Connor, T.M., Dickinson, A., and Everitt, B.J. (2001a) Involvement of the central nucleus of the amygdala and nucleus accumbens core in mediating Pavlovian influences on instrumental behaviour. *European Journal of Neuroscience* 13: 1984–1992.

Hall, J., Thomas, K.L., and Everitt, B.J. (2001b) Cellular imaging of zif268 expression in the hippocampus and amygdala during contextual and cued fear memory retrieval: selective activation of hippocampal CA1 neurons during the recall of contextual memories. *J Neurosci* 21: 2186–2193.

Hall, W., Carter, L., and Morley, K.I. (2004) Neuroscience research on the addictions: a prospectus for future ethical and policy analysis. *Addict Behav* 29: 1481–1495.

Hanson, G.R., Rau, K.S., and Fleckenstein, A.E. (2004) The methamphetamine experience: a NIDA partnership. *Neuropharmacology* 47 Suppl 1: 92–100.

Harmer, C.J. and Phillips, G.D. (1999) Enhanced dopamine efflux in the amygdala by a predictive, but not a non-predictive, stimulus: Facilitation by prior repeated D-amphetamine. *Neuroscience* 90: 119–130.

Harmer, C.J., McTavish, S.F., Clark, L., Goodwin, G.M., and Cowen, P.J. (2001) Tyrosine depletion attenuates dopamine function in healthy volunteers. *Psychopharmacology (Berl)* 154: 105–111.

Harmon-Jones, E. and Devine, P.G. (2003) Introduction to the special section on social neuroscience: promise and caveats. *J Pers Soc Psychol* 85: 589–593.

Harvey, J.A. (2004) Cocaine effects on the developing brain: current status. *Neuroscience and Biobehavioral Reviews* 27: 751.

Haykin, S. (1999) *Neural networks: a comprehensive foundation.* Upper Saddle River, New Jersey: Prentice-Hall.

He, M. and Shippenberg, T.S. (2000) Strain differences in basal and cocaine-evoked dopamine dynamics in mouse striatum. *Journal of Pharmacology And Experimental Therapeutics* 293: 121–127.

Heather, N. (1998) A conceptual framework for explaining drug addiction. *J Psychopharmacol* 12: 3–7.

Heckerman, D.E., Horvitz, E.J., and Nathwani, B.N. (1992) Toward normative expert systems: Part I. The Pathfinder project. *Methods of Information in Medicine* 31: 90–105.

Heidbreder, C.A., Weiss, I.C., Domeney, A.M., Pryce, C., Homberg, J., Hedou, G., Feldon, J., Moran, M.C., and Nelson, P. (2000) Behavioral, neurochemical and endocrinological characterization of the early social isolation syndrome. *Neuroscience* 100: 749–768.

Heidbreder, C.A., Foxton, R., Cilia, J., Hughes, Z.A., Shah, A.J., Atkins, A., Hunter, A.J., Hagan, J.J., and Jones, D.N.C. (2001) Increased responsiveness of dopamine to atypical, but not typical antipsychotics in the medial prefrontal cortex of rats reared in isolation. *Psychopharmacology* 156: 338.

Hellstrom-Lindahl, E. and Norberg, A. (2002) Smoking during pregnancy: a way to transfer the addiction to the next generation? *Respiration* 69: 289–293.

Henricks, K.K., Miner, L.L., and Marley, R.J. (1997) Differential cocaine sensitivity between two closely related substrains of C57BL mice. *Psychopharmacology* 132: 161–168.

Henry, D.J. and White, F.J. (1995) The persistence of behavioral sensitization to cocaine parallels enhanced inhibition of nucleus accumbens neurons. *J Neurosci* 15: 6287–6299.

Hernandez, P.J., Sadeghian, K., and Kelley, A.E. (2002) Early consolidation of instrumental learning requires protein synthesis in the nucleus accumbens. *Nat Neurosci* 5: 1327–1331.

Hernandez-Avila, C.A., Rounsaville, B.J., and Kranzler, H.R. (2004) Opioid-, cannabis- and alcohol-dependent women show more rapid progression to substance abuse treatment. *Drug and Alcohol Dependence* 74: 265–272.

Herrnstein, R.J. and Prelec, D. (1992) A theory of addiction. In: G. Loewenstein and J. Elster (eds), *Choice over time.* New York: Russell Sage Press: 331–361.

Hester, R. and Garavan, H. (2004) Executive dysfunction in cocaine addiction: evidence for discordant frontal, cingulate, and cerebellar activity. *J Neurosci* 24: 11017–11022.

Heyman, G.M. (1996) Resolving the contradictions of addiction. *Behavioral and Brain Sciences* 19: 561–610.

Heyman, G.M. (2000) An economic approach to animal models of alcoholism. *Alcohol Res Health* 24: 132–139.

Heyman, G.M. (2003) Consumption dependent changes in reward value: a framework for understanding addiction. In: N. Heather and R.E. Vuchinich (eds), *Choice, behavioral economics and addiction.* Oxford: Elsevier: 95–121.

Heyman, G.M., Gendel, K., and Goodman, J. (1999) Inelastic demand for alcohol in rats. *Psychopharmacology (Berl)* 144: 213–219.

Higgins, S.T., Alessi, S.M., and Dantona, R.L. (2002) Voucher-based incentives. A substance abuse treatment innovation. *Addict Behav* 27: 887–910.

Higley, J.D., Suomi, S.J., and Linnoila, M. (1991a) CSF monoamine metabolite concentrations vary according to age, rearing, and sex, and are influenced by the stressor of social separation in rhesus monkeys. *Psychopharmacology (Berl)* 103: 551–556.

Higley, J.D., Hasert, M., Suomi, S., and Linnoila, M. (1991b) Nonhuman primate model of alcohol abuse: effects of early experience, personality, and stress on alcohol consumption. *Proc Natl Acad Sci USA* 88: 7261–7265.

Higley, J.D., Suomi, S.J., and Linnoila, M. (1996) A nonhuman primate model of type II excessive alcohol consumption? Part 1. Low cerebrospinal fluid 5-hydroxyindoleacetic acid concentrations and diminished social competence correlate with excessive alcohol consumption. *Alcohol Clin Exp Res* 20: 629–642.

Hiroi, N., Brown, J.R., Haile, C.N., Ye, H., Greenberg, M.E., and Nestler, E.J. (1997) FosB mutant mice: loss of chronic cocaine induction of Fos-related proteins and heightened sensitivity to cocaine's psychomotor and rewarding effects. *Proc Natl Acad Sci USA* 94: 10397–10402.

Holland, P.C. and Gallagher, M. (2004) Amygdala–frontal interactions and reward expectancy. *Curr Opin Neurobiol* 14: 148–155.

Homer (~800 BC) *Odyssey*.

Hooks, M.S., Jones, G.H., Smith, A.D., Neill, D.B., and Justice, J.B., Jr. (1991a) Individual differences in locomotor activity and sensitization. *Pharmacology Biochemistry and Behavior* 38: 467–470.

Hooks, M.S., Jones, G.H., Smith, A.D., Neill, D.B., and Justice, J.B., Jr. (1991b) Response to novelty predicts the locomotor and nucleus accumbens dopamine response to cocaine. *Synapse* 9: 121–128.

Hooks, M.S., Jones, G.H., Liem, B.J., and Justice, J.B., Jr. (1992a) Sensitization and individual differences to IP amphetamine, cocaine, or caffeine following repeated intracranial amphetamine infusions. *Pharmacology, Biochemistry and Behavior* 43: 815–823.

Hooks, M.S., Colvin, A.C., Juncos, J.L., and Justice, J.B., Jr. (1992b) Individual differences in basal and cocaine-stimulated extracellular dopamine in the nucleus accumbens using quantitative microdialysis. *Brain Research* 587: 306–312.

Hooks, M.S., Juncos, J.L., Justice, J.B.J., Meiergard, S.M., Povlock, S.L., Schenk, J.O., and Kalivas, P.W. (1994) Individual locomotor response to novelty predicts selective alterations in D_1 and D_2 receptors and mRNAs. *The Journal of Neuroscience* 14: 6144–6152.

Hooks, M.S., Jones, G.H., Neill, D.B., and Justice, J.B., Jr. (2004) Individual differences in amphetamine sensitization: Dose-dependent effects. *Pharmacology Biochemistry and Behavior* 41: 203–210.

Hope, B.T., Nye, H.E., Kelz, M.B., Self, D.W., Iadarola, M.J., Nakabeppu, Y., Duman, R.S., and Nestler, E.J. (1994) Induction of a long-lasting AP-1 complex composed of altered Fos-like proteins in brain by chronic cocaine and other chronic treatments. *Neuron* 13: 1235–1244.

Horger, B.A., Iyasere, C.A., Berhow, M.T., Messer, C.J., Nestler, E.J., and Taylor, J.R. (1999) Enhancement of locomotor activity and conditioned reward to cocaine by brain-derived neurotrophic factor. *J Neurosci* 19: 4110–4122.

Horvitz, J.C. (2000) Mesolimbocortical and nigrostriatal dopamine responses to salient non-reward events. *Neuroscience* 96: 651–656.

Hou, Y., Tan, Y., Belcheva, M.M., Clark, A.L., Zahm, D.S., and Coscia, C.J. (2004) Differential effects of gestational buprenorphine, naloxone, and methadone on mesolimbic mu opioid and ORL1 receptor G protein coupling. *Developmental Brain Research* 151: 149–157.

Howes, S.R., Dalley, J.W., Morrison, C.H., Robbins, T.W., and Everitt, B.J. (2000) Leftward shift in the acquisition of cocaine self-administration in isolation-reared rats: relationship to extracellular levels of dopamine, serotonin and glutamate in the nucleus accumbens and amygdala-striatal FOS expression. *Psychopharmacology* 151: 55–63.

Hu, M., Crombag, H.S., Robinson, T.E., and Becker, J.B. (2004) Biological basis of sex differences in the propensity to self-administer cocaine. *Neuropsychopharmacology* 29: 81–85.

Hughes, J., Stead, L., and Lancaster, T. (2004) Antidepressants for smoking cessation. *Cochrane Database Syst Rev*: CD000031.

Hull, C.L. (1943) *Principles of behavior*. New York: Appleton-Century-Crofts.

Huot, R.L., Plotsky, P.M., Lenox, R.H., and McNamara, R.K. (2002) Neonatal maternal separation reduces hippocampal mossy fiber density in adult Long Evans rats. *Brain Research* 950: 52–63.

Hurd, Y.L. and Herkenham, M. (1993) Molecular alterations in the neostriatum of human cocaine addicts. *Synapse* 13: 357–369.

Hursh, S.R. (1978) The economics of daily consumption controlling food- and water-reinforced responding. *Journal of the Experimental Analysis of Behavior* 29: 475–491.

Hutcheson, D.M., Parkinson, J.A., Robbins, T.W., and Everitt, B.J. (2001a) The effects of nucleus accumbens core and shell lesions on intravenous heroin self-administration and the acquisition of drug-seeking behaviour under a second-order schedule of heroin reinforcement. *Psychopharmacology (Berl)* 153: 464–472.

Hutcheson, D.M., Everitt, B.J., Robbins, T.W., and Dickinson, A. (2001b) The role of withdrawal in heroin addiction: enhances reward or promotes avoidance? *Nat Neurosci* 4: 943–947.

Hutchison, K.E., McGeary, J., Smolen, A., Bryan, A., and Swift, R.M. (2002) The DRD4 VNTR polymorphism moderates craving after alcohol consumption. *Health Psychology* 21: 139–146.

Hutchison, K.E., Wooden, A., Swift, R.M., Smolen, A., McGeary, J., Adler, L., and Paris, L. (2003) Olanzapine reduces craving for alcohol: a DRD4 VNTR polymorphism by pharmacotherapy interaction. *Neuropsychopharmacology* 28: 1882–1888.

Ikemoto, S. and Panksepp, J. (1999) The role of nucleus accumbens dopamine in motivated behavior: a unifying interpretation with special reference to reward-seeking. *Brain Research Reviews* 31: 6–41.

Iqbal, U., Dringenberg, H.C., Brien, J.F., and Reynolds, J.N. (2004) Chronic prenatal ethanol exposure alters hippocampal GABA(A) receptors and impairs spatial learning in the guinea pig. *Behavioural Brain Research* 150: 117–125.

Ito, R., Dalley, J.W., Howes, S.R., Robbins, T.W., and Everitt, B.J. (2000) Dissociation in conditioned dopamine release in the nucleus accumbens core and shell in response to cocaine cues and during cocaine-seeking behavior in rats. *Journal of Neuroscience* 20: 7489–7495.

Ito, R., Dalley, J.W., Robbins, T.W., and Everitt, B.J. (2002) Dopamine release in the dorsal striatum during cocaine-seeking behavior under the control of a drug-associated cue. *J Neurosci* 22: 6247–6253.

Ito, R., Robbins, T.W., and Everitt, B.J. (2004) Differential control over drug seeking behavior by nucleus accumbens core and shell. *Nature Neuroscience* 17: 389–397.

Jaffe, E.H., De Frias, V., and Ibarra, C. (1993) Changes in basal and stimulated release of endogenous serotonin from different nuclei of rats subjected to two models of depression. *Neurosci Lett* 162: 157–160.

Jaquet, P.E., Ferrer-Alcon, M., Ventayol, P., Guimon, J., and Garcia-Sevilla, J.A. (2001) Acute and chronic effects of morphine and naloxone on the phosphorylation of neurofilament-H proteins in the rat brain. *Neurosci Lett* 304: 37–40.

Jentsch, J.D., Olausson, P., De La Garza, R., 2nd and Taylor, J.R. (2002) Impairments of reversal learning and response perseveration after repeated, intermittent cocaine administrations to monkeys. *Neuropsychopharmacology* 26: 183–190.

Jodogne, C., Marinelli, M., Le Moal, M., and Piazza, P.V. (1994) Animals predisposed to develop amphetamine self-administration show higher susceptibility to develop contextual conditioning of both amphetamine-induced hyperlocomotion and sensitization. *Brain Res* 657: 236–244.

Jones, G.H., Hernandez, T.D., Kendall, D.A., Marsden, C.A., and Robbins, T.W. (1992) Dopaminergic and serotonergic function following isolation rearing in rats: study of behavioural responses and postmortem and in vivo neurochemistry. *Pharmacology, Biochemistry and Behavior* 43: 17–35.

Justice, A.J. and de Wit, H. (1999) Acute effects of d-amphetamine during the follicular and luteal phases of the menstrual cycle in women. *Psychopharmacology* 145: 67–75.

Justice, A.J. and De Wit, H. (2000) Acute effects of d-amphetamine during the early and late follicular phases of the menstrual cycle in women. *Pharmacology Biochemistry and Behavior* 66: 509–515.

Kahneman, D., Slovic, P., and Tversky, A. (eds) (1982) *Judgement under uncertainty: heuristics and biases.* New York: Cambridge University Press.

Kalinichev, M., White, D.A., and Holtzman, S.G. (2004) Individual differences in locomotor reactivity to a novel environment and sensitivity to opioid drugs in the rat. I. Expression of morphine-induced locomotor sensitization. *Psychopharmacology* 177: 61–67.

Kalivas, P.W. and McFarland, K. (2003) Brain circuitry and the reinstatement of cocaine-seeking behavior. *Psychopharmacology (Berl)* 168: 44–56.

Kalivas, P.W., Pierce, R.C., Cornish, J., and Sorg, B.A. (1998) A role for sensitization in craving and relapse in cocaine addiction. *Journal of Psychopharmacology* 12: 49–53.

Kalivas, P.W., McFarland, K., Bowers, S., Szumlinski, K., Xi, Z.X., and Baker, D. (2003) Glutamate transmission and addiction to cocaine. *Ann NY Acad Sci* 1003: 169–175.

Kane, V.B., Fu, Y., Matta, S.G., and Sharp, B.M. (2004) Gestational nicotine exposure attenuates nicotine-stimulated dopamine release in the nucleus accumbens shell of adolescent Lewis rats. *Journal of Pharmacology and Experimental Therapeutics* 308: 521–528.

Kantak, K.M. (2003) Vaccines against drugs of abuse: a viable treatment option? *Drugs* 63: 341–352.

Kaufman, J.N., Ross, T.J., Stein, E.A., and Garavan, H. (2003) Cingulate hypoactivity in cocaine users during a GO-NOGO task as revealed by event-related functional magnetic resonance imaging. *J Neurosci* 23: 7839–7843.

Keller, R.W., LeFevre, R., Raucci, J., and Carlson, J.N. (1996) Enhanced cocaine self-administration in adult rats prenatally exposed to cocaine. *Neuroscience Letters* 205: 153.

Kelley, A.E. and Berridge, K.C. (2002) The neuroscience of natural rewards: relevance to addictive drugs. *J Neurosci* 22: 3306–3311.

Kelley, B.M. and Rowan, J.D. (2004) Long-term, low-level adolescent nicotine exposure produces dose-dependent changes in cocaine sensitivity and reward in adult mice. *International Journal of Developmental Neuroscience* 22: 339–348.

Kelley, A.E., Smith-Roe, S.L., and Holahan, M.R. (1997) Response-reinforcement learning is dependent on N-methyl-D-aspartate receptor activation in the nucleus accumbens core. *Proc Natl Acad Sci USA* 94: 12174–12179.

Kelley, W.M., Macrae, C.N., Wyland, C.L., Caglar, S., Inati, S., and Heatherton, T.F. (2002a) Finding the self? An event-related fMRI study. *J Cogn Neurosci* 14: 785–794.

Kelley, A.E., Bakshi, V.P., Haber, S.N., Steininger, T.L., Will, M.J., and Zhang, M. (2002b) Opioid modulation of taste hedonics within the ventral striatum. *Physiol Behav* 76: 365–377.

Kelley, A.E., Will, M.J., Steininger, T.L., Zhang, M., and Haber, S.N. (2003) Restricted daily consumption of a highly palatable food (chocolate Ensure(R)) alters striatal enkephalin gene expression. *Eur J Neurosci* 18: 2592–2598.

Kelley, A.E., Schochet, T., and Landry, C.F. (2004) Risk taking and novelty seeking in adolescence. *Annals of the New York Academy of Sciences* 1021: 27.

Kelz, M.B. and Nestler, E.J. (2000) deltaFosB: a molecular switch underlying long-term neural plasticity. *Curr Opin Neurol* 13: 715–720.

Kelz, M.B., Chen, J., Carlezon, W.A., Jr., Whisler, K., Gilden, L., Beckmann, A.M., Steffen, C., Zhang, Y.J., Marotti, L., Self, D.W., Tkatch, T., Baranauskas, G., Surmeier, D.J., Neve, R.L., Duman, R.S., Picciotto, M.R., and Nestler, E.J. (1999) Expression of the transcription factor deltaFosB in the brain controls sensitivity to cocaine. *Nature* 401: 272–276.

Kempermann, G. and Kronenberg, G. (2003) Depressed new neurons–adult hippocampal neurogenesis and a cellular plasticity hypothesis of major depression. *Biol Psychiatry* 54: 499–503.

Kenny, P.J., Koob, G.F., and Markou, A. (2003) Conditioned facilitation of brain reward function after repeated cocaine administration. *Behav Neurosci* 117: 1103–1107.

Khantzian, E.J. (1985) The self-medication hypothesis of addictive disorders: focus on heroin and cocaine dependence. *Am J Psychiatry* 142: 1259–1264.

Kheramin, S., Body, S., Ho, M., Velazquez-Martinez, D.N., Bradshaw, C.M., Szabadi, E., Deakin, J.F., and Anderson, I.M. (2003) Role of the orbital prefrontal cortex in choice between delayed and uncertain reinforcers: a quantitative analysis. *Behav Processes* 64: 239–250.

Killcross, A.S. and Coutureau, E. (2003) Coordination of actions and habits in the medial prefrontal cortex of rats. *Cerebral Cortex* 13: 400–408.

Klein, S.B. and Kihlstrom, J.F. (1998) On bridging the gap between social-personality psychology and neuropsychology. *Pers Soc Psychol Rev* 2: 228–242.

Klein, S.B., Rozendal, K., and Cosmides, L. (2002) A social-cognitive neuroscience analysis of the self. *Social Cognition* 20: 105–135.

Knackstedt, L.A., Samimi, M.M., and Ettenberg, A. (2002) Evidence for opponent-process actions of intravenous cocaine and cocaethylene. *Pharmacol Biochem Behav* 72: 931–936.

Knutson, B., Burgdorf, J., and Panksepp, J. (1999) High-frequency ultrasonic vocalizations index conditioned pharmacological reward in rats. *Physiology and Behavior* 66: 639–643.

Knutson, B., Adams, C.M., Fong, G.W., and Hommer, D. (2001) Anticipation of increasing monetary reward selectively recruits nucleus accumbens. *J Neurosci* 21: RC159.

Kolb, B., Gorny, G., Li, Y., Samaha, A.N., and Robinson, T.E. (2003) Amphetamine or cocaine limits the ability of later experience to promote structural plasticity in the neocortex and nucleus accumbens. *Proc Natl Acad Sci USA* 100: 10523–10528.

Konradi, C., Cole, R.L., Heckers, S., and Hyman, S.E. (1994) Amphetamine regulates gene expression in rat striatum via transcription factor CREB. *J Neurosci* 14: 5623–5634.

Koob, G.F. and Bloom, F.E. (1988) Cellular and molecular mechanisms of drug dependence. *Science* 242: 715–723.

Koob, G.F. and Nestler, E.J. (1997) The neurobiology of drug addiction. *Journal of Neuropsychiatry and Clinical Neurosciences* 9: 482–497.

Koob, G.F., Stinus, L., Le Moal, M., and Bloom, F.E. (1989) Opponent process theory of motivation: neurobiological evidence from studies of opiate dependence. *Neuroscience and Biobehavioral Reviews* 13: 135–140.

Koob, G.F., Rocio, M., Carrera, A., Gold, L.H., Heyser, C.J., Maldonado-Irizarry, C., Markou, A., Parsons, L.H., Roberts, A.J., Schulteis, G., Stinus, L., Walker, J.R., Weissenborn, R., and Weiss, F. (1998) Substance dependence as a compulsive behavior. *Journal of Psychopharmacology* 12: 39–48.

Koob, G.F., Caine, S.B., Parsons, L., Markou, A., and Weiss, F. (1997) Opponent process model and psychostimulant addiction. *Pharmacology Biochemistry and Behavior* 57: 513–521.

Koob, G.F., Ahmed, S.H., Boutrel, B., Chen, S.A., Kenny, P.J., Markou, A., O'Dell, L. E., Parsons, L.H., and Sanna, P.P. (2004) Neurobiological mechanisms in the transition from drug use to drug dependence. *Neurosci Biobehav Rev* 27: 739–749.

Kosten, T.A., Miserendino, M.J., Chi, S., and Nestler, E.J. (1994) Fischer and Lewis rat strains show differential cocaine effects in conditioned place preference and behavioral sensitization but not in locomotor activity or conditioned taste aversion. *J Pharmacol Exp Ther* 269: 137–144.

Kosten, T.A., Miserendino, M.J., Haile, C.N., DeCaprio, J.L., Jatlow, P.I., and Nestler, E.J. (1997) Acquisition and maintenance of intravenous cocaine self-administration in Lewis and Fischer inbred rat strains. *Brain Res* 778: 418–429.

Kosten, T.A., Miserendino, M.J., and Kehoe, P. (2000) Enhanced acquisition of cocaine self-administration in adult rats with neonatal isolation stress experience. *Brain Res* 875: 44–50.

Krasnegor, N.A. (1978) Behaviorial tolerance: research and treatment implications: introduction. *NIDA Res Monogr*: 1–3.

Kroll, J. and Egan, E. (2004) Psychiatry, moral worry, and the moral emotions. *J Psychiatr Pract* 10: 352–360.

Kruzich, P.J., Congleton, K.M., and See, R.E. (2001) Conditioned reinstatement of drug-seeking behavior with a discrete compound stimulus classically conditioned with intravenous cocaine. *Behav Neurosci* 115: 1086–1092.

Kuzmin, A. and Johansson, B. (2000) Reinforcing and neurochemical effects of cocaine: differences among C57, DBA, and 129 mice. *Pharmacol Biochem Behav* 65: 399–406.

Lamb, R.J., Preston, K.L., Schindler, C.W., Meisch, R.A., Davis, F., Katz, J.L., Henningfield, J.E., and Goldberg, S.R. (1991) The reinforcing and subjective effects of morphine in post-addicts: a dose-response study. *J Pharmacol Exp Ther* 259: 1165–1173.

Lane-Ladd, S.B., Pineda, J., Boundy, V.A., Pfeuffer, T., Krupinski, J., Aghajanian, G.K., and Nestler, E.J. (1997) CREB (cAMP response element-binding protein) in the locus coeruleus: biochemical, physiological, and behavioral evidence for a role in opiate dependence. *J Neurosci* 17: 7890–7901.

Lawrence, A.D., Evans, A.H., and Lees, A.J. (2003) Compulsive use of dopamine replacement therapy in Parkinson's disease: reward systems gone awry? *Lancet Neurol* 2: 595–604.

Le, A.D., Poulos, C.X., Harding, S., Watchus, J., Juzytsch, W., and Shaham, Y. (1999) Effects of naltrexone and fluoxetine on alcohol self-administration and reinstatement of alcohol seeking induced by priming injections of alcohol and exposure to stress. *Neuropsychopharmacology* 21: 435–444.

LeDoux, J.E. (2000a) The amygdala and emotion: a view through fear. In: J. P. Aggleton (ed.) *The amygdala: a functional analysis.* 2nd edition. New York: Oxford University Press: 289–310.

LeDoux, J.E. (2000b) Emotion circuits in the brain. *Annual Review of Neuroscience* 23: 155–184.

Lee, M.K. and Cleveland, D.W. (1996) Neuronal intermediate filaments. *Annu Rev Neurosci* 19: 187–217.

Lee, J.L., Everitt, B.J., and Thomas, K.L. (2004) Independent cellular processes for hippocampal memory consolidation and reconsolidation. *Science* 304: 839–843.

Leshner, A.I. (1997) Addiction is a brain disease, and it matters. *Science* 278: 45–47.

Levesque, J., Joanette, Y., Mensour, B., Beaudoin, G., Leroux, J.M., Bourgouin, P., and Beauregard, M. (2004) Neural basis of emotional self-regulation in childhood. *Neuroscience* 129: 361–369.

Levin, E.D. (2002) Nicotinic receptor subtypes and cognitive function. *J Neurobiol* 53: 633–640.

Lew, R. and Malberg, J. (1997) Evidence for and mechanism of action of neurotoxicity of amphetamine-related compounds. In: R. Kostrzewa (ed.), *Highly selective neurotoxins: basic and clinical applications.* Totowa, N.J: Human Press Inc: 235–268.

Lex, B. (1991a) Gender differences and substance abuse. *Advances in Substance Abuse* 4: 225.

Lex, B. (1991b) Some gender differences in alcohol and polysubstance users. *Health Psychology* 10: 121–132.

Leyton, M., Boileau, I., Benkelfat, C., Diksic, M., Baker, G., and Dagher, A. (2002) Amphetamine-induced increases in extracellular dopamine, drug wanting, and novelty seeking: a PET/[11C]raclopride study in healthy men. *Neuropsychopharmacology* 27: 1027.

Li, M.D., Konu, O., Kane, J.K., and Becker, K.G. (2002) Microarray technology and its application on nicotine research. *Mol Neurobiol* 25: 265–285.

Licata, S.C. and Pierce, R.C. (2003) The roles of calcium/calmodulin-dependent and Ras/mitogen-activated protein kinases in the development of psychostimulant-induced behavioral sensitization. *J Neurochem* 85: 14–22.

Lieberman, M.D. (2000) Intuition: a social cognitive neuroscience approach. *Psychol Bull* 126: 109–137.

Lieberman, M.D., Schreiber, D., and Ochsner, K.N. (2003) Is political sophistication like riding a bicycle? How cognitive neuroscience can inform research on political attitudes and decision-making. *Political Psychology* 24: 681–704.

Lindgren, J.L., Gallagher, M., and Holland, P.C. (2003) Lesions of basolateral amygdala impair extinction of CS motivational value, but not of explicit conditioned responses, in Pavlovian appetitive second-order conditioning. *European Journal of Neuroscience* 17: 160–166.

Liu, J.G. and Anand, K.J. (2001) Protein kinases modulate the cellular adaptations associated with opioid tolerance and dependence. *Brain Res Brain Res Rev* 38: 1–19.

Loewenstein, G. (1996) Out of control: visceral influences on behavior. *Organizational Behavior and Human Decision Processes* 63: 272–292.

Loewenstein, G.F. and O'Donoghue, T. (2004) *Animal spirits: affective and deliberative processes in economic behavior* [http://ssrn.com/abstract=539843].

Longshore, D., Hsieh, S., and Anglin, M.D. (1993) Ethnic and gender differences in drug users' perceived need for treatment. *International Journal of Addictions* 28: 539–558.

Lovibond, P.F. (1983) Facilitation of instrumental behavior by a Pavlovian appetitive conditioned stimulus. *Journal of Experimental Psychology: Animal Behavior Processes* 9: 225–247.

Lu, B. and Chow, A. (1999) Neurotrophins and hippocampal synaptic transmission and plasticity. *Journal of Neuroscience Research* 58: 76–87.

Lu, Y. and Wehner, J.M. (1997) Enhancement of contextual fear-conditioning by putative (+/−)-alpha-amino-3-hydroxy-5-methylisoxazole-4-propionic acid (AMPA) receptor modulators and N-methyl-D-aspartate (NMDA) receptor antagonists in DBA/2J mice. *Brain Res* 768: 197–207.

Lu, L., Grimm, J.W., Shaham, Y., and Hope, B.T. (2003) Molecular neuroadaptations in the accumbens and ventral tegmental area during the first 90 days of forced abstinence from cocaine self-administration in rats. *J Neurochem* 85: 1604–1613.

Lu, L., Dempsey, J., Liu, S.Y., Bossert, J.M., and Shaham, Y. (2004) A single infusion of brain-derived neurotrophic factor into the ventral tegmental area induces long-lasting potentiation of cocaine seeking after withdrawal. *J Neurosci* 24: 1604–1611.

Lu, L., Hope, B.T., Dempsey, J., Liu, S.Y., Bossert, J.M., and Shaham, Y. (2005) Central amygdala ERK signaling pathway is critical to incubation of cocaine craving. *Nat Neurosci* 8: 212–219.

Lucas, L.R., Angulo, J.A., Le Moal, M., McEwen, B.S., and Piazza, P.V. (1998) Neurochemical characterization of individual vulnerability to addictive drugs in rats. *Eur J Neurosci* 10: 3153–3163.

Lynch, G. (2002) Memory enhancement: the search for mechanism-based drugs. *Nat Neurosci* 5 Suppl: 1035–1038.

Lynch, W.J. and Carroll, M.E. (1999) Sex differences in the acquisition of intravenously self-administered cocaine and heroin in rats. *Psychopharmacology* 144: 77–82.

Lynch, W.J. and Carroll, M.E. (2000) Reinstatement of cocaine self-administration in rats: sex differences. *Psychopharmacology* 148: 196–200.

Lynch, W.J., Roth, M.E., Mickelberg, J.L., and Carroll, M.E. (2001) Role of estrogen in the acquisition of intravenously self-administered cocaine in female rats. *Pharmacology Biochemistry and Behavior* 68: 641–646.

MacCoun, R. (2003a) Is the addiction concept useful for drug policy? In: N. Heather and R.E. Vuchinich (eds), *Choice, behavioral economics and addiction*. Oxford: Elsevier: 383–401, 407.

MacCoun, R. (2003b) Comments on Chaloupka, Emery, and Liang. In: N. Heather and R.E. Vuchinich (eds), *Choice, behavioral economics and addiction*. Oxford: Elsevier: 90–94.

MacDonald, A.W., Cohen, J.D., Stenger, V.A., and Carter, C.S. (2000) Dissociating the role of the dorsolateral prefrontal and anterior cingulate cortex in cognitive control. *Science* 288: 1835–1838.

Mackintosh, N.J. (1974) *The psychology of animal learning*. London: Academic Press.

Madden, G.J. and Bickel, W.K. (1999) Abstinence and price effects on demand for cigarettes: a behavioral-economic analysis. *Addiction* 94: 577–588.

Madden, G.J., Bickel, W.K., and Jacobs, E.A. (1999) Discounting of delayed rewards in opioid-dependent outpatients: exponential or hyperbolic discounting functions? *Exp Clin Psychopharmacol* 7: 284–293.

Maisonneuve, I.M. and Kreek, M.J. (1994) Acute tolerance to the dopamine response induced by a binge pattern of cocaine administration in male rats: an *in vivo* microdialysis study. *Journal of Pharmacology and Experimental Therapeutics* 268: 916–921.

Malberg, J.E. and Duman, R.S. (2003) Cell proliferation in adult hippocampus is decreased by inescapable stress: reversal by fluoxetine treatment. *Neuropsychopharmacology* 28: 1562–1571.

Maldonado, R., Blendy, J.A., Tzavara, E., Gass, P., Roques, B.P., Hanoune, J., and Schutz, G. (1996) Reduction of morphine abstinence in mice with a mutation in the gene encoding CREB. *Science* 273: 657–659.

Marinelli, M. and White, F.J. (2000) Enhanced vulnerability to cocaine self-administration is associated with elevated impulse activity of midbrain dopamine neurons. *J Neurosci* 20: 8876–8885.

Markou, A. and Koob, G.F. (1991) Postcocaine anhedonia. An animal model of cocaine withdrawal. *Neuropsychopharmacology* 4: 17–26.

Markou, A., Kosten, T.R., and Koob, G.F. (1998) Neurobiological similarities in depression and drug dependence: a self-medication hypothesis. *Neuropsychopharmacology* 18: 135–174.

Marshall, J.C., Halligan, P.W., Fink, G.R., Wade, D.T., and Frackowiak, R.S. (1997) The functional anatomy of a hysterical paralysis. *Cognition* 64: B1–8.

Martin, P.D., and Ono, T. (2000) Effects of reward anticipation, reward presentation, and spatial parameters on the firing of single neurons recorded in the subiculum and nucleus accumbens of freely moving rats. *Behav Brain Res* 116: 23–38.

Mattay, V.S., Goldberg, T.E., Fera, F., Hariri, A.R., Tessitore, A., Egan, M.F., Kolachana, B., Callicott, J.H., and Weinberger, D.R. (2003) Catechol O-methyltransferase val158-met genotype and individual variation in the brain response to amphetamine. *Proc Natl Acad Sci USA* 100: 6186–6191.

Matthews, K., Wilkinson, L.S., and Robbins, T.W. (1996a) Repeated maternal separation of preweanling rats attenuates behavioral responses to primary and conditioned incentives in adulthood. *Physiol Behav* 59: 99–107.

Matthews, K., Hall, F.S., Wilkinson, L.S., and Robbins, T.W. (1996b) Retarded acquisition and reduced expression of conditioned locomotor activity in adult rats following repeated early maternal separation: effects of prefeeding, d-amphetamine, dopamine antagonists and clonidine. *Psychopharmacology (Berl)* 126: 75–84.

Matthews, K., Robbins, T.W., Everitt, B.J., and Caine, S.B. (1999) Repeated neonatal maternal separation alters intravenous cocaine self-administration in adult rats [In Process Citation]. *Psychopharmacology (Berl)* 141: 123–134.

Mattson, S.N., Schoenfeld, A.M., and Riley, E.P. (2001) Teratogenic effects of alcohol on brain and behavior. *Alcohol Research and Health* 25: 185.

Mazur, J.E. (1987) An adjusting procedure for studying delayed reinforcement. In: M.L. Commons, J.E. Mazur, J.A. Nevin, and H. Rachlin (eds), *Quantitative analyses of behavior: V. The effect of delay and of intervening events on reinforcement value.* Hillsdale, New Jersey: Lawrence Erlbaum: 55–73.

Mazur, J.E., Stellar, J.R., and Waraczynski, M. (1987) Self-control choice with electrical stimulation of the brain as a reinforcer. *Behavioural Processes* 15: 143–153.

McAllister, A.K., Katz, L.C., and Lo, D.C. (1999) Neurotrophins and synaptic plasticity. *Annual Review of Neuroscience* 22: 295–318.

McCance-Katz, E.F., Carroll, K.M., and Rounsaville, B.J. (1999) Gender differences in treatment-seeking cocaine abusers-implications for treatment and prognosis. *American Journal of Addiction* 8: 300.

McCann, U.D., Szabo, Z., Scheffel, U., Dannals, R.F., and Ricaurte, G.A. (1998) Positron emission tomographic evidence of toxic effect of MDMA ('Ecstasy') on brain serotonin neurons in human beings. *Lancet* 352: 1433–1437.

McClure, S.M., Berns, G.S., and Montague, P.R. (2003) Temporal prediction errors in a passive learning task activate human striatum. *Neuron* 38: 339–346.

McClure, S.M., Laibson, D.I., Loewenstein, G., and Cohen, J.D. (2004) Separate neural systems value immediate and delayed monetary rewards. *Science* 306: 503–507.

McCollister, K.E. and French, M.T. (2003) The relative contribution of outcome domains in the total economic benefit of addiction interventions: a review of first findings. *Addiction* 98: 1647–1659.

McDonald, R.J. and White, N.M. (1993) A triple dissociation of memory systems: hippocampus, amygdala, and dorsal striatum. *Behavioral Neuroscience* 107: 3.

McFarland, K. and Kalivas, P.W. (2001) The circuitry mediating cocaine-induced reinstatement of drug-seeking behavior. *J Neurosci* 21: 8655–8663.

McFarland, K., Davidge, S.B., Lapish, C.C., and Kalivas, P.W. (2004) Limbic and motor circuitry underlying footshock-induced reinstatement of cocaine-seeking behavior. *J Neurosci* 24: 1551–1560.

McGlynn, S.M. and Schacter, D.L. (1989) Unawareness of deficits in neuropsychological syndromes. *J Clin Exp Neuropsychol* 11: 143–205.

Meaney, M.J., Aitken, D.H., van Berkel, C., Bhatnagar, S., and Sapolsky, R.M. (1988) Effect of neonatal handling on age-related impairments associated with the hippocampus. *Science* 239: 766.

Meil, W.M. and See, R.E. (1997) Lesions of the basolateral amygdala abolish the ability of drug associated cues to reinstate responding during withdrawal from self-administered cocaine. *Behavioural Brain Research* 87: 139–148.

Mignot, E., Taheri, S., and Nishino, S. (2002) Sleeping with the hypothalamus: emerging therapeutic targets for sleep disorders. *Nat Neurosci* 5 Suppl: 1071–1075.

Miles, F.J., Everitt, B.J., and Dickinson, A. (2003) Oral cocaine seeking by rats: action or habit? *Behav Neurosci* 117: 927–938.

Minabe, Y., Emori, K., and Ashby, C.R., Jr. (1995) Significant differences in the activity of midbrain dopamine neurons between male Fischer 344 (F344) and Lewis rats: an in vivo electrophysiological study. *Life Sciences* 56: 261.

Minsky, M.L. (1961) Steps towards artificial intelligence. *Proceedings of the Institute of Radio Engineers* 9: 8–30.

Mitchell, S.H. (2003) Discounting the value of commodities according to different types of cost. In: N. Heather and R.E. Vuchinich (eds), *Choice, behavioral economics and addiction.* Oxford: Elsevier: 339–357.

Mitchell, S.H., Laurent, C.L., and de Wit, H. (1996) Interaction of expectancy and the pharmacological effects of d-amphetamine: subjective effects and self-administration. *Psychopharmacology (Berl)* 125: 371–378.

Miyazaki, K., Mogi, E., Araki, N., and Matsumoto, G. (1998) Reward-quality dependent anticipation in rat nucleus accumbens. *Neuroreport* 9: 3943–3948.

Mobini, S., Body, S., Ho, M.Y., Bradshaw, C.M., Szabadi, E., Deakin, J.F., and Anderson, I.M. (2002) Effects of lesions of the orbitofrontal cortex on sensitivity to delayed and probabilistic reinforcement. *Psychopharmacology* 160: 290–298.

Mogenson, G.J., Jones, D.L., and Yim, C.Y. (1980) From motivation to action: functional interface between the limbic system and the motor system. *Progress in Neurobiology* 14: 69–97.

Moratalla, R., Elibol, B., Vallejo, M., and Graybiel, A.M. (1996) Network-level changes in expression of inducible Fos-Jun proteins in the striatum during chronic cocaine treatment and withdrawal. *Neuron* 17: 147–156.

Morgan, M.A. and LeDoux, J.E. (1995) Differential contribution of dorsal and ventral medial prefrontal cortex to the acquisition and extinction of conditioned fear in rats. *Behavioral Neuroscience* 109: 681–688.

Morgan, M.A. and LeDoux, J.E. (1999) Contribution of ventrolateral prefrontal cortex to the acquisition and extinction of conditioned fear in rats. *Neurobiol Learn Mem* 72: 244–251.

Morgan, M.A., Romanski, L.M., and LeDoux, J.E. (1993) Extinction of emotional learning: contribution of medial prefrontal cortex. *Neurosci Lett* 163: 109–113.

Morley-Fletcher, S., Bianchi, M., Gerra, G., and Laviola, G. (2002) Acute and carryover effects in mice of MDMA ('ecstasy') administration during periadolescence. *European Journal of Pharmacology* 448: 31.

Morse, S.J. (2004) Medicine and morals, craving and compulsion. *Subst Use Misuse* 39: 437–460.

Mullainathan, S. (2002) Behavioral economics. In: P.B. Baltes and N.J. Smelser (eds), *International encyclopedia of the social and behavioral sciences*. Oxford: Pergamon.

Murphy, N.P., Lam, H.A., and Maidment, N.T. (2001) A comparison of morphine-induced locomotor activity and mesolimbic dopamine release in C57BL6, 129Sv and DBA2 mice. *Journal of Neurochemistry* 79: 626–635.

Myers, K.M. and Davis, M. (2002) Behavioral and neural analysis of extinction. *Neuron* 36: 567–584.

Nader, K. (2003) Memory traces unbound. *Trends Neurosci* 26: 65–72.

Nader, K., Schafe, G.E., and Le Doux, J.E. (2000) Fear memories require protein synthesis in the amygdala for reconsolidation after retrieval. *Nature* 406: 722–726.

Nader, M.A., Daunais, J.B., Moore, T., Nader, S.H., Moore, R.J., Smith, H.R., Friedman, D.P., and Porrino, L.J. (2002) Effects of cocaine self-administration on striatal dopamine systems in rhesus monkeys: Initial and chronic exposure. *Neuropsychopharmacology* 27: 35–46.

Nestler, E.J. (2001) Molecular basis of long-term plasticity underlying addiction. *Nat Rev Neurosci* 2: 119–128.

Nestler, E.J. (2002) Common molecular and cellular substrates of addiction and memory. *Neurobiol Learn Mem* 78: 637–647.

Nestler, E.J. and Malenka, R.C. (2004) The addicted brain. *Sci Am* 290: 78–85.

Newhouse, P.A., Potter, A., and Singh, A. (2004) Effects of nicotinic stimulation on cognitive performance. *Curr Opin Pharmacol* 4: 36–46.

Newton, S.S., Thome, J., Wallace, T.L., Shirayama, Y., Schlesinger, L., Sakai, N., Chen, J., Neve, R., Nestler, E.J., and Duman, R.S. (2002) Inhibition of cAMP response element-binding protein or dynorphin in the nucleus accumbens produces an antidepressant-like effect. *J Neurosci* 22: 10883–10890.

NHSDA (2001) *Summary of findings from the 2000 National Household Survey on Drug Abuse* [DHHS Publication Number (SMA) 01–3549]. Substance Abuse and Mental Health Services Administration (Department of Health and Human Services, USA).

Niaura, R. (2000) Cognitive social learning and related perspectives on drug craving. *Addiction* 95 Suppl 2: S155–163.

Nixon, K. and Crews, F.T. (2002) Binge ethanol exposure decreases neurogenesis in adult rat hippocampus. *J Neurochem* 83: 1087–1093.

Noonan, L.R., Caldwell, J.D., Li, L., Walker, C.H., Pedersen, C.A., and Mason, G.A. (1994) Neonatal stress transiently alters the development of hippocampal oxytocin receptors. *Developmental Brain Research* 80: 115–120.

Norrholm, S.D., Bibb, J.A., Nestler, E.J., Ouimet, C.C., Taylor, J.R., and Greengard, P. (2003) Cocaine-induced proliferation of dendritic spines in nucleus accumbens is dependent on the activity of cyclin-dependent kinase-5. *Neuroscience* 116: 19–22.

Nye, H.E. and Nestler, E.J. (1996) Induction of chronic Fos-related antigens in rat brain by chronic morphine administration. *Mol Pharmacol* 49: 636–645.

O'Brien, C.P. (1997) A range of research-based pharmacotherapies for addiction. *Science* 278: 66–70.

O'Brien, C.P. and McLellan, A.T. (1996) Myths about the treatment of addiction. *Lancet* 347: 237–240.

O'Brien, C.P., O'Brien, T.J., Mintz, J., and Brady, J.P. (1975) Conditioning of narcotic abstinence symptoms in human subjects. *Drug Alcohol Depend* 1: 115–123.

O'Brien, C.P., Testa, T., O'Brien, T.J., and Greenstein, R. (1976) Conditioning in human opiate addicts. *Pavlov J Biol Sci* 11: 195–202.

O'Brien, C.P., Testa, T., O'Brien, T.J., Brady, J.P., and Wells, B. (1977) Conditioned narcotic withdrawal in humans. *Science* 195: 1000–1002.

O'Brien, C.P., Ehrman, R.N., and Ternes, J.W. (1986) Classical conditioning in human opioid dependence. In: S. R. Goldberg and I. P. Stolerman (eds), *Behavioural analysis of drug dependence*. London: Academic Press: 329–356.

O'Brien, C.P., Childress, A.R., McLellan, T., and Ehrman, R. (1990) Integrating systemic cue exposure with standard treatment in recovering drug dependent patients. *Addict Behav* 15: 355–365.

O'Brien, C., Childress, A.R., Ehrman, R., Robbins, S., and McLellan, A.T. (1992) Conditioning mechanisms in drug dependence. *Clin Neuropharmacol* 15 Suppl 1 Pt A: 66A–67A.

O'Brien, C.P., Childress, A.R., Ehrman, R., and Robbins, S.J. (1998) Conditioning factors in drug abuse: can they explain compulsion? *Journal of Psychopharmacology* 12: 15–22.

O'Doherty, J.P. (2004) Reward representations and reward-related learning in the human brain: insights from neuroimaging. *Curr Opin Neurobiol* 14: 769–776.

O'Doherty, J.P., Dayan, P., Friston, K., Critchley, H., and Dolan, R.J. (2003a) Temporal difference models and reward-related learning in the human brain. *Neuron* 38: 329–337.

O'Doherty, J., Critchley, H., Deichmann, R., and Dolan, R.J. (2003b) Dissociating valence of outcome from behavioral control in human orbital and ventral prefrontal cortices. *J Neurosci* 23: 7931–7939.

O'Doherty, J., Dayan, P., Schultz, J., Deichmann, R., Friston, K., and Dolan, R.J. (2004) Dissociable roles of ventral and dorsal striatum in instrumental conditioning. *Science* 304: 452–454.

O'Donnell, P. and Grace, A.A. (1995) Synaptic interactions among excitatory afferents to nucleus accumbens neurons: hippocampal gating of prefrontal cortical input. *J Neurosci* 15: 3622–3639.

O'Hara, B.F., Smith, S.S., Bird, G., Persico, A.M., and Suarez, B.K. (1993) Dopamine D2 receptor RFLPs, haplotypes and their association with substance use in black and Caucasian research volunteers. *Human Heredity* 43: 209–218.

Ochsner, K.N. (2004) Current directions in social cognitive neuroscience. *Curr Opin Neurobiol* 14: 254–258.

Ochsner, K.N. and Feldman, B.L. (2001) A multiprocess perspective on the neuroscience of emotion. In: T. J. Mayne and G. A. Gonnanno (eds), *Emotions: current issues and future directions*. New York: Guilford Press: 38–81.

Ochsner, K.N. and Lieberman, M.D. (2001) The emergence of social cognitive neuroscience. *Am Psychol* 56: 717–734.

Ochsner, K.N., Bunge, S.A., Gross, J.J., and Gabrieli, J.D. (2002) Rethinking feelings: an FMRI study of the cognitive regulation of emotion. *J Cogn Neurosci* 14: 1215–1229.

Ogawa, T., Mikuni, M., Kuroda, Y., Muneoka, K., Mori, K.J., and Takahashi, K. (1994) Periodic maternal deprivation alters stress response in adult offspring: potentiates the negative feedback regulation of restraint stress-induced adrenocortical response and reduces the frequences of open field-induced behaviors. *Pharmacology Biochemistry and Behavior* 49: 961.

Olausson, P., Jentsch, J.D., and Taylor, J.R. (2003) Repeated Nicotine Exposure Enhances Reward-Related Learning in the Rat. *Neuropsychopharmacology* 28: 1264–1271.

Olds, J. and Milner, P. (1954) Positive reinforcement produced by electrical stimulation of septal area and other regions of rat brain. *Journal of Comparative and Physiological Psychology* 47: 419–427.

Olmstead, M.C., Lafond, M.V., Everitt, B.J., and Dickinson, A. (2001) Cocaine seeking by rats is a goal-directed action. *Behav Neurosci* 115: 394–402.

Orsini, C., Buchini, F., Piazza, P.V., Puglisi-Allegra, S., and Cabib, S. (2004) Susceptibility to amphetamine-induced place preference is predicted by locomotor response to novelty and amphetamine in the mouse. *Psychopharmacology* 172: 264.

Ortiz, J., Fitzgerald, L.W., Charlton, M., Lane, S., Trevisan, L., Guitart, X., Shoemaker, W., Duman, R.S., and Nestler, E.J. (1995) Biochemical actions of chronic ethanol exposure in the mesolimbic dopamine system. *Synapse* 21: 289–298.

Oscar-Berman, M. and Marinkovic, K. (2003) Alcoholism and the brain: an overview. *Alcohol Res Health* 27: 125–133.

Packard, M.G. and McGaugh, J.L. (1996) Inactivation of hippocampus or caudate nucleus with lidocaine differentially affects expression of place and response learning. *Neurobiology of Learning and Memory* 65: 65–72.

Park, S.B., Coull, J.T., McShane, R.H., Young, A.H., Sahakian, B.J., Robbins, T.W., and Cowen, P.J. (1994) Tryptophan depletion in normal volunteers produces selective impairments in learning and memory. *Neuropharmacology* 33: 575–588.

Parkinson, J.A., Olmstead, M.C., Burns, L.H., Robbins, T.W., and Everitt, B.J. (1999a) Dissociation in effects of lesions of the nucleus accumbens core and shell on appetitive Pavlovian approach behavior and the potentiation of conditioned reinforcement and locomotor activity by d-amphetamine. *Journal of Neuroscience* 19: 2401–2411.

Parkinson, J.A., Robbins, T.W., and Everitt, B.J. (1999b) Selective excitotoxic lesions of the nucleus accumbens core and shell differentially affect aversive Pavlovian conditioning to discrete and contextual cues. *Psychobiology* 27: 256–266.

Parkinson, J.A., Cardinal, R.N., and Everitt, B.J. (2000a) Limbic cortical-ventral striatal systems underlying appetitive conditioning. *Progress in Brain Research* 126: 263–285.

Parkinson, J.A., Robbins, T.W., and Everitt, B.J. (2000b) Dissociable roles of the central and basolateral amygdala in appetitive emotional learning. *European Journal of Neuroscience* 12: 405–413.

Parkinson, J.A., Willoughby, P.J., Robbins, T.W., and Everitt, B.J. (2000c) Disconnection of the anterior cingulate cortex and nucleus accumbens core impairs Pavlovian approach behavior: Further evidence for limbic cortical-ventral striatopallidal systems. *Behavioral Neuroscience* 114: 42–63.

Parkinson, J.A., Dalley, J.W., Cardinal, R.N., Bamford, A., Fehnert, B., Lachenal, G., Rudarakanchana, N., Halkerston, K.M., Robbins, T.W., and Everitt, B.J. (2002) Nucleus accumbens dopamine depletion impairs both acquisition and performance of appetitive Pavlovian approach behaviour: implications for mesoaccumbens dopamine function. *Behavioural Brain Research* 137: 149–163.

Parkinson, J.A., Roberts, A.C., Everitt, B.J., and Di Ciano, P. (2005) Acquisition of instrumental conditioned reinforcement is resistant to the devaluation of the unconditioned stimulus. *The Quarterly Journal of Experimental Psychology* 58B: 19–30.

Pavlov, I.P. (1927) *Conditioned reflexes.* Oxford: Oxford University Press.

Peakman, M.C., Colby, C., Perrotti, L.I., Tekumalla, P., Carle, T., Ulery, P., Chao, J., Duman, C., Steffen, C., Monteggia, L., Allen, M.R., Stock, J.L., Duman, R.S., McNeish, J.D., Barrot, M., Self, D.W., Nestler, E.J., and Schaeffer, E. (2003) Inducible, brain region-specific expression of a dominant negative mutant of c-Jun in transgenic mice decreases sensitivity to cocaine. *Brain Res* 970: 73–86.

Pecina, S., Berridge, K.C., and Parker, L.A. (1997) Pimozide does not shift palatability: separation of anhedonia from sensorimotor suppression by taste reactivity. *Pharmacology Biochemistry and Behavior* 58: 801–811.

Pecina, S., Cagniard, B., Berridge, K.C., Aldridge, J.W., and Zhuang, X. (2003) Hyperdopaminergic mutant mice have higher 'wanting' but not 'liking' for sweet rewards. *J Neurosci* 23: 9395–9402.

Pennartz, C.M., McNaughton, B.L., and Mulder, A.B. (2000) The glutamate hypothesis of reinforcement learning. *Prog Brain Res* 126: 231–253.

Peoples, L.L. (2002) Neuroscience. Will, anterior cingulate cortex, and addiction. *Science* 296: 1623–1624.

Petkov, V.V., Konstantinova, E., and Grachovska, T. (1985) Changes in brain opiate receptors in rats with isolation syndrome. *Pharmacology Research Communications* 17: 575–584.

Petry, N.M., Bickel, W.K., and Arnett, M. (1998) Shortened time horizons and insensitivity to future consequences in heroin addicts. *Addiction* 93: 729–738.

Pettit, H.O. and Justice, J.B., Jr. (1989) Dopamine in the nucleus accumbens during cocaine self-administration as studied by in vivo microdialysis. *Pharmacol Biochem Behav* 34: 899–904.

Pettit, H.O., Ettenberg, A., Bloom, F.E., and Koob, G.F. (1984) Destruction of dopamine in the nucleus accumbens selectively attenuates cocaine but not heroin self-administration in rats. *Psychopharmacology (Berl)* 84: 167–173.

Pettit, H.O., Pan, H.T., Parsons, L.H., and Justice, J.B., Jr. (1990) Extracellular concentrations of cocaine and dopamine are enhanced during chronic cocaine administration. *J Neurochem* 55: 798–804.

Phillips, G.D., Robbins, T.W., and Everitt, B.J. (1994a) Bilateral intra-accumbens self-administration of d-amphetamine: antagonism with intra-accumbens SCH-23390 and sulpiride. *Psychopharmacology (Berl)* 114: 477–485.

Phillips, G.D., Howes, S.R., Whitelaw, R.B., Wilkinson, L.S., Robbins, T.W., and Everitt, B.J. (1994b) Isolation rearing enhances the locomotor response to cocaine and a novel environment, but impairs the intravenous self-administration of cocaine. *Psychopharmacology (Berl)* 115: 407–418.

Phillips, G.D., Howes, S.R., Whitelaw, R.B., Robbins, T.W., and Everitt, B.J. (1994c) Isolation rearing impairs the reinforcing efficacy of intravenous cocaine or intraaccumbens

D-amphetamine – impaired response to intraaccumbens D1 and D2/D3 dopamine-receptor antagonists. *Psychopharmacology* 115: 419–429.

Phillips, A.G., Ahn, S., and Howland, J.G. (2003) Amygdalar control of the mesocorticolimbic dopamine system: parallel pathways to motivated behavior. *Neurosci Biobehav Rev* 27: 543–554.

Philpot, R.M. and Kirstein, C.L. (2004) Developmental differences in the accumbal dopaminergic response to repeated ethanol exposure. *Annals of the New York Academy of Sciences* 1021: 422–426.

Piazza, P.V. and Le Moal, M.L. (1996) Pathophysiological basis of vulnerability to drug abuse: role of an interaction between stress, glucocorticoids, and dopaminergic neurons. *Annu Rev Pharmacol Toxicol* 36: 359–378.

Piazza, P.V., Deminiere, J.M., Maccari, S., Mormede, P., Le Moal, M., and Simon, H. (1990) Individual reactivity to novelty predicts probability of amphetamine self-administration. *Behav Pharmacol* 1: 339–345.

Piazza, P.V., Maccari, S., Deminiere, J.M., Le Moal, M., Mormede, P., and Simon, H. (1991a) Corticosterone levels determine individual vulnerability to amphetamine self-administration. *Proc Natl Acad Sci USA* 88: 2088–2092.

Piazza, P.V., Rouge-Pont, F., Deminiere, J.M., Kharoubi, M., Le Moal, M., and Simon, H. (1991b) Dopaminergic activity is reduced in the prefrontal cortex and increased in the nucleus accumbens of rats predisposed to develop amphetamine self-administration. *Brain Res* 567: 169–174.

Piazza, P.V., Deroche, V., Rouge-Pont, F., and Le Moal, M. (1998) Behavioral and biological factors associated with individual vulnerability to psychostimulant abuse. *NIDA Research Monographs* 169: 105–133.

Piazza, P.V., Deroche-Gamonent, V., Rouge-Pont, F., and Le Moal, M. (2000) Vertical shifts in self-administration dose-response functions predict a drug-vulnerable phenotype predisposed to addiction. *The Journal of Neuroscience* 20: 4226–4232.

Pickens, C.L., Saddoris, M.P., Setlow, B., Gallagher, M., Holland, P.C., and Schoenbaum, G. (2003) Different roles for orbitofrontal cortex and basolateral amygdala in a reinforcer devaluation task. *J Neurosci* 23: 11078–11084.

Pierce, R.C., Pierce-Bancroft, A.F., and Prasad, B.M. (1999) Neurotrophin-3 contributes to the initiation of behavioral sensitization to cocaine by activating the Ras/Mitogen-activated protein kinase signal transduction cascade. *J Neurosci* 19: 8685–8695.

Pilla, M., Perachon, S., Sautel, F., Garrido, F., Mann, A., Wermuth, C.G., Schwartz, J.C., Everitt, B.J., and Sokoloff, P. (1999) Selective inhibition of cocaine-seeking behaviour by a partial dopamine D3 receptor agonist. *Nature* 400: 371–375.

Pinder, R.M. and Sandler, M. (2004) Alcohol, wine and mental health: focus on dementia and stroke. *J Psychopharmacol* 18: 449–456.

Pistis, M., Perra, S., Pillolla, G., Melis, M., Muntoni, A.L., and Gessa, G.L. (2004) Adolescent exposure to cannabinoids induces long-lasting changes in the response to drugs of abuse of rat midbrain dopamine neurons. *Biological Psychiatry* 56: 86–94.

Pitkänen, A. (2000) Connectivity of the rat amygdaloid complex. In: J. P. Aggleton (ed.), *The amygdala: a functional analysis.* 2nd edition. New York: Oxford University Press: 31–115.

Pliakas, A.M., Carlson, R.R., Neve, R.L., Konradi, C., Nestler, E.J., and Carlezon, W.A., Jr. (2001) Altered responsiveness to cocaine and increased immobility in the forced swim test associated with elevated cAMP response element-binding protein expression in nucleus accumbens. *J Neurosci* 21: 7397–7403.

Plotsky, P.M. and Meaney, M.J. (1993) Early, postnatal experience alters hypothalamic corticotropin-releasing factor (CRF) mRNA, median eminence CRF content and stress-induced release in adult rats. *Molecular Brain Research* 18: 195–200.

Pollock, J.D. (2002) Gene expression profiling: methodological challenges, results, and prospects for addiction research. *Chem Phys Lipids* 121: 241–256.

Porrino, L.J., Lyons, D., Smith, H.R., Daunais, J.B., and Nader, M.A. (2004) Cocaine self-administration produces a progressive involvement of limbic, association, and sensorimotor striatal domains. *J Neurosci* 24: 3554–3562.

Post, R.M. and Weiss, S.R. (1988) Psychomotor stimulant vs. local anesthetic effects of cocaine: role of behavioral sensitization and kindling. *NIDA Res Monogr* 88: 217–238.

Poulos, C.X., Parker, J.L., and Le, A.D. (1996) Dexfenfluramine and 8-OH-DPAT modulate impulsivity in a delay-of-reward paradigm: implications for a correspondence with alcohol consumption. *Behavioural Pharmacology* 7: 395–399.

Preskorn, S.H. (2001) The human genome project and drug discovery in psychiatry: identifying novel targets. *Journal of Psychiatric Practice* 7: 133–137.

Przybyslawski, J. and Sara, S.J. (1997) Reconsolidation of memory after its reactivation. *Behavioural Brain Research* 84: 241–246.

Przybyslawski, J., Roullet, P., and Sara, S.J. (1999) Attenuation of emotional and nonemotional memories after their reactivation: role of beta adrenergic receptors. *Journal of Neuroscience* 19: 6623–6628.

Quirk, G.J., Likhtik, E., Pelletier, J.G., and Pare, D. (2003) Stimulation of medial prefrontal cortex decreases the responsiveness of central amygdala output neurons. *J Neurosci* 23: 8800–8807.

Rachlin, H. (1997) Four teleological theories of addiction. *Psychonomic Bulletin and Review* 4: 462–473.

Rachlin, H. (2000a) The lonely addict. In: W.K. Bickel and R.E. Vuchinich (eds), *Reframing health behavior change with behavioral economics.* Mahwah, NJ: Lawrence Erlbaum Associates: 145–166.

Rachlin, H. (2000b) *The science of self-control.* Cambridge, Massachusetts: Harvard University Press.

Rachlin, H. (2003) Economic concepts in the behavioral study of addiction. In: N. Heather and R.E. Vuchinich (eds), *Choice, behavioral economics and addiction.* Oxford: Elsevier: 129–149.

Rachlin, H. and Green, L. (1972) Commitment, choice and self-control. *Journal of the Experimental Analysis of Behavior* 17: 15–22.

Rachlin, H., Green, L., Kagel, J., and Battalio, R. (1976) Economic demand theory and psychological studies of choice. In: G. Bower (ed.), *The psychology of learning and motivation.* New York: Academic Press: 129–154.

Ramsey, N.F., Niesink, R.J., and Van ree, J.M. (1993) Prenatal exposure to morphine enhances cocaine and heroin self-administration in drug-naive rats. *Drug and Alcohol Dependence* 33: 41.

Ranaldi, R., Bauco, P., McCormick, S., Cools, A.R., and Wise, R.A. (2001) Equal sensitivity to cocaine reward in addiction-prone and addiction-resistant rat genotypes. *Behavioural Pharmacology* 12: 527.

Rescorla, R.A. (1990a) Evidence for an association between the discriminative stimulus and the response-outcome association in instrumental learning. *Journal of Experimental Psychology: Animal Behavior Processes* 16: 326–334.

Rescorla, R.A. (1990b) The role of information about the response-outcome relation in instrumental discrimination learning. *Journal of Experimental Psychology: Animal Behavior Processes* 16: 262–270.

Reuter, J., Raedler, T., Rose, M., Hand, I., Glascher, J., and Buchel, C. (2005) Pathological gambling is linked to reduced activation of the mesolimbic reward system. *Nat Neurosci* 8: 147–148.

Reynolds, J.N. and Wickens, J.R. (2002) Dopamine-dependent plasticity of corticostriatal synapses. *Neural Netw* 15: 507–521.

Reynolds, J.N., Hyland, B.I., and Wickens, J.R. (2001) A cellular mechanism of reward-related learning. *Nature* 413: 67–70.

Ricaurte, G.A., Martello, A.L., Katz, J.L., and Martello, M.B. (1992) Lasting effects of (+−)-3,4-methylenedioxymethamphetamine (MDMA) on central serotonergic neurons in nonhuman primates: neurochemical observations. *J Pharmacol Exp Ther* 261: 616–622.

Richards, J.B. and Seiden, L.S. (1995) Serotonin depletion increases impulsive behavior in rats. *Society for Neuroscience Abstracts* 21: 1693.

Richards, J.B., Mitchell, S.H., de Wit, H., and Seiden, L.S. (1997) Determination of discount functions in rats with an adjusting-amount procedure. *Journal of the Experimental Analysis of Behavior* 67: 353–366.

Rinn, W., Desai, N., Rosenblatt, H., and Gastfriend, D.R. (2002) Addiction denial and cognitive dysfunction: a preliminary investigation. *J Neuropsychiatry Clin Neurosci* 14: 52–57.

Robbins, T.W. and Everitt, B.J. (1992) Functions of dopamine in the dorsal and ventral striatum. *Seminars in the Neurosciences* 4: 119–127.

Robbins, T.W. and Everitt, B.J. (1999) Drug addiction: bad habits add up [news]. *Nature* 398: 567–570.

Roberts, D.C.S., Bennet, S.A.L., and Vickers, G. (1989) The estrous cycle affects cocaine self-administration on a progressive ratio schedule of reinforcement in rats. *Psychopharmacology* 98: 408–411.

Robinson, T.E. and Berridge, K.C. (1993) The neural basis of drug craving: an incentive-sensitization theory of addiction. *Brain Research Reviews* 18: 247–291.

Robinson, T.E. and Kolb, B. (1999) Alterations in the morphology of dendrites and dendritic spines in the nucleus accumbens and prefrontal cortex following repeated treatment with amphetamine or cocaine. *Eur J Neurosci* 11: 1598–1604.

Rocha, B.A., Mead, A.N., and Kosofsky, B.E. (2002) Increased vulnerability to self-administer cocaine in mice prenatally exposed to cocaine. *Psychopharmacology (Berl)* 163: 221–229.

Rogers, R.D. and Robbins, T.W. (2001) Investigating the neurocognitive deficits associated with chronic drug misuse. *Curr Opin Neurobiol* 11: 250–257.

Rogers, R.D., Everitt, B.J., Baldacchino, A., Blackshaw, A.J., Swainson, R., Wynne, K., Baker, N.B., Hunter, J., Carthy, T., Booker, E., London, M., Deakin, J.F., Sahakian, B.J., and Robbins, T.W. (1999a) Dissociable deficits in the decision-making cognition of chronic amphetamine abusers, opiate abusers, patients with focal damage to prefrontal cortex, and tryptophan-depleted normal volunteers: evidence for monoaminergic mechanisms. *Neuropsychopharmacology* 20: 322–339.

Rogers, R.D., Blackshaw, A.J., Middleton, H.C., Matthews, K., Hawtin, K., Crowley, C., Hopwood, A., Wallace, C., Deakin, J.F., Sahakian, B.J., and Robbins, T.W. (1999b) Tryptophan depletion impairs stimulus-reward learning while methylphenidate disrupts attentional control in healthy young adults: implications for the monoaminergic basis of impulsive behaviour. *Psychopharmacology (Berl)* 146: 482–491.

Rogers, R.D., Tunbridge, E.M., Bhagwagar, Z., Drevets, W.C., Sahakian, B.J., and Carter, C.S. (2003) Tryptophan depletion alters the decision-making of healthy volunteers through altered processing of reward cues. *Neuropsychopharmacology* 28: 153–162.

Roiser, J.P., Cook, L.J., Cooper, J.D., Runinsztein, D., and Sahakian, B.J. (2005) A functional polymorphism in the serotonin transporter gene is associated with abnormal emotional processing in ecstasy users. *American Journal of Psychiatry* 162: 609–612.

Rosenkranz, J.A., Moore, H., and Grace, A.A. (2003) The prefrontal cortex regulates lateral amygdala neuronal plasticity and responses to previously conditioned stimuli. *J Neurosci* 23: 11054–11064.

Roth, M.E. and Carroll, M.E. (2004) Acquisition and maintenance of i.v. self-administration of methamphetamine in rats: effects of sex and estrogen. *Psychopharmacology* 172: 443–449.

Roth, M.E., Cosgrove, K.P., and Carroll, M.E. (2004) Sex differences in the vulnerability to drug abuse: a review of preclinical studies. *Neuroscience and Behavioral Reviews* 28: 533–546.

Rouge-Pont, F., Piazza, P.V., Kharouby, M., leMoal, M., and Simon, H. (1993) Higher and longer stress-induced increase in dopamine concentrations in the nucleus accumbens of animals predisposed to amphetamine self-administration. A microdialysis study. *Brain Research* 602: 169–174.

Rubino, T., Vigano, D., Massi, P., Spinello, M., Zagato, E., Giagnoni, G., and Parolaro, D. (2000) Chronic delta-9-tetrahydrocannabinol treatment increases cAMP levels and cAMP-dependent protein kinase activity in some rat brain regions. *Neuropharmacology* 39: 1331–1336.

Russell, S.J. and Norvig, P.N. (1995) *Artificial intelligence: a modern approach*. Upper Saddle River, New Jersey: Prentice-Hall.

Saffer, H. and Chaloupka, F.J. (1995) *The demand for illicit drugs* [Working Paper 5238]. National Bureau of Economic Research.

Sahakian, B.J. and Robbins, T.W. (1977) Isolation-rearing enhances tail pinch-induced oral behavior in rats. *Physiol Behav* 18: 53–58.

Salamone, J.D. (1994) The involvement of nucleus accumbens dopamine in appetitive and aversive motivation. *Behavioural Brain Research* 61: 117–133.

Salamone, J.D. and Correa, M. (2002) Motivational views of reinforcement: implications for understanding the behavioral functions of nucleus accumbens dopamine. *Behav Brain Res* 137: 3–25.

Salamone, J.D., Correa, M., Mingote, S.M., and Weber, S.M. (2003) Nucleus accumbens dopamine and the regulation of effort in food-seeking behavior: implications for studies of natural motivation, psychiatry, and drug abuse. *J Pharmacol Exp Ther* 305: 1–8.

Salvatore, M.F., Hudspeth, O., Arnold, L.E., Wilson, P.E., Stanford, J.A., Mactutus, C.F., Booze, R.M., and Gerhardt, G.A. (2004) Prenatal cocaine exposure alters postassium-evoked dopamine release dynamics in rat striatum. *Neuroscience* 123: 481–490.

Samhsa (2000) Substance Abuse and Mental Health Services Administration, 2001. *Summary of findings from the 2000 National Household Survey on Drug Abuse.* (SMA) 01–3549.

Samson, D., Apperly, I.A., Chiavarino, C., and Humphreys, G.W. (2004) Left temporoparietal junction is necessary for representing someone else's belief. *Nat Neurosci* 7: 499–500.

Sax, K.W. and Strakowski, S.M. (2001) Behavioral sensitization in humans. *J Addict Dis* 20: 55–65.

Schaler, J.A. (2000) *Addiction is a choice.* Chicago, Illinois: Open Court Publishing.

Schenk, S., Britt, M.D., and Atalay, J. (1982) Isolation rearing decreases opiate receptor binding in rat brain. *Pharmacology Biochemistry and Behavior* 16: 841–842.

Schenk, S., Lacelle, G., Gorman, K., and Amit, Z. (1987) Cocaine self-administration in rats influenced by environmental conditions: implications for the etiology of drug abuse. *Neuroscience Letters* 81: 227–231.

Schinder, A.F. and Poo, M.M. (2000) The neurotrophin hypothesis for synaptic plasticity. *Trends in Neurosciences* 23: 639–645.

Schneider, F., Habel, U., Volkmann, J., Regel, S., Kornischka, J., Sturm, V., and Freund, H.J. (2003) Deep brain stimulation of the subthalamic nucleus enhances emotional processing in Parkinson disease. *Arch Gen Psychiatry* 60: 296–302.

Schochet, T., Kelley, A.E., and Landry, C.F. (2004) Differential behavioral effects of nicotine exposure in adolescent and adult rats. *Psychopharmacology* 175: 265–273.

Schultz, W. (1998) Predictive reward signal of dopamine neurons. *J Neurophysiol* 80: 1–27.

Schultz, W. (2004) Neural coding of basic reward terms of animal learning theory, game theory, microeconomics and behavioural ecology. *Curr Opin Neurobiol* 14: 139–147.

Schultz, W. and Dickinson, A. (2000) Neuronal coding of prediction errors. *Annual Review of Neuroscience* 23: 473–500.

Schultz, W., Apicella, P., Scarnati, E., and Ljungberg, T. (1992) Neuronal activity in monkey ventral striatum related to the expectation of reward. *Journal of Neuroscience* 12: 4595–4610.

Schultz, W., Dayan, P., and Montague, P.R. (1997) A neural substrate of prediction and reward. *Science* 275: 1593–1599.

Schultz, W., Tremblay, L., and Hollerman, J.R. (1998) Reward prediction in primate basal ganglia and frontal cortex. *Neuropharmacology* 37: 421–429.

Schultz, W., Tremblay, L., and Hollerman, J.R. (2000) Reward processing in primate orbitofrontal cortex and basal ganglia. *Cereb Cortex* 10: 272–284.

See, R.E., Kruzich, P.J., and Grimm, J.W. (2001) Dopamine, but not glutamate, receptor blockade in the basolateral amygdala attenuates conditioned reward in a rat model of relapse to cocaine-seeking behavior. *Psychopharmacology (Berl)* 154: 301–310.

Seger, R. and Krebs, E.G. (1995) The MAPK signaling cascade. *Faseb J* 9: 726–735.

Selden, N.R., Everitt, B.J., Jarrard, L.E., and Robbins, T.W. (1991) Complementary roles for the amygdala and hippocampus in aversive conditioning to explicit and contextual cues. *Neuroscience* 42: 335–350.

Self, D.W. and Nestler, E.J. (1998) Relapse to drug-seeking: neural and molecular mechanisms. *Drug Alcohol Depend* 51: 49–60.

Self, D.W., Genova, L.M., Hope, B.T., Barnhart, W.J., Spencer, J.J., and Nestler, E.J. (1998) Involvement of cAMP-dependent protein kinase in the nucleus accumbens in cocaine self-administration and relapse to cocaine-seeking behavior. *Journal of Neuroscience* 18: 1848.

Sell, L.A., Morris, J., Bearn, J., Frackowiak, R.S., Friston, K.J., and Dolan, R.J. (1999) Activation of reward circuitry in human opiate addicts. *Eur J Neurosci* 11: 1042–1048.

Semenova, S. and Markou, A. (2003) Cocaine-seeking behavior after extended cocaine-free periods in rats: role of conditioned stimuli. *Psychopharmacology (Berl)* 168: 192–200.

Shaham, Y. and Stewart, J. (1996) Effects of opioid and dopamine receptor antagonists on relapse induced by stress and re-exposure to heroin in rats. *Psychopharmacology (Berl)* 125: 385–391.

Shaham, Y., Erb, S., and Stewart, J. (2000a) Stress-induced relapse to heroin and cocaine seeking in rats: a review. *Brain Research Reviews* 33: 13.

Shaham, Y., Highfield, D., Delfs, J., Leung, S., and Stewart, J. (2000b) Clonidine blocks stress-induced reinstatement of heroin seeking in rats: an effect independent of locus coeruleus noradrenergic neurons. *Eur J Neurosci* 12: 292–302.

Shaham, Y., Shalev, U., Lu, L., De Wit, H., and Stewart, J. (2003) The reinstatement model of drug relapse: history, methodology and major findings. *Psychopharmacology (Berl)* 168: 3–20.

Shahan, T.A. (2002) The observing-response procedure: a novel method to study drug-associated conditioned reinforcement. *Exp Clin Psychopharmacol* 10: 3–9.

Shahan, T.A., Magee, A., and Dobberstein, A. (2003) The resistance to change of observing. *J Exp Anal Behav* 80: 273–293.

Shalev, U., Morales, M., Hope, B., Yap, J., and Shaham, Y. (2001) Time-dependent changes in extinction behavior and stress-induced reinstatement of drug seeking following withdrawal from heroin in rats. *Psychopharmacology (Berl)* 156: 98–107.

Shaw-Lutchman, T.Z., Impey, S., Storm, D., and Nestler, E.J. (2003) Regulation of CRE-mediated transcription in mouse brain by amphetamine. *Synapse* 48: 10–17.

Shaywitz, A.J. and Greenberg, M.E. (1999) CREB: a stimulus-induced transcription factor activated by a diverse array of extracellular signals. *Annu Rev Biochem* 68: 821–861.

Shen, R.Y., Hannigan, J.H., and Kapatos, G. (1999) Prenatal ethanol reduces the activity of adult midbrain dopamine neurons. *Alcohol Clinical Experimental Research* 23: 1801–1807.

Shepard, J.D., Bossert, J.M., Liu, S.Y., and Shaham, Y. (2004) The anxiogenic drug yohimbine reinstates methamphetamine seeking in a rat model of drug relapse. *Biol Psychiatry* 55: 1082–1089.

Shippenberg, T.S. and Rea, W. (1997) Sensitization to the behavioral effects of cocaine: modulation by dynorphin and kappa-opioid receptor agonists. *Pharmacol Biochem Behav* 57: 449–455.

Shizgal, P. (1997) Neural basis of utility estimation. *Current Opinion in Neurobiology* 7: 198–208.

Shors, T.J., Townsend, D.A., Zhao, M., Kozorovitskiy, Y., and Gould, E. (2002) Neurogenesis may relate to some but not all types of hippocampal-dependent learning. *Hippocampus* 12: 578–584.

Siegel, S. (1975) Evidence from rats that morphine tolerance is a learned response. *J Comp Physiol Psychol* 89: 498–506.

Siegel, S. (1976) Morphine analgesic tolerance: its situation specificity supports a Pavlovian conditioning model. *Science* 193: 323–325.

Siegel, S. (1988) Drug anticipation and the treatment of dependence. *NIDA Res Monogr* 84: 1–24.

Siegel, S. (1999) Drug anticipation and drug addiction. The 1998 H. David Archibald Lecture. *Addiction* 94: 1113–1124.

Siegel, S., Hinson, R.E., Krank, M.D., and McCully, J. (1982) Heroin 'overdose' death: contribution of drug-associated environmental cues. *Science* 216: 436–437.

Sircar, R., Mallinson, K., Goldbloom, L.M., and Kehoe, P. (2001) Postnatal stress selectively upregulates striatal N-methyl-D-aspartate receptors in male rats. *Brain Research* 904: 145–148.

Skinner, B.F. (1938) *The behavior of organisms: an experimental analysis.* New York: Appleton.

Skinner, B.F. (1953) *Science and Human Behavior.* New York: Macmillan.

Skog, O.-J. (2003) Addiction: definitions and mechanisms. In: N. Heather and R.E. Vuchinich (eds), *Choice, behavioral economics and addiction.* Oxford: Elsevier: 157–175, 182.

Slotkin, T.A., Seidler, F.J., and Yanai, J. (2003) Heroin neuroteratogenicity: delayed-onset deficits in catecholaminergic synaptic activity. *Brain Research* 948: 189–197.

Slovic, P., Fischhoff, B., and Lichtenstein, S. (1982) Facts versus fears: understanding perceived risk. In: D. Kahneman, P. Slovic, and A. Tversky (eds), *Judgement under uncertainty: heuristics and biases.* New York: Cambridge University Press: 463-489.

Smith-Roe, S.L. and Kelley, A.E. (2000) Coincident activation of NMDA and dopamine D1 receptors within the nucleus accumbens core is required for appetitive instrumental learning. *J Neurosci* 20: 7737–7742.

Smith, A.M., Fried, P.A., Hogan, M.J., and Cameron, I. (2004) Effects of prenatal marijuana on response inhibition: an fMRI study of young adults. *Neurotoxicology and Teratology* 26: 533–542.

Smith, J.K., Neill, J.C., and Costall, B. (1997) Post-weaning housing conditions influence the behavioural effects of cocaine and d-amphetamine. *Psychopharmacology* 131: 23–33.

Smith, S.S., O'Hara, B.F., Persico, A.M., Gorelick, M.A., Newlin, D.B., and Vlahov, D. (1992) Genetic vulnerability to drug abuse, the D2 dopamine receptor Taq 1 B1 restriction fragment length polymorphism appears more frequently in polysubstance abusers. *Archives of General Psychiatry* 49: 723–727.

Smith, Z. (1999) *The revenue effect of changing alcohol duties.* Institute for Fiscal Studies.

Smits, B.M.G., D'Souza, U.M., Berezikov, E., Cuppen, E., and Sluyter, F. (2004) Identifying polymorphisms in the *Rattus norvegicus*

D3 dopamine receptor gene and regulatory region. *Genes Brain Behavior* 3: 138–148.

Sofuoglu, M., Dudish-Poulsen, S., Nelson, D., Pentel, P.R., and Hatsukami, D.K. (1999) Sex and menstrual cycle differences in the subjective effects from smoked cocaine in humans. *Experimental and Clinical Psychopharmacology* 7: 274–283.

Sokoloff, P., Giros, B., Martres, M.P., Bouthenet, M.L., and Schwartz, J.C. (1990) Molecular cloning and characterization of a novel dopamine receptor (D3) as a target for neuroleptics. *Nature* 347: 146–151.

Solanto, M.V., Arnsten, A.F., and Castellanos, F.X. (2001) *Stimulant drugs and ADHD: Basic and clinical neuroscience.* Oxford University Press, New York.

Solomon, R.L. (1980a) Recent experiments testing an opponent-process theory of acquired motivation. *Acta Neurobiol Exp (Wars)* 40: 271–289.

Solomon, R.L. (1980b) The opponent-process theory of acquired motivation: the costs of pleasure and the benefits of pain. *Am Psychol* 35: 691–712.

Solomon, R.L. and Corbit, J.D. (1973) An opponent-process theory of motivation. II. Cigarette addiction. *J Abnorm Psychol* 81: 158–171.

Solomon, R.L. and Corbit, J.D. (1974) An opponent-process theory of motivation. I. Temporal dynamics of affect. *Psychol Rev* 81: 119–145.

Spear, L.P. (2000) The adolescent brain and age-related behavioral manifestations. *Neuroscience and Biobehavioral Reviews* 24: 417.

Spence, S.A. and Frith, C. (1999) Towards a functional anatomy of volition. *Consciousness Studies* 6: 11–29.

Spence, S.A., Hirsch, S.R., Brooks, D.J., and Grasby, P.M. (1998) Prefrontal cortex activity in people with schizophrenia and control subjects. Evidence from positron emission tomography for remission of 'hypofrontality' with recovery from acute schizophrenia. *Br J Psychiatry* 172: 316–323.

Spence, S.A., Hunter, M.D., Farrow, T.F., Green, R.D., Leung, D.H., Hughes, C.J., and Ganesan, V. (2004) A cognitive neurobiological account of deception: evidence from functional neuroimaging. *Philos Trans R Soc Lond B Biol Sci* 359: 1755–1762.

St Popova, J.S. and Petkov, V.V. (1977) Changes in 5-HT 1 receptors in different brain structures of rats with isolation syndrome. *General Pharmacology* 18: 223–225.

Stansfield, K.H., Philpot, R.M., and Kirstein, C.L. (2004) An animal model of sensation seeking: the adolescent rat. *Annals of the New York Academy of Sciences* 1021: 453.

Stewart, J. and Vezina, P. (1988) A comparison of the effects of intra-accumbens injections of amphetamine and morphine on reinstatement of heroin intravenous self-administration behavior. *Brain Res* 457: 287–294.

Stigler, G. and Becker, G.S. (1977) De gustibus non est disputandum. *American Economic Review* 67: 76–90.

Stone, V.E., Cosmides, L., Tooby, J., Kroll, N., and Knight, R.T. (2002) Selective impairment of reasoning about social exchange in a patient with bilateral limbic system damage. *Proc Natl Acad Sci USA* 99: 11531–11536.

Strecker, R.E., Eberle, C.A., and Ashby, C.R., Jr. (2004) Extracellular dopamine and its metabolites in the nucleus accumbens of Fischer and Lewis rats: basal levels and cocaine-induced changes. *Science* 56: 135.

Stuss, D.T., Gallup, G.G., Jr., and Alexander, M.P. (2001) The frontal lobes are necessary for 'theory of mind'. *Brain* 124: 279–286.

Suomi, S.J., Rasmussen, K.L.R., and Higley, J.D. (1992) Primate models of behavioral and physiological change in adolescence. In: K. McAnarney, R.E. Kreipe, D.P. Orr, and G.D. Comerci (eds), *Textbook of adolescent medicine.* Philadelphia: W.B. Saunders: 135–140.

Suzuki, T., George, F.R., and Meisch, R.A. (1988) Differential establishment and maintenance of oral ethanol reinforced behavior in Lewis and Fisher 344 inbred rat strains. *Journal of Pharmacology And Experimental Therapeutics* 245: 164–170.

Suzuki, T., George, F.R., and Meisch, R.A. (1992) Etonitazene delivered orally serves as a reinforcer for Lewis but not Fischer 344 rats. *Pharmacology Biochemistry and Behavior* 42: 579–586.

Suzuki, T., Otani, Y., Koike, M., and Misawa, M. (1998) Genetic differences in preferences for morphine and codeine in Lewis and Fischer 344 inbred rat strains. *Japanese Journal of Pharmacology* 47: 425–431.

Suzuki, A., Josselyn, S.A., Frankland, P.W., Masushige, S., Silva, A.J., and Kida, S. (2004) Memory reconsolidation and extinction have distinct temporal and biochemical signatures. *Journal of Neuroscience* 24: 4787–4795.

Szerman, N., Peris, L., Mesias, B., Colis, P., Rosa, J., and Prieto, A. (2005) Reboxetine for the treatment of patients with Cocaine Dependence Disorder. *Hum Psychopharmacol* 20: 189–192.

Szumlinski, K.K., Dehoff, M.H., Kang, S.H., Frys, K.A., Lominac, K.D., Klugmann, M., Rohrer, J., Griffin, W., 3rd, Toda, S., Champtiaux, N.P., Berry, T., Tu, J.C., Shealy, S.E., During, M.J., Middaugh, L.D., Worley, P.F., and Kalivas, P.W. (2004) Homer proteins regulate sensitivity to cocaine. *Neuron* 43: 401–413.

Taylor, J.R. and Horger, B.A. (1999) Enhanced responding for conditioned reward produced by intra-accumbens amphetamine is potentiated after cocaine sensitization. *Psychopharmacology* 142: 31–40.

Taylor, J.R. and Robbins, T.W. (1984) Enhanced behavioural control by conditioned reinforcers following microinjections of d-amphetamine into the nucleus accumbens. *Psychopharmacology* 84: 405–412.

Terwilliger, R.Z., Beitner-Johnson, D., Sevarino, K.A., Crain, S.M., and Nestler, E.J. (1991) A general role for adaptations in G-proteins and the cyclic AMP system in mediating the chronic actions of morphine and cocaine on neuronal function. *Brain Res* 548: 100–110.

Thibault, C., Lai, C., Wilke, N., Duong, B., Olive, M.F., Rahman, S., Dong, H., Hodge, C.W., Lockhart, D.J., and Miles, M.F. (2000) Expression profiling of neural cells reveals specific patterns of ethanol-responsive gene expression. *Mol Pharmacol* 58: 1593–1600.

Thoa, N.B., Tizabi, Y., and Jacobowitz, D.M. (1977) The effect of isolation on catecholamine concentration and turnover in discrete areas of the rat brain. *Brain Research* 131: 259–269.

Thomas, M.J. and Malenka, R.C. (2003) Synaptic plasticity in the mesolimbic dopamine system. *Philos Trans R Soc Lond B Biol Sci* 358: 815–819.

Thomas, M.J., Beurrier, C., Bonci, A., and Malenka, R.C. (2001) Long-term depression in the nucleus accumbens: a neural correlate of behavioral sensitization to cocaine. *Nat Neurosci* 4: 1217–1223.

Thomas, K.L., Arroyo, M., and Everitt, B.J. (2003) Induction of the learning and plasticity-associated gene Zif268 following exposure to a discrete cocaine-associated stimulus. *European Journal of Neuroscience* 17: 1964–1972.

Thompson, T.L. (1999) Attenuation of dopamine uptake in vivo following priming with estradiol benzoate. *Brain Research* 834: 164–167.

Thorndike, E.L. (1905) *The elements of psychology.* New York: Seiler.

Thorndike, E.L. (1911) *Animal intelligence: experimental studies.* New York: Macmillan.

Tiffany, S.T. (1990) A cognitive model of drug urges and drug-use-behavior: role of automatic and nonautomatic processes. *Psychological Review* 97: 147–168.

Tiffany, S.T. and Carter, B.L. (1998) Is craving the source of compulsive drug use? *J Psychopharmacol* 12: 23–30.

Tiffany, S.T. and Drobes, D.J. (1990) Imagery and smoking urges: the manipulation of affective content. *Addict Behav* 15: 531–539.

Toates, F. (1986) *Motivational systems.* Cambridge: Cambridge University Press.

Toda, S., McGinty, J.F., and Kalivas, P.W. (2002) Repeated cocaine administration alters the expression of genes in corticolimbic circuitry after a 3-week withdrawal: a DNA macroarray study. *J Neurochem* 82: 1290–1299.

Toni, N., Buchs, P.A., Nikonenko, I., Bron, C.R., and Muller, D. (1999) LTP promotes formation of multiple spine synapses between a single axon terminal and a dendrite. *Nature* 402: 421–425.

Tsuang, M.T., Lyons, M.J., Harley, R.M., Xian, H., Eisen, S., Goldberg, J., True, W. R., and Faraone, S.V. (1999) Genetic and environmental influences on transitions in drug use. *Behavioural Genetics* 29: 473.

Tully, T., Bourtchouladze, R., Scott, R., and Tallman, J. (2003) Targeting the CREB pathway for memory enhancers. *Nat Rev Drug Discov* 2: 267–277.

Turgeon, S.M., Pollack, A.E., and Fink, J.S. (1997) Enhanced CREB phosphorylation and changes in c-Fos and FRA expression in striatum accompany amphetamine sensitization. *Brain Res* 749: 120–126.

Turner, D.C., Clark, L.J., Robbins, T.W., and Sahakian, B.J. (2004) Modafinil improves cognition and response inhibition in adult ADHD. *Biological Psychiatry* 55: 1031–1039.

Tyler, W.J., Alonso, M., Bramham, C.R., and Pozzo-Miller, L.D. (2002) From acquisition to consolidation: on the role of brain-derived neurotrophic factor signaling in hippocampal-dependent learning. *Learning and Memory* 9: 224–237.

Uchtenhagen, A. (1997) *Summary of the synthesis report*. Institute for Social and Preventive Medicine at the University of Zurich.

Uhl, G.R. (1999) Molecular genetics of substance abuse vulnerability: a current approach. *Neuropsychopharmacology* 20: 3–9.

Uhl, G.R. (2004) Molecular genetic underpinnings of human substance abuse vulnerability: likely contributions to understanding addiction as a mnemonic process. *Neuropharmacology* 47: 140.

Uhlenhuth, E.H., Johanson, C.E., Kilgore, K., and Kobasa, S.C. (1981) Drug preference and mood in humans: preference for d-amphetamine and subject characteristics. *Psychopharmacology (Berl)* 74: 191–194.

Unterwald, E.M., Cox, B.M., Kreek, M.J., Cote, T.E., and Izenwasser, S. (1993) Chronic repeated cocaine administration alters basal and opioid-regulated adenylyl cyclase activity. *Synapse* 15: 33–38.

Vaglenova, J., Birru, S., Pandiella, N.M., and Breese, C.R. (2004) An assessment of the long-term developmental and behavioral teratogenicity of prenatal nicotine exposure. *Behavioural Brain Research* 150: 159–170.

Valverde, O., Mantamadiotis, T., Torrecilla, M., Ugedo, L., Pineda, J., Bleckmann, S., Gass, P., Kretz, O., Mitchell, J.M., Schutz, G., and Maldonado, R. (2004) Modulation of anxiety-like behavior and morphine dependence in CREB-deficient mice. *Neuropsychopharmacology* 29: 1122–1133.

Vanderschuren, L.J. and Everitt, B.J. (2004) Drug seeking becomes compulsive after prolonged cocaine self-administration. *Science* 305: 1017–1019.

Vanderschuren, L.J. and Kalivas, P.W. (2000) Alterations in dopaminergic and glutamatergic transmission in the induction and expression of behavioral sensitization: a critical review of preclinical studies. *Psychopharmacology* 151: 99–120.

Ventura, R., Alcaro, A., Cabib, S., Conversi, D., Mandolesi, S., and Puglisi-Allegra, S. (2004) Dopamine in the medial prefrontal cortex controls genotype-dependent effects of amphetamine on mesoaccumbens dopamine release and locomotion. *Neuropsychopharmacology* 29: 72.

Vezina, P. (2004) Sensitization of midbrain dopamine neuron reactivity and the self-administration of psychomotor stimulant drugs. *Neurosci Biobehav Rev* 27: 827–839.

Volkow, N.D. and Li, T.K. (2004) Drug addiction: the neurobiology of behaviour gone awry. *Nat Rev Neurosci* 5: 963–970.

Volkow, N.D. and Li, T.K. (2004) Science and Society: Drug addiction: the neurobiology of behaviour gone awry. *Nat Rev Neurosci* 5: 963–970.

Volkow, N.D., Fowler, J.S., and Wang, G.J. (1999a) Imaging studies on the role of dopamine in cocaine reinforcement and addiction in humans. *J Psychopharmacol* 13: 337–345.

Volkow, N.D., Wang, G.J., Fowler, J.S., Logan, J., Gatley, S.J., Wong, C., Hitzemann, R., and Pappas, N. (1999b) Reinforcing effects of psychostimulants in humans are associated with increases in brain dopamine and occupancy of D2 receptors. *The Journal of Pharmacology and Experimental Therapeutics* 291: 409–415.

Volkow, N.D., Wang, G.J., Fowler, J.S., Logan, J., Gatley, S.J., Gifford, A., Hitzemann, R., Ding, Y.S., and Pappas, N. (1999c) Prediction of reinforcing responses to psychostimulants in humans by brain dopamine D2 receptor levels. *Am J Psychiatry* 156: 1440–1443.

Volkow, N.D., Fowler, J.S., and Wang, G.J. (2003a) Positron emission tomography and single-photon emission computed tomography in substance abuse research. *Semin Nucl Med* 33: 114–128.

Volkow, N.D., Fowler, J.S., and Wang, G.J. (2003b) The addicted human brain: insights from imaging studies. *J Clin Invest* 111: 1444–1451.

von Neumann, J. and Morgenstern, O. (1947) *Theory of games and economic behavior*. Princeton, New Jersey: Princeton University Press.

Vorel, S.R., Liu, X., Hayes, R.J., Spector, J.A., and Gardner, E.L. (2001) Relapse to cocaine-seeking after hippocampal theta burst stimulation. *Science* 292: 1175–1178.

Vorel, S.R., Ashby, C.R., Jr., Paul, M., Liu, X., Hayes, R., Hagan, J.J., Middlemiss, D.N., Stemp, G., and Gardner, E.L. (2002) Dopamine D3 receptor antagonism inhibits cocaine-seeking and cocaine-enhanced brain reward in rats. *J Neurosci* 22: 9595–9603.

Vuchinich, R.E. and Heather, N. (2003) Introduction: overview of behavioural economic perspectives on substance use and addiction. In: N. Heather and R.E. Vuchinich (eds), *Choice, behavioral economics and addiction*. Oxford: Elsevier: 1–31.

Wade, T.R., de Wit, H., and Richards, J.B. (2000) Effects of dopaminergic drugs on delayed reward as a measure of impulsive behavior in rats. *Psychopharmacology* 150: 90–101.

Walker, M.P., Brakefield, T., Hobson, J.A., and Stickgold, R. (2003) Dissociable stages of human memory consolidation and reconsolidation. *Nature* 425: 616–620.

Walter, B.L. and Vitek, J.L. (2004) Surgical treatment for Parkinson's disease. *Lancet Neurol* 3: 719–728.

Walters, C.L. and Blendy, J.A. (2001) Different requirements for cAMP response element binding protein in positive and negative reinforcing properties of drugs of abuse. *J Neurosci* 21: 9438–9444.

Walton, M.E., Bannerman, D.M., and Rushworth, M.F. (2002) The role of rat medial frontal cortex in effort-based decision making. *J Neurosci* 22: 10996–11003.

Walton, M.E., Bannerman, D.M., Alterescu, K., and Rushworth, M.F.S. (2003) Functional specialization within medial frontal cortex of the anterior cingulate for evaluating effort-related decisions. *J Neurosci* 23: 6475–6479.

Wang, S.H., Ostlund, S.B., Nader, K., and Balleine, B.W. (2005) Consolidation and reconsolidation of incentive learning in the amygdala. *J Neurosci* 25: 830–835.

Ward, N.S., Oakely, D.A., Frackowiak, R.S., and Halligan, P.W. (2003) Differential brain activations during intentionally simulated and subjectively experienced paralysis. *Cog Neuropsychiatry* 8: 295–312.

Warner, L.A., Kessler, R.C., Hughes, M., Anthony, J.C., and Nelson, C.B. (1995) Prevalence and correlates of drug use and dependence in the United States. Results from the National Comorbidity Survey. *Arch Gen Psychiatry* 52: 219–229.

Watts, V.J. (2002) Molecular mechanisms for heterologous sensitization of adenylate cyclase. *J Pharmacol Exp Ther* 302: 1–7.

Weinstock, M., Speiser, A., and Ashkenazi, R. (1978) Changes in brain catecholamine turnover and receptor sensitivity induced by social deprivation in rats. *Psychopharmacology* 56: 205.

Weiss, R.D. and Mirin, S.M. (1986) Subtypes of cocaine abusers. *Psychiatr Clin North Am* 9: 491–501.

Weiss, F., Markou, A., Lorang, M.T., and Koob, G.F. (1992) Basal extracellular dopamine levels in the nucleus accumbens are decreased during cocaine withdrawal

after unlimited-access self-administration. *Brain Research* 593: 314–318.

Whitaker-Azmitia, P., Zhou, F., Hobin, J., and Borella, A. (2000) Isolation-rearing of rats produces deficits as adults in the serotonergic innervation of hippocampus. *Peptides* 21: 1755–1759.

White, N.M. (1996) Addictive drugs as reinforcers: multiple partial actions on memory systems. *Addiction* 91(7): 921–949.

White, A.M. and Swartzwelder, H.S. (2004) Hippocampal function during adolescence: a unique target of ethanol effects. *Annals of the New York Academy of Sciences* 1021: 206.

White, T.L., Justice, A.J., and de Wit, H. (2002) Differential subjective effects of D-amphetamine by gender, hormone levels and menstrual cycle phase. *Pharmacology Biochemistry and Behavior* 73: 729–741.

Whitelaw, R.B., Markou, A., Robbins, T.W., and Everitt, B.J. (1996) Excitotoxic lesions of the basolateral amygdala impair the acquisition of cocaine-seeking behaviour under a second-order schedule of reinforcement. *Psychopharmacology* 127: 213–224.

Wigger, A. and Neumann, I.D. (1999) Periodic maternal deprivation induces gender-dependent alterations in behavioral and neuroendocrine responses to emotional stress in adult rats. *Physiology and Behavior* 66: 293–302.

Wikler, A. (1965) Conditioning factors in opiate addiction and relapse. In: D.I. Wilner and G.G. Kessenbaum (eds), *Narcotics*. New York: McGraw-Hill: 85–100.

Wikler, A. (1973) Dynamics of drug dependence: Implications of a conditioning theory for research and treatment. *Archives of General Psychiatry* 28: 611–616.

Wilkins, A.S., Genova, L.M., Posten, W., and Kosofsky, B.E. (1998a) Transplacental cocaine exposure. 1: A rodent model. *Neurotoxicology and Teratology* 20: 215–226.

Wilkins, A.S., Jones, K., and Kosofsky, B.E. (1998b) Transplacental cocaine exposure. 2: Effects of cocaine dose and gestational timing. *Neurotoxicology and Teratology* 20: 227–238.

Wilkins, A.S., Marota, J.J., Tabit, E., and Kosofsky, B.E. (1998c) Transplacental cocaine exposure. 3: Mechanisms underlying altered brain development. *Neurotoxicology and Teratology* 20: 239–249.

Will, M.J., Franzblau, E.B., and Kelley, A.E. (2003) Nucleus accumbens mu-opioids regulate intake of a high-fat diet via activation of a distributed brain network. *J Neurosci* 23: 2882–2888.

Williams, B.A. (1994) Reinforcement and choice. In: N.J. Mackintosh (ed.), *Animal Learning and Cognition*, pp. 81–108. Academic Press, San Diego.

Wilson, C., Nomikos, G.G., Collu, M., and Fibiger, H.C. (1995) Dopaminergic correlates of motivated behavior: importance of drive. *J Neurosci* 15: 5169–5178.

Wilson, J.M., Kalasinsky, K.S., Levey, A.I., Bergeron, C., Reiber, G., Anthony, R.M., Schmunk, G.A., Shannak, K., Haycock, J.W., and Kish, S.J. (1996) Striatal dopamine nerve terminal markers in human, chronic methamphetamine users. *Nat Med* 2: 699–703.

Winstanley, C.A., Theobald, D.E., Cardinal, R.N., and Robbins, T.W. (2004) Contrasting roles of basolateral amygdala and orbitofrontal cortex in impulsive choice. *J Neurosci* 24: 4718–4722.

Winston, G.C. (1980) Addiction and backsliding: a theory of compulsive consumption. *Journal of Economic Behavior and Organization* 1: 295–324.

Wise, R.A. (1981) Brain dopamine and reward. In: S. J. Cooper (ed.), *Theory in psychopharmacology Volume 1*. London: Academic Press: 103-122.

Wise, R.A. (1982) Neuroleptics and operant behavior: the anhedonia hypothesis. *Behavioral and Brain Sciences* 5: 39–87.

Wise, R.A. and Bozarth, M.A. (1985) Brain mechanisms of drug reward and euphoria. *Psychiatr Med* 3: 445–460.

Wogar, M.A., Bradshaw, C.M., and Szabadi, E. (1993) Effect of lesions of the ascending 5-hydroxytryptaminergic pathways on choice between delayed reinforcers. *Psychopharmacology* 111: 239–243.

Wright, I.K., Ismail, H., Upton, N., and Marsden, C.A. (1990) Effect of isolation-rearing on performance in the elevated plus-maze and open field behaviour. *British Journal of Pharmacology* 100: 375P.

Wyvell, C.L. and Berridge, K.C. (2000) Intra-accumbens amphetamine increases the conditioned incentive salience of sucrose reward: enhancement of reward 'wanting' without enhanced 'liking' or response reinforcement. *Journal of Neuroscience* 20: 8122–8130.

Wyvell, C.L. and Berridge, K.C. (2001) Incentive sensitization by previous amphetamine exposure: increased cue-triggered 'wanting' for sucrose reward. *Journal of Neuroscience* 21: 7831–7840.

Yamada, K., Mizuno, M., and Nabeshima, T. (2002) Role for brain-derived neurotrophic factor in learning and memory. *Life Sciences* 70: 735–744.

Yamaguchi, M., Suzuki, T., Seki, T., Namba, T., Juan, R., Arai, H., Hori, T., and Asada, T. (2004) Repetitive cocaine administration decreases neurogenesis in adult rat hippocampus. *Ann N Y Acad Sci* 1025: 351–362.

Yang, X., Diehl, A.M., and Wand, G.S. (1996) Ethanol exposure alters the phosphorylation of cyclic AMP responsive element binding protein and cyclic AMP responsive element binding activity in rat cerebellum. *J Pharmacol Exp Ther* 278: 338–346.

Yin, H.H., Knowlton, B.J., and Balleine, B.W. (2004) Lesions of dorsolateral striatum preserve outcome expectancy but disrupt habit formation in instrumental learning. *Eur J Neurosci* 19: 181–189.

Young, A.M. (2004) Increased extracellular dopamine in nucleus accumbens in response to unconditioned and conditioned aversive stimuli: studies using 1 min microdialysis in rats. *J Neurosci Methods* 138: 57–63.

Zhang, M. and Kelley, A.E. (2000) Enhanced intake of high-fat food following striatal mu-opioid stimulation: microinjection mapping and fos expression. *Neuroscience* 99: 267–277.

Zhang, M. and Kelley, A.E. (2002) Intake of saccharin, salt, and ethanol solutions is increased by infusion of a mu opioid agonist into the nucleus accumbens. *Psychopharmacology (Berl)* 159: 415–423.

Zhang, M., Gosnell, B.A., and Kelley, A.E. (1998) Intake of high-fat food is selectively enhanced by mu opioid receptor stimulation within the nucleus accumbens. *Journal of Pharmacology and Experimental Therapeutics* 285: 908–914.

Zhu, J. (2004) Understanding volition. *Philosophical Psychology* 17: 247–273.

Zink, C.F., Pagnoni, G., Martin-Skurski, M.E., Chappelow, J.C., and Berns, G.S. (2004) Human striatal responses to monetary reward depend on saliency. *Neuron* 42: 509–517.

Zocchi, A., Orsini, C., Cabib, S., and Puglisi-Allegra, S. (1998) Parallel strain-dependent effect of amphetamine on locomotor activity and dopamine release in the nucleus accumbens: an in vivo study in mice. *Neuroscience* 82: 521–528.

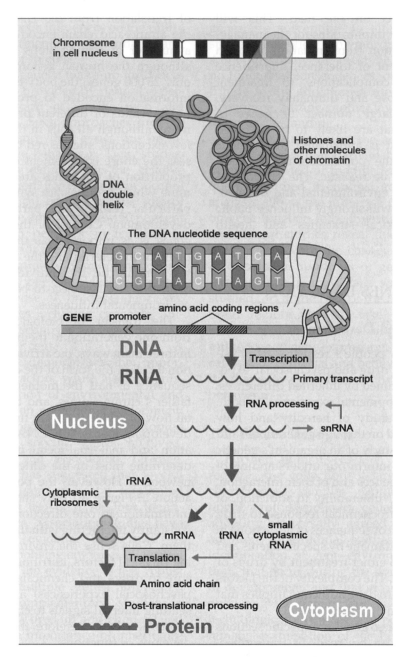

FIGURE 4.1 Basic structure and function of the genome. A schematic summary of the structure of the genome from chromosome (visible under the light microscope) down to the DNA nucleotide sequence, and the function of the genome through transcription of the DNA code of the gene into RNAs with mRNA (messenger RNA) being translated into protein. As emphasised in the text, this figure portrays the action in one direction only, namely gene expression. In response to signals from the internal and external environment, gene expression is triggered by molecular complexes binding to the promoter region of the gene to either activate the gene by promoting transcription, or silence the gene by locking it into tightly packed chromatin.

transcription regulatory factors (molecules or complexes of molecules that bind to DNA and determine gene expression levels) depends on the chromatin state. This in turn can mean that developmental experience can be captured as changes in chromatin state leading to more or less permanent changes in gene expression.

The constant two-way flow of information modulating cell function through changes in gene expression is central to the role of genetics and genomic research in drug addiction and its treatment. This has to be borne in mind throughout the sections of this review that focus on inherited differences between people. In the final analysis, we are usually dealing with differences in response, even if the developmental outcome is a more or less fixed change in gene expression that then contributes to what used to be called a person's 'constitution'.

2.2 Relating Genes to Addiction

We all know what 'addiction' is meant to mean, but when it is discussed, different individuals will emphasise different aspects. Different mechanisms may underlie the propensity to abuse drugs and the propensity to become dependent upon them. Liability to addiction will reflect a mixture of psychological, neurobiological and other biological traits. Thus, certain addictions may be related to a trait of risk taking. But a risk-taking trait will not always reveal itself as a tendency to take drugs. It may appear as promiscuity, free-fall parachute jumping, or investing on the stock exchange.

At a neurobiological level, most drugs of abuse are known to affect, directly or indirectly, neurotransmission in pathways using the neurotransmitter dopamine. These pathways have been long implicated in mediating the ability of rewards (including drugs) to influence behaviour. There is emerging evidence that particular alleles of genes encoding the dopamine D2 receptor (DRD2) may be associated with a reduction in the efficiency of this system and thus a reduced ability to experience reward. Individuals

with such genes may be predisposed to take drugs to restore the activity of these systems. However, even if such a relationship were proven, it is clear that the DRD2 gene is not simply a gene for addiction, but is involved in much wider brain functions. Other genes may encode proteins that are essential for the breakdown of drugs. Variations in such genes will affect the rate of metabolism of the drug, which may make it more or less addictive. This shows that understanding the contribution of genomics to drug addiction will need the integration of evidence from many fields. Identifying variations in genetic constitution between groups of addicts (even if they are very clearly defined) and non-addicts will provide only a glimmer of the knowledge needed to understand the particular role of any gene.

2.3 Inherited Variation

2.3.1 What Contribution do Genetic Variants Make to Behavioural Differences?

A key question in human biomedical research is the contribution of inherited variation to differences between people, including differences in vulnerability to or recovery from addiction, and differences in susceptibility to damage from specific agents or in response to treatment. The primary source of inherited variation is differences in the DNA sequence that alter the gene product or its expression. There is also emerging evidence that certain chromatin states at particular genes may be transmitted from parent to offspring (Rakyan et al., 2003) but it is far too early to know whether this will turn out to be an important determinant of the offspring's health or just a curiosity.

Discovering which DNA-sequence variant contributes to what variation in response is important for two reasons. If the genetic effect is substantial, testing for the DNA-sequence variant might allow people to be forewarned about their vulnerability, or help them select 'tailor-made' therapy. Equally important, a causal link between a gene variant and an aspect of variation in response to psychoactive agents reveals something about the biological mechanisms involved, even if the link is mediated in a complex way. This is true even if the effect is small. So, discovering a specific genetic modulation of a response and showing that it contributes to the differences between people is a powerful, independent way into the physiological and biochemical pathways mediating that difference. Such insights can lead to experimental verification in animals and a more logical development of therapy.

Most behavioural traits are influenced by a number of genes, each of which may exist in different forms called alleles. Variations in a behavioural trait are likely to be the consequence of differences in the contributions of different alleles for different genes. By cross-breeding strains with and without a behavioural trait of interest (such as the tendency to consume large quantities of alcohol), and tracking the trait across generations, it is possible, using DNA-sequence variants as chromosomal markers, to determine the approximate chromosomal location of genes contributing to it. A chromosomal locus that is important in determining a continuous character is called a quantitative trait locus (QTL). Chromosomal mapping of a QTL is only the first step. One is then faced with identifying which of the genes in that region are relevant. This task has been made much easier by the various 'genome projects' that have sequenced the entire genomes of man and several experimental species.

2.3.2 Human Genetic Variation

There is currently a worldwide effort to define the common and less common DNA sequence differences between people, both within and between human populations. The simplest and cheapest DNA variants to analyse are single nucleotide polymorphisms (SNPs). It has been estimated that there are 10–15 million SNPs whose more common allele occurs in at least 1 per cent of genomes

(Botstein and Risch, 2003; Kruglyak and Nickerson, 2001). Much of the international effort to date has been focused on defining these SNPs by sequencing suitable panels of samples – for example, the International HapMap Project (IHMP, 2003), and the work of Perlegen (www.perlegen.com). By 2005, large-scale sequencing studies had trebled the number of markers available, to a total of 8 million SNPs, an average of one for every 360 nucleotide base pairs in the genome, and 1 million deletion–insertion polymorphisms (DIPs) (dbSNP build 121 at www.ncbi.nlm.nih.gov/SNP and Mullikin, personal communication).

Despite these rich resources, our current knowledge of common SNPs in the genome is incomplete and there is much we don't know about other types of genomic variation. There can be chromosomal rearrangements, large-scale gene copy-number variation (Carter, 2004), variation in the length of repeat sequences, including the length of the chromosome end 'caps' (telomeres) (Blackburn, 1991) and insertion/deletion variants beyond single nucleotides. Any of the stable, common DNA polymorphisms can be used as 'markers' of a particular locus on the chromosome and can be used for co-inheritance studies within families with a particular disorder to map a susceptibility locus.

2.3.3 Which Variants are Important in Trait and Disease-risk Differences?

We are still largely ignorant of what classes of genetic variants are likely to be most relevant to human differences. Will common variants with minor allele frequencies of more than 10 per cent be the major players, or are we talking about a combination of multiple rare variants in a gene? Theoretical arguments have been made for both (Lander, 1996; Pritchard, 2001). Clearly, a variant that changes the coding for an amino-acid is a good candidate and by 2005 the sequences of tens of thousands were publicly available (dbSNP release 121; www.ncbi.nlm.nih.gov/SNP/). At least 10 000 of these had been validated. However, variation in the regulatory regions around genes may prove to be more important for common disease (Rockman and Wray, 2002). It is also noteworthy that while transcription-factor binding-site mutations are relatively rare in the monogenic disorders, variants deleting these sites in the normal population seem to be common (Wjst, 2004). It is possible that such deletions will contribute to susceptibility to common diseases.

In terms of genetic influences in common traits and disorders, we are likely to be dealing with the combinatorial effects of variants in the coding region, promoter and other non-coding cis-regulatory DNA sequences, and sequences for functional non-protein-coding RNAs. Furthermore, the transient changes in the level of the activity of a gene in response to some experience is mediated by DNA-binding proteins called transcription factors, which are themselves gene products encoded by genes elsewhere in the genome. An inherited difference in that response may be due to DNA variants in the transcription factors rather than the target gene in question. It is one thing to note inherited variation in a gene's expression, quite another to discover the DNA variant or variants that underlie it.

2.4 Using Genetics to Dissect the Evolved Developmental/ Regulatory Response

2.4.1 Top-down and Bottom-up Approaches

With addiction and other effects of psychoactive agents, like most areas of biomedical research, the ultimate aim must be to understand the underlying evolved regulatory responses. By evolutionary necessity these will be coherent, if complex, sets of gene-gene and gene-environment interactions and therefore their discovery is a tractable task (Pembrey, 2004; Gottesman

and Hanson, 2005). This fact is the starting point for a bottom-up approach to discovery that also allows a very productive shuttling back and forth between laboratory animal experiments and human studies, both observational and interventional, each generating hypotheses to be tested in the other. It is already clear that there are commonalities in the genes underlying addictive behaviours in humans and in animal models.

Human studies most frequently investigate the genetic make-up of populations with a known susceptibility to abuse drugs. Animal studies adopt a variation of this top-down method but also allow bottom-up approaches. Top-down methodologies take a particular characteristic of the animal, such as a trait to consume alcohol, and seek to identify the processes, including genetic influences, that contribute to it. In this respect they are analogous to most human genetic studies. They often require the discovery of the genetic constitution of animal strains selectively bred for a particular behavioural trait, but the same approach can be used to study the consequences of taking a drug, or of withdrawal from a drug, on gene expression. A strength of this approach is that the experimenter deliberately eschews hypotheses regarding the relationship of particular genes to addictive traits. With 25 000 genes potentially contributing to addictive behaviour, which itself has many different aspects, testing the importance of each individual gene in every possible way that might contribute to addiction is an impossible task. Simply studying which gene variations are associated with the addictive trait is more tractable, even though it tells us little about the particular function of any genes that are identified.

In contrast, bottom-up approaches start off with a question about the function of a particular gene, and how modifying it alters an animal's behaviour. The manipulation of an individual's genes is ethically unacceptable (as well as technically intractable) for human studies. Temporary experimental manipulation of gene function with drugs may offer an acceptable approach in humans in some circumstances. Such bottom-up approaches can address hypotheses regarding the importance of individual genes.

There are several methods available for such manipulations. Genes of interest may be deleted in mice using molecular biological techniques called gene knockouts, or extra copies may be inserted into the mouse genome, a technique called transgenics. These techniques have provided new information that is not available using more traditional techniques. A major surprise was the discovery that the dopamine transporter at which cocaine was assumed to act is not necessary for the rewarding properties of cocaine (Rocha *et al.*, 1998; Sora *et al.*, 1998), forcing behavioural neuroscientists to reconsider the mechanisms by which cocaine achieves its effects. The discovery that deleting the gene-encoding receptors for the neuropeptide substance P abolishes the rewarding, but not the analgesic, properties of morphine (Ripley *et al.*, 2002; Murtra *et al.*, 2000; De Felipe *et al.*, 1998) suggests the possibility of producing powerful pain killers without dependence or abuse.

However, it is increasingly recognised that such genetic manipulations may have influences on the broader development of the organism. The resulting test animal may differ in its response to drugs in several ways, some perhaps independent of the role of the targeted gene in the drug response of normal adult animals (Stephens *et al.*, 2002). Knockouts offer an important refinement to this technique. Gene deletion in the germ line will influence development, and perhaps allow related genes to take over parts of the role of the deleted gene, although if the gene is knocked out late in life, it will not affect development, nor are compensatory mechanisms as likely to be activated. Furthermore, the manipulation of genes encoding for proteins that are used in multiple systems may have a range of behavioural effects. Disentangling them will be easier if the genetic manipulation is limited to a single tissue. Conditional knockouts have not yet been used widely in addiction research but are likely to become more frequent in the future.

In keeping with our knowledge that behavioural traits are unlikely to be attributable to single genes, the consequences of manipulating single genes using knockout techniques may differ depending on the genetic background of the mouse strain in which the knockout is made. Thus, deletion of the DAT gene has rather different consequences for cocaine reward, depending upon the mouse strain in which the knockout is created (Morice *et al.*, 2004).

A novel way to increase gene expression in a particular area of the brain, and thus to test that gene's involvement in a particular aspect of addictive behaviour, is to incorporate the gene into the genetic material of a virus modified to make it harmless to humans, and to inject the virus into the area of interest in the brain. Once the virus penetrates a nearby nerve cell, it will produce products of the inserted gene, which the nerve cell will then incorporate in its own machinery, leading to an increase in the levels of that particular protein. This exciting technique has already been used to suggest an association of the DRD2 with reduced alcohol consumption (Thanos *et al.*, 2001), and of the GRIA1 gene encoding GluR1 subunits of glutamate receptors in sensitisation to cocaine (Carlezon and Nestler, 2002). Such gene-transfer technology may be used in the near future to re-insert genes in specific brain areas of mice from which the native genes have been deleted in knockout experiments. If this reinstates a disrupted behaviour, then the causal relationship between the gene and behaviour is firmly established.

In point of fact, the top-down and bottom-up approaches are complementary, so that, for instance, genes identified by microarray studies of chromosomal loci identified by the QTL approach can be tested directly by targeted gene-knockout technologies. It is unlikely, however, that genes identified in this way can be described as genes for addiction. Genes encode proteins, and those proteins are likely to be involved in many different essential bodily processes with very indirect relationships to the processes underlying addiction.

2.4.2 Towards Systematic Bottom-up Approaches in Humans

Individuality can be found at each '-omic' level from genome, through transcriptome, proteome and metabolome (Scriver, 2004; Gottesman and Gould, 2003). One general principle of the bottom-up approach can be applied in humans. The bottom-up approach asks what a particular gene or genetic variant does. This question is independent of any preconceived idea of disease category or phenotypic classification, although data have to be collected on the full range of phenotypic 'outcomes' to answer the question. Such planned approaches, exploiting phenotype-rich cohorts, have been dubbed the 'Human Phenome Project' (Freimer and Sabatti, 2003) or Phenome Scans (Pembrey, 2004). If our current phenotypic labels or measures map poorly onto the evolved biological mechanisms that underlie human response to the availability and use of psychoactive agents, then research designs such as case-control approaches, which start with such labels, may not be optimal for discovering specific genetic influences. Recognising this possibility has led to the incorporation of intermediate phenotypes into case-control types of research on the grounds that these may be closer to sites of gene action (Gottesman and Gould, 2003).

It is also important to recognise that most genes and their genetic variants are likely to have multiple effects that cut across the way we currently carve up disorders into medical specialties based largely on organ systems.

2.4.3 The Relevance of the Timing of Developmental Experience

An important aspect of how people are moulded by developmental experience is whether particular susceptibility periods exist during development and how reversible the effects of certain exposures

during these times may be. On first principles one might expect exposure during foetal life and early childhood to influence development most directly and permanently, a view reflected in our attempt to protect the foetus and infant from drug exposure. The effects of foetal exposure to maternal alcohol consumption (Mukherjee *et al.*, 2005) and cigarette smoking (DiFranza *et al.*, 2004) are obvious examples. In both instances, these effects are likely to be modified by genetic variants in the mother and the foetus. There is also experimental rodent evidence that adolescence may represent a window of vulnerability to the consequences of psychoactive drugs, including addictive behaviour (Adriani and Laviola, 2004). From the genetic perspective, the question is how exposure at these critical times brings about the long-term changes in gene expression that underlie observed changes in brain function and molecular structure. While longitudinal observational studies in humans can look at the behavioural and certain molecular consequences of foetal exposure through maternal use in pregnancy or direct use later in childhood, animal experiments can attempt to define the mechanistic link with changed gene expression.

3 GENETIC ANALYSIS

3.1 Principles, Problems and Potential Solutions

3.1.1 Family and Twins Studies

The traditional starting point for the study of genetic influences is to carry out family studies and twin studies to estimate the 'heritability' of a condition; crudely speaking an attempt at estimating how genetic it is. Just the use of this term is controversial (Guo, 2000) because it is widely misunderstood. Its magnitude is not a reliable measure of the inherited component, especially of complex traits. Even RA Fisher (1951), a founder of heritability studies, called it 'an unfortunate shortcut'. The principle is to compare the occurrence of the condition of interest between two relatives, or unrelated people, in relation to the proportion of genes and genetic variants they would be expected to share by inheritance from a common embryo, parents or ancestors. This is 100 per cent for monozygotic (identical) twins and 50 per cent for dizygotic (non-identical) twins. If a condition has a significant genetic component, provided the environmental factors making them similar or different are approximately the same, the greater concordance in monozygotic twins should be due to their greater genetic similarity. Heritability is essentially a measure of familial aggregation which can be caused by genetic effects alone, by familial aggregation of environmental factors alone, or by a combination of genetic and environmental factors and their interactions. Moreover, the magnitude of the measure is determined not only by the strength of genetic and environmental effects and their interactions, but also by gene and environmental exposure frequencies, so it is a statement about a particular population under a particular set of environmental circumstances (Guo, 2000). Thus, while results from family studies can be consistent with genetic influence, they do not represent proof due to confounding from shared environment, and further support has been derived from adoption studies. These natural experiments provide the opportunity to study individuals reared by unrelated parents.

Both family and twin studies depend on defining the disorder of interest, which immediately raises the difficulty of how to classify a relative or twin who has an overlapping phenotype or a different but similar condition, such as addiction to a different agent. However, this difficulty can sometimes be exploited to raise testable hypotheses on underlying traits linking outcomes to gene effects. Accepting the provisos flagged up above about heritability, multivariate twin modelling has been used to dissect the structure of genetic and environmental risk factors for common psychiatric and substance-use disorders, where co-morbidity

is common (Kendler *et al.*, 2003). Heritability estimates will always have their limitations and will no doubt continue to produce newspaper headlines such as 'the infidelity gene' (BioNews, 2004) or similar misconceptions. Traditionally, a heritability estimate is often the starting point of a family and twin study that goes on to include genetic linkage and genetic association studies, although its magnitude is a poor guide to the chances of success of such studies.

Human studies to elucidate the genetic contribution to complex behaviours and psychiatric disorders have mainly adopted one of these two strategies (see Sham and McGuffin, 2002). A linkage or family study 'maps' a putative gene variant that is causing or contributing to a disorder in a particular chromosomal region. An association study, on the other hand, identifies a gene variant or variants that occur more often in people with the disorder compared with those without the disorder.

3.1.2 Linkage

Thanks to the human genome project and other research, we know the location of all the identified SNPs and other genetic variants along the chromosomes. Analysing a suitable set of such variants ('markers') in families allows the transmission of any chromosomal region to be followed, despite the recombinations that occur during egg and sperm formation. Thus, in linkage approaches, the inheritance of a trait or disorder is tracked through pedigrees in an attempt to identify a co-inheritance between a genetic marker and the condition. If linkage is identified, this would implicate a gene, in the broad region around the marker, in the development of the disorder. Linkage studies are ideal for the systematic identification of genes of major effect, but the regions they identify are large. In addition, many of the approaches require the estimation of several unknown parameters, including penetrance and phenocopy rate, which are essentially best guesses. As such they are less useful for identifying the relatively modest individual genetic contributions that are anticipated in most psychiatric disorders and complex behaviours, such as alcohol dependence.

Genetic linkage studies of simply-inherited, monogenic disorders with a clear-cut phenotype are now straightforward provided enough sufficiently large families can be recruited to the study. The genotyping challenges of genetic linkage studies are essentially solved, whether one is dealing with mendelian disorders or more complex familial disorders where susceptibility loci are likely to exist. However, problems remain with complex traits, the main ones being the expected small effect of individual causal variants and the fact that the chromosomal region identified can be quite large. While there have been notable examples of success in linkage studies of common disease phenotypes (e.g. Calpain-10 and T2D (Horikawa et al., 2000), ALOX5AP and CHD (Helgadottir et al., 2004), DPP10 and asthma (Van Eerdewegh et al., 2002)), there are also many examples of studies that have not yielded robust outcomes (Altmuller et al., 2001). In the absence of prohibitively large samples, the linkage approach is not well suited for complex traits with variants that contribute only modestly to the overall disease risk (Risch, 2000). Attention has turned to the association approach as a preferred genetic strategy for identifying novel aetiological loci via genome-wide scanning (Botstein and Risch, 2003; Risch, 2000).

3.1.3 Association

Genetic association studies usually attempt to detect a difference in the distribution of a genetic variant between a sample of unrelated individuals with a particular phenotype, such as a diagnosis of alcohol dependence, and a matched control sample. As such they have the advantage of not requiring the estimation of unknown parameters. Association studies can also be used to detect genetic associations with a continuous variable or trait. In addition, in contrast to linkage studies, association is capable of detecting gene variants of relatively small effect, such as those that are more likely in alcohol dependence, although many thousands of markers would be required for a systematic approach that could screen the entire human genome. As a consequence, association studies have until now usually adopted the candidate-gene approach, examining DNA variants within genes on the basis of an a priori suspicion of a role in, say, alcohol dependence.

Two strategies have been adopted for association studies – direct and indirect. The former relies on identifying functional variants in the genes such that any association identified is very likely to be due to the DNA change itself and therefore replicable in other comparable studies. The second approach relies on linkage disequilibrium (essentially a co-inheritance of genetic variants close together on the chromosome) between markers such as SNPs, presumed to be non-functional in the condition, and the putative susceptibility or causal variant. Both approaches can be employed simultaneously.

Indirect Association Studies

The great hope has been that linkage disequilibrium (LD) can be exploited in genome-wide association studies to capture most of the human disease associations with relatively little genotyping. The $100 million International HapMap Project was predicated on just such a strategy, but the jury is still out on how much of a short cut this will prove to be in the end. There is, for example, the problem of replication of the initial discovery in a population with different allele frequencies or haplotype structure (Neale and Sham, 2004). Linkage disequilibrium is caused by the co-inheritance of genetic variants close together on the chromosome. In general, the closer alleles are on a chromosome, the less likely they are to be separated during egg and sperm formation. Thus short arrays of alleles on a chromosome, so-called haplotypes, are transmitted intact and become established in populations until they are eventually disrupted by recombination or by a new genetic variant arising. It happens that meiotic recombination tends to occur at specific recombination 'hot spots' along the chromosomes, generating relatively stable 'haplotype blocs' in between. Thus, it was hoped that if a few easily genotyped SNPs could be found that were a reliable signature or 'tag' for each haplotype bloc, these could be used to detect disease associations with any of the functional causal genetic variants within the haplotype bloc. Just the associated haplotype blocs could then be genotyped extensively to find the causal variants. If only haplotype-based association screening was that simple! Haplotypes vary between populations, and haplotype blocs are a (rather arbitrary) matter of degree of LD, the blocs often breaking up into different haplotypes as a greater density of SNPs are typed. Clearly more cost-effective genotyping on more population samples will lead to better and better descriptions of the LD structure of human genomes worldwide. This is fine for 'out of Africa'-style population research into human evolution, diversity and recent migrations, but how relevant it is to disease or trait association studies is still unknown. Any predictions are at the mercy of our ignorance of which classes of genetic variants are most likely to underlie genetic susceptibility or resistance to common disorders.

Some Current Issues in Association Studies

Statistical Issues in Multiple Testing. Association approaches are also very prone to type-1 errors or false positives, hence the importance of replication studies. For example, if a single test identifies an 'association' with a P value of 0.05, we recognise that this result could have occurred by chance once every 20 times. The question then arises of how we know that a positive result is a genuine finding. Buckland (2001) explores this in the context of alcoholism. In his analysis, he assumes that all genes have an equal chance of association, that there are 20 genes truly associated with alcohol dependence, there are 80 000 genes in the human genome (an overestimate according to latest figures) and that the role of each gene can be tested using a single genetic polymorphism. Thus, examining 80 000 genes would result in a true association every 4000 polymorphisms studied. Furthermore, any finding with a P value of 0.05 would have a 20/4000 chance of being true, 0.5 per cent. Conversely that means that it has a 99.5 per cent likelihood of arising by chance. If there are a mere 30 000 genes in the human genome, as currently indicated, this would alter these figures to one true association every 1500 genes studied. And the likelihood of an association with a P value of 0.05 arising by chance is more than 98 per cent. Extrapolating this further, to increase the likelihood of a true positive to more than 95 per cent, a P value of 0.00001 is needed. Clearly, the assumption that one polymorphism can fully assess the role of one gene is not valid and another estimate has set a P value of 0.00000005 for a genome-wide scan for association with a 95 per cent probability of no false positives (Risch and Merikangas, 1996). While the chances of identifying a positive association can be increased by examining strong candidates, it must be admitted that the probability of identifying a novel true gene using an association approach alone is very slim.

The older methods for correcting for multiple testing, e.g. Bonferroni, are overly conservative, and other methods based on false discovery rates (Benjamini and Yekutieli, 2001) and Monte Carlo approaches (Lin, 2004) are being adopted in both genome-wide association studies and microarray expression experiments. As more information on psychoactive drug effects and gene function becomes available, Bayesian approaches to prior probabilities can be incorporated into statistical analysis (Greenland, 2001). In the end, integration of information from clinical studies, pharmacology and basic molecular biology into genetic epidemiology will allow hypotheses with higher prior probability to be tested (Greenland *et al.*, 2004).

Towards definitive studies. In the final analysis, definitive studies will depend on the ability to DNA re-sequence thousands of 'whole' human genomes, thereby eliminating the risk of selecting limited DNA-sequence variations for analysis in the hope that they carry sufficient information to answer the key biomedical questions (see section 5, Future Directions in Research).

In the meantime, there are a number of issues to be tackled with respect to studies of genetic influences in psychoactive drug use, effects and addiction, not least of which is the continuation and establishment of suitable human cohort studies or 'case' collections that combine detailed phenotyping and psychosocial and other exposures with consent for genetic analysis. One worry for the indirect association approach is the recent recognition that meiotic recombination 'hot spots', which are inaccessible to LD approaches, are associated with gene-conversion events (Jeffreys and May, 2004) which could themselves be causal variants.

Population substructure. It is well understood that population stratification for both allele frequencies and disease prevalence can lead to false-positive results in case-control association studies, as well as to false negatives, the failure to detect real effects (Pritchard and Donnelly, 2001). As study sizes grow (both in terms of sample sizes and the number of markers tested), even very small amounts of population substructure can theoretically cause serious difficulties for case-control studies (Marchini *et al.*, 2004; Freedman *et al.*, 2004), if not recognised and corrected for (Devlin and Roeder, 1999; Devlin *et al.*, 2004). Similar issues apply to cryptic relatedness, the phenomenon whereby cases may be more closely (though still very distantly) related than controls (e.g. Devlin and Roeder, 1999). One way of circumventing population stratification problems is to study the differential transmission of alleles to affected offspring using parent–child trios. Such transmission disequilibrium tests (Speilman and Ewens, 1996) add the complication of requiring parental DNA samples and have

been regarded as being relatively underpowered statistically. However, there are recent indications that exhaustive allelic transmission disequilibrium tests can provide a valuable approach to genome-wide association studies exploiting LD to detect association with both common and rare causal variants (Lin *et al.*, 2004). One is still left with actually defining which variants in the region are contributing to disease susceptibility or resistance.

Meta-analyses. Genetic association studies testing functional variants in candidate genes now represent a huge research industry. Because of the difficulties of assembling large, well-defined case collections or phenotypically-rich cohorts, these studies may be too statistically underpowered to detect small effects and often produce conflicting results. A secondary industry has sprung up, namely meta-analysis, where comparable studies are combined in a systematic way to produce valuable composite results (Munafo and Flint, 2004). With cheaper genotyping, there is a current move towards gene-based analysis in which all common variation within a candidate gene is considered jointly. This is repeated in replication studies, although subsequent meta-analyses pose significant statistical challenges (Neale and Sham, 2004).

3.1.4 Gene–Environment Interactions

Given that the ultimate aim is to understand evolved developmental and regulatory responses as they relate to vulnerability to addiction and drug effects, the analysis of gene-environment interactions (GEI) has to be an integral part of future research. Designing and executing suitable studies is a huge challenge, given that 'genetic effects' may be strongly conditional on environmental pressures. Figure 4.2, originally based on the differential risk, by CYPA1A genotype, of lung cancer with increasing lifetime cigarette-smoking dose (Nakachi *et al.*, 1991), illustrates one possible scenario. The point is that the genetic effect in terms of risk

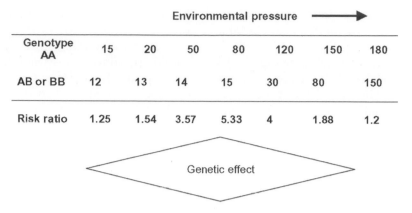

FIGURE 4.2   One model of how the size of the genetic effect is contingent on the level of environmental pressure. In this population of 10 000, 9.29 per cent die from lung cancer due to cigarette smoking. Overall, two-thirds of these cases have the AA genotype (risk ratio ~2). However, the risk ratio varies according to the lifetime dose of cigarettes, peaking at 5.33 with *moderate* exposure. This scenario is developed from data on the effect of a CYPA1A variant on smoking-related lung cancer (Nakachi *et al.*, 1991) where the 'genetic effect' became less with the heaviest exposure. The left-hand side of the curve is supported by the minimal (if any) effect of this CYP1A1 variant on lung cancer risk in non-smokers where exposure environmental to tobacco smoke is minimal (Hung *et al.*, 2003).

could peak at a moderate level of exposure, while all genotypes are 'overwhelmed' at higher levels (Nakachi *et al.*, 1991) and low exposure is barely sufficient to bring out the genetic differences (Hung *et al.*, 2003). Whatever the exact population dynamics of GEI, in many situations stratifying by exposure should help reveal genetic associations, provided the study has sufficient statistical power. This is not only a matter of sample size, but also of the quality of the measures used, since the ability to detect GEI increases as measurement error is reduced. For continuous traits, a sample size of 10 000 provides sufficient power using precise measures (Wong *et al.*, 2003). It is generally, and rightly, assumed that collecting reliable measures of exposure and outcomes across the full range will be more feasible if done prospectively within a general population cohort. Such cohorts of the required size of ~10 000 are feasible, as demonstrated by the Avon Longitudinal Study of Parents and Children (ALSPAC; Golding *et al.*, 2001).

Where one could postulate from existing biological insights that an exposure might only have an adverse outcome in those with a particular genotype, the combined study of exposure and genotype will increase statistical power. However, there tends to be a general assumption that individual genetic variants will only contribute a low or modest risk and situations where a known environmental risk will only apply to those with a specific genotype will be 'unlikely to be frequently encountered in the study of complex disease' (Clayton and McKeigue, 2001). In these circumstances it is argued that for adequate statistical power to detect modest risk ratios, the case-control design is more feasible than the cohort design (Clayton and McKeigue, 2001). However, results over the last few years have shown this to be over-pessimistic. There is now clear evidence that investigating interactions between measured genes and measured environments can be a powerful route to 'genetic' discovery using cohorts (Moffitt *et al.*, 2005). Three studies from the Dunedin cohort in New Zealand (n ~ 1000) have discovered measured GEI in mental disorders, and the first two findings have already been replicated by others (Moffitt *et al.*, 2005). The latest study demonstrates the moderation of the effect of adolescent-onset cannabis use on adult psychosis by a functional variant in the catechol-o-methyltransferase (COMT) gene (Caspi *et al.*, 2005).

3.1.5 Gene Expression Studies

Gene expression results are heavily dependent on the tissue being examined and, for much of the research into drug effects on the brain, tissue from a specific region of the brain is needed. For this reason, much current and future research will be on experimental animals, usually rodents, but also other mammalian species, and invertebrates such as fruit flies or worms, since some of the effects of drugs on gene expression are at fundamental levels of organisation common across the entire animal kingdom.[1] Gene chips can be used directly to study the influence of abused drugs on gene expression. Typically, gene chips contain several thousand genes and expression studies identify changes in a few dozen of them. Such mass screening is subject to errors and any changes observed require confirmation using more rigorous techniques. Sophisticated publicly available databases (e.g. webQTL, www.webqtl.org) allow researchers to search for behavioural traits associated with genes identified by microarray analyses.

Although it is an important first step, such knowledge does not provide an understanding of the mechanisms whereby changes in the expression of one or more genes may contribute to the behavioural change that lies at the heart of addiction. It is likely to take many years of research before we understand the causal relationships between gene expression and cellular function, between cellular function and organ function, and organ function and the whole organism, which will allow us to understand the relationship between gene expression and behaviour.

We have tended to write about genes as inherited material that contributes to, or even determines the occurrence of, behavioural traits, including addictive behaviour. However, genes do not only form the 'blueprint' for behaviour, but are themselves part of the mechanism whereby experience influences bodily, brain and behavioural function. Addictive drugs themselves influence brain plasticity and behaviour by altering the patterns of gene expression, turning on hitherto silent genes, while silencing others. Using microarray techniques,[2] it is possible to study treatment-induced changes in the expression of thousands of genes simultaneously, a method called gene expression profiling. In the short term, the expression of many different genes is altered by a single administration of a drug. In a recent study, we found a single dose of alcohol to alter the expression of over 140 genes in the midbrain of mice, nearly 2 per cent of the genes tested. Some of these genes are transcription factors that in turn control the expression of other genes, some of them perhaps permanently.

Gene array (microarray; gene chip) techniques study changes in the abundance of mRNA in the tissue under investigation. While variations in mRNA will tell us something about which genes are being expressed in the tissue as a result of an experimental manipulation (e.g. feeding alcohol), gene expression at the mRNA level does not correlate well with either the level of the protein that it encodes, or with cellular function. As a result of post-transcription editing of the mRNA, a number of different proteins may be formed, each potentially with a different cellular function. Proteomics (the study of the protein make-up of a tissue) uses various techniques, such as mass spectrometry, to investigate protein levels, but none of them is able to capture the entire wealth of protein expression with the efficiency that gene array studies capture gene expression. Studies of protein expression are usually more limited in their extent, and more likely to be hypothesis-driven, than gene array studies. Techniques such as MALDI-TOF mass spectrometry are more akin to gene array studies, in that the experimenter need not have prior hypotheses as to the nature of the proteins altered by drug experience. But even these allow a sampling of only a subset of proteins (those that are not attached or imbedded in cellular membranes, precisely the proteins that are most likely to interact directly with drugs). Both proteomic and microarray methods are insensitive in identifying changes in levels of expression of those genes that are most active, or those that express at very low levels, and it is usually an arbitrary judgement whether, say, a two-fold increase or decrease in expression of one gene is considered more or less important biologically than a difficult-to-resolve 1.2-fold increase in the expression of another gene. These are difficult issues implicit in the field, and it may take considerable time to resolve them. Finally, current techniques study alterations in gene expression in whole organs, or regions of the brain, both in humans and in animal studies. Yet we know that such tissue samples are likely to be made up of many classes of cell (e.g. neurones and glia) so that some biologically important changes in expression in, say, neurones, may be undetectable against a background of gene expression in glia. When we consider the various functions of different neuronal types, each with its own distinct pattern of gene expression, the technical difficulty of the task facing us becomes clear. How drugs of abuse induce long-term changes in neuronal and other organ function that contribute to their pathological consequences, as well as to future propensity to take drugs, is an area for future research.

3.2 Illustrative Examples of Potential Confounds in Genetic Analysis

It is important to appreciate that all genetic linkage and association studies end up with a similar 'end game'; namely deciding which of several genetic variants in and around a gene is actually causing the difference between people's vulnerability to addiction, organ damage, or response to treatment. If the variants are in strong LD, the question cannot be answered with association studies alone. Direct functional studies are needed using a combination of animal experiments and human cells or tissues. As described elsewhere, variation in DRD2 is of interest in both nicotine and alcohol addiction and their treatment. To this end studies have focused on the Taq1A polymorphism of the DRD2 gene, a C to T substitution located in a noncoding region of the DRD2 locus, which has been suggested to affect DRD2 availability in post-mortem striatal samples (Noble *et al.*, 1991; Thompson *et al.*, 1997). There is also evidence from *in vivo* studies for an association between the A1 (T) allele and lower mean relative glucose metabolic rate in dopaminergic regions in the human brain (Noble *et al.*, 1997), and PET studies have indicated that this allele is also associated with low receptor density (Pohjalainen *et al.*, 1998; Jönsson *et al.*, 1999). However, recent work shows that the Taq1 A site is, in fact, an amino-acid-changing single nucleotide polymorphism in a previously unrecognised protein kinase gene (ANKK1) near the DRD2 locus (Neville *et al.*, 2004). The two genes and therefore probably their variants are in LD, so the question now becomes: is the relevant causal change in the gene product from ANKK1 (e.g. the Taq1 A site itself) or in the DRD2 gene where it just happens to be in strong LD with the Taq1A site? Resolving this type of problem will depend on functional studies of the specific genes and their variants in both animal and human studies.

Where exactly comparable animal models are not available for experimental studies, there are still approaches that can be used with human material. Methods are being developed to detect the effect of specific haplotypes on gene expression (Knight *et al.*, 2003). Furthermore, genetic constructs incorporating 'risk' and 'non-risk' haplotypes into human cell lines can be made for functional analysis (Bochukova *et al.*, 2003; Inoue *et al.*, 2004).

Another issue that is particularly important in addiction is the possibility that the same gene variant is affecting both initiation behaviour and its subsequent biological effects. Alcohol drinking is considered to be a risk factor for oesophageal cancer, and exposure to high levels of acetaldehyde, the principle metabolite of alcohol, is hypothesised to be responsible for the increased cancer risk. The ability to metabolise acetaldehyde is encoded by the aldehyde dehydrogenase (ALDH2) gene, which is polymorphic in some populations. An individual's genotype at this locus may influence their oesophageal cancer risk through two mechanisms, first through influencing alcohol intake and second through influencing acetaldehyde levels. A meta-analysis of studies looking at the ALDH2 genotype and oesophageal cancer found that risk was reduced among *2*2 homozygotes; OR = 0.35 (95%CI 0.17–0.71) and increased among heterozygotes; OR = 3.06 (95%CI 2.55–3.67) relative to *1*1 homozygotes (Lewis and Davey Smith, personal communication, 2005). This provides strong evidence that alcohol intake increases the risk of oesophageal cancer and that individuals whose genotype results in lower alcohol intake (due to the intense side-effects) are thus protected. It also illustrates how the interpretation of genetic associations (in this case, in opposite directions) is relatively easy once the metabolic pathway is well understood. Just imagine trying to make sense of this, if the biology was unknown, from the knowledge that one *2 allele gives the highest risk and two *2 alleles give the lowest risk. It also shows the danger of relying entirely on allele-based, as opposed to genotype-based, statistical tests, particularly where the only model examined is an increasing risk from one to two alleles.

4 CURRENT STATE OF PLAY

4.1 Alcohol

4.1.1 Vulnerability to Alcohol Dependence

Family and Twin Studies

'Ebrii gignunt ebrios', or 'drunkards beget drunkards', is quoted by Robert Burton in *The Anatomy of Melancholy* (1625) and attributed to the Greek historian Plutarch (Burton, [1625] 1972). Dating back to AD 110, it emphasises the long-standing recognition that alcohol dependence runs in families and is hereditary. Interestingly, the original source for this quote invites an environmental interpretation, a timely reminder not to overemphasise the role of genetics (Plutarch, 110).

Such observations have been given scientific credibility by formal family studies. In her review of 39 family studies, representing the families of 6251 alcoholics and 4083 non-alcoholics, Cotton (1979) reported that an alcoholic was six times more likely than a non-alcoholic to report parental alcoholism, although between 47 per cent and 82 per cent of alcoholics did not come from families in which one or both parents were alcoholics. Furthermore, the rates of alcoholism are significantly higher in relatives of individuals with a diagnosis of alcoholism (15.3 per cent) than in non-alcoholic controls (8.7 per cent; Guze et al., 1986). And the odds of developing alcohol dependence increase with the proximity and number of affected relatives such that the risk is increased by 167 per cent in individuals with both a first- and second-degree relative affected, 86 per cent in those with an affected first-degree relative, and 45 per cent among those with a second- or third-degree affected relative (Dawson et al., 1992).

While these family studies are consistent with genetic influence, they do not represent proof, and further support has been derived from adoption studies. These natural experiments provide the opportunity to study individuals reared by unrelated parents. The earliest report was a small negative study by Roe and Burks (1945). However, the subsequent three major adoption series provide strong evidence for the action of genetic factors in males, with weaker support in females (Bohman, 1978, 1981; Bohman et al., 1981; Cadoret et al., 1985; Cadoret and Gath, 1978; Cadoret et al., 1987; Cloninger et al., 1981; Goodwin et al., 1973, 1974, 1977a, 1977b; Roe and Burks, 1945; Sigvardsson et al., 1996; Yates et al., 1996). Furthermore, there was no correlation between drinking behaviour in the adoptees and alcoholism in the adoptive parents and thus no evidence of a protective effect conferred by being raised away from the biological parent (Goodwin *et al.*, 1974, 1977b). Thus, this increased rate of alcoholism in adoptees who have a biological parent who is alcoholic provides strong evidence for a significant genetic contribution to the development of alcoholism.

Further support and an estimate of heritability can be derived from twin studies. In essence, twin studies compare the rates of alcohol dependence in monozygotic and dizygotic twins. If a condition has a significant genetic component, provided the environmental factors making them similar or different are approximately the same, the greater concordance in monozygotic twins should be due to their greater genetic similarity. The results are by and large consistent with the view that genes contribute to familiality and that alcoholism has a significant genetic component. Three basic approaches have been adopted: proband ascertainment with co-twin follow-up; the use of archival records with population-based twin registers; and clinical assessment using population-based twin registers (Prescott, 2001). Estimates of heritability using these approaches range widely from 0.0 to 0.98 with typical figures of 0.5 for males and 0.25 for females (Allgulander *et al.*, 1991; Caldwell and Gottesman, 1991; Gurling *et al.*, 1981; Gurling *et al.*, 1984; Heath *et al.*, 1997; Hrubec and Omenn, 1981; Kaij, 1960; Kendler *et al.*, 1992, 1997; Koskenvuo *et al.*, 1984; McGue *et al.*, 1992; Pickens *et al.*, 1991; Prescott *et al.*, 1999; Reed *et al.*, 1996; Romanov *et al.*, 1991; True *et al.*, 1996).

An analogous approach in animals is the comparison of the addiction-related behaviours of inbred strains, whose individual members are essentially genetically identical. Some strains of mice, selected for qualities independent of addiction liability, such as the C57Bl/6 strain, willingly drink alcohol (Fuller, 1964; Phillips *et al.*, 1998), and may represent animal genetic models of some human types of excess alcohol consumption, while others such as the DBA/2 strain consume practically no alcohol. Several strains of rat have been

purposely bred by selective breeding of the animals in a random population that, for example, consume high (or low) amounts of alcohol (Browman *et al.*, 2000). Such selective breeding leads, over the generations, to strains with marked differences for the selected trait, providing good evidence that several aspects of alcohol-related behaviour are genetically determined. Such traits include sensitivity to alcohol, preference for and aversion to alcohol, and withdrawal severity. In the case of several mouse strains with high alcohol preference, and rats selected for high alcohol preference, the behaviour is associated with low functionality of the brain's serotonin systems, consistent with observations in humans. Within mouse strains, the tendency to drink alcohol, and the severity of acute alcohol withdrawal, were negatively correlated, suggesting that related genes may underlie both abuse and dependence (Metten *et al.*, 1998), though it is important to acknowledge that these genes may influence alcohol-related behaviours as a consequence of broader behavioural influences. Thus, a cross-strain comparison revealed that strains that were capable, in response to a tone signal, of inhibiting an ongoing behaviour directed at obtaining food, also showed low ethanol consumption (Logue *et al.*, 1998). Crabbe (2003) points out that a genetic predisposition to severe withdrawal, and a good ability to inhibit a prepotent behaviour, may lead some mouse strains not to consume alcohol when it is freely available.

Linkage and Association Studies

In spite of the likely genetic complexity of alcohol dependence, two recent linkage studies performed in the United States have reported positive findings and interestingly, several positive linkage regions contain potential candidate genes (see below; Long *et al.*, 1998; Reich *et al.*, 1998). The smaller of the two enhanced the possibility of identifying linkage by using an ethnically homogeneous sample selected from the American-Indian population. Linkage was reported in two chromosomal regions, namely chromosomes 4p and 11 p. The best evidence for linkage was with a marker, D11S1984, on chromosome 11, and there was also good evidence for linkage with D4S3242 on chromosome 4. The linkage region on chromosome 4 is close to the β1 GABA (gamma-aminobutyric acid) receptor gene (GABRB1), while that for chromosome 11 is close to the genes encoding the dopamine D4 receptor and tyrosine hydroxylase.

The larger multi-centre study, COGA (Collaborative Study on the Genetics of Alcoholism) analysed genetic linkage in 105 multigenerational families identified by centres in the United States (Reich et al., 1998). The COGA sample is largely composed of Caucasians (approximately 74 per cent) with smaller numbers of African-Americans (approximately 17 per cent) and Hispanics (6 per cent). The study reports suggestive evidence of linkage on chromosomes 1 and 7, with a protective locus on chromosome 4 near the alcohol dehydrogenase (ADH) gene cluster. Following these initial reports, there have been rigorous re-analyses of the COGA data comparing definitions of phenotype and methods of analysis (Birznieks et al., 1999; Chen et al., 1999b; Comuzzie and Williams, 1999; Curtis et al., 1999; Lin et al., 1999; Turecki et al., 1999). However, the original findings have not been fully confirmed in the replication sample (Hesselbrock et al., 2001).

The first reported genetic association study firmly established the DRD2 as a strong candidate gene. There followed both successful and failed attempts to replicate this finding and more robust association methods have not supported the original report (Edenberg et al., 1998). This highlights one of the fundamental problems with the association approach, i.e. that it is highly prone to false positives, and some argue that the chances of finding a false positive greatly outweigh that of a true positive result (Buckland, 2001).

The most robust and convincing association findings have been reported with the alcohol-metabolising enzymes, primarily in oriental populations. Most ethanol elimination occurs via oxidation to acetaldehyde and acetate and this is mostly catalysed by ADH and aldehyde dehydrogenase 2 (ALDH2; Yin and Agarwal, 2001).

The ADH genes are clustered on the long arm of chromosome 4 and in oriental populations the frequencies of the high-velocity genetic variants of ADH_2 and ADH_3 are significantly decreased in alcoholics when compared with controls (Chen et al., 1996; Higuchi et al., 1995, 1996; Maezawa et al., 1995; Nakamura et al., 1996; Shen et al., 1997; Tanaka et al., 1997; Thomasson et al., 1991, 1994). These genetic variants are associated with a difference of up to 40-fold in the Vmax, the limiting velocity of the reaction that metabolises ethanol to acetaldehyde, in the ADH_2 alleles. However, these associations have been less consistently reported in other populations (Borras et al., 2000; Ehlers et al., 2001; Gilder et al., 1993; Whitfield et al., 1998). Despite this, the fact that these enzymes are clustered in one of the COGA linkage regions indicates that they may also be important determinants in non-oriental populations (Reich et al., 1998). As the greater difference in Vmax is exhibited within the ADH_2 genetic variants, the apparent involvement of the ADH_3 locus may be due to linkage disequilibrium between these two genes as they are closely associated within the cluster (Osier et al., 1999). This suggestion is also supported by the lack of association between ADH_3 and alcohol dependence in Caucasian populations and a multiple logistic regression study of ALDH2, ADH_2 and ADH_3 in a Chinese population (Borras et al., 2000; Chen et al., 1999a; Couzigou et al., 1990; Gilder et al., 1993). At intoxicating levels of alcohol, ADH_4, a class II enzyme, may account for up to 40 per cent of ethanol oxidation. This gene has also been localised to the 4q22 ADH cluster and a functional polymorphism has been reported in the promoter region that doubles the promoter activity, a region involved in gene transcription or expression (Edenberg et al., 1999).

ALDH2, the enzyme responsible for the majority of acetaldehyde oxidation, has been mapped to the long arm of chromosome 12. It exists in two forms that differ dramatically in activity and this is the result of a single nucleotide, or base, difference in exon 12 of the gene sequence (Yoshida *et al.*, 1985). The enzymatic activity is virtually reduced to zero by this change. Following alcohol exposure, individuals carrying this low-activity variant experience high levels of acetaldehyde, with consequent unpleasant and aversive effects including pronounced facial flushing. This is a similar response to that produced by disulfiram (Antabuse), a drug used to aid the maintenance of abstinence. Not surprisingly, this low-activity variant protects against alcohol dependence (Chen *et al.*, 1996; Higuchi *et al.*, 1995; Maezawa *et al.*, 1995; Shen *et al.*, 1997; Thomasson *et al.*, 1991; Yoshida, 1992). However, the low-activity variant is rare in many races, including western Europeans, and does not play a significant protective role in such populations (Goedde *et al.*, 1992).

The parsimonious interpretation of these associations between alcohol dependence and genetic variants in the alcohol-metabolising enzymes is that they exert their influence through an effect on levels of acetaldehyde. Thus, low-activity variants of ADH, namely $ADH_2{}^1$ and possibly $ADH_3{}^2$, and the high-activity 'wild type' allele of ALDH2, both result in lower levels of this aversive compound and this predisposes individuals to alcohol-dependence syndrome. Conversely, protection against alcohol dependence is afforded by high-activity variants of ADH and low-activity variants of ALDH2.

Less robust findings have also been reported using the association approach, primarily implicating genes within the dopaminergic, serotonergic and GABA systems as reported in the review by Dick and Foroud (2003).

4.1.2 Vulnerability to Alcohol Effects

In addition to vulnerability to addiction, genetic factors are also important in the development of addiction-related damage.

It is striking that some individuals with severe alcohol-induced liver disease (ALD) present early in their drinking career, while this complication does not feature in others with more extensive drinking histories. Thus, while up to two-thirds of cases of cirrhosis in the United Kingdom are caused by alcohol abuse, only 8–30 per cent of long-term abusers develop this condition (Grant *et al.*, 1988; Saunders *et al.*, 1981; Saunders and Williams, 1983; Sherman and Williams, 1994). This variation is in part related to genetic factors, demonstrated by twin studies reporting an increased concordance rate for ALD in monozygotic, when compared with dizygotic, twins (Hrubec and Omenn, 1981). Thus, the development of this complication represents a complex interaction of genes and environment, which occurs during a process of disease development and progression.

The search for the genes that underlie this genetic predisposition has primarily focused on the enzymes involved in alcohol metabolism, including ADH, ALDH2 and the cytochrome P450IIE1, part of the microsomal ethanol-oxidising system (MEOS; Ball *et al.*, 1995; Bataller *et al.*, 2003; Hayashi *et al.*, 1991). While some studies have supported a role for these genes in ALD, the findings have not been consistently replicated. Other genes that have also been implicated include those of the cytokine system, ApoE, and superoxide dismutase, an antioxidant (Degoul *et al.*, 2001; Giraud *et al.*, 1998; Grove *et al.*, 1997, 2000; Iron *et al.*, 1994; Takamatsu *et al.*, 2000). Genetic factors have also been implicated in alcohol withdrawal symptoms, including fits and delirium, pancreatitis and Wernicke–Korsakoff syndrome (Hanck *et al.*, 2003; Heap *et al.*, 2002; Matsushita *et al.*, 2000; Muramatsu *et al.*, 1997; Wernicke *et al.*, 2002).

In summary, there is great and growing interest in the elucidation of genetic vulnerability to addiction-related damage. However, in common with those studies that address the predisposition to dependence itself, there is a lack of robust findings.

4.1.3 Genetics of Treatment Response for Alcohol Dependence

Interest in the role of DRD2 was initially focused on vulnerability to alcohol dependence and other addictions, but has now been extended to include treatment response. Thus, the response to bromocriptine, a dopamine agonist, was compared in alcoholics subdivided by DRD2 genotype. Those carrying the A1 allele, previously implicated in predisposition to alcoholism, demonstrated a greater response in terms of both craving and anxiety. Furthermore, the lack of response reported by those homozygous for the A2 allele was such that this study raised the real possibility that this treatment could be targeted on the basis of a simple genetic test (Lawford et al., 1995). Despite such an important finding there do not appear to be any published attempts at replication. More recently, treatment response to naltrexone has been reported to be associated with genetic variation in the μ-opioid receptor (Oslin et al., 2003).

4.1.4 Gene Expression Studies and Alcohol

Genes provide the blueprint that specifies and limits the organism's response to drugs, and also the means by which drugs induce long-term changes in the organism that affect its future behaviour, perhaps including its future predisposition to take drugs. Thus, although we are born with a certain complement of genes inherited from our parents, at any given time in development, many of these genes are switched off, so the proteins they encode are not synthesised and play no part in the organism's physiology. Inactive genes are switched on, and active genes switched off (or, more precisely, their activity is increased or decreased) at determined times in development. Gene expression is also regulated by experience, including exposure to drugs.

There is currently a great effort to understand which genes are activated and inactivated by particular drugs, and under which circumstances, and the mechanisms whereby such induction and suppression of gene activity occurs. Methods used for such studies include northern blots, differential display, realtime reverse transcriptase–polymerase chain reaction (RT-PCR), and in situ hybridisation. More recently, the development of DNA microarrays has facilitated the screening of the genome for actively-expressed genes. Using such methods, over 600 genes have been identified that are regulated in response to alcohol and may contribute to alcohol abuse and alcoholism.

Many of these genes contribute to signalling pathways that are already known to be influenced by alcohol. Thus, we know that alcohol affects neurotransmission by facilitating $GABA_A$ receptors, by blocking glutamatergic N-methyl-D-aspartate (NMDA) receptors, and by increasing the release of opioid peptides. In keeping with this knowledge, a number of genes encoding subunits of $GABA_A$ receptors, subunits of NMDA receptors, opiate receptors and opiate peptide transmitters, as well as genes encoding proteins involved in other neurotransmitter systems (including dopamine and serotonin) have been identified in animal studies as being regulated by ethanol. A second group of alcohol-regulated genes includes a number of transcription factors, including NfkappaB (Rulten et al., 2006), which themselves regulate the expression of other genes (see Worst and Vrana, 2005, for review), and a third group includes various genes encoding proteins likely to be involved in cellular metabolic housekeeping functions that are influenced by alcohol. However, a wide array of other genes have also been identified from diverse biochemical pathways, only some of which have a clear relationship to alcohol's effects. It should be emphasised that there is considerable confusion in the literature at present, with different studies reporting different patterns of changes in gene expression. Different laboratories have used different means of administering alcohol, for different time periods, and these differences undoubtedly contribute to the range of findings. It will be some years before we have a clear appreciation of the most salient effects of alcohol on gene expression that are relevant for alcohol abuse, dependence, and toxicity.

Analysis of rat strains with high and low preference for alcohol has revealed that the high-preference strain has lower levels of serotonin innervation in brain regions including the hippocampus; higher levels of serotonin 1B receptors; and lower levels of opioid δ-receptors (Strother *et al.*, 2001; Wong *et al.*, 1993; Zhou *et al.*, 1994). More recently, using microarray technology, Edenberg and colleagues (2005) have identified a series of genes that differ between alcohol-preferring and non-preferring rats. These include the preferring strain having increased expression of the $GABA_A$ receptor β1 subunit, but lower expression of the enzyme Gad1 which converts glutamate to the neurotransmitter GABA, perhaps indicating lower GABA function, and consistent with the human data reviewed above. However, a number of other genes also differ between the strains, including enzymes involved in aldehyde metabolism, as well as in cellular growth and maintenance, cell survival, and development as well as neurotransmission. In a recent presentation, Edenberg reported that in different brain areas, more than 240 genes differed between the strains. There is clearly much scope here for a genetic influence on ethanol preference in these strains.

In human post-mortem studies of alcoholics, a striking finding has been changes in genes in pathways associated with myelinisation of neurones (Lewohl *et al.*, 2000; Mayfield *et al.*, 2002). This is consistent with our knowledge of the loss of white matter in alcoholism. Nevertheless, a lack of agreement is also found among the several studies of gene expression in human alcoholic post-mortem tissue. Worst and Vrana (2005) compare three important reports (Lewohl *et al.*, 2000; Mayfield *et al.*, 2002; Sokolov *et al.*, 2003) which together identify changes in expression of a few hundred genes in the brains of alcoholics. Strikingly, only six

genes are identified in all three reports. Likewise, a comparison of nine published reports of gene expression in various biological systems, including human alcoholic postmortem tissue, rodent models of high alcohol consumption, and cultured human neuroblastoma cells exposed to alcohol, showed only 13 genes identified by two studies, and no genes in common between any three studies.

4.2 Nicotine

4.2.1 Vulnerability to Nicotine Dependence

Family and Twin Studies

Family studies demonstrate an increased rate of nicotine dependence in relatives of an individual similarly affected, which is consistent with the operation of genetic factors (Niu *et al.*, 2000). Adoption studies provide further evidence for a genetic contribution to smoking (Osler *et al.*, 2001). Estimates of this genetic contribution can be derived from twin studies. The heritability of smoking initiation ranges from 37 per cent to 84 per cent for women and from 28 per cent to 84 per cent in males. The heritability of smoking persistence varies between 53 per cent and 71 per cent for women and 52 per cent and 69 per cent for males (Hall *et al.*, 2002).

Linkage and Association Studies

Three linkage studies have attempted to identify genetic loci implicated in tobacco dependence. Two of these used the COGA families, recruited for the study of alcohol dependence as discussed above, and the third used 130 families recruited from Christchurch, New Zealand. These studies reported little overlap in findings, so regions on almost half of the chromosomes have been implicated; including chromosomes 2, 4, 5, 6, 9, 10, 14, 15, 16, 17 and 18 (Bergen *et al.*, 1999; Duggirala *et al.*, 1999; Straub *et al.*, 1999).

Furthermore, association studies have implicated genes involved in nicotine metabolism including cytochrome P450 2A6 (CYP2A6), 2B6 (CYP2B6) and 2E1 (CYP2E1), genes involved in the monoamine systems including the dopamine receptor 1 (DRD1), DRD2 described previously, dopamine transporter (DAT), dopamine beta-hydroxylase (DBH), monoamine oxidase A (MAOA), tyrosine hydroxylase (TH) and serotonin transporter (5HTT) along with the cholecystokinin (CCK) gene (Munafo et al., 2004; Tyndale, 2003).

4.2.2 Vulnerability to Tobacco Toxicity

In nicotine dependence, attention has focused on elucidating the genes implicated in cancers and coronary heart disease (Bartsch et al., 2000; Humphries et al., 2001; Wang and Mahaney, 2001). Prompted by the conversion of carcinogens originating from tobacco to DNA-reactive metabolites by cytochrome P450 enzymes, Bartsch and colleagues reviewed the effects of genetic variants in these enzymes, alone and in combination with other detoxifying enzymes. They reported an increased risk for cancers of the lung, oesophagus, head and neck associated with some cytochrome P450 variants. In addition, they describe a particularly potent combination of genotypes in CYP1A1 and GSTM1 that results in an increased risk for lung cancer and was also associated with shortened post-operative survival (Goto et al., 1996; Kawajiri et al., 1996).

4.2.3 Pharmacogenetics of Smoking Cessation

Response to nicotine replacement therapy has been reported to be more effective in carriers of the A1 allele of the DRD2 gene (Johnstone et al., 2004). In another study, treatment response was also associated with genetic variation in the μ opioid receptor (Lerman et al., 2004). Treatment response to bupropion has also been reported to be associated with DRD2 – women carrying the A1 allele were more likely to report stopping taking this medication because of side-effects

and after 12 months were more likely to report smoking, although this latter finding did not reach significance (Swan et al., 2005).

4.2.4 Gene Expression Studies and Smoking

Less information is available on the consequences of smoking or nicotine treatment on gene expression than for alcohol. In a rat study (Li et al., 2004), as with similar studies using other abused drugs, some 200–300 genes were modulated in different brain regions, and following different periods of exposure. Within these genes, however, at any particular time, only a handful showed changes in expression in more than two brain regions, and several were up-regulated in one region but down-regulated in another. The dynamic complexity of these changes makes interpretation of the contribution of any particular changes impossible at this stage of knowledge. An added complexity is that nicotine administration early in life may have additional effects (see below).

4.2.5 Developmental 'Programming' and Smoking

One way of exploring developmentally sensitive periods in humans is to look at the effect of prenatal exposure through maternal smoking, as well as childhood onset of smoking. However, such studies need appropriate longitudinal designs that can deal with the main confounders. There is a growing body of evidence suggesting that maternal tobacco consumption during pregnancy may have specific, negative effects on a range of behavioural outcomes expressed in childhood and adolescence, including smoking (Brook et al., 2000; Day et al., 2000; Fergusson et al., 1993; Griesler et al., 1988; Fergusson et al., 1998; Cornelius et al., 2000; Kandel et al., 1994). Two recent studies (Oncken et al., 2004; Roberts et al., 2005)

At least two-generation cohort studies are needed to study transgenerational effects and this is not easy in humans. It is important to appreciate that the mother's genotype, insofar as it modulates her metabolism of drugs, for example, contributes to the foetal environment. Indeed the mother's developmentally 'programmed' metabolism captures information on some of her own early exposures, and this could itself be transmitted to the developing foetus (Bateson *et al.*, 2004). More remarkable is the emerging evidence from historical studies in Sweden that sperm seem to transmit ancestral nutritional information down the male line. For example, the nutrition of the paternal grandfather (specifically) in mid-childhood influences the mortality rate of his grandchildren (Bygren *et al.*, 2001; Kaati *et al.*, 2002). There is unpublished evidence from the ALSPAC study that paternal onset of smoking in mid-childhood is associated with transgenerational effects on both gestational length and obesity in future sons (M. Pembrey and Golding, personal communication). Whether these transgenerational effects represent epigenetic inheritance of an altered chromatin state (Pembrey, 2002) or some other mechanism should be amenable to molecular analysis in the future.

6 THE IMPLICATIONS OF DEFINING GENETIC INFLUENCES IN DRUG USE FOR THE INDIVIDUAL AND SOCIETY

The identification of genes involved in addiction will elucidate the biological underpinning of the natural history of addiction from initiation, through maintenance, tolerance, dependence and the development of complications to recovery. It is anticipated that some genes will be common to addictive behaviours and others specific to a substance or behaviour. For example, genes implicated in reward mechanisms, such as the dopaminergic and opiate systems, may be relevant across substance and behaviour, whereas genes involved in drug metabolism are likely to be substance specific. Thus, the complex choreography that occurs between different genes and the environment, during a process of development, will be clarified.

Such an approach is not without its critics and some have argued that the potential benefits do not justify the investment, given that other treatment methods exist that may ultimately prove to be more effective than any gene-based strategies (Merikangas and Risch, 2003).

6.1 The Biological Basis of Addiction and Treatment Implications

Understanding the biological contributions to addiction will identify biological targets for the development of novel treatments, which are much needed in this field. For example, while medically assisted detoxification from alcohol is highly successful, the rates for maintenance of abstinence are poor, around 20 per cent at 6–12 months (Sass *et al.*, 1996). Such high relapse rates are very common across the addictive behaviour range. Furthermore, genotype–phenotype studies could identify subtypes of addiction, with implications for pharmacological, psychological, spiritual and social treatment strategies, and it may be possible to tailor the management of an individual on the basis of various prognostic indicators including a genetic test (Ball, 2004; Ball and Collier, 2002; Nuffield Council on Bioethics, 1998).

6.2 Predisposition to Addiction

If genes of major effect are found, it may be possible to refine an individual's risk of developing dependence using genetic data. Such predictive genetic testing is most applicable when a single gene confers a high risk, which, as we have seen, is an unlikely scenario in addiction. However, if several genes of relatively modest effect are identified, these could be combined in a multiplex reaction, or on a DNA chip, to provide an indication of risk. But the purpose of identifying individuals at increased risk is uncertain as most addictive behaviours confer no benefit and so the advice in general is to avoid use. Furthermore, the individual interpretation of such testing is unclear. A test result indicating low risk of dependence may encourage naïve individuals to experiment in the belief that they have no risk of progression to dependence. Similarly, a high result might support a fatalistic approach, either for the individual or for treatment services. Finally, it is unlikely that such risk alteration will be extended to population screening. The more genes are involved, the smaller will be the proportion of the population possessing most of the high-risk variants, making screening inefficient (Hall *et al.*, 2002; Hepple and Nuffield Council on Bioethics, 2002; Nuffield Council on Bioethics, 1998).

6.3 Vulnerability to the Consequences of Addictive Behaviour

There may be a greater role for identifying the genes that predispose individuals to the complications of their addictive behaviour, although here again, a reported low risk of associated illness may encourage established users to persist in drug use in the belief that they are safe. This belief may, of course, be valid for some individuals and it is possible that we may eventually understand enough to test for this. As an example, future research may clarify the relationship between cannabis use and the early onset of schizophrenia. At present the jury is out on whether there is a causal link (Veen *et al.*, 2004; Krebs *et al.*, 2005), but it is conceivable that there is a genetically definable subgroup for whom early smoking of cannabis does indeed constitute a significant risk factor for subsequent schizophrenia. Individuals may choose to take this test via the Internet, regardless of what the professional view is of such action. However, it has to be remembered that safety related to one aspect of substance use, for example, cancer in smoking, may confer a sense of security,

not supported and sustained by the exposure to other risks, for example, cardiovascular complications (Hall *et al.*, 2002; Hepple and Nuffield Council on Bioethics, 2002; Nuffield Council on Bioethics, 1998).

In summary, the identification of genes involved in addiction, via their developmental interplay with the environment, will have a profound effect on the understanding of the field. This will inevitably have important implications for the management of patients from initiation, through tolerance, dependence, physical complications and treatment response. Genetic testing *per se* is likely to be of limited use (except perhaps in selecting medical treatments) and further extending such risk modification to population screening would seem even less credible. The pessimistic future portrayed in the film *Gattaca*, in which individuals are given a percentage chance of developing addiction, preimplantation screening of foetuses excludes this risk, and role in society is determined by a DNA test, is highly unlikely to be fulfilled. However, in looking forward to this exciting future, the important moral and ethical lessons of the past should be heeded and the implications considered and widely debated (Müller-Hill, 1998). While developments in this arena may influence public policy, perhaps the most profound effect is likely to be on the public attitude to addiction.

7 THE BRAIN SCIENCE, ADDICTION AND DRUGS PROJECT QUESTIONS

7.1 What will be the Psychoactive Substances of the Future?

The contribution of genomics to this question will be indirect but could be important. Neuropharmacological understanding (to which genomics-based studies will contribute) might be able to predict the addictive potential of new substances and thereby aid the search for safer substitutes. Separating the pathways leading to addiction from other, therapeutic, pharmacological effects might reveal new targets for the development of drugs with defined effects. It has to be recognised that introducing new or existing drugs as novel approaches to serious disorders, as with the development of chromatin therapeutic agents like valproic acid (see above), also introduces a new agent for abuse. The addition of valproic acid as an 'enhancer' in psychoactive substance abuse, for example, could be highly dangerous.

7.2 What are the Effects of Using Psychoactive Substances?

We expect the application of genetics and genomics to make a big contribution to our understanding of the effects of using psychoactive substances, particularly addiction. The consequences of taking drugs for gene expression, leading to possibly permanently altered function, is a major part of understanding both the development of addictions and their long-term consequences for brain function, as well as adverse or beneficial effects on other organs. There is more than a remote chance that drug taking in childhood will have transgenerational consequences in terms of health, through both the female and the male line.

7.3 What Mechanisms do we have to Manage the Use of Psychoactive Substances?

Despite the UK Government White Paper *Our inheritance, our future. Realising the potential of genetics in the NHS* (June 2003) raising the possible role of genetic profiling at birth in health management, we think 'genetic profiling' will have a limited role, if any, in the prevention of drug abuse. The individual genetic effects will be so contingent on other influences that the predictive power of genetic profiles to define vulnerability is likely to be limited. However, pharmacogenomics will lead to more refined, targeted treatment.

8 CONCLUSIONS

- Advances in affordable genotyping and gene expression and epigenetic analysis will not be the limiting factor. Many 'genes' with hitherto unknown function will be characterised.
- Animal research will also not be limiting, as we understand commonalities in the genes underlying addictive behaviours in humans and in animal models.
- The biggest challenge is applying these technologies and biological insights to research on the human population. To supplement clinical and family studies, the optimum design is a large contemporary (two-generation) pre-birth cohort study in which the full range of psychosocial and other environmental exposures have been documented prospectively and the full range of developmental outcomes are being measured.

NOTES

1. Although there are now several studies of the effects of drugs of abuse on gene expression in *Drosophila*, which may tell us something about the kinds of genes influenced by drugs, it must be noted that regulation of gene expression differs in some respects between mammals and invertebrates. On the other hand, it is technically easier, and perhaps ethically more acceptable, to create directed mutations in single genes in flies, so that hypotheses regarding the functions of individual genes in drug-related behaviour can be tested more efficiently. Most importantly, addiction is largely a behavioural disorder, and invertebrates offer little opportunity to model genomic influences on human behaviour.
2. Microarrays contain a large number of an organism's genes individually gridded onto an area less than $2cm^2$. By spotting extract of a tissue on to the array, those genes that are currently active can be detected using a rapid automated screening procedure.

References

Abreu-Villaça, Y., Seidler, F.J., and Slotkin, T.A. (2004a) Does prenatal nicotine exposure sensitize the brain to nicotine-induced neurotoxicity in adolescence? *Neuropsychopharmacology*, 29: 1440–1450.

Abreu-Villaça, Y., Seidler, F.J., Tate, C.A., Cousins, M.M., and Slotkin, T.A. (2004b) Prenatal nicotine exposure alters the response to nicotine administration in adolescence: effects on cholinergic systems during exposure and withdrawal. *Neuropsychopharmacology* 29: 879–890.

Adriani, W. and Laviola, G. (2004) Windows of vulnerability to psychopathology and therapeutic strategy in the adolescent rodent model. *Behav Pharmacol* 15: 341–352.

Adriani, W., Spijker, S., Deroche-Gamonet, V. et al. (2003) Evidence for enhanced neurobehavioral vulnerability to nicotine during periadolescence in rats. *J Neurosci* 23: 4712–4716.

Allgulander, C., Nowak, J., and Rice, J.P. (1991) Psychopathology and treatment of 30,344 twins in Sweden. II. Heritability estimates of psychiatric diagnosis and treatment in 12,884 twin pairs. *Acta Psychiatr Scand* 83: 12–15.

Altmuller, J., Palmer, L.J., Fischer, G., Scherb, H., and Wjst, M. (2001) Genomewide scans of complex human diseases: true linkage is hard to find. *Am J Hum Genet* 69: 936–950.

Ambrosio, E., Goldberg, S.R., and Elmer, G.I. (1995) Behavior genetic investigation of the relationship between spontaneous locomotor activity and the acquisition of morphine self-administration behavior. *Behav Pharmacol* 6: 229–237.

Ball, D. (2004) Genetic approaches to alcohol dependence. *Br J Psychiatry* 185: 449–451.

Ball, D. and Collier, D. (2002) Substance misuse. In: P. McGuffin, et al. (eds), *Psychiatric Genetics and Genomics*. Oxford: Oxford University Press.

Ball, D.M., Sherman, D., Gibb, R. et al. (1995) No association between the c2 allele at the cytochrome P450IIE1 gene and alcohol induced liver disease, alcohol Korsakoff's syndrome or alcohol dependence syndrome. *Drug Alcohol Depend* 39: 181–184.

Bartsch, H., Nair, U., Risch, A., Rojas, M., Wikman, H., and Alexandrov, K. (2000) Genetic polymorphism of CYP genes, alone or in combination, as a risk modifier of tobacco-related cancers. *Cancer Epidemiol Biomarkers Prev* 9: 3–28.

Bataller, R., North, K.E., and Brenner, D.A. (2003) Genetic polymorphisms and the progression of liver fibrosis: a critical appraisal. *Hepatology* 37: 493–503.

Bateson, P., Barker, D., Clutton-Brock, T. et al. (2004) Developmental plasticity and human health. *Nature* 430: 419–421.

Benjamini, Y. and Yekutieli, D. (2001) The control of the false discovery rate in multiple testing under dependency. *The Annals of Statistics* 29: 1165–1188.

Bergen, A.W., Korczak, J.F., Weissbecker, K.A., and Goldstein, A.M. (1999) A genome-wide search for loci contributing to smoking and alcoholism. *Genet Epidemiol* 17 Suppl 1: S55–S60.

Berrettini, W.H., Ferraro, T.N., Alexander, R.C., Buchberg, A.M., and Vogel, W.H. (1994) Quantitative trait loci mapping of three loci controlling morphine preference using inbred mouse strains. *Nat Genet* 7: 54–58.

Bierut, L.J., Dinwiddie, S.H., Begleiter, H. et al. (1998) Familial transmission of substance dependence: alcohol, marijuana, cocaine, and habitual smoking: a report from the Collaborative Study on the Genetics of Alcoholism. *Arch Gen Psychiatry* 55: 982–988.

BioNews (2004) 286 Twin studies shed light on human behaviour. www.BioNews.org.uk/new.lasso?storyid=2362

Birznieks, G., Ghosh, S., Watanabe, R.M., and Mitchell, B.D. (1999) The effect of phenotype variation on detection of linkage in the COGA data. *Genet Epidemiol* 17 Suppl 1: S61–S66.

Blackburn, E.H. (1991) Structure and function of telomeres. *Nature* 350: 569–573.

Bochukova, E.G., Jefferson, A., Francis, M.J., and Monaco, A.P. (2003) Genomic studies of gene expression: regulation of the Wilson's disease gene. *Genomics* 81: 531–542.

Bohman, M. (1978) Some genetic aspects of alcoholism and criminality. A population of adoptees. *Arch Gen Psychiatry* 35: 269–276.

Bohman, M. (1981) The interaction of heredity and childhood environment: some adoption studies. *J Child Psychol Psychiatry* 22: 195–200.

Bohman, M., Sigvardsson, S., and Cloninger, C.R. (1981) Maternal inheritance of alcohol abuse. Cross-fostering analysis of adopted women. *Arch Gen Psychiatry* 38: 965–969.

Borras, E., Coutelle, C., Rosell, A. et al. (2000) Genetic polymorphism of alcohol dehydrogenase in Europeans: the ADH2*2 allele decreases the risk for alcoholism and is associated with ADH3*1. *Hepatology* 31: 984–989.

Botstein, D. and Risch, N. (2003) Discovering genotypes underlying human phenotypes: past successes for mendelian disease, future approaches for complex disease. *Nat Genet* 33 Suppl: 228–237.

Brook, J.S., Brook, D.W., and Whiteman, M. (2000) The influence of maternal smoking during pregnancy on the toddler's negativity. *Arch Pediatr Adolesc Med* 154: 381–385.

Browman, K.E., Crabbe, J.C., and Li, T.K. (2000) Alcohol and genetics: new animal models. In: F.E. Bloom and D.J. Kupfer (eds), *Psychopharmacology: a fourth generation of progress.* New York: Lippincott, Williams and Wilkins.

Buckland, P.R. (2001) Genetic association studies of alcoholism: problems with the candidate-gene approach. *Alcohol Alcohol* 36: 99–103.

Burton, P. (2001) Commentary: Gene-environment interactions: fundamental yet elusive. *Int J Epidemiol* 30: 1040–1041.

Burton, R. (1972) *The anatomy of melancholy.* London: Dent.

Bygren, L.O., Kaati, G., and Edvinsson, S. (2001) Longevity determined by ancestors' overnutrition during their slow growth period. *Acta Biotheoretica* 49: 53–59.

Cadoret, R.J. and Gath, A. (1978) Inheritance of alcoholism in adoptees. *Br J Psychiatry* 132: 252–258.

Cadoret, R.J., O'Gorman, T.W., Troughton, E., and Heywood, E. (1985) Alcoholism and antisocial personality. Interrelationships, genetic and environmental factors. *Arch Gen Psychiatry* 42: 161–167.

Cadoret, R.J., Troughton, E., O'Gorman, T.W., and Heywood, E. (1986) An adoption study of genetic and environmental factors in drug abuse. *Arch Gen Psychiatry* 43: 1131–1136.

Cadoret, R.J., Troughton, E., and O'Gorman, T.W. (1987) Genetic and environmental factors in alcohol abuse and antisocial personality. *J Stud Alcohol* 48: 1–8.

Caldwell, C.B. and Gottesman, I.I. (1991) Sex differences in the risk for alcoholism: a twin study. *Behav Genet* 21: 563.

Campbell, J.H. and Perkins, P. (1988) Transgenerational effects of drug and hormonal treatments in mammals: a review of observations and ideas. *Prog Brain Res* 73: 535–553.

Carlezon, W.A., Jr, and Nestler, E.J. (2002) Elevated levels of GluR1 in the midbrain: a trigger for sensitization to drugs of abuse? *Trends Neurosci* 25: 610–615.

Carter, N. (2004) As normal as normal can be? *Nature Genetics* 36: 931–932.

Caspi, A., McClay, J., Moffitt, T.E. *et al.* (2002) Role of genotype in the cycle of violence in maltreated children. *Science* 297: 851–854.

Caspi, A., Sugden, K., Moffitt, T.E. *et al.* (2003) Influence of life stress on depression: moderation by a polymorphism in the 5-HTT gene. *Science* 301: 386–389.

Caspi, A., Moffit, T.E., Cannon, M., McClay, J., Murray, R., Harrington, H., Taylor, A., Arseneault, L., Williams, B., Braithwaite, A., Poulton, R., and Craig, I.W. (2005) Moderation of the effects of adolescent-onset cannabis use on adult psychosis by a functional polymorphism in the catecho-o-methyltransferase gene: longitudinal evidence of a gene × environment interaction. *Biol Psychiatry* 57: 1117–1127.

Chen, W.J., Loh, E.W., Hsu, Y.P., Chen, C.C., Yu, J.M., and Cheng, A.T. (1996) Alcohol-metabolising genes and alcoholism among Taiwanese Han men: independent effect of ADH2, ADH3 and ALDH2. *Br J Psychiatry* 168: 762–767.

Chen, C.C., Lu, R.B., Chen, Y.C. *et al.* (1999a) Interaction between the functional polymorphisms of the alcohol-metabolism genes in protection against alcoholism. *Am J Hum Genet* 65: 795–807.

Chen, C.H., Finch, S.J., Mendell, N.R., and Gordon, D. (1999b) Comparison of empirical strategies to maximize GENEHUNTER lod scores. *Genet Epidemiol* 17 Suppl1: S103–S108.

Chen, C.K., Hu, X., Lin, S.K. *et al.* (2004) Association analysis of dopamine D2-like receptor genes and methamphetamine abuse. *Psychiatr Genet* 14: 223–226.

Clayton, D. and McKeigue, P.M. (2001) Epidemiological methods in studying genes and environmental factors in complex diseases. *Lancet* 358: 1356–1360.

Cloninger, C.R., Bohman, M., and Sigvardsson, S. (1981) Inheritance of alcohol abuse. Cross-fostering analysis of adopted men. *Arch Gen Psychiatry* 38: 861–868.

Comuzzie, A.G. and Williams, J.T. (1999) Correcting for ascertainment bias in the COGA data set. *Genet Epidemiol* 17 Suppl 1: S109–S114.

Cornelius, M.D., Leech, S.L., Goldschmidt, L., and Day, N.L. (2000) Prenatal tobacco exposure: is it a risk factor for early tobacco experimentation? *Nicotine Tob Res* 2: 45–52.

Cotton, N.S. (1979) The familial incidence of alcoholism: a review. *J Stud Alcohol* 40: 89–116.

Couzigou, P., Fleury, B., Groppi, A., Cassaigne, A., Begueret, J., and Iron, A. (1990) Genotyping study of alcohol dehydrogenase class I polymorphism in French patients with alcoholic cirrhosis. The French Group for Research on Alcohol and Liver. *Alcohol Alcohol* 25: 623–626.

Crabbe, J.C. (2003) Finding genes for complex behaviors: progress in mouse models of the addictions. In: R. Plomin, J.C. Defries, I.W. Craig and P. McGuffin (eds), *Behavioral genetics in the postgenomic era*. Washington, DC: American Psychological Association.

Crabbe, J.C., Phillips, T.J., Buck, K.J., Cunningham, C.L., and Belknap, J.K. (1999) Identifying genes for alcohol and drug sensitivity: recent progress and future directions. *Trends Neurosci* 22: 173–179.

Curtis, D., Zhao, J.H., and Sham, P.C. (1999) Comparison of GENEHUNTER and MFLINK for analysis of COGA linkage data. *Genet Epidemiol* 17 Suppl 1: S115–S120.

Dawson, D.A., Harford, T.C., and Grant, B.F. (1992) Family history as a predictor of alcohol dependence. *Alcohol Clin Exp Res* 16: 572–575.

Day, N.L., Richardson, G.A., Goldschmidt, L., and Cornelius, M.D. (2000) Effects of prenatal tobacco exposure on preschoolers' behavior. *J Dev Behav Pediatr* 21: 180–188.

De Felipe, C., Herrero, J.F., O'Brien, J.A. *et al.* (1998) Altered nociception, analgesia and aggression in mice lacking the receptor for substance P. *Nature* 392: 394–397.

Degoul, F., Sutton, A., Mansouri, A. *et al.* (2001) Homozygosity for alanine in the mitochondrial targeting sequence of superoxide dismutase and risk for severe alcoholic liver disease. *Gastroenterology* 120: 1468–1474.

Devlin, B. and Roeder, K. (1999) Genomic control for association studies. *Biometrics* 55: 997–1004.

Devlin, B., Bacanu, S.A., and Roeder, K. (2004) Genomic control to the extreme. *Nat Genet* 36: 1129–1130.

Dick, D.M. and Foroud, T. (2003) Candidate genes for alcohol dependence: a review of genetic evidence from human studies. *Alcohol Clin Exp Res* 27: 868–879.

DiFranza, J.R., Aligne, C.A., and Weitzman, M. (2004) Prenatal and postnatal environmental tobacco smoke exposure and children's health. *Pediatrics* 113: 1007–1015.

Drake, A.J., Walker, B.R., and Seckl, J.R. (2005) Intergenerational consequences of fetal programming by in utero exposure to glucocorticoids in rats. *Am J Physiol Regul Integr Comp Physiol* 288: R34–R38.

Duggirala, R., Almasy, L., and Blangero, J. (1999) Smoking behavior is under the influence of a major quantitative trait locus on human chromosome 5q. *Genet Epidemiol* 17 Suppl 1: S139–S144.

Edenberg, H.J., Foroud, T., Koller, D.L. *et al.* (1998) A family-based analysis of the association of the dopamine D2 receptor (DRD2) with alcoholism. *Alcohol Clin Exp Res* 22: 505–512.

Edenberg, H.J., Jerome, R.E., and Li, M. (1999) Polymorphism of the human alcohol dehydrogenase 4 (ADH4) promoter affects gene expression. *Pharmacogenetics* 9: 25–30.

Edenberg, H.J., Strother, W.N., McClintick, Jr, *et al.* (2005) Gene expression in the hippocampus of inbred alcohol-preferring and -nonpreferring rats. *Genes Brain Behav* 4: 20–30.

Ehlers, C.L., Gilder, D.A., Harris, L., and Carr, L. (2001) Association of the ADH2*3 allele with a negative family history of alcoholism in African American young adults. *Alcohol Clin Exp Res* 25: 1773–1777.

Fergusson, D.M., Horwood, L.J., and Lynskey, M.T. (1993) Maternal smoking before and after pregnancy: effects on behavioral outcomes in middle childhood. *Pediatrics* 92: 815–822.

Fergusson, D.M., Woodward, L.J., and Horwood, L.J. (1998) Maternal smoking during pregnancy and psychiatric adjustment in late adolescence. *Arch Gen Psychiatry* 55: 721–727.

Fisher, R.A. (1951) The limits of intensive production in animals. *Br Agr Bull* 4: 217–218.

Fisher, P.J., Turic, D., Williams, N.M. *et al.* (1999) DNA pooling identifies QTLs on chromosome 4 for general cognitive ability in children. *Hum Mol Genet* 8: 915–922.

Frank, M.G., Srere, H., Ledezma, C., O'Hara, B., and Heller, H.C. (2001) Prenatal nicotine alters vigilance states and AChR gene expression in the neonatal rat: implications for SIDS. *Am J Physiol Regul Integr Comp Physiol* 280: R1134–R1140.

Freedman, M.L., Reich, D., Penney, K.L. *et al.* (2004) Assessing the impact of population stratification on genetic association studies. *Nature Genetics* 36: 388–393.

Freimer, N. and Sabatti C. (2003) The human phenome project. *Nature Genetics* 34: 15–21.

Fuller, J.L. (1964) Measurement of alcohol preference in genetic experiments. *J Comp Physiol Psychol* 57: 85–88.

Gilder, F.J., Hodgkinson, S., and Murray, R.M. (1993) ADH and ALDH genotype profiles in Caucasians with alcohol-related problems and controls. *Addiction* 88: 383–388.

Giraud, V., Naveau, S., Betoulle, D. *et al.* (1998) Influence of apolipoprotein E polymorphism in alcoholic cirrhosis. *Gastroenterol Clin Biol* 22: 571–575.

Goedde, H.W., Agarwal, D.P., Fritze, G. *et al.* (1992) Distribution of ADH2 and ALDH2 genotypes in different populations. *Hum Genet* 88: 344–346.

Golding, J., Pembrey, M., and Jones, R. (2001) The ALSPAC Study Team. ALSPAC: The Avon Longitudinal Study of Parents and Children. I. Study methodology. *Paediatric and Perinatal Epidemiol* 15: 74–87.

Goodwin, D.W., Schulsinger, F., Hermansen, L., Guze, S.B., and Winokur, G. (1973) Alcohol problems in adoptees raised apart from alcoholic parents. *Arch Gen Psychiatry* 28: 238–243.

Goodwin, D.W., Schulsinger, F., Moller, N., Hermansen, L., Winokur, G., and Guze, S.B. (1974) Drinking problems in adopted and nonadopted sons of alcoholics. *Arch Gen Psychiatry* 31: 164–169.

Goodwin, D.W., Schulsinger, F., Knop, J., Mednick, S., and Guze, S.B. (1977a) Alcoholism and depression in adopted-out daughters of alcoholics. *Arch Gen Psychiatry* 34: 751–755.

Goodwin, D.W., Schulsinger, F., Knop, J., Mednick, S., and Guze, S.B. (1977b) Psychopathology in adopted and nonadopted daughters of alcoholics. *Arch Gen Psychiatry* 34: 1005–1009.

Goto, I., Yoneda, S., Yamamoto, M., and Kawajiri, K. (1996) Prognostic significance of germ line polymorphisms of the CYP1A1 and glutathione S-transferase genes in patients with non-small cell lung cancer. *Cancer Res* 56: 3725–3730.

Gottesman, I.I. and Gould, T.D. (2003) The endophenotype concept in psychiatry: etymology and strategic Intentions. *Am J Psychiatry* 160: 636–645.

Gottesman, I.I. and Hanson, D.R. (2005) Human development: biological and genetic processes. *Annu Rev Psychol* 56: 263–286.

Gottlicher, M., Minucci, S., Zhu, P. *et al.* (2001) Valproic acid defines a novel class of HDAC inhibitors inducing differentiation of transformed cells. *EMBO J* 20: 6969–6978.

Grant, B.F., Dufour, M.C., and Harford, T.C. (1988) Epidemiology of alcoholic liver disease. *Semin Liver Dis* 8: 12–25.

Greenland, S. (2001) Sensitivity analysis, Monte Carlo risk analysis, and Bayesian uncertainty assessment. *Risk Analysis* 21: 579–583.

Greenland, S., Gago-Dominduez, M., and Castelao, J.E. (2004) Value of risk-factor ('black box') epidemiology. *Epidemiology* 15: 529–535.

Griesler, P.C., Kandel, D.B., and Davies, M. (1988) Maternal smoking in pregnancy, child behaviour problems, and adolescent smoking. *J Res Adolesc* 8: 159–185.

Grove, W.M., Eckert, E.D., Heston, L., Bouchard, T.J., Jr, Segal, N., and Lykken, D.T. (1990) Heritability of substance abuse and antisocial behavior: a study of monozygotic twins reared apart. *Biol Psychiatry* 27: 1293–1304.

Grove, J., Daly, A.K., Bassendine, M.F., and Day, C.P. (1997) Association of a tumor necrosis factor promoter polymorphism with susceptibility to alcoholic steatohepatitis. *Hepatology* 26: 143–146.

Grove, J., Daly, A.K., Bassendine, M.F., Gilvarry, E., and Day, C.P. (2000) Interleukin 10 promoter region polymorphisms and susceptibility to advanced alcoholic liver disease. *Gut* 46: 540–545.

Guitart, X., Beitner-Johnson, D., Marby, D.W., Kosten, T.A., and Nestler, E.J. (1992) Fischer and Lewis rat strains differ in basal levels of neurofilament proteins and their regulation by chronic morphine in the mesolimbic dopamine system. *Synapse* 12: 242–253.

Guo, S.W. (2000) Gene-environment interaction and the mapping of complex traits: some statistical models and their implications. *Hum Hered* 50: 286–303.

Gurling, H.M., Murray, R.M., and Clifford, C.A. (1981) Investigations into the genetics of alcohol dependence and into its effects on brain function. *Prog Clin Biol Res* 69 Pt C: 77–87.

Gurling, H.M., Oppenheim, B.E., and Murray, R.M. (1984) Depression, criminality and psychopathology associated with alcoholism: evidence from a twin study. *Acta Genet Med Gemellol* (Roma) 33: 333–339.

Guze, S.B., Cloninger, C.R., Martin, R., and Clayton, P.J. (1986) Alcoholism as a medical disorder. *Compr Psychiatry* 27: 501–510.

Gynther, L.M., Carey, G., Gottesman, I.I., and Vogler, G.P. (1995) A twin study of non-alcohol substance abuse. *Psychiatry Res* 56: 213–220.

Hall, W., Madden, P., and Lynskey, M. (2002) The genetics of tobacco use: methods, findings and policy implications. *Tob Control* 11: 119–124.

Hanck, C., Schneider, A., and Whitcomb, D.C. (2003) Genetic polymorphisms in alcoholic pancreatitis. *Best Pract Res Clin Gastroenterol* 17: 613–623.

Hayashi, S., Watanabe, J., and Kawajiri, K. (1991) Genetic polymorphisms in the 5′-flanking region change transcriptional regulation of the human cytochrome P450IIE1 gene. *J Biochem* (Tokyo) 110: 559–565.

Heap, L.C., Pratt, O.E., Ward, R.J. *et al.* (2002) Individual susceptibility to Wernicke-Korsakoff syndrome and alcoholism-induced cognitive deficit: impaired thiamine utilization found in alcoholics and alcohol abusers. *Psychiatr Genet* 12: 217–224.

Heath, A.C., Bucholz, K.K., Madden, P.A. *et al.* (1997) Genetic and environmental contributions to alcohol dependence risk in a national twin sample: consistency of findings in women and men. *Psychol Med* 27: 1381–1396.

Helgadottir, A., Manolescu, A., Thorleifsson, G. *et al.* (2004) The gene encoding 5-lipoxygenase activating protein confers risk of myocardial infarction and stroke. *Nat Genet* 36: 233–239.

Hepple, B.A., Nuffield Council on Bioethics. (2002) *Genetics and human behaviour: the ethical context.* London: Nuffield Council on Bioethics.

Hesselbrock, V., Foroud, T., Edenberg, H.J., Nurnberger, J., Jr, Reich, T., and Rice, J. (2001) Genetics and alcoholism: the COGA project. In: D.P. Agarwal, and H.K. Seitz (eds), *Alcohol in health and disease.* New York: Marcel Dekker: 103–124.

Higuchi, S., Matsushita, S., Murayama, M., Takagi, S., and Hayashida, M. (1995) Alcohol and aldehyde dehydrogenase polymorphisms and the risk for alcoholism. *Am J Psychiatry* 152: 1219–1221.

Higuchi, S., Muramatsu, T., Matsushita, S., Murayama, M., and Hayashida, M. (1996) Polymorphisms of ethanol-oxidizing enzymes in alcoholics with inactive ALDH2. *Hum Genet* 97: 431–434.

Hill, L., Craig, I.W., Asherson, P. *et al.* (1999) DNA pooling and dense marker maps: a systematic search for genes for cognitive ability. *Neuroreport* 10: 843–848.

Horikawa, Y., Oda, N., Cox, N.J. *et al.* (2000) Genetic variation in the gene encoding calpain-10 is associated with type 2 diabetes mellitus. *Nat Genet* 26: 163–175.

Hrubec, Z. and Omenn, G.S. (1981) Evidence of genetic predisposition to alcoholic cirrhosis and psychosis: twin concordances for alcoholism and its biological end points by zygosity among male veterans. *Alcohol Clin Exp Res* 5: 207–215.

Humphries, S.E., Talmud, P.J., Hawe, E., Bolla, M., Day, I.N., and Miller, G.J. (2001) Apolipoprotein E4 and coronary heart disease in middle-aged men who smoke: a prospective study. *Lancet* 358: 115–119.

Hung, R.J., Boffetta, P., Brockmoller, J. *et al.* (2003) CYP1A1 and GSTM1 genetic polymorphisms and lung cancer risk in Caucasian non-smokers: a pooled analysis. *Carcinogenesis* 24: 875–882.

Inoue, R., Moghaddam, K.A., Ranasinghe, M., Saeki, Y., Chiocca, E.A., and Wade-Martins, R. (2004) Infectious delivery of the 132 kb CDKN2A/CDKN2B genomic DNA region results in correctly spliced gene expression and growth suppression in glioma cells. *Gene Ther* 11: 1195–1204.

International HapMap Consortium. (2003) The International HapMap Project. *Nature* 426: 786–796.

Iron, A., Richard, P., Pascual, D.Z., Dumas, F., Cassaigne, A., and Couzigou, P. (1994) Genetic polymorphism of apolipoprotein E in Caucasian alcoholic cirrhotics. *Alcohol Alcohol* 29: 715–718.

Jang, K.L., Livesley, W.J., and Vernon, P.A. (1995) Alcohol and drug problems: a multivariate behavioural genetic analysis of co-morbidity. *Addiction* 90: 1213–1221.

Jeffreys, A.J. and May, C.A. (2004) Intense and highly localized gene conversion activity in human meiotic crossover hot spots. *Nature Genetics* 36: 151–156.

Johnstone, E.C., Yudkin, P.L., Hey, K. *et al.* (2004) Genetic variation in dopaminergic pathways and short-term effectiveness of the nicotine patch. *Pharmacogenetics* 14: 83–90.

Jonsson, E.G., Nothen, M.M., Grunhage, F. et al. (1999) Polymorphisms in the dopamine D2 receptor gene and their relationships to striatal dopamine receptor density of healthy volunteers. *Mol Psychiatry* 4: 290–296.

Kaati, G., Bygren, L.O., and Edvinsson, S. (2002) Cardiovascular and diabetes mortality determined by nutrition during parents' and grandparents' slow growth period. *Eur J Hum Genet* 10: 682–688.

Kaij, L. (1960) *Alcoholism in twins.* Stockholm: Almquist and Wiksell.

Kandel, D.B., Wu, P., and Davies, M. (1994) Maternal smoking during pregnancy and smoking by adolescent daughters. *Am J Public Health* 84: 1407–1413.

Karkowski, L.M., Prescott, C.A., and Kendler, K.S. (2000) Multivariate assessment of factors influencing illicit substance use in twins from female-female pairs. *Am J Med Genet* 96: 665–670.

Kawajiri, K., Eguchi, H., Nakachi, K., Sekiya, T., and Yamamoto, M. (1996) Association of CYP1A1 germ line polymorphisms with mutations of the p53 gene in lung cancer. *Cancer Res* 56: 72–76.

Kendler, K.S. (2001) Twin studies of psychiatric illness: an update. *Arch Gen Psychiatry* 58: 1005–1014.

Kendler, K.S. and Prescott, C.A. (1998) Cannabis use, abuse, and dependence in a population-based sample of female twins. *Am J Psychiatry* 155: 1016–1022.

Kendler, K.S., Heath, A.C., Neale, M.C., Kessler, R.C., and Eaves, L.J. (1992) A population-based twin study of alcoholism in women. *JAMA* 268: 1877–1882.

Kendler, K.S., Prescott, C.A., Neale, M.C., and Pedersen, N.L. (1997) Temperance board registration for alcohol abuse in a national sample of Swedish male twins, born 1902 to 1949. *Arch Gen Psychiatry* 54: 178–184.

Kendler, K.S., Karkowski, L., and Prescott, C.A. (1999a) Hallucinogen, opiate, sedative and stimulant use and abuse in a population-based sample of female twins. *Acta Psychiatr Scand* 99: 368–376.

Kendler, K.S., Karkowski, L.M., Corey, L.A., Prescott, C.A., and Neale, M.C. (1999b) Genetic and environmental risk factors in the aetiology of illicit drug initiation and subsequent misuse in women. *Br J Psychiatry* 175: 351–356.

Kendler, K.S., Karkowski, L.M., Neale, M.C., and Prescott, C.A. (2000) Illicit psychoactive substance use, heavy use, abuse, and dependence in a US population-based sample of male twins. *Arch Gen Psychiatry* 57: 261–269.

Kendler, K.S., Prescott, C.A., Myers, J., and Neale, M.C. (2003) The structure of genetic and environmental risk factors for common psychiatric and substance use disorders in men and women. *Arch Gen Psychiatry* 60: 929–937.

Klein, L.C., Stine, M.M., Pfaff, D.W., and Vandenbergh, D.J. (2003) Maternal nicotine exposure increases nicotine preference in periadolescent male but not female C57B1/6J mice. *Nicotine Tob Res* 5: 117–124.

Knight, J.C., Keating, B.J., Rockett, K.A., and Kwiatkowski, D.P. (2003) In vivo characterization of regulatory polymorphisms by allele-specific quantification of RNA polymerase loading. *Nature Genet* 33: 469–475.

Koskenvuo, M., Langinvainio, H., Kaprio, J., Lonnqvist, J., and Tienari, P. (1984) Psychiatric hospitalization in twins. *Acta Genet Med Gemellol* (Roma) 33: 321–332.

Kosten, T.A., Miserendino, M.J., Chi, S., and Nestler, E.J. (1994) Fischer and Lewis rat strains show differential cocaine effects in conditioned place preference and behavioral sensitization but not in locomotor activity or conditioned taste aversion. *J Pharmacol Exp Ther* 269: 137–144.

Kosten, T.A., Miserendino, M.J., Haile, C.N., DeCaprio, J.L., Jatlow, P.I., and Nestler, E.J. (1997) Acquisition and maintenance of intravenous cocaine self-administration in Lewis and Fischer inbred rat strains. *Brain Res* 778: 418–429.

Krebs, M.-O., Goldberger, C., and Dervaux, A. (2005) Cannabis use and schizophrenia. *Am J Psychiatry* 162: 401–402.

Kreek, M.J., Bart, G., Lilly, C., LaForge, K.S., and Nielsen, D.A. (2005) Pharmacogenetics and human molecular genetics of opiate and cocaine addictions and their treatments. *Pharmacol Rev* 57: 1–26.

Kruglyak, L. and Nickerson, D.A. (2001) Variation is the spice of life. *Nat Genet* 27: 234–236.

Lander, E.S. (1996) The new genomics: global views of biology. *Science* 274: 536–539.

Lawford, B.R., Young, R.M., Rowell, J.A. et al. (1995) Bromocriptine in the treatment of alcoholics with the D2 dopamine receptor A1 allele. *Nat Med* 1: 337–341.

Lerman, C., Wileyto, E.P., Patterson, F. et al. (2004) The functional mu opioid receptor (OPRM1) Asn40Asp variant predicts short-term response to nicotine replacement therapy in a clinical trial. *Pharmacogenomics J* 4: 184–192.

Lewohl, J.M., Wang, L., Miles, M.F., Zhang, L., Dodd, P.R., and Harris, R.A. (2000) Gene expression in human alcoholism: microarray analysis of frontal cortex. *Alcohol Clin Exp Res* 24: 1873–1882.

Li, M.D., Kane, J.K., Wang, J., and Ma, J.Z. (2004) Time-dependent changes in transcriptional profiles within five rat brain regions in response to nicotine treatment. *Brain Res Mol Brain Res* 132: 168–180.

Lin, D.Y. (2005) An efficient Monte Carlo approach to assessing statistical significance in genomic studies. *Bioinformatics* 21: 781–787.

Lin, S., Irwin, M.E., and Wright, F.A. (1999) A multiple locus analysis of the collaborative study on the genetics of alcoholism data set. *Genet Epidemiol* 17 Suppl 1: S229–S234.

Lin, S., Chakravarti, A., and Cutler, D. (2004) Exhaustive allelic transmission disequilibrium tests as a new approach to genome-wide association studies. *Nature Genetics* 36: 1181–1188.

Logue, S.F., Swartz, R.J., and Wehner, J.M. (1998) Genetic correlation between performance on an appetitive-signaled nosepoke task and voluntary ethanol consumption. *Alcohol Clin Exp Res* 22: 1912–1920.

Long, J.C., Knowler, W.C., Hanson, R.L. *et al.* (1998) Evidence for genetic linkage to alcohol dependence on chromosomes 4 and 11 from an autosome-wide scan in an American Indian population. *Am J Med Genet* 81: 216–221.

Lowinson, J.H., Ruiz, P., and Millman, R.B. (1992) *Substance abuse: a comprehensive handbook.* Baltimore: Williams and Wilkins.

McGue, M., Pickens, R.W., and Svikis, D.S. (1992) Sex and age effects on the inheritance of alcohol problems: a twin study. *J Abnorm Psychol* 101: 3–17.

Maezawa, Y., Yamauchi, M., Toda, G., Suzuki, H., and Sakurai, S. (1995) Alcohol-metabolizing enzyme polymorphisms and alcoholism in Japan. *Alcohol Clin Exp Res* 19: 951–954.

Marchini, J., Cardon, L.R., Phillips, M.S., and Donnelly, P. (2004) The effects of human population structure on large genetic association studies. *Nature Genetics* 36: 512–517.

Matsushita, S., Kato, M., Muramatsu, T., and Higuchi, S. (2000) Alcohol and aldehyde dehydrogenase genotypes in Korsakoff syndrome. *Alcohol Clin Exp Res* 24: 337–340.

Mayfield, R.D., Lewohl, J.M., Dodd, P.R., Herlihy, A., Liu, J., and Harris, R.A. (2002) Patterns of gene expression are altered in the frontal and motor cortices of human alcoholics. *J Neurochem* 81: 802–813.

Merikangas, K.R. and Risch, N. (2003) Genomic priorities and public health. *Science* 302: 599–601.

Merikangas, K.R., Stolar, M., Stevens, D.E. *et al.* (1998) Familial transmission of substance use disorders. *Arch Gen Psychiatry* 55: 973–979.

Metten, P., Phillips, T.J., Crabbe, J.C. *et al.* (1998) High genetic susceptibility to ethanol withdrawal predicts low ethanol consumption. *Mamm Genome* 9: 983–990.

Moffitt, T.E., Caspi, A., and Rutter, M. (2005) Strategy for investigating interactions between measured genes and measured environments. *Arch Gen Psychiatry* 62: 473–481.

Morice, E., Denis, C., Giros, B., and Nosten-Bertrand, M. (2004) Phenotypic expression of the targeted null-mutation in the dopamine transporter gene varies as a function of the genetic background. *Eur J Neurosci* 20: 120–126.

Mukherjee, R.A.S., Hollins, S., Abou-Saleh, M.T., and Turk, J. (2005) Low level alcohol consumption and the foetus. *BMJ* 330: 375–376.

Müller-Hill, B. (1998) *Murderous science: elimination by scientific selection of Jews, Gypsies, and others in Germany, 1933–1945.* Plainview, NY: Cold Spring Harbor Laboratory Press.

Munafo, M.R. and Flint, J. (2004) Meta-analysis of genetic association studies. *Trends Genet* 20: 439–444.

Munafo, M., Clark, T., Johnstone, E., Murphy, M., and Walton, R. (2004) The genetic basis for smoking behavior: a systematic review and meta-analysis. *Nicotine Tob Res* 6: 583–597.

Muramatsu, T., Kato, M., Matsui, T. *et al.* (1997) Apolipoprotein E epsilon 4 allele distribution in Wernicke-Korsakoff syndrome with or without global intellectual deficits. *J Neural Transm* 104: 913–920.

Murtra, P., Sheasby, A.M., Hunt, S.P., and De Felipe, C. (2000) Rewarding effects of opiates are absent in mice lacking the receptor for substance P. *Nature* 405: 180–183.

Nakachi, K., Imai, K., Hayashi, S., Watanabe, J., and Kawajiri, K. (1991) Genetic susceptibility to squamous cell carcinoma of the lung in relation to cigarette smoking dose. *Cancer Res* 51: 5177–5180.

Nakamura, K., Iwahashi, K., Matsuo, Y., Miyatake, R., Ichikawa, Y., and Suwaki, H. (1996) Characteristics of Japanese alcoholics with the atypical aldehyde dehydrogenase 2*2. I. A comparison of the genotypes of ALDH2, ADH2, ADH3, and cytochrome P-4502E1 between alcoholics and nonalcoholics. *Alcohol Clin Exp Res* 20: 52–55.

Neale, B.M. and Sham, P.C. (2004) The future of association studies: gene-based analysis and replication. *Am J Hum Genet* 75: 353–362.

Neville, M.J., Johnstone, E.C., and Walton, R.T. (2004) Identification and characterization of ANKK1: a novel kinase gene closely linked to DRD2 on chromosome band 11q23.1. *Hum Mutat* 23: 540–545.

Niu, T., Chen, C., and Ni, J. *et al.* (2000) Nicotine dependence and its familial aggregation in Chinese. *Int J Epidemiol* 29: 248–252.

Noble, E.P., Blum, K., Ritchie, T., Montgomery, A., and Sheridan, P.J. (1991) Allelic association of the D2 dopamine receptor gene with receptor-binding characteristics in alcoholism. *Arch Gen Psychiatry* 48: 648–654.

Noble, E.P., Gottschalk, L.A., Fallon, J.H., Ritchie, T.L., and Wu, J.C. (1997) D2 dopamine receptor polymorphism and brain regional glucose metabolism. *Am J Med Genet* 74: 162–166.

Nuffield Council on Bioethics. (1998) *Mental disorders and genetics: the ethical context.* London: Nuffield Council on Bioethics.

Oliff, H.S. and Gallardo, K.A. (1999) The effect of nicotine on developing brain catecholamine systems. *Front Biosci* 4: D883–D897.

Oncken, C., McKee, S., Krishnan-Sarin, S., O'Malley, S., and Mazure, C. (2004) Gender effects of reported in utero tobacco exposure on smoking initiation, progression and nicotine dependence in adult offspring. *Nicotine Tob Res* 6: 829–833.

Osier, M., Pakstis, A.J., Kidd, J.R. *et al.* (1999) Linkage disequilibrium at the ADH2 and ADH3 loci and risk of alcoholism. *Am J Hum Genet* 64: 1147–1157.

Osler, M., Holst, C., Prescott, E., and Sorensen, T.I. (2001) Influence of genes and family environment on adult smoking behavior assessed in an adoption study. *Genet Epidemiol* 21: 193–200.

Oslin, D.W., Berrettini, W., Kranzler, H.R. *et al.* (2003) A functional polymorphism of the mu-opioid receptor gene is associated with naltrexone response in alcohol-dependent patients. *Neuropsychopharmacology* 28: 1546–1552.

Pedersen, N. (1981) Twin similarity for usage of common drugs. *Prog Clin Biol Res* 69 Pt C: 53–59.

Pembrey, M.E. (2002) Time to take epigenetic inheritance seriously. *Eur J Hum Genet* 10: 669–671.

Pembrey, M.E. (2004) Genetic epidemiology: some special contributions of birth cohorts. *Paediatr Perinat Epidemiol* 18: 3–7.

Phiel, C.J., Zhang, F., Huang, E.Y., Guenther, M.G., Lazar, M.A., and Klein, P.S. (2001) Histone deacetylase is a direct target of valproic acid, a potent anticonvulsant, mood stabilizer and teratogen. *J Biol Chem* 276: 36734–36741.

Phillips, T.J., Belknap, J.K., Buck, K.J., and Cunningham, C.L. (1998) Genes on mouse chromosomes 2 and 9 determine variation in ethanol consumption. *Mamm Genome* 9: 936–941.

Pickens, R.W. and Svikis, D.S. (1991) Genetic influences in human substance abuse. *J Addict Dis* 10: 205–213.

Pickens, R.W., Svikis, D.S., McGue, M., Lykken, D.T., Heston, L.L., and Clayton, P.J. (1991) Heterogeneity in the inheritance of alcoholism. A study of male and female twins. *Arch Gen Psychiatry* 48: 19–28.

Plutarch. *The Training of Children.* 110.

Pohjalainen, T., Rinne, J.O., Nagren, K. *et al.* (1998) The A1 allele of the human D2 dopamine receptor gene predicts low D2 receptor availability in healthy volunteers. *Mol Psychiatry* 3: 256–260.

Prescott, C.A. (2001) The genetic epidemiology of alcoholism. In: D.P. Agarwal and H.K. Seitz (eds), *Alcohol in health and disease.* New York: Marcel Dekker: 125–149.

Prescott, C.A., Aggen, S.H., and Kendler, K.S. (1999) Sex differences in the sources of genetic liability to alcohol abuse and dependence in a population-based sample of US twins. *Alcohol Clin Exp Res* 23: 1136–1144.

Pritchard, J.K. (2001) Are rare variants responsible for susceptibility to complex disease? *Am J Hum Genet* 69: 124–137.

Pritchard, J.K. and Donnelly P. (2001) Case-control studies of association in structured or admixed populations. *Theor Popul Biol* 60: 227–237.

Rakyan, V.K., Chong, S., Champ, M.E. *et al.* (2003) Transgenerational inheritance of epigenetic states at the murine $Axin^{Fu}$ allele occurs following maternal and paternal transmission. *Proc Nat Acad Sci* 100: 2538–2543.

Reed, T., Page, W.F., Viken, R.J., and Christian, J.C. (1996) Genetic predisposition to organ-specific endpoints of alcoholism. *Alcohol Clin Exp Res* 20: 1528–1533.

Reich, T., Edenberg, H.J., Goate, A. *et al.* (1998) Genome-wide search for genes affecting the risk for alcohol dependence. *Am J Med Genet* 81: 207–215.

Ripley, T.L., Gadd, C.A., De Felipe, C., Hunt, S.P., and Stephens, D.N. (2002) Lack of self-administration and behavioural sensitisation to morphine, but not cocaine, in mice lacking NK1 receptors. *Neuropharmacology* 43: 1258–1268.

Risch, N.J. (2000) Searching for genetic determinants in the new millennium. *Nature* 405: 847–856.

Risch, N. and Merikangas, K. (1996) The future of genetic studies of complex human diseases. *Science* 273: 1516–1517.

Roberts, K.H. Munafò, M.R., and Rodriguez, D. *et al.* (2005) Longitudinal analysis of prenatal nicotine exposure on offspring's subsequent smoking behaviour. *Nicotine Tob Res* 7: 801–808.

Rocha, B.A., Fumagalli, F., Gainetdinov, R.R. *et al.* (1998) Cocaine self-administration in dopamine-transporter knockout mice. *Nat Neurosci* 1: 132–137.

Rockman, M.V. and Wray, G.A. (2002) Abundant raw material for *cis*-regulatory evolution in humans. *Mol Biol Evol* 19: 1991–2004.

Roe, A. and Burks B. (1945) Adult adjustment of foster-children of alcoholic and psychotic parentage and the influence of the foster home. In: *Memoirs of the section on alcohol studies.* No 3. New Haven: Yale University Press: 1–164.

Roloff, T.C. and Nuber, U.A. (2005) Chromatin, epigenetics and stem cells. *Eur J Cell Biol* 84: 123–135.

Romanov, K., Kaprio, J., Rose, R.J., and Koskenvuo, M. (1991) Genetics of alcoholism: effects of migration on concordance rates among male twins. *Alcohol Alcohol* Suppl 1: 137–140.

Rulten, S.L., Ripley, T.L., Hunt, C.L., Stephens, D.N., and Mayne, L.V. (2006) Expression profiling reveals roles for Sp1 and NfkappaB in the mouse brain acute response to ethanol. *Genes Brain Behav* 5: 257–273.

Sass, H., Soyka, M., Mann, K., and Zieglgansberger, W. (1996) Relapse prevention by acamprosate. Results from a placebo-controlled study on alcohol dependence. *Arch Gen Psychiatry* 53: 673–680.

Saunders, J.B. and Williams, R. (1983) The genetics of alcoholism: is there an inherited susceptibility to alcohol related problems? *Alcohol Alcohol* 18: 189–217.

Saunders, J.B., Walters, J.R., Davies, A.P., and Paton, A. (1981) A 20-year prospective study of cirrhosis. *Br Med J (Clin Res Ed)* 282: 263–266.

Scriver, C.R. (2004) After the genome – the phenome? *J Inherit Metab Dis* 27: 305–317.

Sham, P. and McGuffin, P. (2002) Linkage and association. In: P. McGuffin, M. Owen, and I.I. Gottesman (eds), *Psychiatric genetics and genomics.* Oxford: Oxford University Press: 55–73.

Sharma, R.P. (2005) Schizophrenia, epigenetics and ligand-activated nuclear receptors: A framework for chromatin therapeutics. *Schizophrenia Research* 72: 79–90.

Shen, Y.C., Fan, J.H., Edenberg, H.J. *et al.* (1997) Polymorphism of ADH and ALDH genes among four ethnic groups in China and effects upon the risk for alcoholism. *Alcohol Clin Exp Res* 21: 1272–1277.

Sherman, D.I. and Williams, R. (1994) Liver damage: mechanisms and management. *Br Med Bull* 50: 124–138.

Sigvardsson, S., Bohman, M., and Cloninger, C.R. (1996) Replication of the Stockholm Adoption Study of Alcoholism. Confirmatory cross-fostering analysis. *Arch Gen Psychiatry* 53: 681–687.

Slotkin, T.A., Pinkerton, K.E., Auman, J.T., Qiao, D. and Seidler F.J. (2002) Perinatal exposure to environmental tobacco smoke upregulates nicotinic cholinergic receptors in monkey brain. *Brain Res Dev Brain Res* 133: 175–179.

Sokolov, B.P., Jiang, L., Trivedi, N.S., and Aston, C. (2003) Transcription profiling reveals mitochondrial, ubiquitin and signaling systems abnormalities in postmortem brains from subjects with a history of alcohol abuse or dependence. *J Neurosci Res* 72: 756–767.

Sora, I., Wichems, C., Takahashi, N. *et al.* (1998) Cocaine reward models: conditioned place preference can be established in dopamine- and in serotonin-transporter knockout mice. *Proc Natl Acad Sci USA* 95: 7699–7704.

Speilman, R.S. and Ewens, W.J. (1996) The TDT and other family-based tests for linkage disequilibrium and association. *Am J Hum Genet* 59: 983–989.

Stephens, D.N., Mead, A.N., and Ripley, T.L. (2002) Studying the neurobiology of stimulant and alcohol abuse and dependence in genetically manipulated mice. *Behav Pharmacol* 13: 327–345.

Stohr, T., Schulte Wermeling, D., Weiner, I., and Feldon, J. (1998) Rat strain differences in open-field behavior and the locomotor stimulating and rewarding effects of amphetamine. *Pharmacol Biochem Behav* 59: 813–818.

Straub, R.E., Sullivan, P.F., Ma, Y. *et al.* (1999) Susceptibility genes for nicotine dependence: a genome scan and follow-up in an independent sample suggest that regions on chromosomes 2, 4, 10, 16, 17 and 18 merit further study. *Mol Psychiatry* 4: 129–144.

Strother, W.N., Chernet, E.J., Lumeng, L., Li, T.K., and McBride, W.J. (2001) Regional central nervous system densities of delta-opioid receptors in alcohol-preferring P, alcohol-nonpreferring NP, and unselected Wistar rats. *Alcohol* 25: 31–38.

Suzuki, T., George, F.R., and Meisch, R.A. (1988) Differential establishment and maintenance of oral ethanol reinforced behavior in Lewis and Fischer 344 inbred rat strains. *J Pharmacol Exp Ther* 245: 164–170.

Suzuki, T., George, F.R., and Meisch, R.A. (1992) Etonitazene delivered orally serves as a reinforcer for Lewis but not Fischer 344 rats. *Pharmacol Biochem Behav* 42: 579–586.

Swan, G.E., Valdes, A.M., Ring, H.Z., Khroyan, T.V., Jack, L.M., and Ton, C.C. *et al.* (2005) Dopamine receptor DRD2 genotype and smoking cessation outcome following treatment with bupropion, SR. *Pharmacogenomics J* 5: 21–29.

Takamatsu, M., Yamauchi, M., Maezawa, Y., Saito, S., Maeyama, S., and Uchikoshi, T. (2000) Genetic polymorphisms of interleukin-1beta in association with the development of alcoholic liver disease in Japanese patients. *Am J Gastroenterol* 95: 1305–1311.

Tanaka, F., Shiratori, Y., Yokosuka, O., Imazeki, F., Tsukada, Y., and Omata, M. (1997) Polymorphism of alcohol-metabolizing genes affects drinking behavior and alcoholic liver disease in Japanese men. *Alcohol Clin Exp Res* 21: 596–601.

Thanos, P.K., Volkow, N.D., and Freimuth, P. *et al.* (2001) Overexpression of dopamine D2 receptors reduces alcohol self-administration. *J Neurochem* 78: 1094–1103.

Thomasson, H.R., Edenberg, H.J., Crabb, D.W. *et al.* (1991) Alcohol and aldehyde dehydrogenase genotypes and alcoholism in Chinese men. *Am J Hum Genet* 48: 677–681.

Thomasson, H.R., Crabb, D.W., Edenberg, H.J. *et al.* (1994) Low frequency of the ADH2*2 allele among Atayal natives of Taiwan with alcohol use disorders. *Alcohol Clin Exp Res* 18: 640–643.

Thompson, J., Thomas, N., Singleton, A. *et al.* (1997) D2 dopamine receptor gene (DRD2) Taq1 A polymorphism: reduced dopamine D2 receptor binding in the human striatum associated with the A1 allele. *Pharmacogenetics* 7: 479–484.

Tremolizzo, L., Carboni, G., Ruzicka, W.B. *et al.* (2002) An epigenetic mouse model for molecular and behavioural neuropathologies related to schizophrenia vulnerability. *Proc Natl Acad Sci USA* 99: 17095–17100.

True, W.R., Heath, A.C., Bucholz, K. *et al.* (1996) Models of treatment seeking for alcoholism: the role of genes and environment. *Alcohol Clin Exp Res* 20: 1577–1581.

Tsuang, M.T., Bar, J.L., Harley, R.M., and Lyons, M.J. (2001) The Harvard Twin Study of Substance Abuse: what we have learned. *Harv Rev Psychiatry* 9: 267–279.

Turecki, G., Rouleau, G.A., and Alda, M. (1999) Family density of alcoholism and linkage information in the analysis of the COGA data. *Genet Epidemiol* 17 Suppl 1: S361–S366.

Tyndale, R.F. (2003) Genetics of alcohol and tobacco use in humans. *Ann Med* 35: 94–121.

Tyndale, R.F., Droll, K.P., and Sellers, E.M. (1997) Genetically deficient CYP2D6 metabolism provides protection against oral opiate dependence. *Pharmacogenetics* 7: 375–379.

Van den Bree, M.B., Svikis, D.S., and Pickens, R.W. (1998) Genetic influences in antisocial personality and drug use disorders. *Drug Alcohol Depend* 49: 177–187.

Van Eerdewegh, P., Little, R.D., Dupuis, J. *et al.* (2002) Association of the ADAM33 gene with asthma and bronchial hyperresponsiveness. *Nature* 418: 426–430.

Veen, N.D., Selton J.-P., van der Tweed, I., Feller, W.G., Hoek, H.W., and Kahn, R.S. (2004) Cannabis use and age of onset of schizophrenia. *Am J Psychiatry* 161: 501–506.

Von Knorring, A.L., Cloninger, C.R., Bohman, M., and Sigvardsson, S. (1983) An adoption study of depressive disorders and substance abuse. *Arch Gen Psychiatry* 40: 943–950.

Wang, X.L. and Mahaney, M.C. (2001) Genotype-specific effects of smoking on risk of CHD. *Lancet* 358: 87–88.

Waterland, R.A. and Jirtle, R.L. (2003) Transposable elements: targets for early nutritional effects on sepigenetic gene regulation. *Mol Cell Biol* 23: 5293–5300.

Weaver, I.C.G., Cervoni, N., Champagne, F.A. *et al.* (2004) Epigenetic programming by maternal behaviour. *Nat Neurosci* 7: 847–854.

Wernicke, C., Smolka, M., Gallinat, J., Winterer, G., Schmidt, L.G., and Rommelspacher, H. (2002) Evidence for the importance of the human dopamine transporter gene for withdrawal symptomatology of alcoholics in a German population. *Neurosci Lett* 333: 45–48.

Whitfield, J.B., Nightingale, B.N., Bucholz, K.K., Madden, P.A., Heath, A.C., and Martin, N.G. (1998) ADH genotypes and alcohol use and dependence in Europeans. *Alcohol Clin Exp Res* 22: 1463–1469.

Wjst, M. (2004) Target SNP selection in complex disease association studies. *BMC Bioinformatics* 5: 92.

Wong, D.T., Reid, L.R., Li, T.K., and Lumeng, L. (1993) Greater abundance of serotonin 1A receptor in some brain areas of alcohol-preferring (P) rats compared to nonpreferring (NP) rats. *Pharmacol Biochem Behav* 46: 173–177.

Wong, M.Y., Day, N.E., Luan, J.A., Chan, K.P., and Wareham, N.J. (2003) The detection of gene-environment interaction for continuous traits: should we deal with measurement error by bigger studies or better measurement? *Int J Epidemiol* 32: 51–57.

Worst, T.J. and Vrana, K.E. (2005) Alcohol and gene expression in the central nervous system. *Alcohol Alcohol* 40: 63–75.

Yates, W.R., Cadoret, R.J., Troughton, E., and Stewart, M.A. (1996) An adoption study of DSM-IIIR alcohol and drug dependence severity. *Drug Alcohol Depend* 41: 9–15.

Yin, S.J. and Agarwal, D.P. (2001) Functional polymorphism of ADH and ALDH. In: D.P. Agarwal and H.K. Seitz (eds), *Alcohol in health and disease.* New York: Marcel Dekker: 1–26.

Yoshida, A. (1992) Molecular genetics of human aldehyde dehydrogenase. *Pharmacogenetics* 2: 139–147.

Yoshida, A., Ikawa, M., Hsu, L.C., and Tani, K. (1985) Molecular abnormality and cDNA cloning of human aldehyde dehydrogenases. *Alcohol* 2: 103–106.

Zhou, F.C., Pu, C.F., Murphy, J., Lumeng, L., and Li, T.K. (1994) Serotonergic neurons in the alcohol preferring rats. *Alcohol* 11: 397–403.

Experimental Psychology and Research into Brain Science, Addiction and Drugs

Theodora Duka, Barbara Sahakian and Danielle Turner

1 EXECUTIVE SUMMARY

Experimental psychology is ideally placed to determine the cognitive and emotional effects of psychoactive substances, and the contribution of cognition and emotion to addiction. We are beginning to understand the neurobiological and genetic contributions to altered cognition, emotion and motivation, all of which contribute to addictive behaviour.

This report illustrates the advances that have been made in exploring the effects of psychoactive substance use, using tools and techniques that focus on our understanding of learning, reward, motivation and cognition. This understanding is central to preventing and treating the devastating effects of psychoactive drug addiction and improving the quality of life for patients suffering from cognitive impairment, and helps us develop robust theories of human behaviour in the context of psychoactive substance use.

This report focuses mainly on drugs, but it is possible that in the future many of the same considerations will apply to non-chemical approaches such as transcranial magnetic stimulation (based on the use of pulsed magnetic fields) or neural prosthetics (the intracranial implantation of computer chips modelling brain function to replace damaged or dysfunctional brain tissue).

2 INTRODUCTION

Experimental psychology uses controlled laboratory experiments to study the role of attentional, cognitive and emotional processing in human behaviours, and aims to understand the inner workings of the mind from inferences based on experimental observation. It contributes to, and draws on, a number of related disciplines including clinical psychology, anatomy, pharmacology, neuroimaging and genetics. Experimental psychology uses techniques that have made it possible to experimentally target the reward pathways in the brain in such a way as to provide insight into addictions such as drug taking and gambling. It is now possible to explore the cognitive effects of psychoactive substances in healthy volunteers and, in combination with other techniques such as neurobiological and neuroimaging advances, determine the neural basis of these processes. This report focuses on the contributions of experimental psychology to our understanding of psychotropic drug use, but refers to related areas where these have contributed to advancing our understanding of the brain and addiction.

The major strength of experimental psychology is that it provides objective, precise and testable explanations of behaviour by systematically deconstructing complex human behaviours such as drug addiction and eliminating the extraneous uncontrolled factors that are found in more naturalistic observations. Equally beneficially, clinical observations can be transferred into a laboratory environment to define the processes involved in observed behaviours such as dependence and withdrawal. The identification of the processes involved may facilitate targeting for treatment.

Exciting recent developments in the creation of computer-based psychometric tasks and learning procedures allow similar aspects of behaviour in animals and humans to be tested (Robbins et al., 1994). Paradigms have been developed that allow observations in humans to be modelled in animals, and for animal observations to be tested directly in humans. This cross-species translational approach has been particularly fruitful in the area of cognitive psychopharmacology. For example, there are versions of the Cambridge Neuropsychological Test Automated Battery (CANTAB) intradimensional–extradimensional (IDED) attentional set shifting test, a computerised test of cognitive flexibility akin to the well-used Wisconsin Card Sorting Test (WCST), for rat, monkey and man (Birrell and Brown, 2000; Dias et al., 1996; Ornstein et al., 2000). This test is crucial for assessing the ability to shift attention and learn new rules (Figure 5.1a). Ornstein et al. (2000) found that chronic amphetamine abusers could be discriminated from heroin users on performance of this test. The chronic amphetamine abusers were significantly impaired in their performance on the extra-dimensional shift (a core component of the WCST) whereas, in contrast, the heroin abusers were impaired in learning the normally easier intradimensional shift component. Neuroimaging studies in humans and neurobiological studies in animals indicate that the frontal lobes are key areas for the successful performance of tasks requiring cognitive flexibility.

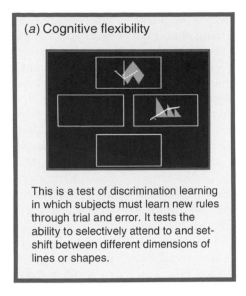

(a) Cognitive flexibility

This is a test of discrimination learning in which subjects must learn new rules through trial and error. It tests the ability to selectively attend to and set-shift between different dimensions of lines or shapes.

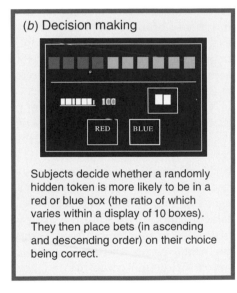

(b) Decision making

Subjects decide whether a randomly hidden token is more likely to be in a red or blue box (the ratio of which varies within a display of 10 boxes). They then place bets (in ascending and descending order) on their choice being correct.

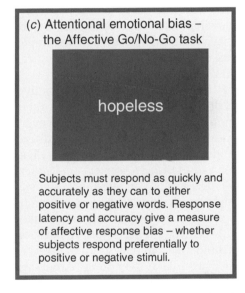

(c) Attentional emotional bias – the Affective Go/No-Go task

hopeless

Subjects must respond as quickly and accurately as they can to either positive or negative words. Response latency and accuracy give a measure of affective response bias – whether subjects respond preferentially to positive or negative stimuli.

FIGURE 5.1 Computerised testing. Computerised testing is ideal for the comparative assessment of cognitive performance across different groups of patients and volunteers, even in different countries, and for assessing the processes underlying particular forms of cognitive function, as well as determining individual strengths or weaknesses in comparison to normative data. Tests can be designed to be sensitive to the effects of neurochemical manipulations, and have good test–retest reliability. A further advantage of certain tests is their close association with tests used in the determination of neural models of cognition in non-human primates and rodents.

The development of brain imaging techniques is an important recent technology that allows the experimenter to draw parallels between a specific behaviour and changes in activation in precise brain areas in healthy volunteers and different patient groups. The use of cognitive psychological tests in combination with functional magnetic resonance imaging has enabled the identification of the neural basis for human reward systems. These discoveries have enormous potential for identifying abnormal reward circuits in people suffering from drug addiction and for identifying effective mechanisms for correcting these changes.

Research using learned behaviours in animals has helped achieve significant progress in determining the processes involved in maintaining drug taking and those aspects that lead to relapse during abstinence. In animals, it has been shown that the attentional processing of drug-related cues can lead to changes in an animal's motivational state and that this can produce the behavioural responses required to obtain the drug. Analogous methods are now available to test these components of drug taking in humans (Hogarth et al., 2003a, 2005). There is a need for a translational medicine approach to drug development which uses these experimental psychological measures to determine the effects of drugs, including neurological effects, in man.

People traditionally take psychoactive drugs in order to feel better, enhance their mood or improve their memory. However, with repeated use, many of these drugs produce dependence and addiction. The Diagnostic and Statistical Manual 4th Edition (DSM-IV) description of substance dependence refers to continuing drug use despite awareness of the long-term negative consequences, repeated attempts to cut back or quit substance use, and a gradual exacerbation of drug intake over time (American Psychiatric Association, 1994). It is well recognised that addiction is characterised by a long-lasting risk of relapse (often initiated by exposure to drug-related cues), although good-quality drug treatment can be highly effective (Gossop et al., 2003). There is still a large amount of work to be done in understanding the behavioural and neural substrates of compulsive drug use.

There are several frameworks within which experimental psychologists can approach the study of addiction. One interesting proposal, which integrates several psychological indices mapped onto neural networks, has been put forward by Volkow and colleagues (2003) (Figure 5.2). Four neural networks, all of them modulated by drugs of abuse, have been proposed to be instrumental in drug abuse and addiction (Volkow et al., 2003). These include brain circuits of reward (including the nucleus accumbens and ventral pallidum areas of the brain), motivation and drive (including the orbitofrontal cortex and subcallosal cortex), memory and learning (including the amygdala and hippocampus) and control (including the prefrontal cortex and anterior cingulate gyrus). These four circuits all receive direct innervations from dopamine neurones, but they are also connected to each other through various direct and indirect projections, mostly involving the neurochemical glutamate. This means that a large number of brain regions may be involved in each circuit. In addition, one region may participate in more than one circuit. Patterns of activity in this four-circuit network may be at the core of behavioural choice.

Volkow and colleagues have proposed that the decision to take a drug will depend on the expected positive feelings (the reward) to be had from taking it, which in turn will be affected by previous knowledge and memories, as well as a person's internal needs or motivation. The cognitive decision to act (or not) to procure the drug would be processed in part by brain areas such as the prefrontal cortex and the anterior cingulate gyrus. Addiction could occur when disruptions to these circuits by agents (most likely dopaminergic) produce a greater and longer-lasting activation of the reward circuit than that obtained with non-drug stimuli, and this could overcome the inhibitory control exerted by the prefrontal cortex.

This framework is perhaps too simplistic to explain some of the more sophisticated aspects of addiction. Nevertheless, it provides a useful basis for conceptualising some of the processes and structures that are important in understanding addictive behaviour. This report highlights developments in our understanding of the scientific

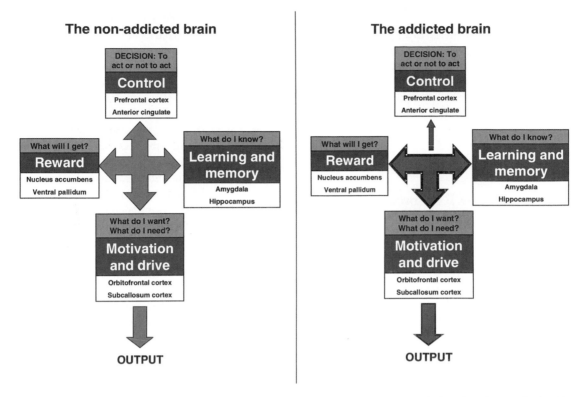

FIGURE 5.2 Four fully interactive circuits have been proposed by Volkow *et al.* (2003) to be involved with addiction: reward (saliency), motivation/drive (internal state), memory (learned associations) and control (conflict resolution). During addiction, it is suggested that greater activity in the dopamine-regulated reward circuit and the motivational/drive and memory circuits overcomes the inhibitory control normally exerted by the prefrontal cortex, resulting in compulsive drug taking. Figure adapted from Volkow *et al.* (2003).

basis of drug addiction and the effects of psychoactive substance use in terms of these core psychological components. This is followed by a description of some of the psychoactive substances that we believe will feature in the future, and potential interventions to manage their use. We conclude with several visions of the future and how experimental psychology will impact on these.

3 SCIENTIFIC BASIS OF DRUG ADDICTION

Experimental psychology has approached the analysis of drug addiction with research into several main areas, which are largely incorporated into Volkow's model. Five main areas – reward and reinforcement, motivation, emotion, learning, and cognition and cognitive control – form this part of the report.

Advances in neurobiology have enabled neuroscientists to manipulate specific brain molecules, neurons and systems. This has led to major advances in the neuroscience of reward, which is the key to our understanding of addiction. An understanding of how humans respond to reward is central to providing insights into disorders involving psychoactive substances and also into conditions such as obsessive–compulsive disorder, depression and eating disorders.

Reward consists of numerous psychological components and is often considered in terms of the processes of emotion, motivation and learning (Berridge and Robinson, 2003; Robbins and Everitt, 1999). The challenge is to identify how different brain circuits mediate different psychological components of reward, and how these components interact.

3.1 Reward and Reinforcement

Addictive drugs can be both rewarding (interpreted by the brain as intrinsically positive) and reinforcing (behaviours associated with such drugs tend to be repeated) (White, 1989). A large amount of work using classical pavlovian conditioning paradigms has shown that it is possible for a number of effects of a drug to become conditioned. This occurs when a previously neutral stimulus becomes an incentive when paired with the acute reinforcing effects of a drug (Altman et al., 1996). Another striking phenomenon observed as part of addictive behaviour is the response of the individual to the presence of drug-related cues. Appetitive pavlovian theories of drug addiction (Hogarth et al., 2003a, 2005; Stewart et al., 1984), for example, argue that stimuli associated with drug reinforcement (such as feeling high, and a reduction of anxiety or tension) acquire the capacity to elicit conditioned responses that lead to drug-seeking and drug-taking behaviour and become reinforcers in their own right.

One important consequence of such a property is that the drug's initial rewarding effects (such as a desirable taste, or feelings of warmth), or even expectancies related to the drug consumption, become conditioned stimuli that come to control behaviour. This phenomenon, known as the 'priming effect', has been studied with alcohol in the laboratory. Studies on the priming effects of alcohol in social, non-alcoholic, drinkers showed that priming will lead to an increase in choosing alcohol over an alcohol-free beverage (de Wit and Chutuape, 1993) or over money (Fillmore and Rush, 2001; Kirk and de Wit, 2000), as well as an increase in the desire to drink (de Wit and Chutuape, 1993; Duka et al., 1999) and the amount of drinking (Duka et al., 1998). Similar effects have been shown with alcoholics (Hodgson et al., 1979; for a review see Stockwell, 1991). Since the priming effect is associated with relapse in alcoholics ('one drink, one drunk'), understanding the phenomenon is of major importance. Similarly, data from research on humans and rodents has shown that re-exposure to the drug itself, exposure to stress or the presentation of drug-associated cues are all effective at triggering relapse or causing reinstatement of the behaviour (Wang et al., 2000).

Molecular changes in the brain can promote continued drug taking that becomes increasingly difficult for the individual to control (reviewed in Hyman and Malenka, 2001). Imaging studies in drug abusers have shown that drugs of abuse increase extracellular concentrations of dopamine in the striatum (where the nucleus accumbens is located) and that these increases are associated with the reinforcing effects of the drugs (Volkow et al., 2003). Studies examining the reinforcing and rewarding effects of drugs have shown that these effects are associated not only with the magnitude, but also with the abruptness, of dopamine increase in the brain. Thus, for an equivalent increase in dopamine, intravenous administration of methylphenidate (Ritalin) – which results in a rapid uptake of the drug and a corresponding rapid alteration in dopamine concentrations – is considerably more reinforcing than oral administration (Volkow et al., 1999a, 2001).

Indeed, there is strong evidence that the dopaminergic system that projects from the ventral tegmental area of the midbrain to the nucleus accumbens, and to other forebrain sites, is the major substrate of reward and reinforcement for both natural rewards (such as food and sexual opportunities) and addictive drugs (Robbins and Everitt, 1996; Wise and Bozarth, 1987). Drugs can stimulate brain reward circuitry with a strength, time course and reliability that exceeds almost any natural stimulus, powerfully consolidating responses to drug-associated stimuli (Berke and Hyman, 2000). Drug-induced synaptic changes in the nucleus accumbens and dorsal striatum may therefore contribute to addiction by consolidating drug-wanting, drug-seeking and drug-taking behaviours. The nucleus accumbens is involved in responding to the motivational significance of stimuli, and the dorsal striatum is involved in the learning and execution of behavioural sequences in order to ensure an efficient response to the cue. Addictive drugs increase the levels of synaptic dopamine in the nucleus accumbens while pharmacological antagonism and lesion studies have shown that dopamine is generally required for reward and reinforcement (Di Chiara and Imperato, 1988; Koob and Bloom, 1988; Wise and Bozarth, 1987). Opiates, such as heroin and morphine, represent a partial exception to the central role of dopamine. Although opiates can produce reinforcement by dopamine release, they can also interact directly with opioid receptors on nucleus accumbens neurones (Nestler, 1996).

However, increases in dopamine concentrations during intoxication can occur in both drug-addicted and non-addicted volunteers. This means that addiction might arise not so much from dopamine increases as from repeated marked increases and decreases in dopamine in the reward circuits, which in turn disrupt motivational, memory and higher cognitive circuits. For example, drug-addicted volunteers display longer-lasting decreases in the number of dopamine D2 receptors than controls (Volkow et al., 2002a). It is possible that this results in a decreased sensitivity of the reward circuits, leading to reduced interest in ordinary environmental stimuli, apathy or anhedonia, which could predispose a person to seek drugs to enhance the importance of these stimuli. Thus dopamine-regulated reward circuitry in tobacco smokers fails to activate in response to monetary reward compared with non-smokers (Martin-Solch et al.,

2001). Decreased sensitivity of reward circuits to acute alcohol administration has also been documented in cocaine abusers compared with control subjects (Volkow et al., 2000). These findings suggest an overall reduction in the sensitivity of reward circuits in drug-addicted individuals to natural reinforcers and to drugs, including others in addition to the one to which they are addicted.

3.2 Motivation

Motivation and decision making are also implicated in determining how rewarding a substance is. Drugs have the potential to be much greater reinforcers than natural rewards. One area of the brain involved in rating the relative value of reinforcers is thought to be the orbitofrontal cortex (Rolls, 2000; Schultz et al., 2000). Chronic amphetamine abusers are known to make suboptimal decisions, which correlates with years of drug abuse, as well as deliberating for far longer before making their choices during tests of decision making (Figure 5.1b) (Rogers et al., 1999). In contrast, in the same study, opiate abusers were shown to have intact decision-making abilities, although they also deliberated far longer than controls. What is particularly interesting is that this study included patients with focal damage to the prefrontal cortex, with the suggestion that chronic amphetamine abusers show similar decision-making deficits to patients with focal damage to the orbitofrontal cortex, although these findings are awaiting replication.

Imaging studies support this behavioural evidence of involvement of the orbitofrontal cortex in the deficits associated with addiction. The orbitofrontal cortex has been shown to be underactive in drug-addicted volunteers tested during withdrawal, possibly as a result of the lack of brain stimulation by salient stimuli during detoxification (Volkow et al., 2003). In contrast, in active cocaine abusers, the orbitofrontal cortex has been shown to be overactive – in proportion to the intensity of the craving experienced by the volunteers (Volkow *et al.*, 1991). It is therefore possible that, in the withdrawal state, exposure to the drug or drug-related stimuli reactivates the orbitofrontal cortex, resulting in compulsive drug taking.

There are several other avenues of research that implicate the orbitofrontal cortex in motivation. Increased orbitofrontal cortex activation has been associated with compulsive disorders (Insel, 1992), and it is known that tobacco users show greater impairment on neuropsychological measures sensitive to orbitofrontal function, and that tobacco use is correlated with the degree of impairment (Spinella, 2005). It is also known that nicotine activates orbitofrontal–striatal and limbic circuits (Stein *et al.*, 1998), and that cigarette-related cues cause activation of orbitofrontal cortex (Brody *et al.*, 2002). This is consistent with the accounts of drug addicts who claim that once they start taking the drug they cannot stop, even when the drug is no longer pleasurable. Since the orbitofrontal cortex also processes information associated with associative learning and the prediction of reward (Schultz *et al.*, 2000), its activation during cue exposure could indicate changes in signal reward prediction, which could then be experienced as craving by the addicted subject.

Motivated action, or instrumental conditioning, is the process whereby behaviour is altered in the presence of an association between the behaviour and a reinforcing outcome (Cardinal and Everitt, 2004). Motivation to take the drug cannot be dissociated from the behaviour to seek and consume it, that is, 'we will work for what we value'. Rescorla and Solomon's (1967) two-process learning theory proposes that appetitive behaviour is controlled by two associative learning processes. The first involves pavlovian stimulus-reinforcer contingencies resulting in the stimulus acquiring the capacity to elicit physiological conditioned responses that prepare for, and support, the motor activity of seeking and consuming the reinforcer.

The second process involves response–reinforcer contingencies, which endow the agent with the repertoire of motor responses to acquire and consume the reinforcer. These two processes interact so that the stimulus acquires the capacity to elicit instrumental responses trained with the same reinforcer. This final prediction is demonstrated in the pavlovian-to-instrumental-transfer effect (Borchgrave *et al.*, 2002; Hall *et al.*, 2001; Lovibond, 2003), where pavlovian conditioned stimuli augment instrumental responses trained separately with the same reinforcer.

All three predictions of Rescorla and Solomon's (1967) two-process learning theory are supported, albeit sometimes indirectly, by the human tobacco addiction literature. For example, conditioned stimuli, paired with tobacco-smoke reinforcement and stimuli related to smoking, have been shown to elicit greater excitatory physiological responses than control stimuli (Carter and Tiffany, 2001; Field and Duka, 2001). These excitatory physiological conditioned responses could conceivably prepare for, and support, the motor activity of reinforcer acquisition and consumption (see Obrist *et al.*, 1970).

Evidence for a pavlovian-to-instrumental-transfer effect in human tobacco addiction is indirect. Smoking-related cues have been shown to augment aspects of human smoking behaviour relative to control cues including naturalistic cues (Droungas *et al.*, 1995; Niaura *et al.*, 1992; Payne *et al.*, 1991; Perkins *et al.*, 1994) and arbitrary cues that have been associated with the reinforcer in the laboratory (Mucha *et al.*, 1998; Payne *et al.*, 1990).

3.3 Emotion

In contrast to many other drugs of abuse, ecstasy (MDMA) has been shown to cause permanent reductions in serotonin axons and receptors in rats (McKenna and Peroutka, 1990; Ricaurte *et al.*, 1987), non-human primates (Hatzidimitriou *et al.*, 1999) and humans (Kish *et al.*, 2000; Reneman *et al.*, 2001; Semple *et al.*, 1999), in addition to effects on dopamine. Because of the important role of serotonin in modulating mood and emotion, it might be expected that such long-lasting depletions may cause vulnerability to depression in chronic ecstasy users. Consistent with this hypothesis, a number of studies have demonstrated that ecstasy users report higher levels of depression than controls, both in the days following ecstasy use (Curran and Travill, 1997; Parrott and Lasky, 1998; Verheyden *et al.*, 2002) and following a period of abstinence (Gamma *et al.*, 2001; Gerra *et al.*, 2000; MacInnes *et al.*, 2001; Thomasius *et al.*, 2003).

However, not all studies have found evidence to support a relationship between depression and ecstasy use (Parrott *et al.*, 2000, 2001; Verkes *et al.*, 2001). This discrepancy was recently clarified using advances in genetic subtyping (Roiser *et al.*, 2005). Specific genetic subtypes of drug users were shown to be more susceptible to the emotional and cognitive effects of ecstasy than others. For example, ecstasy users who were homozygous for the *s*-allele of the serotonin transporter gene showed higher subjective depression ratings, increased affective lability (see Figure 5.1*c* – the Affective Go/No-Go test, for an objective, computerised test of emotional bias) and less rational betting behaviour on a decision-making test than others.

Patients who suffer from depression show a similar affective bias and respond more rapidly to sad as opposed to happy stimuli (see Figure 5.1*c*) compared with healthy control subjects, thus providing validation for this task in mood disorders (Murphy *et al.*, 1999). This test is sensitive to detecting first episode depression in adolescents (Kyte *et al.*, 2004) and might provide a useful mechanism for detecting vulnerability to mood changes in ecstasy users. This task has also been shown to be sensitive in healthy volunteers to manipulations of the dopamine and serotonin neurotransmitter systems in tyrosine and tryptophan depletion studies

respectively (McLean *et al.*, 2004; Murphy *et al.*, 2002).

3.4 Learning

Learning and the formation of habits are enormously important in addiction. Seeing certain people, places and paraphernalia can trigger an intense desire for the drug in addicts, and this can often result in relapse. Drug addiction has been considered in terms of normal learning and memory systems of the brain which, through the actions of chronically self-administered drugs, are pathologically subverted, leading to the establishment of compulsive drug-seeking habits (Everitt *et al.*, 2001). Many forms of learning are mediated by different brain systems, with multiple memory systems having been implicated in drug addiction (Berridge and Robinson, 2003; Lee *et al.*, 2004a). As described above, exposure to a drug may sensitise the incentive-motivational system, producing compulsive drug-seeking behaviour (or 'craving'), even though the drug has ceased to give pleasure. Much of this work has been explored using the phenomenon of 'second-order schedules', in which animals will work for a long period to obtain access to a drug, providing that their operant behaviour is maintained by the response-contingent presentation of conditioned reinforcing stimuli paired with the eventual drug infusions (Kelleher and Goldberg, 1977). Similarly, it is known that addicts will work under a 'second-order' schedule to produce eventual injections of opiates, provided there is intermittent presentation of drug-associated cues. Learnt knowledge is thus extremely useful for making predictions about rewards, anticipating outcomes, and performing goal-directed actions. All of these can be studied in the laboratory in both humans and animals.

Humans are exquisitely able to evaluate relationships between events with great accuracy and adapt behaviour rapidly in response to unexpected occurrences (Shanks, 1995). This ability to learn about whether an action will lead to a rewarding outcome or not, and to use knowledge of causal relationships between our actions and their consequences on the world, is critical for the behavioural expression of cognition (Dickinson, 2001). However, the process by which selective attention to drug-associated cues relates to learning stimulus–response associations that support drug acquisition and consumption is not yet fully understood. According to certain attentional theories of both pavlovian and instrumental learning (Mackintosh, 1975; Pearce and Hall, 1980; Sutherland and Mackintosh, 1971), stimuli that signal that an instrumental response will be drug-reinforced should acquire the capacity to command the focus of attention and bring about the instrumental response. Although these learning theories all agree that attention for discriminative stimuli plays a crucial role in the acquisition of discriminative control, thereafter they assume that attentional processing of the discriminative stimuli varies with knowledge of the stimulus-reinforcer contingencies. Mackintosh (1975; Sutherland and Mackintosh, 1971) predicts that attention to a rewarded stimulus should increase to the extent that the stimulus is the best predictor of the reinforcer. Similarly, according to incentive salience theories (Bindra, 1978; Robinson and Berridge, 1993; Sokolov, 1963; Stewart et al., 1984), as the relationship between the stimulus and the drug reinforcer is learned, the amount of attention allocated to the reinforced stimulus increases to asymptote. These theories regard the attentional orienting response elicited by the stimulus as being like other conditioned responses, such as salivation and skin conductance, which increase with training.

By contrast, alternative attentional learning theories (Kaye and Pearce, 1984; Pearce and Hall, 1980) propose that, although attention for the reinforced stimulus is necessary for learning about the predictive relationship between the stimulus and the reinforcer, once this relationship is well learned the processing of the stimulus becomes efficient. As a consequence, the attentional orienting

response towards the reinforced stimulus might well decrease when the stimulus is established as a good predictor of the reinforcer. Dual-process theories predict that, as exposure to a drug reinforcer increases, the mechanisms that control addictive behaviour change from being controlled, cognitively mediated and goal-directed, to being automatic and habitual. At this stage, the circle of reward–motivation–drive and learning must become self-sufficient and does not require mental representations or control input.

A further important consequence of drug-related cues acquiring incentive properties is that the cues can capture the attention of the addict and control the addict's behaviour. There is a vast amount of evidence supporting the presence of attentional bias towards drug-related stimuli in addiction-related disorders, as seen during the performance of tasks of attentional orienting (for example, using MacLeod's dot-probe task; or eye tracking), disruption with a secondary task and adverse interference (e.g. the Stroop task). This type of attentional bias has been demonstrated for dependence on alcohol (Bauer and Cox, 1998; Stetter et al., 1995; Townshend and Duka, 2001), nicotine (Droungas et al., 1995; Glad and Adesso, 1976; Herman, 1974; Hogarth et al., 2003b; Niaura et al., 1994; Payne et al., 1991; Surawy et al., 1985), cocaine (Rosse et al., 1997) and opiates (Lubman et al., 2000). Changes in the motivational state of the individual, either by priming with the drug (Duka and Townshend, 2004) or by deprivation from the drug (Sayette and Hufford, 1994) can also alter attentional bias to substance-related stimuli. A significant number of studies with human volunteers in the laboratory using arbitrary cues have provided evidence that attentional bias is the result of the conditioning of incentive associations between the drug-reinforcing properties and the cues, including alcohol (Field and Duka, 2002) and nicotine (Hogarth et al., 2003a, 2005).

By experimentally modulating the learning of stimulus-reinforcer contingencies either by instruction (Hogarth et al., 2005; Lovibond, 2003) or by over-training, we can understand how the capture of attention by drug-related cues relates to the response to obtain them. In one such study, explicit knowledge of stimulus-reinforcer contingencies was accompanied by a decrease in attentional orienting towards the stimulus (Hogarth *et al.*, 2005), demonstrating that behaviour, through learning, became more efficient. Eye-tracking techniques that have become available are now applied to investigate the role of attention in the development of addiction (Field *et al.*, 2004; Mogg *et al.*, 2003).

In terms of the neural basis of learning, some theories of reward-dependent learning suggest that learning is driven by the unpredictability of the association between the cue and the reward (Pearce and Hall, 1980; Rescorla and Wagner, 1972). Error-driven learning only advances when prediction errors occur, with single dopamine neurones coding reward prediction error in a signed (positive or negative) bidirectional fashion (Schultz, 2002). Neural manipulation could influence rewarded behaviour by altering one of many forms of learning. The activation of regions linked with memory has been reported during drug intoxication (Breiter *et al.*, 1997; Stein *et al.*, 1998) and during craving induced by drug references (Wang *et al.*, 1999). For example, studies of drug abusers experiencing withdrawal have shown decreased dopamine D2 receptor expression and dopamine release in the dorsal striatum (Volkow *et al.*, 1997). The dorsal striatum is associated with habit learning and it is possible that, in addiction, the routine associated with drug consumption may be triggered automatically by exposure to the drug or drug-related cues (Ito *et al.*, 2002). Drug addiction may be an aberrant form of learning, possibly mediated by the maladaptive recruitment of particular memory systems in the brain (for review, see Robbins and Everitt, 1999).

3.5 Cognition and Cognitive Control

Effective cognitive functioning typically involves numerous neuronal pathways and neurotransmitter systems, with several distinct neurotransmitters being implicated in the alteration of cognitive function (Robbins *et al.*, 1997). In particular, executive functions, such as attention, planning, problem solving, adapting behaviour and attending to relevant stimuli while ignoring distracting ones, are crucial for the successful performance of many everyday procedures such as prioritising tasks and remembering important information while performing an action (Stuss and Levine, 2002). Frontostriatal neural networks in the brain have been shown to subserve many of these crucial functions and to be modulated by neurochemicals, such as the catecholamines dopamine and noradrenaline (Solanto *et al.*, 2001). It has been suggested that alterations in brain dopamine activity might lead to a reduced sensitivity to natural reinforcers, such as food and sex, as well as disrupting frontal cortical functions implicated in inhibitory control. It is hoped that a clearer understanding of the neural mechanisms of substance abuse will help drive effective strategies for treatment.

Drug addicts are known to display abnormalities in the prefrontal cortex, including the anterior cingulate gyrus (Goldstein and Volkow, 2002). The prefrontal cortex is involved in decision making and in inhibitory control. Its disruption could lead to inadequate decisions that favour immediate rewards over delayed but more favourable responses. It could also account for impaired control over the intake of the drug, even when the addicted subject expresses a desire to refrain from taking the drug (Goldstein and Volkow, 2002).

An extensive literature has pointed to frontal lobe dysfunction in alcoholic patients (Joyce and Robbins, 1993; for a review see also Moselhy *et al.*, 2001). Studies in animals (Dias *et al.*, 1996) and neurological patients (Owen *et al.*, 1995, 1996) have been able to inform human laboratory testing with addicts so that conclusions can be drawn as to the damaged or dysfunctional area of the brain. Studying cognitive dysfunction in addicts in relation to the history of their addiction can indicate the critical factors contributing to its development. For example, repeated detoxifications from alcohol leads to an increased severity of withdrawal often accompanied by seizures (Duka *et al.*, 2004). Evidence has now accumulated that other aspects of brain function can also deteriorate, resulting in altered motivation. For example, cravings have been shown to be increased (Malcolm *et al.*, 2000), together with impairments in emotional processing (Townshend and Duka, 2003) and executive functions (Duka *et al.*, 2003). The latter has also been associated with binge drinking (Weissenborn and Duka, 2003). Feeling emotions and perceiving emotions in others forms the basis of social encounters and everyday relationships. Similarly, executive functions such as the ability to plan, follow goals, be flexible, and inhibit habitual tendencies all reflect virtues that are essential for controlling excessive drinking. If binge drinking, leading abruptly to high amounts of alcohol in the brain, interacts with withdrawal from alcohol to intensify anxiety, emotional and cognitive disturbances, then it becomes clearer how alcoholics become sensitised to experiencing more intensified withdrawal and are susceptible to relapse.

Repeated detoxifications from alcohol or alcohol binges can impair new learning of both aversive and appetitive associations in animals (Ripley *et al.*, 2004; Stephens *et al.*, 2001) as well as impairing the ability to relearn items such as a new path to escape (Obernier *et al.*, 2002a). More importantly, once aversive learning has been established, stimulus generalisation can also occur (Stephens *et al.*, in press). Such a phenomenon (currently only observed in animals) might underlie the increased incidence of panic attacks noted in alcoholics as a result of inappropriate responses to innocuous stimuli. The identification in animals that structures such as the amygdala, hippocampus or cortical structures might be dysfunctional or sensitised as a result of bingeing or withdrawal from alcohol (Duka *et al.*, 2004; George *et al.*, 1999; Obernier *et al.*, 2002b) provides the beginning of an understanding of the neuropsychology of withdrawal-induced and binge-drinking-related change in emotional and cognitive functions.

With respect to other drugs of abuse, preclinical studies have shown that chronic administration of cocaine or amphetamine results in a significant increase in dendritic branching and the density of dendritic spines in the prefrontal cortex (Robinson *et al.*, 2001). These changes could be involved in the changes in decision-making, judgement, and cognitive control that occur during addiction. Imaging studies have shown evidence of changes in prefrontal activation during a working memory task in smokers compared with ex-smokers (Ernst *et al.*, 2001). It has been proposed that disruption of the prefrontal cortex could lead to loss of self-directed behaviour in favour of automatic sensory-driven behaviour (Goldstein and Volkow, 2002). Moreover, the disruption of self-controlled behaviour is likely to be exacerbated during drug intoxication by the loss of inhibitory control which the prefrontal cortex exerts. The inhibition of top-down control would release behaviours that are normally kept under close monitoring and would simulate stress-like reactions in which control is inhibited and stimulus-driven behaviour is facilitated (Goldstein and Volkow, 2002). Indeed, a recent review has suggested that, in addition to the brain's reward system, two frontal cortical regions (anterior cingulate and orbitofrontal cortices) that are critical in inhibitory control are dysfunctional in addicted individuals (Lubman *et al.*, 2004). These same regions have been implicated in other compulsive conditions characterised by deficits in inhibitory control over maladaptive behaviours, such as obsessive–compulsive disorder (Chamberlain *et al.*, 2005). It is hoped that a better understanding of the neurochemical basis of prefrontal inhibitory control might enable the development of drugs and psychotherapies that selectively activate this function and prevent the general trend for substance-dependent individuals to relapse a few months after quitting.

4 CURRENT PSYCHOACTIVE SUBSTANCES – EFFECTS AND HARMS

The increasing availability of potentially beneficial psychoactive substances demands research to establish the full effects of their use. Psychoactive substances can be taken for a wide range of reasons, including mood-altering or cognitive enhancing purposes. Preclinical, cognitive, imaging and genetic studies are furthering our understanding of the potential benefits and harms of these agents. This section describes our current understanding of the effects of certain of the most commonly used recreational drugs, cognitive enhancers and addictive non-chemical behaviours. Many of these effects are an essential feature of the cycle of abuse, and will apply to new substances as they are introduced in the future.

4.1 'Recreational' Drugs

Recreational drug use usually begins because of a drug's beneficial effects on mood or cognition. However, the defining characteristic of addiction is compulsive, out-of-control drug use that persists despite serious negative consequences. Indeed, the high risk of relapse to drug use that persists even in abstinent addicts long after the cessation of withdrawal symptoms has led some to consider addiction as a chronic medical illness (McLellan *et al.*, 2000). This section focuses on some of the physiological and behavioural effects of drugs of abuse, and in particular highlights findings with respect to some major classes of drugs such as alcohol and the opiates.

4.1.1 Tolerance, Dependence and Withdrawal

Several effects are commonly seen in drug addiction. Tolerance often develops to the desired pleasurable effects of drugs, leading to dosage increases that can exacerbate the molecular changes that lead to addiction (Hyman and Malenka, 2001).

Depending on the pattern of use, some drugs, such as cocaine and amphetamine, can also produce sensitisation (or enhancement) of some drug responses where a smaller dose produces an equivalent effect (Anagnostaras and Robinson, 1996; Badiani *et al.*, 1995). Dependence (which is not considered scientifically equivalent to addiction, Hyman and Malenka, 2001) can also develop. Dependence, narrowly defined, refers to the adapted state of cells, circuits or organ systems that occurs in response to excessive drug stimulation. On drug cessation, this adapted state can result in the production of cognitive, emotional and 'physical' withdrawal symptoms. However, it is possible to experience tolerance, dependence or withdrawal without producing compulsive use, prompting researchers to search for other explanations for addiction.

Mechanisms of dependence, withdrawal and sensitisation have been studied extensively. In particular, the neural and molecular basis of physical opiate dependence and withdrawal has been thoroughly investigated as a model of drug action in the brain. By contrast, convincing animal models of addiction – compulsive use despite negative consequences – are lacking (O'Brien *et al.*, 1998). Robinson and Berridge (1993) have proposed an incentive-sensitisation theory of addiction, which suggests that brain systems normally involved in incentive motivation (but not pleasure) become hypersensitive to drugs and drug-associated stimuli, markedly increasing their incentive salience. However, the motivation of drug-induced pleasure does not fully explain compulsive use, because of the presence of effects such as habituation. Some people have argued that compulsive drug taking might continue in an effort to avoid the negative effects of drug withdrawal.

4.1.2 Relapse

Clinical evidence in drug addicts has shown that relapse can occur even a long time after withdrawal symptoms have cleared, arguing against drug addiction continuing solely from the desire to avoid negative withdrawal symptoms. Researchers have identified other factors that also impair an addict's ability to remain independent of substance abuse. Cues associated with previous drug use can initiate craving and conditioned emotional responses in addicts, and are associated clinically with relapse, both during active drug use and after a period of abstinence (O'Brien *et al.*, 1998). Cues can elicit drug-related behaviour in animal models, including sensitised responses to psychostimulants (Hyman and Malenka, 2001). Importantly, sensitisation in animal models has been shown to be context-dependent, raising the possibility of its providing a good model of relapse in humans (Robinson and Berridge, 2000). In rodent models, stress has been shown to produce resumption of drug self-administration (Piazza and Le Moal, 1996). Its role in relapse in human addicts seems to be significant and deserves further study. Drug-associated cues can elicit conditioned emotional responses, including drug urges, in human addicts (Ehrman *et al.*, 1992). Studies of responses to drug-conditioned cues using positron emission tomography (PET) and functional magnetic resonance imaging (fMRI) have shown activation of prefrontal cortex regions and the amygdala, a brain region involved in the consolidation of stimulus-reward associations (Hyman and Malenka, 2001). Some of these imaging studies have also found activation of the nucleus accumbens and other regions. The cue-induced brain activations observed with PET and fMRI correlate with the onset of subjective drug urges and physiological responses, such as activation of the autonomic nervous system (Hyman and Malenka, 2001). Robbins and Everitt (1999) have suggested that conditioning and memory retrieval may represent useful targets for the treatment of addicts and relapse prevention.

4.1.3 *Cognition and Emotion*

Long-term drug abuse is known to induce cognitive and emotional impairments, detectable using psychological methods.

Alcohol-related, long-term dysfunction of the frontal lobe, and alcohol-related amnesia, including the devastating Korsakoff's syndrome, are examples of the harm that can result from this most common recreational drug. Even moderate consumption of alcohol has been shown to attenuate the brain's capacity to detect errors in performance, potentially explaining alcohol's detrimental effects on tasks such as driving a car and operating machinery (Ridderinkhof *et al.*, 2002). Similarly, ecstasy has been studied in the laboratory with sophisticated neuropsychological methods and it is now generally accepted that it produces memory impairments (Curran and Verheyden, 2003; Daumann *et al.*, 2004; Fox *et al.*, 2002; Morgan, 1999; Morgan, *et al.*, 2002a). Amphetamine-induced psychosis, and the recent data on cannabis-induced psychosis (Henquet *et al.*, 2005), as well as Ecstasy-induced depression (McCardle *et al.*, 2004; Roiser *et al.*, 2005), demonstrate the spectrum of harm that recreational drugs can produce. Ornstein *et al.* (2000) reported deficits across a range of cognitive functions including verbal fluency, pattern and spatial recognition memory, and executive functions such as planning. Heavy ecstasy use has been shown to result in selective executive deficits (Fox *et al.*, 2001), although it is difficult to ascribe the deficits definitively to ecstasy in this particular study as all participants also consumed a range of other illicit drugs.

Robinson and Berridge (2000) have suggested that some drugs of abuse may weaken the 'rational break' of cognitive regulatory processes, which are necessary to inhibit motivational impulses, and could impact on other psychological factors such as decision-making. Numerous studies support the observation of impaired decision making or altered neural activation in substance users (Bechara *et al.*, 2001; Clark and Robbins, 2002; Ersche *et al.*, 2005; Grant *et al.*, 2000; Rogers *et al.*, 1999). Clark *et al.* (2006) have suggested that reduced reflection may represent a cognitive marker for substance abuse that may be associated with vulnerability to substance use or the neurotoxic effects of drug exposure. Only a detailed study in the laboratory of the psychological factors that underlie these phenomena will allow us to further explore these cognitive effects and ultimately help prevent or treat them. These studies must control for polydrug use in order that we can better understand the differences in effects between the individual drugs.

4.2 Cognitive Enhancers

Any discussion on the effects of psychoactive substances must include both their harms and their benefits. Many of the agents mentioned already, such as amphetamine and methylphenidate, bridge both camps, with recognised harmful side effects in addition to their cognitive-enhancing properties. There is a huge need for effective cognitive enhancers and it is anticipated that an increasing number of compounds will be developed to target cognition while reducing the potential for addiction.

4.2.1 Cognitive Enhancers in Patients

Major mental illnesses are extremely common and their effects on behaviour, perception, emotion and cognition are an enormous factor in worldwide disability. Numerous neuropsychiatric disorders, such as attention-deficit hyperactivity disorder (ADHD), schizophrenia, frontal dementia and Parkinson's disease are characterised by cognitive impairments. The potential public health benefit of improving current treatments for cognitive disabilities in patients is largely undisputed (Meltzer, 2003). However, cognitive difficulties are not confined to psychiatric disorders, but are also endured by a much wider sector of society, including those whose deficits arise from sleep deprivation, head injury or age-related cognitive decline. With the increase in use of ecstasy and other recreational drug use as well as alcohol binge drinking, there will be additional groups of people who suffer from cognitive decline who might benefit

from cognition enhancers. Their possible use raises many considerations in terms of their effects on the individual concerned and the ethical implications of their use (discussed in Section 5.2).

The global impact of cognitive impairment has only recently been recognised. The disorder of schizophrenia provides a particularly good illustration of the potential benefits to be had from exploring new options for the treatment of cognitive dysfunction. It is estimated that 24 million people worldwide suffer from schizophrenia, which ranks third in terms of the global burden of neuropsychiatric conditions following depression and alcohol dependence (Murray and Lopez, 1996). Its economic impact alone is enormous. In 2000 in the United States it was suggested that the direct and indirect costs of schizophrenia could have been as much as $40 billion (Fuller Torrey, 2001). In many patients, cognitive difficulties have been shown to be the main factor in limiting full rehabilitation (such as returning to work) and quality of life, even after the clinical symptoms have remitted (Goldberg *et al.*, 1993; Mitchell *et al.*, 2001).

Schizophrenia is an important example in the context of drug use. Cannabis use is a risk indicator for schizophrenia, but its causal effects are not yet established. Stimulant drugs and cannabis can cause transient psychotic symptoms and precipitate relapse of an existing psychotic illness (Degenhardt, 2003). Andreasson *et al.* (1987) showed (in a study of over 45 000 conscripts to the Swedish army) that those who abused cannabis at 18 years of age were more likely to be admitted to hospital with schizophrenia over the next decade and a half than those who did not, and that there was a dose–response relationship so that the more cannabis was consumed, the greater was the likelihood of schizophrenia. The active metabolite of cannabis, delta-9 tetrahydrocannabinol (THC), raises the levels of cerebral dopamine (Tanda *et al.*, 1997) and might precipitate the illness through this mechanism. However, as McDonald and Murray (2000) point out, it is also possible that

Debiec, J., LeDoux, J.E., and Nader, K. (2002). Cellular and systems reconsolidation in the hippocampus. *Neuron* 36: 527–538.

Degenhardt, L. (2003) The link between cannabis use and psychosis: furthering the debate. *Psychol Med* 33: 3–6.

Di Chiara, G. and Imperato, A. (1988) Drugs abused by humans preferentially increase synaptic dopamine concentrations in the mesolimbic system of freely moving rats. *Proc Natl Acad Sci USA* 85: 5274–5278.

Dias, R., Robbins. T.W., and Roberts, A.C. (1996) Dissociation in prefrontal cortex of affective and attentional shifts. *Nature* 380: 69–72.

Dickinson, A. (2001) The 28th Bartlett Memorial Lecture. Causal learning: an associative analysis. *Q J Exp Psychol B* 54: 3–25.

Drevets, W.C., Gautier, C., Price, J.C., Kupfer, D.J., Kinahan, P.E., Grace, A.A., Price, J.L. and Mathis, C.A. (2001) Amphetamine-induced dopamine release in human ventral striatum correlates with euphoria. *Biol Psychiatry* 49: 81–96.

Droungas, A., Ehrman, R.N., Childress, A.R., and O'Brien, C.P. (1995) Effect of smoking cues and cigarette availability on craving and smoking behavior. *Addict Behav* 20: 657–673.

Duka, T. and Townshend, J.M. (2004) The Priming effect of alcohol preload on attentional bias to alcohol-related stimuli. *Psychopharmacology (Berl)*. Advance online publication 26 May 2004 doi: 10.1007/s00213-004-1906-7.

Duka, T., Tasker, R., and Stephens, D.N. (1998) Alcohol choice and outcome expectancies in social drinkers. *Behav Pharmacol* 9: 643–653.

Duka, T., Jackson, A., Smith, D.C. and Stephens, D.N. (1999) Relationship of components of an alcohol interoceptive stimulus to induction of desire for alcohol in social drinkers. *Pharmacol Biochem Behav* 64: 301–309.

Duka, T., Weissenborn, R., and Dienes, Z. (2001) State-dependent effects of alcohol on recollective experience, familiarity and awareness of memories. *Psychopharmacology (Berl)* 153: 295–306.

Duka, T., Townshend, J.M., Collier, K., and Stephens, D.N. (2003) Impairment in cognitive functions after multiple detoxifications in alcoholic inpatients. *Alcohol Clin Exp Res* 27: 1563–1572.

Duka, T., Gentry, J., Malcolm, R., Ripley, T.L., Borlikova, G., Stephens, D.N., Veatch, L.M., Becker, H.C., and Crews, F.T. (2004) Consequences of multiple withdrawals from alcohol. *Alcohol Clin Exp Res* 28: 233–246.

Egan, M.F., Goldberg, T.E., Kolachana, B.S., Callicott, J.H., Mazzanti, C.M., Straub, R.E., Goldman, D., and Weinberger, D.R. (2001) Effect of COMT Val 108/158 Met genotype on frontal lobe function and risk for schizophrenia. *Proc Natl Acad Sci USA* 98: 6917–6922.

Ehrman, R.N., Robbins, S.J., Childress, A.R., and O'Brien, C.P. (1992) Conditioned responses to cocaine-related stimuli in cocaine abuse patients. *Psychopharmacology (Berl)* 107: 523–529.

Elliott, R., Sahakian, B.J., Matthews, K., Bannerjea, A., Rimmer, J., and Robbins, T.W. (1997) Effects of methylphenidate on spatial working memory and planning in healthy young adults. *Psychopharmacology (Berl)* 131: 196–206.

Ernst, M., Matochik, J.A., Heishman, S.J., Van Horn, J.D., Jons, P.H., Henningfield, J.E., and London, E.D. (2001) Effect of nicotine on brain activation during performance of a working memory task. *Proc Natl Acad Sci USA* 98: 4728–4733.

Ersche, K.D., Fletcher, P.C., Lewis, S.J.G., Clark, L., Stocks-Gee, G., London, M., Deakin, J.B., Robbins, T.W., and Sahakian, B.J. (2005). Abnormal frontal activations related to decision-making in current and former amphetamine and opiate dependent individuals. *Psychopharmacology*. Advance online publication 15 March 2005 doi: 10.1007/s00213-005-2205-7.

Everitt, B.J., Dickinson, A., and Robbins, T.W. (2001) The neuropsychological basis of addictive behaviour. *Brain Res Brain Res Rev* 36: 129–138.

Farah, M.J. (2002) Emerging ethical issues in neuroscience. *Nat Neurosci* 5: 1123–1129.

Farah, M.J., Illes, J., Cook-Deegan, R., Gardner, H., Kandel, E., King, P., Parens, E., Sahakian, B., and Wolpe, P.R. (2004) Neurocognitive enhancement: what can we do and what should we do? *Nat Rev Neurosci* 5: 421–425.

Field, M. and Duka, T. (2001) Smoking expectancy mediates the conditioned responses to arbitrary smoking cues. *Behav Pharmacol* 12: 183–194.

Field, M. and Duka, T. (2002) Cues paired with a low dose of alcohol acquire conditioned incentive properties in social drinkers. *Psychopharmacology* 159:325–334.

Field, M., Mogg, K., and Bradley, B.P. (2004) Eye movements to smoking-related cues: effects of nicotine deprivation. *Psychopharmacology (Berl)* 173: 116–123.

Fillmore, M.I. and Rush, C.R. (2001) Alcohol effects on inhibitory and activational response strategies in the acquisition of alcohol and other reinforcers: priming the motivation to drink. *J Stud Alcohol* 62: 646–656.

Fox, H.C., Parrott, A.C., and Turner, J.J. (2001) Ecstasy use: cognitive deficits related to dosage rather than self-reported problematic use of the drug. *J Psychopharmacol* 15: 273–281.

Fox, H.C., McLean, A., Turner, J.J., Parrott, A.C., Rogers, R., and Sahakian, B.J. (2002) Neuropsychological evidence of a relatively selective profile of temporal dysfunction in drug-free MDMA ('Ecstasy') polydrug users. *Psychopharmacology (Berl)* 162: 203–214.

Franklin, T.R., Acton, P.D., Maldjian, J.A., Gray, J.D., Croft, J.R., Dackis, C.A., O'Brien, C.P., and Childress, A.R. (2002) Decreased gray matter concentration in the insular, orbitofrontal, cingulate, and temporal cortices of cocaine patients. *Biol Psychiatry* 51: 134–142.

Fuller Torrey, E. (2001) *Surviving schizophrenia: manual for families, consumers, and providers.* 4th edition. New York: Perennial-Harper Collins Publishers.

Furey, M.L., Pietrini, P., and Haxby, J.V. (2000) Cholinergic enhancement and increased selectivity of perceptual processing during working memory. *Science* 290: 2315–2319.

Gamma, A., Buck, A., Berthold, T., and Vollenweider, F.X. (2001) No difference in brain activation during cognitive performance between Ecstasy (3,4-methylenedioxymethamphetamine) users and control subjects: A [H2(15)O]-positron emission tomography study. *J Clin Psychopharmacol* 21: 66–71.

George, M.S., Teneback, C.C., Malcolm, R.J., Moore, J., Stallings, L.E., Spicer, K.M., Anton, R.F., and Ballenger, J.C. (1999) Multiple previous alcohol detoxifications are associated with decreased medial temporal and paralimbic function in the postwithdrawal period. *Alcohol Clin Exp Res* 23: 1077–1084.

Gerra, G., Zaimovic, A., Ferri, M., Zambelli, U., Timpano, M., Neri, E., Marzocchi, G.F., Delsignore, R., and Brambilla, F.

(2000). Long-lasting effects of (+/−)3,4-methylenedioxymethamphetamine (Ecstasy) on serotonin system function in humans. *Biol Psychiatry* 47: 127–136.

Glad, W. and Adesso, V.J. (1976) The relative importance of socially induced tension and behavioral contagion for smoking behavior. *J Abnorm Psychol* 85: 119–121.

Goff, D.C., Leahy, L., Berman, I., Posever, T., Herz, L., Leon, A.C., Johnson, S.A., and Lynch, G. (2001) A placebo-controlled pilot study of the ampakine CX516 added to clozapine in schizophrenia. *J Clin Psychopharmacol* 21: 484–487.

Goldberg, T.E., Greenberg, R.D., Griffin, S.J., Gold, J.M., Kleinman, J.E., Pickar, D., Schulz, S.C., and Weinberger, D.R. (1993) The effect of clozapine on cognition and psychiatric symptoms in patients with schizophrenia. *Br J Psychiatry* 162: 43–48.

Goldstein, R.Z. and Volkow, N.D. (2002) Drug addiction and its underlying neurobiological basis: neuroimaging evidence for the involvement of the frontal cortex. *Am J Psychiatry* 159: 1642–1652.

Gossop, M., Marsden, J., Stewart, D., and Kidd, T. (2003) The National Treatment Outcome Research Study (NTORS): 4-5 year follow-up results. *Addiction* 98: 291–303.

Grant, S., Contoreggi, C., and London, E.D. (2000) Drug abusers show impaired performance in a laboratory test of decision making. *Neuropsychologia* 38: 1180–1187.

Grasby, P.M. (2003) Positron emission tomography (PET) neurochemistry: where are we now and where are we going? In: T.W. Robbins (ed.), *Disorders of brain and mind 2.* Cambridge: Cambridge University Press: 181–194.

Hada, M., Porjesz, B., Chorlian, D.B., Begleiter, H., and Polich, J. (2001) Auditory P3a deficits in male subjects at high risk for alcoholism. *Biol Psychiatry* 49: 726–738.

Hall, J., Parkinson, J.A., Connor, T.M., Dickinson, A., and Everitt, B.J. (2001) Involvement of the central nucleus of the amygdala and nucleus accumbens core in mediating pavlovian influences on instrumental behaviour. *Eur J Neurosci* 13: 1984–1992.

Hasman, A. and Holm, S. (2004) Nicotine conjugate vaccine: is there a right to a smoking future? *J Med Ethics* 30: 344–345.

Hatzidimitriou, G., McCann, U.D., and Ricaurte, G.A. (1999) Altered serotonin innervation patterns in the forebrain of monkeys treated with (+/−)3,4-methylenedioxymethamphetamine seven years previously: factors influencing abnormal recovery. *J Neurosci* 19: 5096–5107.

Henquet, C., Krabbendam, L., Spauwen, J., Kaplan, C., Lieb, R., Wittchen, H.U., and van Os, J. (2005) Prospective cohort study of cannabis use, predisposition for psychosis, and psychotic symptoms in young people. *BMJ:* 330: 11.

Herman, C.P. (1974) External and internal cues as determinants of the smoking behavior of light and heavy smokers. *J Pers Soc Psychol* 30: 664–672.

Hesselbrock, V., Begleiter, H., Porjesz, B., O'Connor, S., and Bauer, L. (2001) P300 event-related potential amplitude as an endophenotype of alcoholism: evidence from the collaborative study on the genetics of alcoholism. *J Biomed Sci* 8: 77–82.

Hill, S.Y., De Bellis, M.D., Keshavan, M.S., Lowers, L., Shen, S., Hall, J., and Pitts, T. (2001) Right amygdala volume in adolescent and young adult offspring from families at high risk for developing alcoholism. *Biol Psychiatry* 49: 894–905.

Hodgson, R., Rankin, H., and Stockwell, T. (1979) Alcohol dependence and the priming effect. *Behav Res Ther* 17: 379–387.

Hogarth, L., Dickinson, A., and Duka, T. (2003a) Discriminative stimuli that control instrumental tobacco-seeking by human smokers also command selective attention. *Psychopharmacology* 168: 435–445.

Hogarth, L., Mogg, K., Bradley, B.P., Duka, T., and Dickinson, A. (2003b) Attentional orienting towards smoking-related stimuli. *Behav Pharmacol* 14: 153–160.

Hogarth, L., Dickinson, A., and Duka, T. (2005) Explicit knowledge of stimulus-outcome contingencies and stimulus control of selective attention and instrumental action in human smoking behaviour. *Psychopharmacology (Berl)* 177: 428–437.

Honey, G. and Bullmore, E. (2004) Human pharmacological MRI. *Trends Pharmacol Sci* 25: 366–374.

Hyman, S.E. and Malenka, R.C. (2001) Addiction and the brain: the neurobiology of compulsion and its persistence. *Nat Rev Neurosci* 2: 695–703.

Insel, T.R. (1992) Toward a neuroanatomy of obsessive-compulsive disorder. *Arch Gen Psychiatry* 49: 739–744.

Ito, R., Dalley, J.W., Robbins, T.W., and Everitt, B.J. (2002) Dopamine release in the dorsal striatum during cocaine-seeking behavior under the control of a drug-associated cue. *J Neurosci* 22: 6247–6253.

Joyce, E.M. and Robbins, T.W. (1993) Memory deficits in Korsakoff and non-Korsakoff alcoholics following alcohol withdrawal and the relationship to length of abstinence. *Alcohol Suppl* 2: 501–505.

Kabbaj, M., Evans, S., Watson, S.J., and Akil, H. (2004) The search for the neurobiological basis of vulnerability to drug abuse: using microarrays to investigate the role of stress and individual differences. *Neuropharmacology* 47 (Suppl 1): 111–122.

Katsnelson, A. (2004) Ethical quagmire awaits vaccine for cocaine addiction. *Nat Med* 10: 1007.

Kaye, H. and Pearce, J.M. (1984) The strength of the orienting response during pavlovian conditioning. *J Exp Psychol Anim Behav Process* 10: 90–109.

Kelleher, R.T. and Goldberg, S.R. (1977) Fixed-interval responding under second-order schedules of food presentation or cocaine injection. *J Exp Anal Behav* 28: 221–231.

Kirk, J.M. and de Wit, H. (2000) Individual differences in the priming effect of ethanol in social drinkers. *J Stud Alcohol* 61: 64–71.

Kish, S.J., Furukawa, Y., Ang, L., Vorce, S.P., and Kalasinsky, K.S. (2000) Striatal serotonin is depleted in brain of a human MDMA (Ecstasy) user. *Neurology* 55: 294–296.

Koepp, M.J., Gunn, R.N., Lawrence, A.D., Cunningham, V.J., Dagher, A., Jones, T., Brooks, D.J., Bench, C.J., and Grasby, P.M. (1998) Evidence for striatal dopamine release during a video game. *Nature* 393: 266–268.

Koob, G.F. and Bloom, F.E. (1988) Cellular and molecular mechanisms of drug dependence. *Science* 242: 715–723.

Kyte, Z.A., Goodyer, I.M., and Sahakian, B.J. (2004) Selected executive skills in adolescents with recent first episode major depression. *J Child Psychol Psychiatry.* Advance online publication 2 December 2004 doi: 10.1111/j.1469–7610.2004.00400.x.

Lee, J., Everitt, B.J., and Thomas, K.L. (2004a) Independent cellular processes for hippocampal memory consolidation and reconsolidation. *Science* 304: 839–843.

Lee, J., Lim, Y., Graham, S.J., Kim, G., Wiederhold, B.K., Wiederhold, M.D., Kim, I.Y., and Kim, S.I. (2004b) Nicotine craving and cue exposure therapy by using virtual environments. *Cyberpsychol Behav* 7: 705–713.

Lovibond, P.F. (2003) Causal beliefs and conditioned responses: retrospective revaluation induced by experience and by instruction. *J Exp Psychol Learn Mem Cogn* 29: 97–106.

Lubman, D.I., Peters, L.A., Mogg, K., Bradley, B.P., and Deakin, J.F. (2000) Attentional bias for drug cues in opiate dependence. *Psychol Med* 30: 169–175.

Lubman, D.I., Yucel, M., and Pantelis, C. (2004) Addiction, a condition of compulsive behaviour? Neuroimaging and neuropsychological evidence of inhibitory dysregulation. *Addiction* 99: 1491–1502.

MacInnes, N., Handley, S.L., and Harding, G.F. (2001) Former chronic methylenedioxymethamphetamine (MDMA or Ecstasy) users report mild depressive symptoms. *J Psychopharmacol* 15: 181–186.

Mackintosh, N.J. (1975). A theory of attention: variations in the associability of stimuli with reinforcement. *Psychol Rev* 82: 276–298.

Malcolm, R., Herron, J.E., Anton, R.F., Roberts, J., and Moore, J. (2000) Recurrent detoxification may elevate alcohol craving as measured by the obsessive compulsive drinking scale. *Alcohol* 20: 181–185.

Martin-Solch, C., Magyar, S., Kunig, G., Missimer, J., Schultz, W., and Leenders, K.L. (2001) Changes in brain activation associated with reward processing in smokers and nonsmokers. A positron emission tomography study. *Exp Brain Res* 139: 278–286.

Mattay, V.S., Callicott, J.H., Bertolino, A., Heaton, I., Frank, J.A., Coppola, R., Berman, K.F., Goldberg, T.E., and Weinberger, D.R. (2000) Effects of dextroamphetamine on cognitive performance and cortical activation. *Neuroimage* 12: 268–275.

Mattay, V.S., Goldberg, T.E., Fera, F., Hariri, A.R., Tessitore, A., Egan, M.F., Kolachana, B., Callicott, J.H., and Weinberger, D.R. (2003) Catechol O-methyltransferase Val158-Met genotype and individual variation in the brain response to amphetamine. *Proc Natl Acad Sci USA* 100: 6186–6191.

McCardle, K., Luebbers, S., Carter, J.D., Croft, R.J., and Stough, C. (2004) Chronic MDMA (Ecstasy) use, cognition and mood. *Psychopharmacology (Berl)* 173: 434–439.

McDonald, C. and Murray, R.M. (2000) Early and late environmental risk factors for schizophrenia. *Brain Res Brain Res Rev* 31: 130–137.

McDowell, S., Whyte, J., and D'Esposito, M. (1998) Differential effect of a dopaminergic agonist on prefrontal function in traumatic brain injury patients. *Brain* 121: 1155–1164.

McKenna, D.J. and Peroutka, S.J. (1990) Neurochemistry and neurotoxicity of 3,4-methylenedioxymethamphetamine (MDMA, 'Ecstasy'). *J Neurochem* 54: 14–22.

McKinney, E.F., Walton, R.T., Yudkin, P., Fuller, A., Haldar, N.A., Mant, D., Murphy, M., Welsh, K.I. and Marshall, S.E. (2000) Association between polymorphisms in dopamine metabolic enzymes and tobacco consumption in smokers. *Pharmacogenetics* 10: 483–491.

McLean, A., Rubinsztein, J.S., Robbins, T.W., and Sahakian, B.J. (2004) The effects of tyrosine depletion in normal healthy volunteers: implications for unipolar depression. *Psychopharmacology (Berl)* 171: 286–297.

McLellan, A.T., Lewis, D.C., O'Brien, C.P., and Kleber, H.D. (2000) Drug dependence, a chronic medical illness: implications for treatment, insurance, and outcomes evaluation. *JAMA* 284: 1689–1695.

Mehta, M.A., Owen, A.M., Sahakian, B.J., Mavaddat, N., Pickard, J.D., and Robbins, T.W. (2000) Methylphenidate enhances working memory by modulating discrete frontal and parietal lobe regions in the human brain. *J Neurosci* 20: RC65(1–6).

Mehta, M.A., Goodyer, I.M., and Sahakian, B.J. (2004) Methylphenidate improves working memory and set-shifting in AD/HD: relationships to baseline memory capacity. *J Child Psychol Psychiatry* 45: 293–305.

Meltzer, H.Y. (2003) Beyond control of acute exacerbation: enhancing affective and cognitive outcomes. *CNS Spectr* 8: 16–8, 22.

Mitchell, R.L., Elliott, R., and Woodruff, P.W. (2001 FMRI and cognitive dysfunction in schizophrenia. *Trends Cogn Sci* 5: 71–81.

Mogg, K., Bradley, B.P., Field, M., and De Houwer, J. (2003) Eye movements to smoking-related pictures in smokers: relationship between attentional biases and implicit and explicit measures of stimulus valence. *Addiction* 98: 825–836.

Morgan, M.J. (1999) Memory deficits associated with recreational use of 'Ecstasy' (MDMA). *Psychopharmacology (Berl)* 141: 30–36.

Morgan, M.J., McFie, L., Fleetwood, H., and Robinson, J.A. (2002a) Ecstasy (MDMA): are the psychological problems associated with its use reversed by prolonged abstinence? *Psychopharmacology (Berl)* 159: 294–303.

Morgan, D., Grant, K.A., Gage, H.D., Mach, R.H., Kaplan, J.R., Prioleau, O., Nader, S.H., Buchheimer, N., Ehrenkaufer, R.L., and Nader, M.A. (2002b) Social dominance in monkeys: dopamine d2 receptors and cocaine self-administration. *Nat Neurosci* 5: 169–174.

Moselhy, H.F., Georgiou, G., and Kahn, A. (2001) Frontal lobe changes in alcoholism: a review of the literature. *Alcohol* 36: 357–368.

Mucha, R.F., Pauli, P., and Angrilli, A. (1998) Conditioned responses elicited by experimentally produced cues for smoking. *Can J Physiol Pharmacol* 76: 259–268.

Murphy, F.C., Sahakian, B.J., Rubinsztein, J.S., Michael, A., Rogers, R.D., Robbins, T.W., and Paykel, E.S. (1999) Emotional bias and inhibitory control processes in mania and depression. *Psychol Med* 29: 1307–1321.

Murphy, F.C., Smith, K.A., Cowen, P.J., Robbins, T.W., and Sahakian, B.J. (2002) The effects of tryptophan depletion on cognitive and affective processing in healthy volunteers. *Psychopharmacology (Berl)* 163: 42–53.

Murray, C.J.L. and Lopez, A.D. (1996) *The global burden of disease: a comprehensive assessment of mortality and disability from diseases, injuries and risk factors in 1990 and projected to 2020.* Geneva: World Health Organisation.

Nestler, E.J. (1996) Under siege: the brain on opiates. *Neuron* 16: 897–900.

Niaura, R., Abrams, D.B., Pedraza, M., Monti, P., and Rosenhow, D.J. (1992) Smokers' reactions to interpersonal interactions and presentation of smoking cues. *Addictive Behaviors* 17: 557–566.

Niaura, R., Goldstein, M.G., and Abrams, D.B. (1994) Matching high- and low-dependence smokers to self-help treatment with or without nicotine replacement. *Prev Med* 23: 70–77.

Obernier, J.A., White, A.M., Swartzwelder, H.S., and Crews, F.T. (2002a). Cognitive deficits and CNS damage after a 4-day binge ethanol exposure in rats. *Pharmacol Biochem Behav* 72: 521–532.

Obernier, J.A., Bouldin, T.W., and Crews, F.T. (2002b). Binge ethanol exposure in adult rats causes necrotic cell death. *Alcohol Clin Exp Res* 26: 547–557.

O'Brien, C.P., Childress, A.R., Ehrman, R., and Robbins, S.J. (1998) Conditioning factors in drug abuse: can they explain compulsion? *J Psychopharmacol* 12: 15–22.

Obrist, P., Webb, R., Sutterer, J., and Howard, J. (1970) The cardia-somatic relationship: some reformulations. *Psychophysiology* 6: 569–587.

Office for National Statistics (2000) *Drug use, smoking and drinking among young teenagers in 1999.* London: HMSO.

O'Malley, S.S., Krishnan-Sarin, S., Farren, C., Sinha, R., and Kreek, J. (2002) Naltrexone decreases craving and alcohol self-administration in alcohol-dependent subjects and activates the hypothalamo-pituitary-adrenocortical axis. *Psychopharmacology (Berl)* 160: 19–29.

Ornstein, T.J., Iddon, J.L., Baldacchino, A.M., Sahakian, B.J., London, M., Everitt, B.J., and Robbins, T.W. (2000) Profiles of cognitive dysfunction in chronic amphetamine and heroin abusers. *Neuropsychopharmacology* 23: 113–126.

Owen, A.M., Sahakian, B.J., Semple, J., Polkey, C.E., and Robbins, T.W. (1995) Visuospatial short-term recognition memory and learning after temporal lobe excisions, frontal lobe excisions or amygdalo-hippocampectomy in man. *Neuropsychologia* 33: 1–24.

Owen, A.M., Morris, R.G., Sahakian, B.J., Polkey, C.E., and Robbins, T.W. (1996) Double dissociations of memory and executive functions in working memory tasks following frontal lobe excisions, temporal lobe excisions or amygdalo-hippocampectomy in man. *Brain* 119: 1597–1615.

Parrott, A.C. and Lasky, J. (1998) Ecstasy (MDMA) effects upon mood and cognition: before, during and after a Saturday night dance. *Psychopharmacology (Berl)* 139: 261–268.

Parrott, A.C., Sisk, E., and Turner, J.J. (2000) Psychobiological problems in heavy 'Ecstasy' (MDMA) polydrug users. *Drug Alcohol Depend* 60: 105–110.

Parrott, A.C., Milani, R.M., Parmar, R., and Turner, J.D. (2001) Recreational Ecstasy/MDMA and other drug users from the UK and Italy: psychiatric symptoms and psychobiological problems. *Psychopharmacology (Berl)* 159: 77–82.

Payne, T., Etscheidt, M., and Corrigan, S. (1990) Conditioning arbitrary stimuli to cigarette smoke intake: a preliminary study. *J Subst Abuse* 2: 113–119.

Payne, T.J., Schare, M.L., Levis, D.J., and Colletti, G. (1991) Exposure to smoking-relevant cues: effects on desire to smoke and topographical components of smoking behavior. *Addict Behav* 16: 467–479.

Pearce, J.M. and Hall, G. (1980) A model for pavlovian learning: variations in the effectiveness of conditioned but not unconditioned stimuli. *Psychological Review* 87: 532–552.

Perkins, K.A., Epstein, L.H., Grobe, J., and Fonte, C. (1994). Tobacco abstinence, smoking cues, and the reinforcing value of smoking. *Pharmacol Biochem Behav* 47: 107–112.

Piazza, P.V. and Le Moal, M.L. (1996) Pathophysiological basis of vulnerability to drug abuse: role of an interaction between stress, glucocorticoids, and dopaminergic neurons. *Annu Rev Pharmacol Toxicol* 36: 359–378.

Plomin, R. (2003) Genes and behaviour: cognitive abilities and disabilities in normal populations. In: T.W. Robbins (ed.), *Disorders of brain and mind 2*. Cambridge: Cambridge University Press: 1–58.

Rahman, S. (2001) Executive and mnemonic functions in the frontal lobe dementias. PhD thesis, University of Cambridge.

Rangaswamy, M., Porjesz, B., Ardekani, B.A., Choi, S.J., Tanabe, J.L., Lim, K.O., and Begleiter, H. (2004) A functional MRI study of visual oddball: evidence for frontoparietal dysfunction in subjects at risk for alcoholism. *Neuroimage* 21: 329–339.

Redish, A.D. (2004) Addiction as a computational process gone awry. *Science* 306: 1944–1947.

Reneman, L., Booij, J., de Bruin, K., Reitsma, J.B., de Wolff, F.A., Gunning, W.B., den Heeten, G.J., and van den Brink, W. (2001) Effects of dose, sex, and long-term abstention from use on toxic effects of MDMA (Ecstasy) on brain serotonin neurons. *Lancet* 358: 1864–1869.

Rescorla, R.A. and Solomon, R.L. (1967) Two-process learning theory: relationships between pavlovian conditioning and instrumental learning. *Psychol Rev* 74: 151–182.

Rescorla, R.A. and Wagner, A.R. (1972) A theory of pavlovian conditioning: variations in the effectiveness of reinforcement and non-reinforcement. In: W.F. Prokasy (ed.), *Classical conditioning II: current theory and research.* New York: Appleton-Century-Crofts: 64–69.

Ricaurte, G.A., Finnegan, K.F., Nichols, D.E., DeLanney, L.E., Irwin, I., and Langston, J.W. (1987) 3,4-methylenedioxyethylamphetamine (MDE), a novel analogue of MDMA, produces long-lasting depletion of serotonin in the rat brain. *Eur J Pharmacol* 137: 265–268.

Ridderinkhof, K.R., de Vlugt, Y., Bramlage, A., Spaan, M., Elton, M., Snel, J., and Band, G.P.H. (2002) Alcohol consumption impairs detection of performance errors in mediofrontal cortex. *Science* 298: 2209–2211.

Ripley, T.L., Borlikova, G., Lyons, S., and Stephens, D.N. (2004) Selective deficits in appetitive conditioning as a consequence of ethanol withdrawal. *Eur J Neurosci* 19: 415–425.

Robbins, T.W. and Everitt, B.J. (1996) Neurobehavioural mechanisms of reward and motivation. *Curr Opin Neurobiol* 6: 228–236.

Robbins, T.W. and Everitt, B.J. (1999) Drug addiction: bad habits add up. *Nature* 398: 567–570.

Robbins, T.W., James, M., Owen, A.M., Sahakian, B.J., McInnes, L., and Rabbitt, P. (1994) Cambridge neuropsychological test automated battery (CANTAB): a factor analytic study of a large sample of normal elderly volunteers. *Dementia* 5: 266–281.

Robbins, T.W., McAlonan, G., Muir, J.L., and Everitt, B.J. (1997) Cognitive enhancers in theory and practice: studies of the cholinergic hypothesis of cognitive deficits in Alzheimer's disease. *Behav Brain Res* 83: 15–23.

Robinson, T.E. and Berridge, K.C. (1993) The neural basis of drug craving: an incentive-sensitization theory of drug addiction. *Brain Res Rev* 18: 247–291.

Robinson, T.E. and Berridge, K.C. (2000) The psychology and neurobiology of addiction: an incentive-sensitization view. *Addiction* 95(Suppl 2): S91–117.

Robinson, T.E., Gorny, G., Mitton, E., and Kolb, B. (2001) Cocaine self-administration alters the morphology of dendrites and dendritic spines in the nucleus accumbens and neocortex. *Synapse* 39: 257–266.

Rogers, R.D., Everitt, B.J., Baldacchino, A., Blackshaw, A.J., Swainson, R., Wynne, K., Baker, N.B., Hunter, J., Carthy, T., Booker, E., London, M., Deakin, J.F., Sahakian, B.J., and Robbins, T.W. (1999) Dissociable deficits in the decision-making cognition of chronic amphetamine abusers, opiate abusers, patients with focal damage to prefrontal cortex, and tryptophan-depleted normal volunteers: evidence for monoaminergic mechanisms. *Neuropsychopharmacology* 20: 322–339.

Roiser, J.P., Cook, L.J., Cooper, J.D., Rubinsztein, D.C., and Sahakian, B.J. (2005) Association of a functional polymorphism in the serotonin transporter gene with abnormal emotional processing in Ecstasy users. *Am J Psychiatry* 162: 609–612.

Rolls, E.T. (2000) The orbitofrontal cortex and reward. *Cereb Cortex* 10: 284–294.

Rosse, R.B., Johri, S., Kendrick, K., Hess, A.L., Alim, T.N., Miller, M., and Deutsch, S.I. (1997) Preattentive and attentive eye movements during visual scanning of a cocaine cue: correlation with intensity of cocaine cravings. *J Neuropsychiatry Clin Neurosci* 9: 91–93.

Salmond, C.H., Chatfield, D.A., Menon, D.K., Pickard, J.D., and Sahakian, B.J. (2005) Cognitive sequelae of head injury: involvement of basal forebrain and associated structures. *Brain* 128: 189–200.

Sayette, M.A. and Hufford, M.R. (1994) Effects of cue exposure and deprivation on cognitive resources in smokers. *J Abnorm Psychol* 103: 812–818.

Schultz, W. (2002) Getting formal with dopamine and reward. *Neuron* 36: 241–263.

Schultz, W., Tremblay, L., and Hollerman, J.R. (2000) Reward processing in primate orbitofrontal cortex and basal ganglia. *Cereb Cortex* 10: 272–284.

Semple, D.M., Ebmeier, K.P., Glabus, M.F., O'Carroll, R.E., and Johnstone, E.C. (1999) Reduced in vivo binding to the serotonin transporter in the cerebral cortex of MDMA ('Ecstasy') users. *Br J Psychiatry* 175: 63–69.

Sententia, W. (2004) Neuroethical considerations: cognitive liberty and converging technologies for improving human cognition. *Ann NY Acad Sci* 1013: 221–228.

Shanks, D.R. (1995) *The psychology of associative learning*. Cambridge: Cambridge University Press.

Sokolov, Y.N. (1963) *Perception and the conditioned reflex*. Oxford: Pergamon Press.

Solanto, M.V., Arnsten, A.F., and Castellanos, F.X. (2001) The neuroscience of stimulant drug action in ADHD. In: F.X. Castellanos (ed.), *Stimulant drugs and ADHD: basic and clinical neuroscience.* New York: Oxford University Press: 355–379.

Sora, I., Hall, F.S., Andrews, A.M., Itokawa, M., Li, X.F., Wei, H.B., Wichems, C., Lesch, K.P., Murphy, D.L., and Uhl, G.R. (2001) Molecular mechanisms of cocaine reward: combined dopamine and serotonin transporter knockouts eliminate cocaine place preference. *Proc Natl Acad Sci USA* 98: 5300–5305.

Spinella, M. (2005) Compulsive behavior in tobacco users. *Addict Behav* 30: 183–186.

Stein, E.A., Pankiewicz, J., Harsch, H.H., Cho, J.K., Fuller, S.A., Hoffmann, R.G., Hawkins, M., Rao, S.M., Bandettini, P.A., and Bloom, A.S. (1998) Nicotine-induced limbic cortical activation in the human brain: a functional MRI study. *Am J Psychiatry* 155: 1009–1015.

Stephens, D.N., Brown, G., Duka, T., and Ripley, T.L. (2001) Impaired fear conditioning but enhanced seizure sensitivity in rats given repeated experience of withdrawal from alcohol. *Eur J Neurosci* 14: 2023–2031.

Stephens, D.N., Ripley, T.L., Borlikova, G., Schubert, M., Albrecht, D., Hogarth, L., and Duka, T. (2005) Alcohol bingeing impairs synaptic plasticity and aversive conditioning. *Biol Psychiatry* 58: 392–400.

Stetter, F., Ackermann, K., Bizer, A., Straube, E.R., and Mann, K. (1995) Effects of disease-related cues in alcoholic inpatients: results of a controlled 'alcohol stroop' study. *Alcohol Clin Exp Res* 19: 593–599.

Stewart, J., de Wit, H., and Eikelboom, R. (1984) Role of conditioned and unconditioned drug effects in self-administration of opiates and stimulants. *Psycholog Rev* 63: 251–268.

Stockwell, T. (1991) *Experimental analogues of loss of control: a review of human drinking studies.* Sydney: Macmillan.

Stuss, D.T. and Levine, B. (2002) Adult clinical neuropsychology: lessons from studies of the frontal lobes. *Annu Rev Psychol* 53: 401–433.

Surawy, C., Stepney, R., and Cox, T. (1985) Does watching others smoke increase smoking? *Br J Addict* 80: 207–210.

Sutherland, N.S. and Mackintosh, N.J. (1971) *Mechanisms of animal discrimination learning.* New York: Academic Press.

Tanda, G., Pontieri, F.E., and Di Chiara, G. (1997) Cannabinoid and heroin activation of mesolimbic dopamine transmission by a common Mu1 opioid receptor mechanism. *Science* 276: 2048–2050.

Thanos, P.K., Volkow, N.D., Freimuth, P., Umegaki, H., Ikari, H., Roth, G., Ingram, D.K., and Hitzemann, R. (2001) Overexpression of dopamine D2 receptors reduces alcohol self-administration. *J Neurochem* 78: 1094–1103.

Thomasius, R., Petersen, K., Buchert, R., Andresen, B., Zapletalova, P., Wartberg, L., Nebeling, B., and Schmoldt, A. (2003) Mood, cognition and serotonin transporter availability in current and former Ecstasy (MDMA) users. *Psychopharmacology (Berl)* 167: 85–96.

Townshend, J.M. and Duka, T. (2001) Attentional bias associated with alcohol cues: differences between heavy and occasional social drinkers. *Psychopharmacology (Berl)* 157: 67–74.

Townshend, J.M. and Duka, T. (2003) Mixed emotions: alcoholics' impairments in the recognition of specific emotional facial expressions. *Neuropsychologia* 41: 773–782.

Turner, D.C., Robbins, T.W., Clark, L., Aron, A.R., Dowson, J., and Sahakian, B.J. (2003) Cognitive enhancing effects of modafinil in healthy volunteers. *Psychopharmacology (Berl)* 165: 260–269.

Turner, D.C., Clark, L., Dowson, J., Robbins, T.W., and Sahakian, B.J. (2004a) Modafinil improves cognition and response inhibition in adult attention-deficit/hyperactivity disorder. *Biol Psychiatry* 55: 1031–1040.

Turner, D.C., Clark, L., Pomarol-Clotet, E., McKenna, P., Robbins, T.W., and Sahakian, B.J. (2004b) Modafinil improves cognition and attentional set shifting in patients with chronic schizophrenia. *Neuropsychopharmacology* 29: 1363–1373.

Turner, D.C., Blackwell, A.D., Dowson, J.H., McLean, A., and Sahakian, B.J. (2005) Neurocognitive effects of methylphenidate in adult attention-deficit/hyperactivity disorder. *Psychopharmacology (Berl)*. 178: 286–295.

Vaidya, C.J., Austin, G., Kirkorian, G., Ridlehuber, H.W., Desmond, J.E., Glover, G.H., and Gabrieli, J.D. (1998) Selective effects of methylphenidate in attention deficit hyperactivity disorder: a functional magnetic resonance study. *Proc Natl Acad Sci USA* 95: 14494–14499.

Verheyden, S.L., Hadfield, J., Calin, T., and Curran, H.V. (2002) Sub-acute effects of MDMA (+/-3,4-methylenedioxymethamphetamine, 'Ecstasy') on mood: evidence of gender differences. *Psychopharmacology (Berl)* 161: 23–31.

Verkes, R.J., Gijsman, H.J., Pieters, M.S., Schoemaker, R.C., de Visser, S., Kuijpers, M., Pennings, E.J., de Bruin, D., Van de Wijngaart, G., Van Gerven, J.M., and Cohen, A.F. (2001) Cognitive performance and serotonergic function in users of Ecstasy. *Psychopharmacology (Berl)* 153: 196–202.

Volkow, N.D., Fowler, J.S., Wolf, A.P., Hitzemann, R., Dewey, S., Bendriem, B., Alpert, R., and Hoff, A. (1991) Changes in brain glucose metabolism in cocaine dependence and withdrawal. *Am J Psychiatry* 148: 621–626.

Volkow, N.D., Wang, G.J., Fowler, J.S., Logan, J., Gatley, S.J., Hitzemann, R., Chen, A.D., Dewey, S.L., and Pappas, N. (1997) Decreased striatal dopaminergic responsiveness in detoxified cocaine-dependent subjects. *Nature* 386: 830–833.

Volkow, N.D., Wang, G.J., Fowler, J.S., Logan, J., Gatley, S.J., Wong, C., Hitzemann, R., and Pappas, N.R. (1999a) Reinforcing effects of psychostimulants in humans are associated with increases in brain dopamine and occupancy of D(2) receptors. *J Pharmacol Exp Ther* 291: 409–415.

Volkow, N.D., Wang, G.J., Fowler, J.S., Logan, J., Gatley, S.J., Gifford, A., Hitzemann, R., Ding, Y.S., and Pappas, N. (1999b) Prediction of reinforcing responses to psychostimulants in humans by brain dopamine D2 receptor levels. *Am J Psychiatry* 156: 1440–1443.

Volkow, N.D., Wang, G.J., Fowler, J.S., Franceschi, D., Thanos, P.K., Wong, C., Gatley, S.J., Ding, Y.S., Molina, P., Schlyer, D., Alexoff, D., Hitzemann, R., and Pappas, N. (2000) Cocaine abusers show a blunted response to alcohol intoxication in limbic brain regions. *Life Sci* 66: PL161–7.

Volkow, N.D., Wang, G., Fowler, J.S., Logan, J., Gerasimov, M., Maynard, L., Ding, Y., Gatley, S.J., Gifford, A., and Franceschi, D. (2001) Therapeutic doses of oral methylphenidate significantly increase extracellular dopamine in the human brain. *J Neurosci* 21: RC121.

Volkow, N.D., Fowler, J.S., and Wang, G.J. (2002a). Role of dopamine in drug reinforcement and addiction in humans: results from imaging studies. *Behav Pharmacol* 13: 355–366.

Volkow, N.D., Wang, G.J., Fowler, J.S., Thanos, P.K., Logan, J., Gatley, S.J., Gifford, A., Ding, Y.S., Wong, C., and Pappas, N. (2002b) Brain DA D2 receptors predict reinforcing effects of stimulants in humans: replication study. *Synapse* 46: 79–82.

Volkow, N.D., Fowler, J.S., and Wang, G.J. (2003) The addicted human brain: insights from imaging studies. *J Clin Invest* 111: 1444–1451.

Wang, G.J., Volkow, N.D., Fowler, J.S., Cervany, P., Hitzemann, R.J., Pappas, N.R., Wong, C.T., and Felder, C. (1999) Regional brain metabolic activation during craving elicited by recall of previous drug experiences. *Life Sci* 64: 775–784.

Wang, B., Luo, F., Xia, Y.Q., and Han, J.S. (2000) Peripheral electric stimulation inhibits morphine-induced place preference in rats. *Neuroreport* 11: 1017–1020.

Wang, G.J., Volkow, N.D., Thanos, P.K., and Fowler, J.S. (2004) Similarity between obesity and drug addiction as assessed by neurofunctional imaging: a concept review. *J Addict Dis* 23: 39–53.

Wang, S.H., Ostlund, S.B., Nader, K., and Balleine, B.W. (2005) Consolidation and reconsolidation of incentive learning in the amygdala. *J Neurosci* 25: 830–835.

Weinshilboum, R. and Wang, L. (2004) Pharmacogenomics: bench to bedside. *Nat Rev Drug Discov* 3: 739–748.

Weissenborn, R. and Duka, T. (2000) State-dependent effects of alcohol on explicit memory: the role of semantic associations. *Psychopharmacology (Berl)* 149: 98–106.

Weissenborn, R. and Duka, T. (2003) Acute alcohol effects on cognitive function in social drinkers: their relationship to drinking habits. *Psychopharmacology (Berl)* 165: 306–312.

Wesensten, N.J., Belenky, G., Kautz, M.A., Thorne, D.R., Reichardt, R.M., and Balkin, T.J. (2002) Maintaining alertness and performance during sleep deprivation: modafinil versus caffeine. *Psychopharmacology (Berl)* 159: 238–247.

White, N.M. (1989) Reward or reinforcement: what's the difference? *Neurosci Biobehav Rev* 13: 181–186.

Wise, R.A. and Bozarth, M.A. (1987) A psychomotor stimulant theory of addiction. *Psychol Rev* 94: 469–492.

Yerkes, R.M. and Dodson, J.D. (1908) The relation of strength of stimulus to rapidity of habit-formation. *Journal of Comparative Neurology and Psychology* 18: 459–482.

CHAPTER

6

Pharmacology and Treatments

Leslie Iversen, Kelly Morris and David Nutt

1 EXECUTIVE SUMMARY

Science has provided a close-up view of the way in which psychoactive substances, whether illicit, pharmaceutical, or legal and used for recreational purposes, alter brain functioning. In the past four decades, advances in our understanding of the molecular basis of brain functioning have enabled the investigation and the development of psychoactive substances, and neurotransmitter theory and the production of novel psychoactive drugs have expanded almost in parallel. The rate of these advances is now accelerating.

This progress has been accompanied by an increase in problematic psychoactive substance use, mainly substance use disorders that until recently were not usually amenable to drug treatment. Now we are entering an era of multiple drug treatments for substance use disorders – safer alternatives to drugs, agents that block problem drug actions, substances that do both, and therapies to treat the consequences of substance use disorders – which can be administered in conjunction with greater options for psychosocial support and behavioural intervention.

The next two decades could witness a dramatic increase in the number, type, and range of effects of known psychoactive substances. Individuals may employ tailored drug regimens for therapy, prevention, pleasure and enhancement, and combine various types of agents to novel effect. New substances will be developed from various known and possibly novel sources such as the pharmaceutical, chemical and other industries, academic institutions, ethnobotanical sources and illicit and 'underground' sources. These are likely to deliver new products that will increasingly vary in chemical make-up, and potentially in quality and availability. Increased use of psychoactive drugs could be accompanied by increased sophistication in individual and societal attitudes towards alterations in consciousness, such as aspiring to optimise brain functioning.

New treatments and other psychoactive agents promise expanded benefits and harms to society. The advent of effective treatments for substance use disorders will expand available interventions, and may facilitate earlier intervention in problematic drug use. Depending on social perceptions and legal policy, new treatments for substance use disorders (eg vaccines) could also raise the question of whether society is justified in imposing them in a compulsory fashion on affected individuals. The balance of risk in the use of psychoactive substances will depend on external factors (eg controls, availability) and on the properties of individual agents and users. Increased investment of resources and changes in regulatory mechanisms are likely to be needed to maximise the benefits and minimise the harms of current and future psychoactive substances for individuals and society. Despite this, new knowledge will undoubtedly bring unanticipated developments, problems and solutions. The key challenge will continue to be how to use this expansion of psychopharmacology for the most creative and least destructive effects.

2 DEFINITIONS AND SCOPE OF REVIEW

Human psychoactive substance use dates from prehistoric times, and a desire for intoxication may be an innate drive. Although other animals take intoxicants, widespread psychoactive substance use may be a defining feature of humankind (Phillips and Lawton, 2004). This overview focuses on the potential for psychoactive drugs to lead to substance use disorders, and includes illicit, pharmaceutical, legal recreational and other substances. Thus, antidepressants and other psychoactive agents whose adverse effects do not include substance use disorders are not included. The remainder of the review covers biological mechanisms of substance use disorders, and the ways this knowledge informs known and potential treatments for such disorders. We include a summary of the state-of-the-art treatment recommendations from the British Association for Psychopharmacology (BAP; Lingford-Hughes, *et al.*, 2004). Finally, we propose an educated view of the future of problematic drug use, plus possible technologies and other strategies for management.

Terminology in this area is confused, since terms like 'addiction' and 'addicts' are poorly defined and in some quarters stigmatising. Other terms, like 'substance dependence', are better defined and are often used interchangeably. In reality, a spectrum of drug-taking behaviours exists including: appropriate therapeutic use; diversion (non-prescribed use) or other inappropriate use of prescribed agents; self-medication (informal use of drugs to mitigate symptoms); non-problematic recreational use (which may encompass regular use); hazardous drug use and substance misuse; harmful drug use and substance abuse; dependency and addiction (Altman *et al.*, 1996; Meyer, 1996). We have used terminology as indicated in Figure 6.1.

Reward and reinforcement: Drugs taken for pleasure are considered 'rewards' that activate brain reward systems similarly to

may be neuronal or molecular, or psychological and behavioural (Altman *et al.*, 1996).
Withdrawal: Withdrawal encompasses behavioural, psychological and physical symptoms and signs on stopping a drug or with pharmacological blocking of drug action (Altman *et al.*, 1996). Usually withdrawal is an expression of processes that underlie tolerance, but the two states may be differentiated (Nutt, 1994). Physical withdrawal is not a necessary criterion of dependency (American Psychiatric Association, 2000), since some agents, such as antidepressants, are linked with withdrawal symptoms but not dependence (Nutt, 2003a). However, the negative reinforcing aspects of withdrawal often perpetuate or worsen drug-seeking behaviours.
Sensitisation: Several agents engender a progressive increase in effects with repeated administration (also called reverse tolerance) or persistent hypersensitivity due to previous exposure (Altman *et al.*, 1996).
Craving and relapse: These two processes are inter-related, although craving is not essential for relapse, the resumption of drug seeking and use after abstinence. The term 'craving' encompasses subjective desire for the drug, motivation towards drug seeking and avoidance of withdrawal, and behavioural changes. The neurochemical basis of craving is poorly understood, but craving can become conditioned to and elicited by environmental cues related to drug use (eg pubs for alcoholics; injection equipment for heroin users; Altman *et al.*, 1996).

Abuse potential: This is a qualitative measure of the likelihood of a specific agent to lead to dependency and cause harm. Thus, caffeine use is often dependent but usually causes little harm and has low abuse potential. Abuse potential is related to drug factors – agents with faster entry to and exit from the brain plus high efficacy (strong action) have higher abuse potential (Nutt, 1994). Figure 6.2 shows how the form in which the same or similar drugs are taken affects rewarding properties and thus the risk of dependency. The optimum method for determining abuse potential is not known (Kelly *et al.*, 2003), but includes the ability of a drug to maintain self-administration by animals.
Neurotransmitter: any chemical that is released from a neuron into a gap between neurons (synapse) or between a neuron and other cell type to communicate a change in state (excitation or inhibition) to the adjacent cell.

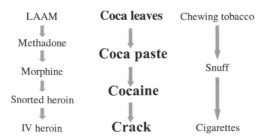

Improving drug effects through applied clinical pharmacology

Faster onset of drug effect = 'better rush'

LAAM	**Coca leaves**	Chewing tobacco
Methadone	**Coca paste**	
Morphine		Snuff
Snorted heroin	**Cocaine**	
IV heroin	**Crack**	Cigarettes

Smoking and IV most rapid = most addictive

...se potential is related to the form of the drug. The chemical make-up and formulation dictate ...o the brain.

Psychoactive drugs: substances that affect brain function through neurotransmitter systems. Actions are described in terms of effects on the synthesis, storage, release, reuptake and metabolism of neurotransmitters and/or by their action at neurotransmitter receptors as follows:

- **Agonist:** any agent that mimics the action of an endogenous neurotransmitter, including the neurotransmitter itself, is an agonist.
- **Antagonist:** an antagonist blocks agonist action but has no intrinsic action itself.
- **Partial agonist:** such substances partly mimic the effects of the neurotransmitter, but in the presence of agonists with greater efficacy, they act as antagonists.
- **Inverse agonist:** for receptor systems that have ongoing (agonist-independent) activity, an inverse agonist will reduce such activity.
- **Ligand:** this is the term for any substance that binds to a receptor.
- **Analogues:** this pharmacological term describes structural relatives of a parent compound.
- **Set and setting:** these lay terms respectively describe aspects of an individual and their environment that impact on psychoactive drug effects.

3 BACKGROUND

Over the past four decades, major advances have occurred in our understanding of brain mechanisms such as the role of neurotransmitters (Snyder, 2002), including those associated with substance use disorders (Robbins *et al.*, 2005). This knowledge has paralleled and influenced psychoactive substance use of all types, with an unprecedented increase in availability of all types of substances. Meanwhile, online technology has enhanced access to both substances and related knowledge of their use, effects and manufacture. Thus, overall drug use is increasing worldwide, with few exceptions. Use of multiple drugs (polypharmacy) is increasing and novel agents are appearing. These changes accompany increases in other excess appetitive behaviours such as overeating and 'Internet addiction' (Orford, 2005).

Already, the concurrent use of several psychoactive substances seems the norm in many populations, and may involve legal recreational substances, illicit drugs, prescription drugs, and other agents (eg herbs and nutrients). Problematic use of multiple substances ('polydrug abuse') seems common in individuals who both do and do not access treatment services. Polydrug abuse may reflect a range of processes, from an individual tendency towards drug taking to the combining of certain substances for specific effects, including alleviation of withdrawal. Common examples include: alcohol with cocaine (synergistic effects); illicit heroin use with prescription methadone (additive); 'speedballs' of heroin plus cocaine (offsetting sedative and stimulant effects); alcohol, cannabis or prescription sedatives taken with or after stimulants and ecstasy (alleviation of overstimulation or 'come-down' effects).

Multiple substance use may also be sequential, with some individuals showing a progression in use through different classes of substances, which also may overlap. For example, alcohol use in young people may predict illicit drug use in later life, while many individuals who abuse illicit drugs in younger years switch to alcohol later, especially if illicit drug use stops. Such patterns could perhaps reflect an underlying neurochemical imbalance (eg untreated anxiety or ADHD). Multiple and sequential drug use are likely to increase harms, complicate treatments and worsen the user's long-term prognosis (Lingford-Hughes *et al.*, 2004; Sumnall *et al.*, 2004).

Internationally, the response to these trends has been diverse and variable according to the substance. Some increased controls have been developed related to tobacco use but not for alcohol. Instead, the availability and relative cheapness of alcoholic drinks has increased, combined with youth marketing (Room, 2005; McKeganey, 2005). For illicit drugs, the UK has until the recent formation of the National Treatment Agency and the Drugs Intervention Programme, focused on reduction of supply as the main means of reducing prevalence, with changes in criminal law enforcement – this is now accompanied by an increasing focus on problematic illicit drug use as a health issue (Room, 2005).

Meanwhile, advances in pharmacology have expanded the drug treatments available for substance use disorders (Lingford-Hughes *et al.*, 2004), including development of partial agonists (eg buprenorphine) and long-acting formulations of known drugs (eg naltrexone). Now, a realisation that treatments developed to target one problem drug may 'cross over' to prove beneficial for other drugs offers new possibilities for treatments. Already, a recognition exists of the potential for tailoring treatments to subgroups and individuals (eg for levels of dependency).

3.1 Psychopharmacology

Psychoactive drugs are known to act through different brain neurotransmitter systems (Figure 6.3).

Currently, at least eight neurotransmitter systems are definitely implicated in drug actions, but the importance of monoamines, particularly dopamine, as a final common pathway underlying drug seeking and craving has become prominent through research (Robbins *et al.*, 2005; Snyder, 2002). Many other systems will probably be found to be involved in drug actions (Snyder, 2002). In addition, some 200 genes in the human genome seem to code for receptors, with functions and ligands that remain to be discovered, known as orphan receptors.

Already, some of the roles of different neurotransmitters in substance use disorders have been disentangled (Nutt *et al.*, 2003; Lingford-Hughes and Nutt, 2003; Lingford-Hughes *et al.*, 2003), although this view is simplistic compared with that likely to be available in 2025 (Robbins *et al.*, 2005). Currently, dependency is viewed as a form of aberrant learning that hijacks brain reward systems formed of two major dopamine pathways (Figure 6.4). Release of mesolimbic dopamine seems to be primarily involved in the anticipation and salience of, and appetite for, rewards such as food or sex and many abused drugs (Schultz, 2001). This system also seems involved in the opposite state, aversion – eg to stressful stimuli. Low function (tone) in this system is a feature of withdrawal (Volkow *et al.*, 1999), and might underpin craving (Lingford-Hughes and Nutt, 2003; Franken, 2003). Mesolimbic nigrostriatal dopamine could be specifically

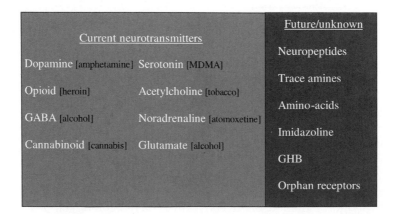

FIGURE 6.3 State of scientific understanding on neurotransmitter targets for psychoactive substances. Examples are given of prototype drugs that act via each known neurotransmitter system, though most psychoactive substances are likely to act via more than one system (eg alcohol acts via GABA, glutamate, and many other systems).

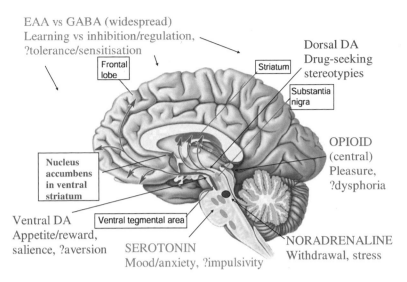

EAA vs GABA (widespread)
Learning vs inhibition/regulation,
?tolerance/sensitisation

Frontal lobe

Striatum

Dorsal DA
Drug-seeking
stereotypies

Substantia nigra

OPIOID
(central)
Pleasure,
?dysphoria

Nucleus
accumbens
in ventral
striatum

Ventral DA
Appetite/reward,
salience, ?aversion

Ventral tegmental area

SEROTONIN
Mood/anxiety, ?impulsivity

NORADRENALINE
Withdrawal, stress

FIGURE 6.4 Pharmacology of dependence – putative neurotransmitter roles. The key neurotransmitter systems are represented stylistically on this brain section, with labels that describe putative roles in symptoms of substance use disorders. For example, dorsal mesolimbic dopamine [= dorsal DA] might be more involved in drug-seeking and other stereotyped actions towards rewards whereas ventral mesolimbic dopamine [= ventral DA] and its cortical projections seem to mediate associative aspects of drug use such as craving elicited by cues.

important in generating drug-seeking stereotyped behaviours.

However, various lines of evidence indicate that the involvement of dopaminergic neurons, receptors and the transporter in drug actions is not as straightforward as previously thought (Bonci *et al.*, 2003; Xu and Zhang, 2004; Budygin *et al.*, 2004; Rocha, 2003). The latest human research suggests that this system could be involved in the ability to generate cycles of learning and consequent behaviour according to beneficial or adverse outcomes (Frank *et al.*, 2004).

Other systems suspected to have key roles in dependency include neural pathways that release opioid neuropeptides, which modulate other neurotransmitter systems, and which may form part of brain pleasure circuits. Three brain receptors recognise opioids – mu, delta and kappa – and recent evidence suggests that these receptors might have distinguishable properties, including enhancement or lack of pleasure and reward-related learning (reinforcement) (Franken, 2003; Contet *et al.*, 2004; Kieffer, 1999).

The balance between diffuse excitatory neurotransmitters like glutamate, and inhibitory ones like GABA and cannabinoids, seems likely to impact on whether an individual learns from an experience or is inhibited from doing so. These systems interact with reward and pleasure systems. So forms of aberrant reward-based learning may underlie symptoms such as craving, tolerance, sensitisation and reinstatement of drug-seeking behaviour (Lingford-Hughes and Nutt, 2003; Lingford-Hughes *et al.*, 2003; Martin *et al.*, 2000). Various neuropeptides that act in emotion-related areas of the brain might have longer-lasting roles in substance use disorders, eg substance P, which seems to mediate some of the pleasurable aspects of opiates and some effects of psychostimulants (Loonam *et al.*, 2003).

The causes and consequences of substance use disorders are becoming clearer. For example, the stress hormone and neurotransmitter noradrenaline and the neuropeptide CRF have been linked with symptoms of withdrawal and the impact that withdrawal and other stressors have on the likelihood of relapse (Shepard *et al.*, 2004; Sinha *et al.*, 2003; Jacobsen *et al.*, 2001). Serotonin is involved in mood and anxiety, and has also been linked with impulsivity, including sensation seeking, as has dopamine (Lingford-Hughes and Nutt, 2003; Lingford-Hughes *et al.*, 2003; Cardinal *et al.*, 2004; Patkar *et al.*, 2003).

4 CURRENT PSYCHOACTIVE DRUGS

4.1 Prevalence

An important step in drafting any response to current and future problematic drug use is to estimate the prevalence of drug use and its associated harms. However, estimation of drug use is difficult, in part because many measures exist, including various crime statistics, seizures of illicit drugs, alcohol and tobacco sales, self-report from several surveys, plus estimates from health services data and death certification. In addition, many data estimates are not sufficiently accurate or responsive, while prevalence is not directly related to the extent of harms and costs (Room, 2005; Godfrey and Cave, 2005).

From available data, cigarette smoking remains stable at 26 per cent of adults in Britain (Office for National Statistics, 2004), with the gap between men and women narrowing. At least 100 000 UK deaths per year are attributed to smoking (Twigg *et al.*, 2004), while lung cancer represents one in five cancer deaths in Europe (Boyle and Ferlay, 2005). Overall, alcohol consumption is rising somewhat, especially in young people and women. Roughly 25 per cent of the English population drink over weekly limits (40 per cent of men and 23 per cent of women in Britain), at least 5 per cent are heavy drinkers, and 7 per cent or more are dependent, with dependent men outnumbering women by more than four to one (Department of Health, 2004; Prime Minister's Strategy Unit, 2004; Lader and Meltzer, 2002). Estimates of directly alcohol-related deaths in England and Wales vary from 5000 to 40 000 per year (Department of Health, 2004; www.drugscope.org.uk), while rates have risen dramatically (Department of Health, 2004). Between 1980 and 2000,

the UK death rate from alcohol-related diseases more than doubled among men and almost doubled among women (Department of Health, 2004).

The British Crime Survey 2002/2003 estimates around four million illicit drug users and around one million Class A drug users, with the majority of people using one type of illicit drug (Condon and Smith, 2003). In 2000, average estimates suggested at least 300 000 problem Class A drug users and under 300 000 injecting opiate users (Godfrey *et al.*, 2002). In 2003 in England and Wales, 2445 deaths related to drugs other than alcohol and tobacco were reported, including 1338 deaths related to illicit drugs, 424 deaths involving antidepressants, 466 involving paracetamol-containing medication, 211 involving benzodiazepine sedatives, and 66 involving other sedatives (Office for National Statistics, 2005). Some deaths involved multiple substances (Office for National Statistics, 2005). Some comparative death statistics are given in Table 6.1.

4.2 Problematic Psychoactive Substances

4.2.1 Tobacco

Cigarette smoking is probably the most harmful use of all psychoactive drugs. Harms extend to those passively exposed to smoke, including the developing foetus. Most smokers are dependent and have a long history of use. Harms include chronic

TABLE 6.1 Drug-related deaths 1997–2002 (www.drugscope.org.uk; England and Wales except where stated).

Tobacco (UK, approximate)	500 000
Alcohol (approximate)	25 000–200 000
Opiates (heroin, morphine and methadone)	6194
Cocaine	508
Amphetamine	436
Solvents (UK)	361
Ecstasy	200

lung disease, increased risk of several cancers, cardiovascular disease, and stroke. Pipe and cigar smoking and oral use of tobacco are also linked with oropharyngeal cancers.

Smoking rates and dependency are greater in people with alcohol problems, and such use negates any health benefits of alcohol and increases many health risks (Romberger and Grant, 2004). Smoking is increased in other substance use disorders, and in several psychiatric disorders – eg schizophrenia, depression – which might represent self-medication with nicotine. Maintenance of high levels of smoking rates in young women has been linked to the appetite suppressant action of tobacco. Any cognitive benefits of nicotine in non-smokers are debatable (Morris *et al.*, 2005a).

Smokeless tobacco products are less harmful than smoked products and induce less dependency – eg snus (snuff placed under the upper lip) has been linked with smoking reduction in Sweden (Tomar *et al.*, 2003). However, these products are not risk-free and may facilitate use of more harmful products, especially when started in childhood (Hatsukami *et al.*, 2004). Medicinal nicotine products are less harmful than smokeless tobacco and have low abuse potential, although dependency has been reported.

Nicotine is widely considered the key addictive substance of some 4000 compounds in cigarette smoke (Harvey *et al.*, 2004). However, other substances in smoke, such as monoamine oxidase inhibitors, are also implicated (Herraiz and Chaparro, 2005; Fowler *et al.*, 2003). Recent research in rodents suggests that acetaldehyde, present in high amounts in tobacco smoke, increases the risk of dependency in adolescent animals (Belluzzi *et al.*, 2004). Menthol, the only publicised additive in cigarettes, increases breath-holding and thus exposure to nicotine, tar, carbon monoxide, and other compounds (Garten and Falkner, 2004). This action increases the likelihood of dependency and the risk of disease.

Nicotine acts on nicotinic acetylcholine receptors, which in turn modulate other neurotransmitter systems, such as dopamine, noradrenaline, and glutamate (Lingford-Hughes and Nutt, 2003; Lingford-Hughes *et al.*, 2003). Changes in mesolimbic dopamine and possibly the release of endogenous opioids are thought to be responsible for the rewarding and pleasurable effects of smoking. Modulation of dopamine circuitry in the prefrontal cortex might be important in learning and in psychiatric diseases such as schizophrenia (George *et al.*, 2000). A role for cannabinoid mechanisms in nicotine craving is suggested by the reported success of a cannabinoid antagonist for smoking cessation (LeFoll and Goldberg, 2004; Lange and Kruse, 2004).

4.2.2 Alcohol

The brain actions of alcohol are numerous and complex (Nutt, 2003b; Oswald and Wand, 2004, Cowen *et al.*, 2004). Binding to certain GABA-A receptors reduces anxiety and motor co-ordination, while effects at NMDA glutamate receptors lead to amnesia and sedation. The rewarding, stimulating and pleasurable effects of alcohol are thought to be due respectively to indirect stimulation of dopamine and noradrenaline circuits plus release of endogenous opioids. CRF is involved in stress-related alcohol consumption, while evidence suggests roles for other neuropeptides, such as urocortin, stresscopin and neuropeptide Y.

In overdose, alcohol causes prolonged opening of the GABA-A receptor, which can paralyse respiratory drive neurons, causing respiratory arrest and death (Nutt, 1999). Long-term alcohol use leads to an imbalance in excitatory and inhibitory systems (Nutt, 1999; De Witte, 2004). In withdrawal, the GABA system is left underfunctioning and the glutamate system is over-excited. GABA hypofunction causes increased anxiety and restlessness, while glutamate over-excitation causes neurons to lose magnesium and gain excess calcium, which can prompt neuronal death, irritability and seizures. This process is exacerbated on subsequent withdrawals, and might if repeated contribute to alcohol-induced brain damage (Nutt, 1999; De Witte, 2004).

Alcohol is considered a 'social lubricant', so it is often (over)used by people with anxiety disorders, such as social phobia, for its anxiolytic effects. However, the overall effect of ongoing use can be an increase in anxiety due to withdrawal effects. Small amounts of alcohol are linked by some studies to reduced cardiovascular disease and overall mortality, especially from middle age onwards. Any excess alcohol is associated with increased cardiovascular disease, liver disease and neurological problems, including cognitive decline (Morris *et al.*, 2005a). Pregnant women who drink more than modest amounts of alcohol increase the risk of miscarriage, while alcohol use can lead to foetal effects, including the most severe form, foetal alcohol syndrome (Farber and Olney, 2003; Mukherjee *et al.*, 2005). Intoxication is associated with large social costs, including accidents, antisocial behaviour, sexual disinhibition or loss of functioning, and relationship breakdown. Alcohol is the drug most associated with aggressive behaviour (Hoaken and Stewart, 2003) and is a key cofactor in deaths from illicit drug use (Office for National Statistics, 2005; Gable, 2004).

4.2.3 Opioids and Opiates

Opiates from *Papaver somniferum* have been found to act on the brain's opioid system. Several synthetic and semi-synthetic agents (eg heroin, fentanyl, pethidine) plus naturally occurring substances (eg codeine, morphine) are available as medicines, mainly for their effective painkilling properties. Analgesia results from rapid, strong binding to μ-opioid brain receptors, which also leads to narcosis (sleepiness) and euphoria, while stimulation of κ receptors produces other adverse effects, such as hallucinations. With repeated use, peaks and troughs of opiate action lead to withdrawal, craving, and drug-seeking behaviour, depending on the rapidity of onset and offset of

drug action (Nutt, 2002). Withdrawal can be severe and can involve marked stress responses, which lead to further drug seeking. Fast-acting opiates or routes of administration (eg intravenous, smoking) reliably lead to dependency when used recreationally, whereas orally ingested opium products and prescription opiate painkillers have less potential for dependency and abuse. When opiates are used in therapeutic contexts, dependency is uncommon.

Exogenous opiates mimic the actions of brain endorphins, which act on opioid receptors, but due to a process known as agonist-directed signalling, regulatory mechanisms to terminate endorphin signalling are less effective with exogenous opiate binding (Contet *et al.*, 2004). The opioid system interacts with many other neurotransmitters, including noradrenaline, acetylcholine, glutamate, GABA and dopamine. Opiates seem to increase the sensitivity of noradrenaline systems to stress responses (Xu *et al.*, 2004), psychostimulants can potentiate the effects of opiates (Dalal and Melrack, 1998), while endogenous cannabinoid (CB1) receptors seem important to mediate the effects of opiates (Solinas *et al.*, 2003). The neuropeptide nociceptin/orphanin FQ seems to be a functional inhibitor of opiate actions (Meis, 2003), while galanin reverses signs of morphine withdrawal (Zachariou *et al.*, 2003).

Potent full opioid agonists such as heroin and methadone can kill in overdose due to respiratory depression, and intravenous heroin has the greatest acute toxicity of common psychoactive drugs (Gable, 2004). Slower-onset agonists (eg codeine) and partial agonists (eg buprenorphine) have lower potential for overdose. Methadone is used as a long-acting heroin substitute in treatment but is implicated in similar numbers of deaths in overdose to heroin (Gable, 2004; Blakemore, 2003) – coadministration of both substances is often a key factor in overdose. Other harms from illicit opiates are mainly related to the use of non-sterile injection syringes and needles, which carry risks including septicaemia, HIV and hepatitis C.

Use in pregnancy can lead to withdrawal in the neonate.

The use of prescription opiates for non-medical purposes is thought to be possibly as common as illicit heroin use in the US (Zacny et al., 2003). Rates are thought to be far lower in the UK but are probably rising, in part due to online availability. Risk of dependency is related to action and formulation – patches (eg fentanyl), longer-acting or partial agonists (eg buprenorphine) and slower-delivery formulations (eg of oxycodone) are less likely to produce euphoria and thus lead to dependency, but such drugs may be administered in non-indicated ways (eg by being crushed and then snorted or injected intravenously) to enhance their euphoric effects.

4.2.4 Cocaine and Other Psychostimulants

Cocaine, including crack, and other classes of psychostimulants such as amphetamines, directly interact with brain dopamine systems to produce psychomotor stimulation and rewarding properties (Everitt, 2002). Amphetamines enhance dopamine release by reversing the action of the dopamine transporter (DAT), while cocaine and others block DAT and thus dopamine reuptake (Kahlig and Galli, 2003). Psychostimulants also interact with noradrenaline and serotonin, which might explain psychostimulant effects in the absence of DAT (Budygin et al., 2004; Raha, 2003). Some responses to these drugs can increase with repeated exposure (sensitisation), perhaps due to aberrant glutamate signalling.

Psychostimulant effects, which can be exploited for therapeutic effects (Morris et al., 2005a), include increased wakefulness, attention, increased energy and reduced appetite, while various classes have other properties, for example, cocaine is a local anaesthetic. Acute psychostimulant toxicity includes hyperthermia, cardiovascular problems, and seizures, especially in vulnerable individuals. Longer-term, high-dose

amphetamines in particular are linked with possible neurotoxicity, cognition disorders and psychosis (Reneman, 2003; Nordahl et al., 2003). Long-term toxicity also includes cardiovascular and cerebrovascular disease, including stroke. Use in pregnancy can lead to withdrawal in the neonate and possibly birth defects.

Psychostimulants are found more rewarding by people with lower brain levels of dopamine-D2 receptors (Volkow et al., 1999). Long-term use reduces DAT levels and prefrontal cortex activity (Everitt, 2002; Kahlig and Galli, 2003), which may enhance risk taking and drug seeking and cause cognitive changes such as reduced decision-making ability. These changes might also increase sexual and other risk taking. Psychostimulant withdrawal leads to disruptions in mood, motivation and potentially hostility, although the relation with aggression is not straightforward (Hoaken and Stewart, 2003). These effects may be mediated in part by increased neuronal excitability and neurotoxicity (Cadet et al., 2003; McCann and Ricaurte, 2004).

The potential for dependency is increased with intravenous use or with smokable forms (eg crack cocaine and methamphetamine ('ice')). Psychostimulants with slower onset of actions such as oral methylphenidate and atomoxetine are less rewarding, and are used for beneficial cognitive and behavioural effects in disorders such as ADHD (Morris et al., 2005a; Kollins et al., 2001; Kollins, 2003). Use of such substances in ADHD is likely to reduce rather than increase subsequent illicit drug use (Wilens, 2001; Biederman, 2003; Faraone and Wilens, 2003; Fischer and Barkley, 2003). However, use of such agents in rodents without ADHD-type deficits has variable and sometimes deleterious effects on brain reward systems, emphasising the need to use such treatments only in people who fit ADHD diagnostic criteria (Bolanos et al., 2003, Carlezon et al., 2003; Brandon et al., 2003; Morris, 2004). The abuse potential of legal psychostimulants depends on the potency and rapidity of drug action, with dopamine releasers more of a concern than reuptake inhibitors. Increasing diversion of medical supplies with use via non-indicated routes is another concern (eg injection or intranasal use of methylphenidate). Newer formulations (eg gel-filled methylphenidate capsules) are designed to reduce such problems.

4.2.5 Ecstasy (MDMA) and Other 'Designer Drugs'

The many so-called designer drugs related to ecstasy (often grouped together as amphetamine-type substances) are taken for their stimulant and mild hallucinogenic properties (Shulgin and Shulgin, 1991). Their effects range from those with mostly psychostimulant properties to those with mostly hallucinogenic properties, presumably dependent on their individual underlying mechanisms. MDMA is most extensively researched, and acts predominantly to block serotonin uptake and enhance release, but also via the dopamine, noradrenaline and possibly other systems (Shulgin and Shulgin, 1991; Liechti and Vollenweider, 2000; Vollenweider and Liechti, 2000; Simantov, 2004).

Use of MDMA and some analogues is widespread though few harmful effects are reported, with notable exceptions such as idiosyncratic toxicity, hyperthermia and effects due to excess serotonin, called serotonin syndrome, liver damage and post-intoxication mood instability (Iversen, 2002). Rare deaths have occurred with MDMA, MDEA, MDA, PMA, and 2CT7, although the extensive usage of these drugs with few mishaps plus other data indicate they are less acutely toxic than classic psychostimulants, opiates or alcohol (Office for National Statistics, 2005; Gable, 2004; Cole and Sumnall, 2003). Notably, the majority of deaths related to ecstasy have been associated with other psychoactive drug use, particularly opiates (Schifano et al., 2003). Physical harms of ecstasy and other designer drugs are likely to be related to the degree of their psychostimulant effects together with

pre-existing vulnerability. Other factors that might increase risk of harms include overheating, extreme exercise, dehydration or, rarely, water intoxication, and concomitant use of other drugs, especially opiates or alcohol (Morris, 1998).

MDMA has been the cause of much debate over its potential for long-term neurotoxicity of brain serotonin neurons, as seen with high doses in animal models (Morris, 1998, 2003a; Boot et al., 2000). Such studies have implicated hyperthermia, loss of temperature regulation and dosing interval in determining neurotoxicity (Green et al., 2004; Sanchez et al., 2004; Saadat et al., 2005; O'shea et al., 2005). Imaging studies in human users have produced varied results, from minor deficits that resolve within weeks to substantial long-term effects (Reneman, 2003), while the psychological symptoms that occur in current and abstinent users often predate MDMA use (Lieb et al., 2002; Lyle and Cadet, 2003). Nevertheless, it seems probable that a minority of heavy, frequent users with vulnerability (eg women) could experience long-term neurotoxicity, though a substantial public-health risk seems unlikely. Use in pregnancy might lead to emotional changes in children, if rodent studies are confirmed in humans (Lyle and Cadet, 2003) – this effect is also seen with SSRIs (Ansorge et al., 2004). Other potential harms include immunosuppression (Connor, 2004) and possible increased sexual risk behaviours (Lyle and Cadet, 2003).

MDMA was used in the 1960s as a tool to aid psychotherapy – and, recently, two trials on its use have been approved in the USA – to investigate use in conjunction with psychotherapy for post-traumatic stress disorder, and for anxiety in terminal cancer patients (Phillips and Lawton, 2004; Check, 2004; Morgan, 2005).

4.2.6 Dissociative Anaesthetics

Certain substances combine anaesthetic with hallucinogenic properties; eg non-competitive NMDA antagonists ketamine and PCP, which produce states similar to schizophrenia (Pietraszek, 2003). The use of ketamine as a club drug may be increasing, especially in combination with other substances such as cocaine. Dissociative anaesthetics have potential for dependency, while other harms are related to reduced levels of consciousness during acute intoxication such as their use to facilitate sexual assault. PCP intoxication also has a possible relationship to violence (Hoaken and Stewart, 2003). Both agents may be harmful to the developing foetal brain (Farber and Olney, 2003). Ketamine has been used therapeutically to treat alcohol dependence, especially in Russia, and is now used in healthy volunteers as an experimental model of schizophrenia.

4.2.7 Gamma-hydroxybutyrate (GHB) and Precursors

GHB is an endogenous molecule synthesised from GABA, while exogenous GHB can be produced from solvent precursors 1-butanediol and butyrolactone. Exogenous GHB appears to affect inhibitory brain neurotransmitter systems over a short timescale, probably via GABA production, GABA-B receptor binding, and the putative GHB system (Wong et al., 2004). Acute use leads in a dose-dependent fashion to relaxation, euphoria and increased disinhibition, poor co-ordination, amnesia, sleep and then coma. Acute toxicity in overdose is high, especially with concomitant alcohol use (Gable, 2004; Gonzales and Nutt, 2005). The drug has been utilised, especially with alcohol, to facilitate sexual assault. GHB has dependency potential, leading to a withdrawal syndrome similar to and sometimes more severe than that of alcohol (Gonzales and Nutt, 2005; McDonough et al., 2004). Sold as sodium oxybate, the agent has been used for anaesthesia and now is used to promote night-time sleep for patients with narcolepsy. GHB has been used as a treatment for alcohol and opiate dependence and might be neuroprotective.

4.2.8 Inhalants

Various substances are inhaled for psychoactive effects, including solvents (eg lighter fuel, toluene and petrol), gases (eg nitrous oxide) and nitrites (eg amyl nitrite). Intermittent use may be widespread but dependency occurs mainly in certain subpopulations, including 'antisocial' young men sniffing glue, nitrite use in gay culture, and petrol abuse among marginalised aboriginal populations. These subpopulations may be overlooked yet at risk of psychiatric disorders, abuse of other drugs, and possibly crime (d'Abbs and Brady, 2004; Sakai et al., 2004; Walker et al., 2004; Putnins, 2003). One concern is that inhalant use may increase in situations where other drugs are unavailable or unaffordable. All substances carry risks of unpredictable acute and more predictable long-term toxicity. For example, solvent use carries risks such as accidents, including fires, and liver and neurological damage, while any prolonged exposure might be harmful to the developing foetus. Nitrous oxide is available in 'gas and air' for obstetric use, and has been used in alcohol withdrawal.

4.2.9 Other Hallucinogens

Numerous natural products such as peyote and 'magic mushrooms', and synthetic substances (eg LSD) are used traditionally (including for religious purposes) and recreationally to alter psychological functioning in ways described as psychedelic – 'mind-manifesting' – and hallucinogenic – 'mind-wandering'. Actions may include the enhancement as well as distortion of perceptions and other cognitive and emotional processes, which vary greatly according to set and setting. The physical toxicity of many of these compounds is very low, while tolerance is often rapid and profound, though short-lived (Gable, 2004; Nicholls, 2004; Hasler et al., 2004).

Anxiety, panic attacks and other psychological distress may occur during intoxication in vulnerable people, though effects rarely persist. Unknown ingestion is almost always a distressing experience. Other harms can result from loss of self-protective abilities during severe intoxication, and toxicity may occur, most often due to mistaken identification (eg *Amanita* species) or the use of plants from the Deadly Nightshade family such as species of *Datura*. Rarely, use has been linked with intermittent or persistent perceptual changes in the absence of the drug, termed 'flashbacks,' and hallucinogen persisting perceptual disorder, although their existence is controversial since such state-specific recall can occur in non-drug-related circumstances (Halpern and Pope, 2003).

Many hallucinogens act as serotonin-2A receptor partial agonists, while specific cellular molecules and other neurotransmitter systems seem likely to be involved in their effects (Nicholls, 2004; Shulgin and Shulgin, 1997; Aghajanian and Marek, 1999). Known and novel hallucinogens are a potential source for development of new psychoactive agents for therapeutic, research and recreational purposes (Nicholls, 2004). A trial of *psilocybin* for anxiety in terminal cancer patients was recently approved by the FDA while a trial of its use for obsessive-compulsive disorder is ongoing (Phillips and Lawton, 2004; Morgan, 2005).

4.2.10 Cannabis

Products from plants of the *Cannabis* genus are widely ingested, usually as smoke and sometimes as food products. The status of such products in the Misuse of Drugs Act 1971 was recently down-scheduled to Class C, reflecting the extensive evidence that suggests lower potential for harms with moderate usage than most other recreational psychoactive drugs (Iversen, 2001, 2003; Hall and Pacula, 2003). Cannabis products have low acute toxicity (Gable, 2004), although panic and anxiety or acute psychosis can sometimes occur. Cannabis use early in life is linked with subsequent psychotic symptoms and psychosis, especially in heavy users and people with predisposed vulnerability (Henquet *et al.*, 2005; Smit *et al.*, 2004; Verdoux and Tournier, 2004). People with certain psychological symptoms might also self-medicate with cannabis (Degenhardt *et al.*, 2003a; Nowak, 2004).

Young, heavy users of cannabis may experience reduced motivation and achievement, plus mood disorders (Patton *et al.*, 2002; Degenhardt *et al.*, 2003b) although the causality in this relation is uncertain (Iversen, 2002; MacLeod *et al.*, 2004). Cannabis use might increase the likelihood of smoking tobacco in youth (Amos *et al.*, 2004) but does not seem to be a 'gateway' to other drug use. In humans, a minority of individuals who use cannabis heavily will develop other substance use disorders, probably reflecting a common predisposition (Amos *et al.*, 2004; Agrawal *et al.*, 2004) plus the fact that cannabis is often sold alongside other illicit drugs. Dependency may occur in around one in ten users (Iversen, 2002), or 1.5 per cent or more of adults (Swift *et al.*, 2001) and withdrawal is characterised by labile mood and hostility (Hoaken and Stewart, 2003). Many dependent cannabis users do not desire to completely stop use of the drug.

The main active principle in cannabis, THC, acts on endogenous cannabinoid receptors – CB1 receptors in the brain, and CB2 receptors in immune cells and other peripheral sites. Endogenous cannabinoids occur naturally in the brain and inhibit neurotransmitter release directly or indirectly – eg via hippocampal GABA neurons that also contain the neuropeptide cholecystokinin (Iversen, 2003). Cannabinoid receptor stimulation probably has reciprocal effects on opioid and monoamine systems (Chichewicz, 2004; Maldonado and Fonseca, 2002; Van der Stelt and Di Marzo, 2003). In addition, a study in adolescent rats suggests that regular adolescent cannabinoid use might encourage neuronal adaptation that leads to cross-tolerance to morphine, cocaine and amphetamine (Pistis *et al.*, 2004). Together such studies could indicate that cannabis use at a vulnerable age might alter pleasure/reward signalling.

The therapeutic benefits of cannabis have been documented regularly, and many people with multiple sclerosis (MS) and epilepsy, in particular, use cannabis (British Medical Association, 1997; Joy *et al.*, 1999; Wingerchuck, 2004). A herbal cannabis extract in a sublingual spray is being considered for approval as a medicine for the treatment of MS and chronic pain in the UK. Current research focuses on the function of individual natural and synthetic cannabinoids, which could include analgesia, anti-inflammatory and anti-allergy effects, sedation, improvement of mood, neuroprotection, and anti-cancer effects. THC is available as the approved drug dronabinol for the treatment of nausea and weight loss, while other natural cannabinoids such as cannabidiol may prove useful for neuroprotection, stroke and seizures. Cannabinoids might prove helpful for selective forgetting. (Morris *et al.*, 2005a; Marsicano *et al.*, 2002; Wilson and Nicoll, 2002). Synthetic cannabinoids aim to isolate therapeutic properties without problematic effects, eg ajulemic acid, a novel painkiller (Burstein *et al.*, 2004).

4.2.11 Benzodiazepine Agonists and Other Sedatives

Benzodiazepines and other drugs that act on GABA-A receptors tend to have both anxiolytic and sedative properties (Nutt and Malizia, 2001). Prescription of these agents fell after their potential for dependency was revealed and stricter controls introduced. However, long-term prescription use, especially of hypnotics (Mendelson *et al.*, 2004), and problematic use, including self-medication via diversion or online pharmacies, seem likely to be increasing, despite the potential for rapid tolerance and dependency with these agents. Acute toxicity, which can lead to death in overdose, may be linked with intravenous administration and coadministration with other drugs, especially sedatives such as opiates and alcohol. With long-term use, resurgence of original cognitive and other symptoms can occur despite continued ingestion of the drug, which can prompt dosage increases and other sedative use. Withdrawal is often unpleasant, involving insomnia, exaggerated stress responses, cognitive difficulties, and possibly aggression (Hoaken and Stewart,

2003; Wichniak *et al.*, 2004; Barker *et al.*, 2004). The non-benzodiazepine hypnotics (i.e. zaleplon, zolpidem, zopiclone) also act at GABA-A receptors and can lead to tolerance and dependency, though less often than benzodiazepines. Barbiturates are rarely prescribed but are highly toxic in overdose.

4.2.12 Other Agents

Various other agents that can be abused have psychoactive properties. One key class is hormone-based agents such as anabolic steroids, which are used widely (eg by bodybuilders) outside of medical contexts. Although not traditionally considered psychoactive, such agents may have problematic psychoactive effects in addition to adverse physical effects. Anabolic steroids may increase aggression and lead to other symptoms, such as fatigue, on withdrawal.

A growing diversity of psychoactive plant products are increasingly available, partly because of globalisation. Such 'herbal highs' show a similar variety of properties to other psychoactive substances (Carlini, 2003), eg stimulants such as khat (*Catha edulis*) and Ephedra species, psychedelics such as morning glory (Ipomoea species) and *Salvia divinorum*, sedatives such as kratom (*Mitragyna speciosa*) and Valeriana species, and others including some with mood-altering or aphrodisiac properties. Such products may interact with other drugs and can differ widely in safety aspects. For example, plant psychostimulants can induce dependency but range in toxicity and abuse potential from low (eg caffeine) to potentially high in vulnerable individuals (eg khat). Psychoactive plants are a likely source of novel compounds (Nicholls, 2004; Sheffler and Roth, 2003).

5 DRUG TREATMENTS FOR SUBSTANCE USE DISORDERS

Drug treatments for substance use disorders are relatively recent, partly due to concerns over giving drugs to people with drug problems. In any case, few treatments have been available until recently (Lingford-Hughes et al., 2004; Pouletty, 2004). However, increased understanding of problem drug mechanisms has led to an expansion in potential pharmacological treatments. Current treatments work mainly as agonists, substituting a less hazardous compound that acts similarly to the problem drug, or antagonists, which block the effects of a drug, thus leading to reduced use by a process called extinction. By contrast, disulfiram disrupts a step in the breakdown of the problem drug (alcohol), leading to symptoms of intolerance. Bupropion and buprenorphine act at key receptors, in different ways, to stabilise the tone of the neurotransmitter system and to block the action of the problem drug if administered. Harms of drug treatment include side-effects of agents, plus the diversion and misuse of agents, which occur mainly with benzodiazepines, methadone and buprenorphine. Agonist activity can lead to abuse of the treatment agent whereas antagonist action can precipitate withdrawal from the problem drug.

The BAP has published guidelines on the treatment of common substance use disorders (Lingford-Hughes et al., 2004). The mainstay of much treatment is psychosocial and behavioural intervention (Drummond and Curran, 2005). Pharmacological treatment is likely to be best delivered in the context of such support since it may improve drug treatment compliance and outcomes. Conversely, drug treatments might facilitate the effectiveness of psychosocial treatments – for example, to provide a window of opportunity from craving or withdrawal to allow psychosocial interventions and behaviour change to take effect.

Evidence-based drug treatments recommended by the BAP are summarised in Table 6.2 (Lingford-Hughes et al., 2004). This summary does not reflect the complete guidelines, which need to be interpreted within the context of new evidence, specific services and individual patients. For example, treatment of alcohol withdrawal

needs adjustment according to local formularies and estimation of individual liver capacity. For treatment of opiate dependency, patients prefer agonist and partial agonist effects rather than antagonists (Nutt, 2002) although these are often beneficial in restricted groups whose members have access to the drug, such as doctors or pharmacists. Other treatments are used for selected patients, particularly for treatment of comorbid psychiatric disorders, eg SSRIs. Drug treatments not shown in Table 6.2 lack a suitable evidence base. However, preliminary evidence points to efficacy of injectable heroin (diamorphine) for opiate dependency; disulfiram, amphetamines and bromocriptine for psychostimulant dependency; buprenorphine for polydrug dependency (eg opiates and cocaine); antiepileptic agents for various drugs, including sedatives, opiates, cocaine and GHB; SSRIs to block acute effects of MDMA, and possibly treat subsequent mood instability; and serotonin-3 antagonists (eg ondansetron) for alcohol dependency (Lingford-Hughes et al., 2004; Franken, 2003; Liechti and Vollenweider, 2000; Johnson et al., 2000).

The aims of treatment services (Lingford-Hughes et al., 2004) usually include:

- management of withdrawal symptoms;
- reduction of harms associated with drug use promotion and maintenance of absence;
- management of complications of drug use.

Since dependency is a chronic, relapsing condition, interventions too usually need to be chronic or repeated, if necessary for use of other agents. Although such treatments can be characterised by poor compliance and high rates of relapse, substantial beneficial outcomes both on drug-taking and related problem behaviours such as crime are now documented (Gossop et al., 2001). Rates of improvement, remission and relapse are comparable to those seen with other psychiatric disorders. Moreover, poor treatment compliance and relapse are seen in many chronic illnesses (eg hypertension, diabetes), and service frameworks for substance use

TABLE 6.2 Evidence-based drug treatments for substance use disorders – based on British Association of Psychopharmacology guidelines (Lingford-Hughes *et al.*, 2004)

Target drug	Therapeutic agent and mechanism	Indications
Alcohol	Benzodiazepines, eg chlordiazepoxide, diazepam – direct GABA agonists	1. Withdrawal symptoms 2. Seizures – prevention and treatment 3. Delirium – prevention and treatment
	Antiepileptic agents, eg carbamazepine – GABA promoters and other less well-characterised mechanisms	1. Withdrawal symptoms 2. Seizure prevention
	Acamprosate – effects on glutamate receptors that reduce withdrawal-related neuronal excitation and neurotoxicity	Maintenance of abstinence/relapse prevention
	Naltrexone – opioid antagonist	Maintenance of abstinence/relapse prevention (though not licensed for this use in the UK)
	Disulfiram – aldehyde dehydrogenase inhibitor that allows build-up of the toxic breakdown product acetaldehyde	Supervised use for maintenance of abstinence/relapse prevention
	Selective serotonin reuptake inhibitors (SSRIs)	1. Maintenance of abstinence/relapse prevention in late-onset alcoholics 2. Treatment of co-morbid depression in selected patients
	Thiamine – vitamin supplement	1. Prevention of neurological complications 2. Treatment of Wernicke's encephalopathy
Benzo-diazepines	Carbamazepine – modulates sodium channels and affects neurotransmission	Prevention and treatment of withdrawal in selected patients
Nicotine	Nicotine replacement therapy – nicotine agonists	Smoking cessation – maintenance therapy
	Bupropion – monoamine, especially dopamine, reuptake inhibitor	Smoking cessation
Opiates	Methadone – opioid agonist	1. Withdrawal symptoms 2. Maintenance therapy
	Buprenorphine – opioid μ receptor partial agonist, κ antagonist	Withdrawal symptoms
	Clonidine and lofexidine – alpha2-adrenoreceptor agonists	Withdrawal symptoms
	Naltrexone	Relapse prevention in selected patients

disorders could benefit from being based on those used for other chronic disorders. This recognition may also reduce the stigma associated with dependency and its treatment.

6 FUTURE PSYCHOACTIVE SUBSTANCES

If current trends continue until 2025, we can expect the expansion of neurosciences and related technologies to be coupled with increasing public interest in altering brain functioning for the treatment of impairments, for pleasure and recreation, and for enhancement. There will probably be more psychoactive substances, while the boundaries between categories of usage – pleasure and recreation, therapeutic use, and enhancement – are likely to become more blurred than they are already. Developments in knowledge will probably be rapid and profound, while its application will be dependent on the context in which this knowledge is applied.

6.1 Scientific and Clinical Context

The following trends are under way and seem likely to continue:

- knowledge of neurotransmitter and receptor systems and their correlates in terms of cognition, mood, behaviour etc., will expand (Robbins *et al.*, Chapter 3; Sahakian *et al.*, Chapter 5)
- increasing sophistication in understanding actions of drugs on the brain will expand development of the new speciality of psychopharmacology
- identification of genes important in drug actions, drug metabolism, substance use disorders and therapeutic responses will offer hope of tailoring therapies to individuals (pharmacogenomics); gaining further insights into biological mechanisms of dependency; and developing new therapies (Ball *et al.*, Chapter 4)
- improved imaging of function, including drug actions, in living human brains

will permit research on the brain circuitry and changes in receptor and transporter densities linked with dependency and other symptoms. Such technology could eventually be used to tailor treatments to their associated neurochemical deficits (Garavan *et al.*, Chapter 9)
- wider availability of drug testing and psychological screening are already mooted and could permit identification of those engaging in or at risk of problematic use (Curran and Drummond, Chapter 7; Cowan *et al.*, Chapter 10)
- services for substance use disorders are anticipating improved use of existing interventions, including medications, and the development of new treatments. The hope is that this broadening array of interventions will be available within higher-quality treatment services that can combine the most effective medications with psychosocial support and behavioural therapy regimes (Chapter 7).

6.2 Socioeconomic Drivers

A broader discussion of social and economic drivers of changing drug use and its management is covered elsewhere (Room, Chapter 11; McKeganey *et al.*, Chapter 12; Cave and Godfrey, Chapter 13). Important trends are related directly to psychoactive substances:

- Overall, prevalence is rising worldwide, with known abusive drugs remaining the key problem. If current UK trends and policies continue for 20 years, smoking prevalence and deaths may fall somewhat, while alcohol consumption could reach among the highest in Europe (Prime Minister's Strategy Unit, 2004), with effects on health and other consequences. Bloodborne infections from intravenous drug use also will continue to rise. Prevalence of other drug use is likely to continue to vary, both up and down in different time periods, depending on the substance, though with current trends, deaths due to other drugs could fall further (Office for

National Statistics, 2005). However, such trends can change rapidly (Bush *et al.*, 2004).

- Increased online availability of prescription drugs and other substances plus information on the use and manufacture of drugs is making control of supply increasingly difficult. Rising off-label use of prescription drugs and illicit diversion seem likely to continue (Room, Chapter 9; McKeganey, this volume).

- Concomitant use of several psychoactive substances is becoming increasingly common and can involve all types of substances. Such polypharmacy may make successful treatment more difficult and increases the likelihood of adverse interactions. In the future, a widening range of novel psychoactive agents plus increasing polypharmacy will present new challenges to health services.

- The availability of a range of cognition-enhancing drugs and other enhancement techniques, such as the wider use of performance enhancers in sport, could lead to increased acceptance of enhancement, which could alter attitudes to recreational psychoactive substance use (Jones *et al.*, Chapter 8).

- Psychoactive substance development and production is a growth area that is likely to continue to expand. Markets for herbs and other plant-based products are expanding, while pharmaceutical companies are seeking markets for their products beyond standard therapeutic markets (eg with 'lifestyle agents' for baldness, obesity and sexual dysfunction). These industries are likely to want to target the potential market of healthy consumers with recreational and enhancement techniques.

6.3 Substances and Sources

The number of psychoactive substances in human use has expanded at growing rates throughout history (Shulgin, 2004). Thus by 2025, a large number of new psychoactive substances are likely to be discovered. The probable sources of these substances are similar to those of today (Figure 6.5) but there may be unanticipated sources.

Approaches to the development of new psychoactive substances will include known and developing technologies, such as the isolation of new natural products, including neurotransmitters; synthesis of analogues or combinations of known compounds; agents selected or designed for specific functions (eg receptor binding by rational drug design); and new strategies, such as protein- and peptide-based agents, cellular products, and proteomic and genomic interventions (eg gene therapy, anti-sense approaches

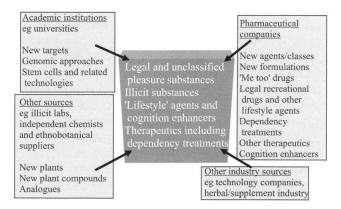

FIGURE 6.5 Predicted future sources for knowledge and development of psychoactive substances. Novel sources might also arise (eg food and chemical industries).

to inactivate cellular material containing instructions to make proteins) (Robbins *et al.*, 2005; Pembury *et al.*, 2005; Williams *et al.*, 2004). Developers of psychoactive drugs will continue to look to developments in other fields to inform drug development, a process encouraged by information technology.

Future drug development is likely to follow similar models to today. Novel psychoactive plants and other substances will be investigated, including those used by indigenous peoples, new psychoactive compounds will be isolated or synthesised and new analogues derived, which may be combined with known substances or components. Recreational drug manufacture is likely to occur in illicit laboratories, but therapeutic agents will continue to be diverted for recreational purposes from pharmaceutical and other companies, which could begin to manufacture pleasure agents. Illicit manufacture might increasingly occur in small laboratories, with growing diversity of products and quality, and potential for environmental damage. Pharmaceutical companies will expand their portfolios with new targets, new agents for old targets, and whole new areas such as cognition-enhancing drugs. Academic institutions will continue to identify new targets and strategies. Major developments in gene-related and stem-cell technologies seem likely, which ultimately may be brought to market by 'spin-off' technology companies.

New forms of known agents such as antidepressants, painkillers and pleasure drugs, and novel classes, are likely to be described and used, perhaps according to their effects on neurotransmitter systems (Robbins *et al.*, 2005; Morris *et al.*, 2005a). One prominent underground chemist has predicted that around 2000 psychedelic compounds alone will be available by 2050 (Shulgin, 2004). New drugs will include effective analogues that can be anticipated to some extent from current pharmacology (eg Shulgin and Shulgin, 1991, 1997) and new psychoactive agents. New pharmaceutical leads already include appetite modulators, for weight loss and enhancement of sexual functioning, and skin-tanning agents; one drug class in development – the melanocortins – seem to promote weight loss, enhance libido, and tan skin simultaneously (Morris, 2003b).

The publication pattern of drug-development knowledge means that it is hard to predict what agents will be available by 2025. We can anticipate developments in where data are published, plus some developments from current science on neuropeptides, genomic approaches, stem cells, neurogenesis and nanotechnology. We cannot predict unexpected successes or failures that are likely to occur in development, but we can predict that only a minority of pharmaceutical drug leads will reach the market, as is the norm for drug development. The current aim and thus the future likelihood is that new therapeutic, lifestyle and pleasure drugs will be better designed to minimise toxicity, dependency and abuse potential.

7 FUTURE THERAPEUTICS

Trends in psychopharmacological research suggest that the next 20 years are likely to bring a large expansion in the types of strategies to prevent and treat substance use disorders, some specific to a problem drug and some generic. Developments in related fields will mean that such therapies are likely to be delivered in the context of an increased understanding of appropriate psychosocial and behavioural interventions and the targeting of treatments to individual symptoms (Drummond and Curran, 2005). New classes of drug treatments will be produced, in terms of action (eg partial inverse agonists, stem-cell replacement), targets (eg neuropeptides, genomic targets) and new formulations (eg patches, nasal sprays, nanoparticles). Increased understanding of the 'downstream' events that occur after receptor binding may allow different molecular pathways inside neurons to be exploited (Robbins *et al.*, 2005).

High-throughput technologies, such as genomics and proteomics, promise to revolutionise the pace and breadth of scientific investigation into the causes, consequences and treatment of substance use disorders (Pembury *et al.*, 2005; Williams *et al.*, 2004). Since individuals vary in their responses to abused drugs and treatments, due in part to genetic variations in key enzymes, pharmacogenomics is likely to prove helpful to tailor certain drug treatments to individuals by 2025 (Pembury *et al.*, 2004). Other techniques developed to manipulate matter at molecular scale and below (nanotechnology) could bring unanticipated developments.

Therapeutic strategies will probably include:

- Agents targeted at specific drug use, including:

  o *alcohol* – eg GABA-A and GABA-B enhancing agents,
  o *tobacco* – eg nicotinic antagonists,
  o *opiates* – eg new formulations of opioid-modulating drugs.
  o *cocaine and other psychostimulants* – eg dopamine-D3 receptor antagonists and partial agonists, dopamine-reuptake inhibitors,
  o *cannabis*– eg CB1 receptor blockers,
  o *other approaches* including active vaccination against nicotine, cocaine and possibly other drugs.

- Interventions with generic actions to modify excess appetitive behaviour, including:

  o learning and anti-learning agents that undo conditioning to external cues (eg association of alcohol with pubs, heroin with needles),
  o drugs acting on inhibitory systems, such as GABA and cannabinoids, that might regulate the switch from normal to dependent states,
  o anti-stress/anxiety drugs, which might reduce important factors in relapse,
  o agents that target and modulate brain reward and pleasure circuits,
  o gene-silencing or turn-on agents (eg for endorphins, dynorphins and other

peptides involved in drug dependency; Pembury *et al.*, 2005),
  o brain stimulation (Robbins *et al.*, 2005) and psychological approaches (Drummond and Curran, 2005; Sahakian *et al.*, 2005).

7.1 Specific Targets

This overview of treatments includes agents in development for specific substance use indications (Pouletty, 2004; www.phrma. org/newmedicines). Many of these may ultimately be found to act on generic circuitry involved in substance use disorders, and thus may cross over for use in other abused drugs.

7.1.1 Tobacco

In addition to known medications (Roddy, 2004; George and O'Malley, 2004), three novel strategies are in clinical studies for tobacco smoking cessation – vaccines, rimonabant and varenicline. Nicotine vaccines produce antibodies that bind nicotine in the bloodstream and thus reduce entry to the brain (Bunce *et al.*, 2003). This 'blockade' is thought to reduce the subjective effects of smoking. The vaccine TA-NIC now is in a phase II trial of 60 smokers, with promising early findings. The nicotine partial agonist varenicline currently is in phase III trials, with about 50 per cent cessation rates in earlier trials.

The cannabinoid-1 receptor antagonist rimonabant (SR141716) has shown promise as an anti-smoking treatment in late clinical trials (LeFoll *et al.*, 2004; Lange and Kruse, 2004; Nutt, 2005). This strategy is also one of several generic approaches that have been proposed for smoking (Cryan *et al.*, 2003). Others include dopamine-D3 receptor partial agonists, noradrenaline reuptake inhibitors, GABA-B receptor agonists, metabotropic glutamate-5 receptor (mGluR5) antagonists, and CRF1 receptor antagonists.

7.1.2 Alcohol

Improvements in abstinence from drinking with acamprosate and naltrexone have prompted further investigation of their use, alone and in combination (Carmen *et al.*, 2004; Soyka and Chick, 2003; Mann *et al.*, 2004; Kiritze-Topor *et al.*, 2004; Kiefer and Wiedemann, 2004). Since naltrexone seems to block the pleasurable effects of alcohol, its use may be warranted in problem drinkers who continue to use alcohol intermittently (Soyka and Chick, 2003). Long-acting formulations of naltrexone that can be administered monthly are in development to improve compliance compared with oral naltrexone (Pouletty, 2004). A naltrexone depot injection (Kranzler, 2000; Modesto-Lowe, 2002) and sustained-release oral naltrexone are both in phase III trials (Pouletty, 2004; www.phrma.org/newmedicines).

Agents that act at NMDA and other glutamate receptors seem to have specific beneficial actions in alcohol dependence to ameliorate the effects of withdrawal, in addition to generic effects on learning and sensitisation. Acamprosate may act via binding to NMDA and mGluR5 receptors to reduce withdrawal-induced excitation of glutamate neurons (Popp and Lovinger, 2000; Harris *et al.*, 2003). Treatment with acamprosate alone and in combination with naltrexone is effective in maintaining abstinence and preventing relapse (Carmen *et al.*, 2004; Soyka and Chick, 2003; Mann *et al.*, 2004; Kiritze-Topor *et al.*, Kiefer and Wiedemann, 2004), perhaps through effects on craving mediated by excess neuronal excitation (De Witte, 2004; Harris *et al.*, 2003). In addition, acamprosate given before withdrawal may prevent glutamate excitation and consequent neurotoxicity (De Witte, 2004). Other NMDA antagonists that selectively target the NR2B receptor subunit also inhibit alcohol-withdrawal neurotoxicity in animal studies (Nagy *et al.*, 2004). These subunit-selective NMDA antagonists (eg CP101606, RG1103) may prove useful to promote withdrawal and abstinence (Nagy, 2004).

Potential new GABA-based strategies for alcohol-use disorders have been proposed using selective GABA-A agonists and other agents. Use of the GABA antagonist flumazenil might be beneficial in certain circumstances. GABA-A binding to the alpha5 receptor subtype is thought to mediate the reinforcing properties of alcohol (June *et al.*, 2003), so GABA (benzodiazepine) alpha5-subunit inverse agonists in development might reduce alcohol effects and related pleasure (Lopes *et al.*, 2004; Szekeres *et al.*, 2004). GABA-B binding induces mesolimbic dopamine release, so potential exists for treatment with agents such as baclofen (GABA-B agonist), tiagabine (GABA uptake blocker) and topiramate, which enhances GABA neurotransmission without affecting GABA receptors and has effects on glutamate signalling (Cousins *et al.*, 2002; Ashton and Young, 2003). Any efficacy of these compounds might be due to generic inhibitory effects on reward-related circuitry (Cousins *et al.*, 2002; Johnson *et al.*, 2004). Other novel targets implicated in alcohol dependency include the inhibition of neuropeptide Y (Schroeder *et al.*, 2003), protein kinase-C epsilon (Choi *et al.*, 2002) and adenosine (Choi *et al.*, 2004; Mailliard and Diamond, 2004).

Strategies that target acute alcohol intoxication are of interest given that the effects of intoxication vary from potentially hazardous to life-threatening. Metadoxine is a coenzyme precursor that alleviates symptoms of acute alcohol intoxication via complex mechanisms that include accelerated breakdown and preservation of brain and liver cellular energy stores (Diaz Martinez *et al.*, 2002; Shpilenya *et al.*, 2002; Bono *et al.*, 1991; Addolorato *et al.*, 2003). The implications of availability beyond medical contexts encapsulate some wider issues surrounding socially available pharmacology. Off-label use could increase harms by allowing further ingestion of alcohol, or facilitate harm reduction, for example, if it permits safe driving.

7.1.3 Opiates

Various opioid-acting drugs are in development to improve withdrawal symptoms and abstinence in heroin dependence. A sublingual buprenorphine tablet with added naloxone to prevent intravenous abuse has been recently approved by the FDA. Injectable or implantable formulations of known treatments seem promising to improve compliance (Foster *et al.*, 2003; Sobel *et al.*, 2004). Monthly depot naltrexone is in phase III trials, while a depot formulation that releases naltrexone for six months is in development (www.phrma.org/newmedicines; Carreno *et al.*, 2003; Hulse *et al.*, 2004). A buprenorphine depot is also in development.

Other agents in clinical trials are the oral opiate dihydrocodeine, alpha-noradrenergic agonist lofexidine in phase III trials, and nicotinic antagonist mecamylamine in phase II (www.phrma.org/newmedicines; Oldham *et al.*, 2004). An accelerated lofexidine regimen and a naloxone/lofexidine combination both show advantages over the standard lofexidine regimen (Bearn *et al.*, 1998; Buntwal *et al.*, 2000; Beswick *et al.*, 2003). The use of nicotinic antagonists is prompted by reports of cross-tolerance between morphine and nicotine and other animal studies (Zarrindast *et al.*, 2003; Glick *et al.*, 2002). Other potential agents include the NMDA and nicotinic antagonist dextromethorphan (Zhu *et al.*, 2003) and agents developed to act via the neuropeptides galanin (Zachariou *et al.*, 2003) and nociceptin (Meis, 2003).

7.1.4 Cocaine

Cocaine dependency has the highest number of potential treatments in development (Pouletty, 2004; Gorelick *et al.*, 2004; www.phrma.org/newmedicines). Many clinical trials are being conducted by the US National Institute on Drug Abuse Clinical Research Efficacy Screening Trial (NIDA CREST) programme, which rapidly screens existing medications. CREST has five medications in phase II trials that directly or indirectly affect dopamine levels: cabergoline (dopamine agonist), reserpine (depletes presynaptic monoamine stores), sertraline (SSRI), tiagabine (GABA uptake blocker), and NS2359 (inhibitor of dopamine, noradrenaline, and serotonin transporters). Ondansetron, a serotonin-3 receptor

antagonist, is in phase II for combined cocaine and methamphetamine dependency. Disulfiram and selegiline, which inhibit dopamine breakdown in different ways, were effective and well tolerated in phase II trials, but selegiline was found ineffective in a recent phase III trial. Agents in NIDA phase I trials include modafinil, cyclazocine (mixed opioid agonist and antagonist), metyrapone (corticosteroid synthesis inhibitor), and vanoxerine (GBR12909, a long-acting dopamine reuptake inhibitor).

The rationale for the investigation of these and other agents is their direct or indirect effects on dopamine neurotransmission. Other direct-acting agents include the dopamine-1 receptor agonist DAS431 in phase II trials. Methylphenidate (a dopamine reuptake inhibitor), amphetamine (a dopamine releaser), adrogolide (a selective D1 receptor agonist), and BP897 (a D3 partial agonist) have reached clinical studies. Further agents that show potential are SB277011 (a D3 antagonist) and various other known and novel compounds that act in different ways on dopamine receptors, transporters or breakdown inhibitors (Gorelick *et al.*, 2004; Lindsey *et al.*, 2004; Dutta *et al.*, 2003). Such strategies are likely to be refined when the role of different dopamine receptors is more fully defined (Milivojevic *et al.*, 2004; Vorel *et al.*, 2002; Gal and Gyertyan, 2003; Campiani *et al.*, 2003).

Another specific strategy is active immunisation with a vaccine that 'mops up' cocaine before it can enter the brain (Bunce *et al.*, 2003; Kosten *et al.*, 2002). Phase II trials found good short-term abstinence rates in abstinent and using cocaine users. Another vaccine strategy in animal studies involves the intranasal delivery of a bacterial virus designed to produce cocaine antibodies within the brain (Carrera *et al.*, 2004).

Other agents showing promise include gabapentin and drugs that target serotonin, noradrenaline, opioid receptors, glutamate, endocannabinoids, neuropeptides and neurohormones (Gorelick *et al.*, 2004; Myrick *et al.*, 2001; Brodie *et al.*, 2003; Hart *et al.*, 2004; Raby and Coomaraswamy, 2004; Maurice *et al.*, 2002; Matsumoto *et al.*, 2003).

Since alterations in serotonin and dopamine neurotransmission seem to be required for the reinforcing effect of cocaine, agents that affect both these neurotransmitters might show specific benefits for cocaine use (Rocha, 2003; Czoty et al., 2002).

7.1.5 Other Psychostimulants

Fewer agents are in development for other psychostimulants such as amphetamines. However, in theory, some successful agents for cocaine dependency, especially dopamine modulators, will also show benefits for other psychostimulants. For example, vanoxerine has shown promise in animal studies, though it may be rewarding itself (Baumann et al., 2002; Holtzman, 2001). Currently, NIDA is testing bupropion and selegiline in phase I trials, and ondansetron for cocaine and methamphetamine use in phase II (www.phrma.org/newmedicines).

7.1.6 Cannabis

The discovery of cannabinoid receptors and the development of antagonists such as rimonabant offer promise for the treatment of cannabis dependency since cannabinoid-1 receptor antagonists block the effects of cannabis in humans and animals and precipitate withdrawal in dependent animals (LeFoll and Goldberg, 2004; Lange and Kruse, 2004; Nutt, 2005). Long-acting agonists and partial agonists might provide additional benefit.

7.2 Generic Strategies

7.2.1 Learning and Anti-learning Agents

In theory, agents that promote learning could either facilitate the extinction of the aberrant learning thought to underlie dependency, or facilitate new learning, eg to associate drug cues with abstinence. D-cycloserine, a partial agonist at glutamate NMDA receptors, has been shown to facilitate the extinction of learned fear in animal studies (Walker et al., 2002)

and to prevent reinstatement of extinguished behaviour (Ledgerwood et al., 2004). D-cycloserine consolidates human neuroplasticity (Nitsche et al., 2004) and has shown potential in combination with naloxone in a small experimental study of opiate-dependent people (Oliveto et al., 2003).

Importantly, NMDA receptor binding seems to mediate sensitisation, a possible initial step in dependence, although glutamate is also implicated in tolerance, craving and withdrawal (Nutt et al., 2003; De Witte, 2004; Camarini et al., 2000; Wolf, 1998). The role of glutamate may also partly explain the success of anticonvulsants in substance use disorders since agents that act as agonists and antagonists at NMDA receptors possess anti-convulsant activity (Wlaz, 1998). Agents such as memantine, and drugs that modulate AMPA and metabotropic glutamate receptor functioning, seem likely to show benefits over older drugs and some are under study for dependency (Cryan et al., 2003; Nagy, 2004; Gorelick et al., 2004).

Agents shown to play similar roles include the alpha2-adrenoreceptor antagonist yohimbine (Cain et al., 2004) and a novel serotonin-4 receptor agonist RS67333 (Lelong et al., 2001). Other cognition enhancers might have beneficial properties in this respect, including cholinesterase inhibitors and calcium-channel blockers (Morris et al., 2005a; Hikida et al., 2003). Effects on calcium channels might also underlie the potential antidependency mechanism of gabapentin. The timing of use and other effects of drugs that affect learning might be crucial, since yohimbine has also been found to reinstate drug-seeking behaviour while D-cycloserine can facilitate tolerance at least to alcohol (Shepard et al., 2004; Lee et al., 2004; Khanna et al., 1993).

7.2.2 Drugs Acting on Inhibitory Systems

GABA neurotransmission in particular is suggested to regulate a switch from normal to drug-dependent states (Laviolette *et al.*, 2004). Possible agents that promote GABA include approved drugs, especially vigabatrin, a GABA-transaminase inhibitor, that has already shown promise in reducing animal consumption of cocaine (Kushner *et al.*, 1999), nicotine (Dewey *et al.*, 1999), alcohol (Stromberg *et al.*, 2001), and heroin (Paul *et al.*, 2001). In animal studies, the GABA-B agonist baclofen has effects on usage of alcohol (Broadbent and Harless, 1999), nicotine (Fadda *et al.*, 2003), morphine (Fadda *et al.*, 2003), cocaine (Fadda *et al.*, 2003; Roberts and Andrews, 1997), amphetamine (Bartoletti *et al.*, 2004), methamphetamine (Ranaldi and Poeggel, 2002), and GHB (Fattore *et al.*, 2001). Clinical trials of baclofen have been promising for opiates (Assadi *et al.*, 2003) and cocaine (Shoptaw *et al.*, 2003). Other agents include tiagabine, topiramate, etifoxine, ganoxolone, and retigabine. Analogues of vigabatrin are in development (Choi and Silverman, 2002), while new analogues of GHB might target both GABA and GIIB inhibitory systems (Waszkielewicz and Bojarski, 2004).

Endocannabinoids have indirect effects on reinforcing dopamine release (Van der Stelt and Di Marzo, 2003), though the link is less well researched than for GABA. However, CB1 receptors have been found to be important in alcohol consumption, including stress-related drinking, and in opiate and amphetamine effects (Solinas *et al.*, 2003; Hungund *et al.*, 2003; Racz *et al.*, 2003; Ledent *et al.*, 1999; Murtra *et al.*, 2000; Huang *et al.*, 2003). Moreover, the cannabinoid antagonist rimonabant has shown benefits in trials as an anti-smoking agent and as a weight-loss agent (LeFoll and Goldberg, 2004; Lange and Kruse, 2004; Nutt, 2005).

7.2.3 Agents to Ameliorate Stress and Anxiety

Stress is a major factor in drug seeking and relapse, while withdrawal is also considered a stressor (Weiss *et al.*, 2001; Lee *et al.*, 2003). Moreover, anxiety is one of the pre-existing conditions thought to predispose individuals to use both sedatives and stimulants. CRF (Cook, 2004) and related neuropeptides (eg neuropeptides Y and S) are known to mediate effects of stress in the brain. So CRF antagonists, such as antalarmin, are being developed as potential dependency treatments. The role of CRF and the potential for CRF-antagonists have been demonstrated in animal models of cocaine (CP154526) (Lu *et al.*, 2003), cannabis withdrawal (Rodriguez de Fonseca *et al.*, 1997), alcohol [D-Phe-CRF(12-41)] (Valdez *et al.*, 2003) and opiates (antalarmin) (Stinus *et al.*, 2004). Recent findings suggest that alcohol directly induces release of CRF (Nie *et al.*, 2004). Thus, CRF antagonists may show particular promise in the treatment of alcohol withdrawal, as may other anxiolytics like GABA agonists and serotonin-1A partial agonists such as buspirone (Breese *et al.*, 2004). Finally, CRF2-receptor agonists such as urocortin may produce similar effects to CRF-1 receptor antagonists (Valdez *et al.*, 2004).

7.2.4 Agents that Target Reward and Pleasure Circuits

Many agents now used or in development as dependency treatments act directly or indirectly on the dopamine, opioid, serotonin and/or endocannabinoid systems. Since these systems seem to be involved in most appetitive behaviours, various agents that act on reward/pleasure circuits might prove beneficial in disorders related to excessive appetitive behaviours. These include buprenorphine, naltrexone and other opioid-acting agents such as the antagonist clocinnamox and methoclocinnamox, a partial agonist with delayed, long-lasting antagonist effects, dopamine modulators, serotonergic agents like ondansetron, and cannabinoid antagonists. This generic approach has already borne fruit, although combination treatments might be required for full efficacy. Thus, buprenorphine was not found very effective for cocaine dependency, but might be efficacious in combination with disulfiram.

The molecular effects of drugs that activate reward/pleasure circuits is beginning to be elucidated. Such effects range from short-term activation of intracellular signalling pathways after receptor binding, through longer-lasting changes in molecules that underlie learning and memory (eg CREB) in brain reward/pleasure regions, to long-term effects mediated by neurotrophic factors (eg BDNF) that alter nerve complexity and growth (Robbins *et al.*, 2005; Morris *et al.*, 2005a; Nestler, 2004; Russo-Ncustadt, 2003). Intracellular and other molecular targets represent challenging but important future targets for therapy of substance use disorders (Robbins *et al.*, 2005; Nestler, 2004).

Neuropeptides are another category of agents that might influence reward/pleasure circuits. Little is known about most neuropeptides, but tools for their manipulation are becoming increasingly available. For example, agents that target cholecystokinin might be beneficial for dependency, while CRF antagonists might help alleviate withdrawal. Manipulation of neuropeptide systems is likely to broaden possibilities for altering brain functioning and behaviour, including for substance use disorders (DiLeone *et al.*, 2003; Cowen *et al.*, 2004). It seems possible that many different types of agents for therapy, pleasure and enhancement will be produced from increasing knowledge of neuropeptide functioning.

7.2.5 Agents that Reduce Availability of Drugs

Several therapeutic strategies have been proposed that neutralise a drug in the bloodstream before it reaches the brain. Such strategies might be useful for prompting or maintaining abstinence and also to treat overdose. Active vaccination is under study and may have potential against many substances, except alcohol and endogenous molecules like GHB. Other strategies include infusion of drug-binding antibodies (passive immunotherapy), use of enzyme accelerators to speed up drug metabolism, and a combination of the two (catalytic antibody therapy) (Vetulani, 2001).

7.2.6 Plant-based Substances

Various medicines based on plant products are traditionally reported to be useful anti-addiction measures, including *Hypericum perforatum*, *Pueraria lobata*, *Lobelia inflata*, *Sceletium tortuosum*, *Passiflora incarnata* and ibogaine from *Tabernanthe iboga*. All might have actions on several neurotransmitter systems (Rezvani *et al.*, 2003; Dwoskin and Crooks, 2002; Baumann *et al.*, 2001; Maisonneuve and Glick, 2003). While virtually no rigorous clinical data exist, ethical investigation of plants with traditional use might inform research on anti-addictive compounds and mechanisms.

8 CONTEXT OF FUTURE TREATMENTS

Advances in drug treatments are likely to bring the capability to genuinely tackle problematic drug use and reduce the demand side of the 'drugs problem'. However, very few strategies are in development specifically for substance use disorders. Strategies are often developed for other conditions and companies then may seek to license them as treatments for dependency. Thus far, drug dependency has not been a priority area for pharmaceutical companies, since aside from problematic alcohol use and smoking, markets are small, while people with dependency attract negative perceptions (Pouletty, 2004). Currently, up to 10 times as many leads are in development for cognition enhancement as for dependency and addiction (Morris *et al.*, 2005a; www.phrma.org/newmedicines). Thus, responsibility for the conduct of trials to ensure a good evidence base may fall to UK funding bodies, the

National Health Service, and academic institutions, to prove and implement the promise of better treatments. Research on problem drugs including alcohol seems to be a low government priority (Joseph Rowntree Foundation, 2000; HM Treasury, 2004).

The success of attempts to reduce the burden of substance use disorders will depend not only on good treatments and services (Lingford-Hughes *et al.*, 2004), but also on the social, legal, ethical and personal contexts of psychoactive substance use and treatment over the next 25 years (Room *et al.*, 2005; McKeganey, 2005; Capps *et al.*, 2005; Hurwitz, 2005). Few data exist to help estimate the impact that broader social, legal and other changes might have on the prevalence of drug use, while effects of such changes on treatment access and outcomes could be complex. For example, access to treatment could be easier for legal drugs (as with tobacco smoking), except if disordered use of the substance is normalised or stigmatised as with alcohol. Illegal status seems likely to represent a barrier to accessing treatment services. Enforcement of treatment, as with current drug testing and treatment orders, has not resulted in improved levels of abstinence compared with voluntary services, and raises ethical issues (Capps *et al.*, 2005).

9 PROSPECTS

9.1 What will be the Psychoactive Substances of the Future?

Most societies are likely to continue to experience a rise in overall psychoactive substance use, together with an increase in the number and type of psychoactive substances available over the next 20 years. The current key problematic drugs are likely to remain in society, while a minority of new drugs will potentially lead to substance use disorders.

Development of psychoactive substances is likely to be a growth area in the next 20 years. Future psychoactive substances will probably be developed by pharmaceutical and other industries, academic institutions, plus 'underground' and illicit sources. The production of new psychoactive substances is likely to include current and novel methods. Advance knowledge of future psychoactive substances is unlikely to be accessible from most commercial and other sources, unless reported in scientific literature or via the Internet.

9.2 What will be the Effects of Using Psychoactive Substances in the Future?

Future psychoactive substances will probably be used for various therapeutic purposes, disease prevention, health maintenance and the enhancement of aspects of functioning such as performance, cognition, mood and pleasure, but may also be abused and lead to dependency. The majority of new psychoactive drugs are likely to have potential benefits and harms – very few future psychoactive drugs will be entirely safe or wholly without benefits. Although the potential for new agents to cause adverse effects or lead to substance use disorders may be largely predictable from their pharmacology, a minority will present unexpected challenges. The expected increase in polypharmacy could well increase interactions between agents, which may result in additional effects that are useful or harmful.

New uses and misuses of psychoactive substances are likely to develop alongside alternate or new classifications of these substances. Future classification will depend on changes in societal attitudes and in legal and regulatory frameworks, but will probably include nutrients and foodstuffs, herbal medicines, therapeutics, legal recreational drugs, other lifestyle and enhancement drugs including cognition enhancers, and illicit drugs. An increased blurring of boundaries is anticipated within current categories. Nutrients may be used in high doses as drugs, cognition enhancers as anti-addiction measures, psychiatric drugs as 'lifestyle' agents, and current illicit drugs used or under study as therapeutics. New types of classification could be based on neurotransmitter actions, actions on gross central nervous system functions, or both.

Psychoactive substances are likely to have an increasing impact on individuals who take them, their communities, and wider society, although the wider effects of increasing psychoactive substance use do not seem predictable at present. The use of psychoactive substances may well become increasingly acceptable and desirable overall.

9.3 What Mechanisms do we have to Manage the Use of Psychoactive Substances?

Prevalence and treatment of problematic use will depend on resources invested, wider social perceptions and social policies. Mechanisms used to manage psychoactive substances in the future will almost certainly include education and other measures aimed at prevention and harm reduction, use of treatments and regulatory mechanisms. Through education and experience, a wider understanding will probably arise in society of the mechanisms of psychoactive drugs, dependency and related problems, plus increasing recognition of the non-abusive use of recreational and other 'lifestyle' or enhancement drugs.

The prevalent view of dependency as a moral weakness is likely to be abandoned and instead will incorporate other elements (eg neurobiological and genetic influences with psychosocial elements). Individuals will tend to become more informed over drug use, and may also seek greater autonomy in choices over substance use and the treatment and prevention of drug use problems. Increasingly sophisticated public attitudes and changes in social policy could facilitate better use of psychoactive substances and encourage entry into treatment services for problematic use.

The treatment of drug dependency and the minimisation of its consequences are likely to become more effective, with more options that allow targeting of therapy. More effective and earlier intervention in the course of substance use disorders could be possible, with expanded treatments and services, including dedicated drug services and others including peer-led education initiatives, and GP and psychiatric services. Prevention might become a realistic possibility. If voluntary entry to treatment or prevention initiatives becomes more acceptable, more available, and associated with better outcomes, society may be less accepting of continued drug dependency that leads to related problems, such as ill health, crime or antisocial behaviour.

Current regulations are likely to be revised to encompass a broader spectrum of psychoactive substances than today, and increased resources will be required to maximise benefits and minimise harms of future agents. More sophisticated regulatory assessments of individual agents could represent the most rational future approach to inform society of novel risks. Properties of psychoactive drugs that will remain important for assessment include abuse potential, potency and efficacy, other safety aspects, history of use and accessibility. Education and research on new and existing agents will probably remain valuable measures. Regulatory authorities are likely to be most effective if they can respond flexibly, rapidly and scientifically to the introduction of new agents and new research findings on known drugs. Continued and long-term assessment after regulatory approval or other release into society of psychoactive agents will probably be increasingly important.

Efforts to eradicate drug abuse seem unlikely to be successful. However, social policy at one extreme could evolve to emphasise prohibition, with coercion as an element of prevention and treatment, or at the other, universal availability with market and other controls. The effects of such policies on the prevalence and treatment of substance use disorders are not predictable since no simple relationship exists between prohibition, availability, usage and harm. A more likely alternative to these extremes is a stratified approach that incorporates different levels of regulatory control for different substances according to potential for harm (Blakemore, 2003).

Directing resources towards a reduction in demand rather than supply is an under-utilised strategy that may be effective at min-imising harm from substance use disorders. Ultimately, fewer resources may be required to enforce avoidance of substance use dis-orders through legal frameworks if more sophisticated use of psychoactive substances is promoted and more effective treatments for substance use disorders are available.

References

Addolorato, G., Ancona, C., Capristo, E., and Gasbarrini, G. (2003) Metadoxine in the treat-ment of acute and chronic alcoholism: a review. *Int J Immunopathol Pharmacol* 16: 207–214.

Aghajanian, G.K. and Marek, G.J. (1999) Serotonin and hallucinogens. *Neuropsychopharmacology* 21: S16–23.

Agrawal, A., Neale, M.C., Prescott, C.A., and Kendler, K.S. (2004) Cannabis and other illicit drugs: comorbid use and abuse/dependence in males and females. *Behav Genet* 34(3): 217–228.

Altman, J., Everitt, B.J., Glautier, S., *et al.* (1996) The biological, social and clinical bases of drug addiction: commentary and debate. *Psy-chopharmacology* 125: 285–345.

American Psychiatric Association. (2000) *Diagnos-tic and statistical manual of mental disorders*, 4th edition (text revision). Washington DC: APA.

Amos, A., Wiltshire, S., Bostock, Y., Haw, S., and McNeill, A. (2004) 'You can't go without a fag . . . you need it for your hash' – a qualitative exploration of smoking, cannabis and young people. *Addiction*. Jan. 99(1): 77–81.

Ansorge, M.S., Zhou, M., Lira, A., Hen, R., Gingrich, J.A. (2004) Early-life blockade of the 5-HT transporter alters emotional behavior in adult mice. *Science* 306(5697): 879–881.

Ashton, H. and Young, A.H. (2003) GABA-ergic drugs: exit stage left, enter stage right. *J Psy-chopharmacol* 17(2): 174–178.

Assadi, S.M., Radgoodarzi, R., and Ahmadi-Abhari, S.A. (2003) Baclofen for maintenance treatment of opioid dependence: a randomized double-blind placebo-controlled clinical trial. *BMC Psychiatry* 3(1): 16.

Barker, M.J., Greenwood, K.M., Jackson, M. and Crowe, S.F. (2004) Persistence of cognitive effects after withdrawal from long-term ben-zodiazepine use: a meta-analysis. *Arch Clin Neuropsychol*. Apr. 19(3): 437–454.

Bartoletti, M., Gubellini, C., Ricci, F., and Gaiardi, M. (2004) The GABAB agonist baclofen blocks the expression of sensitisa-tion to the locomotor stimulant effect of amphetamine. *Behav Pharmacol* 15(56): 397–401.

Baumann, M.H., Rothman, R.B., Pablo, J.P., and Mash, D.C. (2001) In vivo neurobiological effects of ibogaine and its o-desmethyl metabo-lite, 12-hydroxyibogamine (noribogaine), in rats. *J Pharmacol Exp Ther* 297: 531–539.

Baumann, M.H., Phillips, J.M., Ayestas, M.A., Ali, S.F., Rice, K.C., and Rothman, R.B. (2002) Preclinical evaluation of GBR12909 decanoate as a long-acting medication for metham-phetamine dependence. *Ann N Y Acad Sci* 965: 92–108.

Bearn, J., Gossop, M., and Strang, J. (1998) Accel-erated lofexidine treatment regimen compared with conventional lofexidine and methadone treatment for in-patient opiate detoxification. *Drug Alcohol Depend* (3): 227–232.

Belluzzi, J.D., Wang, R., and Leslie, F.M. (2004) Acetaldehyde enhances acquisition of nicotine self-administration in adolescent rats. *Neu-ropsychopharmacology* 20 Oct. Epub ahead of print.

Beswick, T., Best, D., Bearn, J., Gossop, M., Rees, S., and Strang, J. (2003) The effective-ness of combined naloxone/lofexidine in opi-ate detoxification: results from a double-blind randomized and placebo-controlled trial. *Am J Addict* 12(4): 295–305.

Biederman, J. (2003) Pharmacotherapy for attention-deficit/hyperactivity disorder decreases the risk for substance abuse: find-ings from a longitudinal follow-up of youths with and without ADHD. *J Clin Psychiatry* 64 (Suppl II): 3–8.

Blakemore, C. (2003) A scientifically based scale of harm for all social drugs. In: *Proceedings of seminar III: alcohol and other recreational drugs*. Oxford: Beckley Foundation.

Bolanos, C.A., Barrot, M., Bertob, O. Wallace-Black, D., and Nestler, E.J. (2003) Methylphenidate treatment during pre- and periadolescence alters behavioral responses to emotional stimuli at adulthood. *Biol Psychiatry* 54: 1317–1329.

Bonci, A., Bernardi, G., Grillner, P., and Mercuri, N.B. (2003) The dopamine-containing neuron: maestro or simple musician in the orchestra of addiction? *Trends Pharm Sci* 24(4): 172–177.

Bono, G., Sinforiani, E., Merlo, P., Belloni, G., Soldati, M., and Gelso, E. (1991) Alcoholic abstinence syndrome: short-term treatment with metadoxine. *Int J Clin Pharmacol Res* 11: 35–40.

Boot, B.P., McGregor, I.S., and Hall, W. (2000) MDMA (Ecstasy) neurotoxicity: assessing and communicating the risks. *Lancet* 355: 1818–1821.

Boyle, P. and Ferlay, J. (2005) Cancer incidence and mortality in Europe, 2004. *Ann Oncol* Epub 15 February. doi:10.1093/annonc/mdi098.

Brandon, C.L., Marinelli, M., and White, F.J. (2003) Adolescent exposure to methylphenidate alters the activity of rat midbrain dopamine neurons. *Biol Psychiatry* 54: 1338–1344.

Breese, G.R., Knapp, D.J., and Overstreet, D.H. (2004) Stress sensitization of ethanol withdrawal-induced reduction in social interaction: inhibition by CRF-1 and benzodiazepine receptor antagonists and a 5-HT1A-receptor agonist. *Neuropsychopharmacology* 29(3): 470–482.

British Medical Association. (1997) *Therapeutic uses of cannabis*. Netherlands: Harwood.

Broadbent, J. and Harless, W.E. (1999) Differential effects of GABA (A) and GABA (B) agonists on sensitization to the locomotor stimulant effects of ethanol in DBA/2 J mice. *Psychopharmacology* 141(2): 197–205.

Brodie, J.D., Figueroa, E., and Dewey, S.L. (2003) Treating cocaine addiction: from preclinical to clinical trial experience with γ-vinyl GABA. *Synapse* 50: 261–265.

Budygin, E.A., Brodie, M.S., Sotnikova, T.D., et al. (2004) Dissociation of rewarding and dopamine transporter-mediated properties of amphetamine. *Proc Natl Acad Sci USA* 101(20): 7781–7786.

Bunce, C.J., Loudon, P.T., Akers, C., Dobson, J., and Wood, D.M. (2003) Development of vaccines to help treat drug dependence. *Curr Opin Mol Ther* 5(1): 58–63.

Buntwal, N., Bearn, J., Gossop, M., and Strang, J. (2000) Naltrexone and lofexidine combination treatment compared with conventional lofexidine treatment for in-patient opiate detoxification. *Drug Alcohol Depend* 59(2): 183–188.

Burstein, S.H., Karst, M., Schneider, U., and Zurier, R.B. (2004) Ajulemic acid: A novel cannabinoid produces analgesia without a 'high'. *Life Sci* 75: 1513–1522.

Bush, W., Roberts, M., and Trace, M. (2004) *Upheavals in the Australian drug market: heroin drought, stimulant flood*. Oxford: Beckley Foundation.

Cadet, J.L., Jayanthi, S., and Deng, X. (2003) Speed kills: cellular and molecular bases of methamphetamine-induced nerve terminal degeneration and neuronal apoptosis. *FASEB J* 17: 1775–1788.

Cain, C.K., Blouin, A.M., and Barad, M. (2004) Adrenergic transmission facilitates extinction of conditional fear in mice. *Learn Mem* 11(2): 179–187.

Camarini, R., Frussa-Filho, R., Monteiro, M.G., and Calil, H.M. (2000) MK-801 blocks the development of behavioral sensitization to the ethanol. *Alcohol Clin Exp Res* 24(3): 285–290.

Campiani, G., Butini, S., Trotta, F., et al. (2003) Synthesis and pharmacological evaluation of potent and highly selective D3 receptor ligands: inhibition of cocaine-seeking behavior and the role of dopamine D3/D2 receptors. *J Med Chem* 46(18): 3822–3839.

Capps, B., Campbell, A., and Ashcroft, R. (2005) *Foresight state of science review – ethical aspects of developments on neuroscience and drug addiction*. London: Department of Trade and Industry.

Cardinal, R.N., Winstanley, C.A., Robbins, T.W., and Everitt, B.J. (2004) Limbic corticostriatal systems and delayed reinforcement. *Ann NY Acad Sci* 1021: 33–50.

Carlezon W.A., Jr., Mague, S.D., and Anderson, S.L. (2003) Enduring behavioral effects of early exposure to methylphenidate in rats. *Biol Psychiatry* 54: 1330–1337.

Carlini, E.A. (2003) Plants and the central nervous system. *Pharmacol Biochem Behav* 75: 501–512.

Carmen, B., Angeles, M., Ana, M., and Maria, A.J. (2004) Efficacy and safety of naltrexone and acamprosate in the treatment of alcohol dependence: a systematic review. *Addiction* 99: 811–828.

Carreno, J.E., Alvarez, C.E., Narciso, G.I., Bascaran, M.T., Diaz, M., and Bobes, J. (2003) Maintenance treatment with depot opioid antagonists in subcutaneous implants: an alternative in the treatment of opioid dependence. *Addict Biol* 8(4): 429–438.

Carrera, M.R.A., Kaufmann, G.F., Mee, J.M., Meijler, M., Koob, G.F., and Janda, K.D. (2004) Treating cocaine addiction with viruses. *Proc Natl Acad Sci USA* 101: 10416–10421. Epub 28 June. doi: 10.1073/pnas.0403795101

Check, E. (2004) The ups and downs of ecstasy. *Nature* 429: 126–128.

Chichewicz, D.L. (2004) Synergistic interactions between cannabinoid and opioid analgesics. *Life Sci* 74: 1317–1324.

Choi, S., and Silverman, R.B. (2002) Inactivation and inhibition of gamma-aminobutyric acid aminotransferase by conformationally restricted vigabatrin analogues. *J Med Chem* 45 (20): 4531–4539.

Choi, D.S., Wang, D., Dadgar, J., Chang, W.S., and Messing, R.O. (2002) Conditional rescue of protein kinase C epsilon regulates ethanol preference and hypnotic sensitivity in adult mice. *J Neurosci* 22(22): 9905–9011.

Choi, D.S., Cascini, M.G., Mailliard, W., *et al.* (2004) The type 1 equilibrative nucleoside transporter regulates ethanol intoxication and preference. *Nat Neurosci* 18 July. Epub ahead of print. doi:10.1038/nn1288

Cole, J.C. and Sumnall, H.R. (2003) Altered states: the clinical effects of Ecstasy. *Pharm Ther* 98: 35–58.

Condon, J. and Smith, N. (2003) Prevalence of drug use: key findings from the 2002/2003 *British Crime Survey. Findings* 229. London: Home Office.

Connor, T.J. (2004) Methylenedioxymethamphetamine (MDMA, 'Ecstasy'): a stressor on the immune system. *Immunology* 111: 357–367.

Contet, C., Kieffer, B.L., and Befort, K. (2004) Mu opioid receptor: a gateway to drug addiction. *Curr Opin Neurobiol* 14: 370–378.

Cook, C.J. (2004) Stress induces CRF release in the paraventricular nucleus, and both CRF and GABA release in the amygdala. *Physiol Behav* 82(4): 751–762.

Cousins, M.S., Roberts, D.C., and de Wit, H. (2002) GABA (B) receptor agonists for the treatment of drug addiction: a review of recent findings. *Drug Alcohol Depend* 65(3): 209–220.

Cowen, M.S., Chen, F., and Lawrence, A.J. (2004) Neuropeptides: implications for alcoholism. *J Neurochem* 89(2): 273–285.

Cryan, J.F., Gasparini, F., van Heeke, G., and Markou, A. (2003) Non-nicotinic neuropharmacological strategies for nicotine

dependence: beyond buproprion. *Drug Discov Today* 8(22): 1025–1034.

Czoty, P.W., Ginsburg, B.C., and Howell, L.L. (2002) Serotonergic attenuation of the reinforcing and neurochemical effects of cocaine in squirrel monkeys. *J Pharmacol Exp Ther* 300(3): 831–887.

d'Abbs, P., and Brady, M. (2004) Other people, other drugs: the policy response to petrol sniffing among indigenous Australians. *Drug Alcohol Rev* 23(3): 253–260.

Dalal, S. and Melrack, R. (1998) Potentiation of opioid analgesia by psychostimulant drugs: a review. *J Pain Symptom Manage* 16: 245–253.

De Witte, P. (2004) Imbalance between neuroexcitatory and neuroinhibitory amino acids causes craving for ethanol. *Addictive Behaviors* 29: 1325–1339.

Degenhardt, L., Hall, W., and Lynskey, M. (2003a) Testing hypotheses about the relationship between cannabis use and psychosis. *Drug Alcohol Depend* 71(1): 37–48.

Degenhardt, L., Hall, W., and Lynskey, M. (2003b) Exploring the association between cannabis use and depression. *Addiction* 98(11): 1493–1504.

Department of Health. (2004) CMO update May: 8–9. http://www.dh.gov.uk/cmo/

Dewey, S.L., Brodie, J.D., Gerasimov, M., Horan, B., Gardner, E.L., and Ashby, C.R., Jr. (1999) A pharmacologic strategy for the treatment of nicotine addiction. *Synapse* 31(1): 76–86.

Diaz Martinez, M.C., Diaz Martinez, A., Villamil Salcedo, V., and Cruz Fuentes, C. (2002) Efficacy of metadoxine in the management of acute alcohol intoxication. *J Int Med Res* 30: 44–51.

DiLeone, R.J., Georgescu, D., and Nestler, E.J. (2003) Lateral hypothalamic neuropeptides in reward and drug addiction. *Life Sci* 73(6): 759–768.

Drugscope. How many people die from using drugs? http://www.drugscope.org.uk

Drummond, C., and Curran, V. (2005) *Foresight state of science review – psychological treatments of substance abuse*. London: Department of Trade and Industry.

Dutta, A.K., Zhang, S., Kolhatkar, R., and Reith, M.E.A. (2003) Dopamine transporter as target for drug development of cocaine dependence medications. *Eur J Pharmacol* 479: 93–106.

Dwoskin, L.P. and Crooks, P.A. (2002) A novel mechanism of action and potential use for lobeline as a treatment for psychostimulant abuse. *Biochem Pharmacol* 63(2): 89–98.

Everitt, B. (2002) Amphetamine and cocaine – mechanisms and hazards. In: *Proceedings of seminar I: Drugs and the brain.* Oxford: Beckley Foundation.

Fadda, P., Scherma, M., Fresu, A., Collu, M., and Fratta, W. (2003) Baclofen antagonizes nicotine-, cocaine-, and morphine-induced dopamine release in the nucleus accumbens of rat. *Synapse* 50(1): 1–6.

Faraone, S.V. and Wilens, T. (2003) Does stimulant treatment lead to substance use disorders? *J Clin Psychiatry* 64 (Suppl 11): 9–13.

Farber, N.B. and Olney, J.W. (2003) Drugs of abuse that cause developing neurons to commit suicide. *Developmental Brain Res* 147: 37–45.

Fattore, L., Cossu, G., Martellotta, M.C., Deiana, S., and Fratta, W. (2001) Baclofen antagonises intravenous self-administration of gamma-hydroxybutyric acid in mice. *Neuroreport* 12(10): 2243–2246.

Fischer, M. and Barkley, R.A. (2003) Childhood stimulant treatment and risk for later substance abuse. *J Clin Psychiatry* 64 (Suppl II): 19–23.

Foster, J., Brewer, C., and Steele, T. (2003) Naltrexone implants can completely prevent early (1-month) relapse after opiate detoxification: a pilot study of two cohorts totalling 101 patients with a note on naltrexone blood levels. *Addict Biol* 8(2): 211–217.

Fowler, J.S., Logan, J., Wang, G.J., and Volkow, N.D. (2003) Monoamine oxidase and cigarette smoking. *Neurotoxicology* 24(1): 75–82.

Frank, M.J., O'Reilly, R.C., and Seeberger, L.C. (2004) By carrot or by stick: cognitive reinforcement learning in parkinsonism. *Science Express* 4 Nov. doi: 10.1126/science.1102941

Franken, I.H. (2003) Drug craving and addiction: integrating psychological and neuropsychopharmacological approaches. *Prog Neuropsychopharmacol Biol Psychiatry* 27(4): 563–579.

Gable, R.S. (2004) Comparison of acute lethal toxicity of commonly abused psychoactive substances. *Addiction* 99: 686–696.

Gal, K. and Gyertyan, I. (2003) Targeting the dopamine D3 receptor cannot influence continuous reinforcement cocaine self-administration in rats. *Brain Res Bull* 61(6): 595–601.

Garten, S. and Falkner, R.V. (2004) Role of mentholated cigarettes in increased nicotine dependence and greater risk of tobacco-attributable disease. *Prev Med* 38: 793–798.

George, T.P. and O'Malley, S.S. (2004) Current pharmacological treatments for nicotine dependence. *Trends Pharmacol Sci* Jan; 25(1): 42–48.

George, T.P., Verrico, C.D., Picciotto, M.R., and Roth, R.H. (2000) Nicotinic modulation of mesoprefrontal dopamine neurons: pharmacologic and neuroanatomic characterization. *J Pharm Exp Ther* 295: 58–66.

Glick, S.D., Maisonneuve, I.M., Kitchen, B.A., and Fleck, M.W. (2002) Antagonism of alpha 3 beta 4 nicotinic receptors as a strategy to reduce opioid and stimulant self-administration. *Eur J Pharmacol* 438(1–2): 99–105.

Godfrey, C. and Cave, J. (2005) *Foresight state of science review – Economics of Addiction and Drugs.* London: Department of Trade and Industry.

Godfrey, C., Eaton, G., McDougall, C., and Culyer, A. (2002) *Home Office Research Study 249: The economic and social costs of Class A drug use in England and Wales, 2000.* London: Home Office.

Gonzales, M. and Nutt, D.J. (2005) Gamma-hydroxybutyrate (GHB) abuse and dependency. *J Psychopharmacol* 19: 219–220.

Gorelick, D.A., Gardner, E.L., and Xi, Z.X. (2004) Agents in development for management of cocaine abuse. *Drugs* 64(14): 1547–1573.

Gossop, M., Marsden, J., and Stewart, D. (2001) *The National Treatment Outcome Research Study: changes in substance use, health and criminal behaviour during the five years after intake.* London: National Addiction Centre.

Green, A.R., O'Shea, E., and Colado, M.I. (2004) A review of the mechanisms involved in the acute MDMA (ecstasy)-induced hyperthermic response. *Eur J Pharmacol* 500(1–3): 3–13.

Gyertyan, I. and Gal, K. (2003) Dopamine D3 receptor ligands show place conditioning effect but do not influence cocaine-induced place preference. *Neuroreport* 14(1): 93–98.

Hall, W. and Pacula, R.L. (2003) *Cannabis use and dependence: public health and public policy.* Cambridge: Cambridge University Press.

Halpern, J.H., and Pope, H.G. Jr. (2003) Hallucinogen persisting perception disorder: what do we know after 50 years? *Drug Alcohol Depend* 69: 109–119.

Harris, B.R., Gibson, D.A., and Prendergast, M.A., *et al.* (2003) The neurotoxicity induced by ethanol withdrawal in mature organotypic hippocampal slices might involve cross-talk between metabotropic glutamate type 5 receptors and N-methyl-D-aspartate receptors. *Alcohol Clin Exp Res* 27(11): 1724–1735.

Hart, C.L., Ward, A.S., Collins, E.D., Haney, M., and Foltin, R.W. (2004) Gabapentin maintenance decreases smoked cocaine-related subjective effects, but not self-administration by humans. *Drug Alcohol Depend* 73(3): 279–287.

Harvey, D.M., Yasar, S., Heishman, S.J., Panlilio, L.V., Henningfield, J.E., and Goldberg, S.R. (2004) Nicotine serves as an effective reinforcer of intravenous drug-taking behavior in human cigarette smokers. *Psychopharmacology* 175(2): 134–142. Epub 2 March.

Hasler, F., Grimberg, U., Benz, M.A., Huber, T., and Vollenweider, F.X. (2004) Acute psychological and physiological effects of psilocybin in healthy humans: a double-blind, placebo-controlled dose–effect study. *Psychopharmacology* 172: 145–156.

Hatsukami, D.K., Lemmonds, C., and Tomar, S.L. (2004) Smokeless tobacco use: harm reduction or induction approach? *Prev Med* 38: 309–317.

Henquet, C., Krabbendam, L., Spauwen, J., et al. (2005) Prospective cohort study of cannabis use, predisposition for psychosis, and psychotic symptoms in young people. *BMJ* 330(7481): 11–15. Epub 1 December 2004.

Herraiz, T. and Chaparro, C. (2005) Human monoamine oxidase is inhibited by tobacco smoke: beta-carboline alkaloids act as potent and reversible inhibitors. *Biochem Biophys Res Commun* 326(2): 378–386.

Hikida, T., Kitabatake, Y., Pastan, I., and Nakanishi, S. (2003) Acetylcholine enhancement in the nucleus accumbens prevents addictive behaviors of cocaine and morphine. *Proc Natl Acad Sci USA* 100(10): 6169–6173. Epub 29 April.

HM Treasury (2004) *Spending Review 2004: Public Service Agreements 2005–2008*. Chapter 21 – Action against illegal drugs. London: HM Treasury.

Hoaken, P.N.S. and Stewart, S.H. (2003) Drugs of abuse and the elicitation of human aggressive behavior. *Addictive Behaviors* 28: 1533–1554.

Holtzman, S.G. (2001) Differential interaction of GBR 12909, a dopamine uptake inhibitor, with cocaine and methamphetamine in rats discriminating cocaine. *Psychopharmacology* 155(2): 180–186.

Horgan, J. (2005) The electric kool-aid clinical trial. *New Scientist* 185: 36–39.

Huang, Y.C., Wang, S.J., Chiou, L.C., and Gean, P.W. (2003) Mediation of amphetamine-induced long-term depression of synaptic transmission by CB1 cannabinoid receptors in the rat amygdala. *J Neurosci* 23(32): 10311–10320.

Hulse, G.K., Arnold-Reed, D.E., O'Neil, G., Chan, C.T., Hansson, R., and O'Neil, P. (2004) Blood naltrexone and 6-beta-naltrexol levels following naltrexone implant: comparing two naltrexone implants. *Addict Biol* 9(1): 59–65.

Hungund, B.L., Szakall, I., Adam, A., Basavarajappa, B.S., and Vadasz, C. (2003) Cannabinoid CB1 receptor knockout mice exhibit markedly reduced voluntary alcohol consumption and lack alcohol-induced dopamine release in the nucleus accumbens. *J Neurochem* 84(4): 698–704.

Hurwitz, B (2005) *Foresight state of science review – life histories and narratives of addiction*. London: Department of Trade and Industry.

Iversen, L.L. (2001) *The science of marijuana*. Oxford: Oxford University Press.

Iversen, L. (2002) Cannabis and Ecstasy – soft drugs? In: *Proceedings of seminar I: Drugs and the brain*. Oxford: Beckley Foundation.

Iversen, L. (2003) Cannabis and the brain. *Brain* 126(6): 1252–1270.

Jacobsen, L.K., Southwick, S.M., and Kosten, T.R. (2001) Substance use disorders in patients with posttraumatic stress disorder: a review of the literature. *Am J Psychiatry* 158(8): 1184–1190.

Johnson, B.A., Roche, J.D., and Javors, M.A. (2000) Ondansetron for reduction of drinking among biologically predisposed alcoholic patients: a randomized controlled trial. *JAMA* 284(8): 963–971.

Johnson, B.A., Swift, R.M., Ait-Daoud, N., DiClemente, C.C., Javors, M.A., and Malcolm, R.J. Jr. (2004) Development of novel pharmacotherapies for the treatment of alcohol dependence: focus on antiepileptics. *Alcohol Clin Exp Res* 28(2): 295–301.

Joseph Rowntree Foundation (2000) *Drugs: dilemmas, choices, and the law*. London: Joseph Rowntree Foundation.

Joy, J.E., Watson, J., and Benson, J.A. (eds). (1999) *Marijuana and medicine*. Institute of Medicine. Washington DC: National Academy Press.

June, H.L., Foster, K.L., McKay, P.F., et al. (2003) The reinforcing properties of alcohol are mediated by GABA(A1) receptors in the ventral pallidum. *Neuropsychopharmacology* 28(12): 2124–2137.

Kahlig, K.M. and Galli, A. (2003) Regulation of dopamine transporter function and plasma membrane expression by dopamine, amphetamine, and cocaine. *Eur J Pharmacol* 479: 153–158.

Kelly, T.H., Stoops, W.W., Perry, A.S., Prendergast, M.A., and Rush, C.R. (2003) Clinical neuropharmacology of drugs of abuse: a comparison of drug-discrimination and subject-report measures. *Behav Cog Neurosci Rev* 2(4): 227–260.

Khanna, J.M., Kalant, H., and Shah, G., Chau, A. (1993) Effect of D-cycloserine on rapid tolerance to ethanol. *Pharmacol Biochem Behav* 45(4): 983–986.

Kiefer, F. and Wiedemann, K. (2004) Combined therapy: what does acamprosate and naltrexone combination tell us? *Alcohol Alcohol* 39(6): 542–547. Epub 29 September.

Kieffer, B.L. (1999) Opioids: first lessons from knockout mice. *Trends Pharm Sci* 20: 19–26.

Kiritze-Topor, P., Huas, D., Rosenzweig, C., Comte, S., Paille, F., and Lehert, P. (2004) A pragmatic trial of acamprosate in the treatment of alcohol dependence in primary care. *Alcohol Alcohol* 39(6): 520–527. Epub 10 August.

Kollins, S.H. (2003) Comparing the abuse potential of methylphenidate versus other stimulants: a review of available evidence and relevance to the ADHD patient. *J Clin Psych* 64 (Suppl II): 14–18.

Kollins, S.H., MacDonald, E.K., and Rush, C.R. (2001) Assessing the abuse potential of methylphenidate in nonhuman and human subjects – a review. *Pharm Biochem Behav* 68: 611–627.

Kosten, T.R., Rosen, M., Bond, J., *et al.* (2002) Human therapeutic cocaine vaccine: safety and immunogenicity. *Vaccine* 20: 1196–1204.

Kranzler, H.R. (2000) Pharmacotherapy of alcoholism: gaps in knowledge and opportunities for research. *Alcohol Alcohol* 35(6): 537–547.

Kushner, S.A., Dewey, S.L., and Kornetsky, C. (1999) The irreversible gamma-aminobutyric acid (GABA) transaminase inhibitor gamma-vinyl-GABA blocks cocaine self-administration in rats. *J Pharmacol Exp Ther* 290(2): 797–802.

Lader, D. and Meltzer, H. (2002) *Drinking: adults' behaviour and knowledge in 2002.* London: Office for National Statistics.

Lange, J.H. and Kruse, C.G. (2004) Recent advances in CB1 cannabinoid receptor antagonists. *Curr Opin Drug Discov Dev* 7(4): 498–506.

Laviolette, S.R., Gallegos, R.A., Henriksen, S.J., and van der Kooy, D. (2004) Opiate state controls bi-directional reward signaling via GABAA receptors in the ventral tegmental area. *Nat Neurosci* 7(2): 160–169. Epub 18 January.

Ledent, C., Valverde, O., Cossu, G., *et al.* (1999) Unresponsiveness to cannabinoids and reduced addictive effects of opiates in CB1 receptor knockout mice. *Science* 283(5400): 401–404.

Ledgerwood, L., Richardson, R., and Cranney, J. (2004) D-cycloserine and the facilitation of extinction of conditioned fear: consequences for reinstatement. *Behav Neurosci* 118(3): 505–513.

Lee, B., Tiefenbacher, S., Platt, D.M., and Spealman, R.D. (2003) Role of the hypothalamic-pituitary-adrenal axis in reinstatement of cocaine-seeking behavior in squirrel monkeys. *Psychopharmacology* 168(1–2): 177–183. Epub 22 March.

Lee, B., Tiefenbacher, S., Platt, D.M., and Spealman, R.D. (2004) Pharmacological blockade of alpha2-adrenoceptors induces reinstatement of cocaine-seeking behavior in squirrel monkeys. *Neuropsychopharmacology* 29(4): 686–693.

LeFoll, B. and Goldberg, S.R. (2004) Cannabinoid CB1 antagonists as promising new medications for drug dependence. *J Pharmacol Exp Ther* 3 November. Epub ahead of print.

Lelong, V., Dauphin, F., and Boulouard, M. (2001) RS 67333 and D-cycloserine accelerate learning acquisition in the rat. *Neuropharmacology* 41(4): 517–522.

Lieb, R., Schuetz, C.D., Pfister, C.H., von Sydow, K., and Wittchen, H. (2002) Mental disorders in ecstasy users: a prospective-longitudinal investigation. *Drug Alcohol Depend* 68(2): 195–207.

Liechti, M.E. and Vollenweider, F.X. (2000) The serotonin uptake inhibitor citalopram reduces acute cardiovascular and vegetative effects of 3,4-methylenedioxymethamphetamine ('Ecstasy') in healthy volunteers. *J Psychopharmacol* 14(3): 269–274.

Lindsey, K.P., Wilcox, K.M., Votaw, J.R., *et al.* (2004) Effects of dopamine transporter inhibitors on cocaine self-administration in rhesus monkeys: relationship to transporter occupancy determined by positron emission tomography neuroimaging. *J Pharmacol Exp Ther* 309(3): 959–969. Epub 24 February.

Lingford-Hughes, A. and Nutt, D. (2003) Neurobiology of addiction and implications for treatment. *Br J Psychiatry* 182: 97–100.

Lingford-Hughes, A.R., Davies, S.J., McIver, S., Williams, T.M., Daglish, M.R., and Nutt, D.J. (2003) Addiction. *Br Med Bull* 65: 209–222.

Lingford-Hughes, A.R., Welch, S., and Nutt, D.J. (2004) British Association for Psychopharmacology. Evidence-based guidelines for the pharmacological management of substance misuse, addiction and comorbidity: recommendations from the British Association for Psychopharmacology. *J Psychopharmacol* 18(3): 293–335.

Loonam, T.M., Noailles, P.A.H., Yu, J., Zhu, J.P.Q., and Angulo, J.A. (2003) Substance P and cholecystokinin regulate neurochemical responses to cocaine and methamphetamine in the striatum. *Life Sci* 73: 727–739.

Lopes, D.V.S., Caruso, R.R.B., Castro, N.G., Costa, P.R.R., da Silva, A.J.M., and Noel, F. (2004) Characterization of a new synthetic isoflavonoid with inverse agonist activity at the central benzodiazepine receptor. *Eur J Pharmacol* 495: 87–96.

Lu, L., Liu, Z., Huang, M., and Zhang, Z. (2003) Dopamine-dependent responses to cocaine depend on corticotropin-releasing factor receptor subtypes. *J Neurochem* 84(6): 1378–1386.

Lyle, J. and Cadet, J.L. (2003) Methylenedioxymethamphetamine (MDMA, Ecstasy) neurotoxicity: cellular and molecular mechanisms. *Brain Res Rev* 42: 155–168.

MacLeod, J., Oakes, R., Copello, A., *et al.* (2004) Psychological and social sequelae of cannabis and other illicit drug use by young people: a systematic review of longitudinal, general population studies. *Lancet* 363: 1579–1588.

Mailliard, W.S. and Diamond, I. (2004) Recent advances in the neurobiology of alcoholism: the role of adenosine. *Pharm Ther* 101: 39–46.

Maisonneuve, I.M. and Glick, S.D. (2003) Anti-addictive actions of an iboga alkaloid congener: a novel mechanism for a novel treatment. *Pharmacol Biochem Behav* 75(3): 607–618.

Maldonado, R. and Fonseca, R. (2002) Cannabinoid addiction: behavioral models and neural correlates. *J Neurosci* 22: 1326–1331.

Mann, K., Lehert, P., and Morgan, M.Y. (2004) The efficacy of acamprosate in the maintenance of abstinence in alcohol-dependent individuals: results of a meta-analysis. *Alcohol Clin Exp Res* 28(1): 51–63.

Marsicano, G., Wotjak, C.T., Azad, S.C., *et al.* (2002) The endogenous cannabinoid system controls extinction of aversive memories. *Nature* 418: 530–534.

Martin, M., Ledent, C., Parmentier, M., Maldonado, R., and Valverde, O. (2000) Cocaine, but not morphine, induces conditioned place preference and sensitization to locomotor responses in CB1 knockout mice. *Eur J Neurosci* 12(11): 4038–4046.

Matsumoto, R.R., Liu, Y., Lerner, M., Howard, E.W., and Brackett, D.J. (2003) Sigma receptors: potential medications development target for anti-cocaine agents. *Eur J Pharmacol* 469(1–3): 1–12.

Maurice, T., Martin-Fardon, R., Romieu, P., and Matsumoto, R.R. (2002) Sigma(1) (sigma(1)) receptor antagonists represent a new strategy against cocaine addiction and toxicity. *Neurosci Biobehav Rev* 26(4): 499–527.

McCann, U.D. and Ricaurte, G.A. (2004) Amphetamine neurotoxicity: accomplishments and remaining challenges. *Neurosci Biobehav Rev* 27: 821–826.

McDonough, M., Kennedy, N., Glasper, A., and Bearn, J. (2004) Clinical features and management of gamma-hydroxybutyrate (GHB) withdrawal: a review. *Drug Alcohol Depend* 75: 3–9.

McKeganey, N. (2005) *Foresight state of science review – sociology*. London: Department of Trade and Industry.

Meis, S. (2003) Nociceptin/orphanin FQ: actions within the brain. *Neuroscientist* 9(2): 158–168. doi: 10.1177/1073858403252231

Mendelson, W.B., Roth, T., Cassella, J., *et al.* (2004) The treatment of chronic insomnia: drug indications, chronic use and abuse liability. Summary of a 2001 New Clinical Drug Evaluation Unit meeting symposium. *Sleep Med Rev* 8(1): 7–17.

Meyer, R.E. (1996) The disease called addiction: emerging evidence in a 200-year debate. *Lancet* 347: 162–166.

Milivojevic, N., Krisch, I., Sket, D., and Zivin, M. (2004) The dopamine D1 receptor agonist and D2 receptor antagonist LEK-8829 attenuates reinstatement of cocaine-seeking in rats.

Naunyn Schmiedebergs Arch Pharmacol 369(6): 576–582. Epub 7 May.

Modesto-Lowe, V. (2002) Naltrexone depot (Drug Abuse Sciences). *IDrugs* 5(8): 835–838.

Morris, K. (1998) Ecstasy users face consequences of neurotoxicity. *Lancet* 352: 1911.

Morris, K. (2003a) Research reawakens ecstasy neurotoxicity debate. *Lancet Neurology* 2: 650.

Morris, K. (2003b) Melanocortins key to trigger sex on the brain. *Lancet Neurology* 2: 140.

Morris, K. (2004) Rat studies of Ritalin emphasise need for proper ADHD diagnosis. *Lancet Neurol* 3: 75.

Morris, K.A., Jones, R., and Nutt, D.J. (2005a) *Foresight state of science review – cognition enhancers*. London: Department of Trade and Industry.

Morris, P., Jones, T., and Lingford-Hughes, A. (2005b) *Foresight state of science review – Neuroimaging*. London: Department of Trade and Industry.

Mukherjee, R.A.S., Hollins, S., Abou-Saleh, M.T., and Turk, J. (2005) Low level alcohol consumption and the fetus. *BMJ* 330: 375–376. doi:10.1136/bmj.330.7488.375.

Murtra, P., Sheasby, A.M., Hunt, S.P., and De Felipe, C. (2000) Rewarding effects of opiates are absent in mice lacking the receptor for substance, P. *Nature* 405: 180–183.

Myrick, H., Henderson, S., Brady, K.T., and Malcolm, R. (2001) Gabapentin in the treatment of cocaine dependence: a case series. *J Clin Psychiatry* 62(1): 19–23.

Nagy, J. (2004) Renaissance of NMDA receptor antagonists: do they have a role in the pharmacotherapy for alcoholism? *IDrugs* 7(4): 339–350.

Nagy, J., Horvath, C., Farkas, S., Kolok, S., and Szombathelyi, Z. (2004) NR2B subunit selective NMDA antagonists inhibit neurotoxic effect of alcohol-withdrawal in primary cultures of rat cortical neurones. *Neurochem Int* 44(1): 17–23.

Nestler, E.J. (2004) New treatments for drug addiction: intracellular targets for drug discovery. *Neuropsychopharmacology* Suppl 1 (ACNP annual meeting): S60.

Nicholls, D. (2004) Hallucinogens. *Pharm Ther* 101: 131–181.

Nie, Z., Schweitzer, P., Roberts, A.J., Madamba, S.G., Moore, S.D., and Siggins, G.R. (2004) Ethanol augments GABAergic transmission in the central amygdala via CRF1 receptors. *Science* 303: 1512–1514.

Nitsche, M.A., Jaussi, W., Liebetanz, D., Lang, N., Tergau, F., and Paulus, W. (2004) Consolidation of human motor cortical neuroplasticity by D-cycloserine. *Neuropsychopharmacology* 29(8): 1573–1578.

Nordahl, T.E., Salo, R., and Leamon, M. (2003) Neuropsychological effects of chronic methamphetamine use on neurotransmitters and cognition: a review. *J Neuropsych Clin Neurosci* 15: 317–325.

Nowak, R. (2004) How our brains fend off madness. *New Scientist* 184: 13.

Nutt, D. (1994) In: G. Edwards and M. Lader (eds), *Addiction: processes of change*. Oxford: Oxford Medical Publications.

Nutt, D. (1999) Alcohol and the brain: pharmacological insights for psychiatrists. *Br J Psych* 175: 114–119.

Nutt, D. (2002) Heroin and related opiates. In: *Proceedings of seminar I: Drugs and the brain*. Oxford: Beckley Foundation.

Nutt, D.J. (2003a) Death and dependence: current controversies over the selective serotonin reuptake inhibitors. *J Psychopharmacol* 17(4): 355–364.

Nutt, D. (2003b) Alcohol and the brain. In: *Proceedings of seminar III: Alcohol and other recreational drugs*. Oxford: Beckley Foundation.

Nutt, D. (2005) Cannabis antagonists: a new era of social psychopharmacology? *J Psychopharmacol* 19: 3–4.

Nutt, D.J. and Malizia, A.L. (2001) New insights into the role of the GABA(A)-benzodiazepine receptor in psychiatric disorder. *Br J Psychiatry* 179: 390–396.

Nutt, D., Lingford-Hughes, A., and Dalglish, M. (2003) Future directions in substance dependence research. *J Neural Transm* 64(Suppl): 95–103.

O'Shea, E., Escobedo, I., Orio, L., et al. (2005) Elevation of ambient room temperature has differential effects on MDMA-induced 5-HT and dopamine release in striatum and nucleus accumbens of rats. *Neuropsychopharmacology* Jan 26. Epub ahead of print.

Office for National Statistics. (2004) *Results from the General Household Survey 2003/4*. London: Office for National Statistics.

Office for National Statistics. (2005) Deaths related to drug poisoning: England and Wales, 1999–2003. *Health Statistics Quarterly* 25: 52–59.

Oldham, N.S., Wright, N.M., Adams, C.E., Sheard, L., and Tompkins, C.N. (2004)

The Leeds Evaluation of Efficacy of Detoxification Study (LEEDS) project: an open-label pragmatic randomised control trial comparing the efficacy of differing therapeutic agents for primary care detoxification from either street heroin or methadone. *BMC Fam Pract* 5(1): 9.

Oliveto, A., Benios, T., Gonsai, K., Feingold, A., Poling, J., and Kosten, T.R. (2003) D-cycloserine-naloxone interactions in opioid-dependent humans under a novel-response naloxone discrimination procedure. *Exp Clin Psychopharmacol* 11(3): 237–246.

Orford, J. (1988) In: Lader, M. (ed), *The psychopharmacology of addiction.* Oxford: Oxford Medical Publications.

Orford, J. (2005) *Foresight state of science review – problem gambling and other behavioural addictions.* London: Department of Trade and Industry.

Osselton, D., Cowan, D., and Robinson, S. (2005) *Foresight state of science review – drug testing.* London: Department of Trade and Industry.

Oswald, L.M. and Wand, G.S. (2004) Opioids and alcoholism. *Phys Behav* 81: 339–358.

Patkar, A.A., Gottheil, E., Berrettini, W.H., Hill, K.P., Thornton, C.C., and Weinstein, S.P. (2003) Relationship between platelet serotonin uptake sites and measures of impulsivity, aggression, and craving among African-American cocaine abusers. *Am J Addict* 12(5): 432–447.

Patton, G.C., Coffey, C., Carlin, J.B., Degenhardt, L., Lynskey, M., and Hall, W. (2002) Cannabis use and mental health in young people: cohort study. *BMJ* 325(7374): 1195–1198.

Paul, M., Dewey, S.L., Gardner, E.L., Brodie, J.D., Ashby, C.R., Jr. (2001) Gamma-vinyl, GABA(GVG) blocks expression of the conditioned place preference response to heroin in rats. *Synapse* 41(3): 219–220.

Pembrey, M., Ball, D., and Stephens, D. (2005) *Foresight state of science review – genomics.* London: Department of Trade and Industry.

Phillips, H. and Lawton, G. (2004) The intoxication instinct. *New Scientist* 184: 32–41.

Pietraszek, M. (2003) Significance of dysfunctional glutamatergic transmission for the development of psychotic symptoms. *Pol J Pharmacol* 55: 133–154.

Pistis, M., Perra, S., Pillolla, G., Melis, M., Muntoni, A.L., and Gessa, G.L. (2004) Adolescent exposure to cannabinoids induces long-lasting changes in the response to drugs of abuse of rat midbrain dopamine neurons. *Biol Psychiatry* 15 July, 56(2): 86–94.

Popp, R.L. and Lovinger, D.M. (2000) Interaction of acamprosate with ethanol and spermine on NMDA receptors in primary cultured neurons. *Eur J Pharmacol* 394(2–3): 221–231.

Pouletty, P. (2004) Drug addictions as treatable diseases. *Euro Biotech News* 3(5): 44–46.

Prime Minister's Strategy Unit. (2004) *Alcohol harm reduction strategy for England.* London: Strategy Unit.

Putnins, A. (2003) Substance use and the prediction of young offender recidivism. *Drug Alcohol Rev* 22(4): 401–408.

Raby, W.N. and Coomaraswamy, S. (2004) Gabapentin reduces cocaine use among addicts from a community clinic sample. *J Clin Psychiatry* 65(1): 84–86.

Racz, I., Bilkei-Gorzo, A., Toth, Z.E., Michel, K., Palkovits, M., and Zimmer, A. (2003) A critical role for the cannabinoid CB1 receptors in alcohol dependence and stress-stimulated ethanol drinking. *J Neurosci* 23(6): 2453–2458.

Ranaldi, R. and Poeggel, K. (2002) Baclofen decreases methamphetamine self-administration in rats. *Neuroreport* 13(9): 1107–1010.

Reneman, L. (2003) Designer drugs: how dangerous are they? *J Neural Transm* 66(Suppl): 61–83.

Rezvani, A.H., Overstreet, D.H., Perfumi, M., and Massi, M. (2003) Plant derivatives in the treatment of alcohol dependency. *Pharmacol Biochem Behav* 75(3): 593–606.

Robbins, T.W., Cardinal, R., and Everitt, B. (2005) *Foresight state of science review – neuroscience.* London: Department of Trade and Industry.

Roberts, D.C. and Andrews, M.M. (1997) Baclofen suppression of cocaine self-administration: demonstration using a discrete trials procedure. *Psychopharmacology* 131(3): 271–277.

Rocha, B.A. (2003) Stimulant and reinforcing effects of cocaine in monoamine transporter knockout mice. *Eur J Pharmacol* 479(1–3): 107–115.

Roddy, E. (2004) Bupropion and other non-nicotinic pharmacotherapies. *BMJ* 328: 509–11. Epub 18 October. doi:10.1136/bmj.328.7438.509.

Rodriguez de Fonseca, F., Carrera, M.R., Navarro, M., Koob, G.F., and Weiss, F. (1997) Activation of corticotropin-releasing factor in the limbic system during cannabinoid withdrawal. *Science* 276(5321): 2050–2054.

Romberger, D.J. and Grant, K. (2004) Alcohol consumption and smoking status: the role of smoking cessation. *Biomed Pharmacotherapy* 58: 77–83.

Room, R. (2005) *Foresight state of science review – social policy*. London: Department of Trade and Industry.

Russo-Neustadt, A. (2003) Brain-derived neurotrophic factor, behavior, and new directions for the treatment of mental disorders. *Semin Clin Neuropsychiatry* 8(2): 109–118.

Saadat, K.S., O'Shea, E., Colado, M.I., Elliott, J.M., and Green, A.R. (2005) The role of 5-HT in the impairment of thermoregulation observed in rats administered MDMA ('ecstasy') when housed at high ambient temperature. *Psychopharmacology*. Epub ahead of print.

Sahakian, B., Turner, D., and Duka, T. (2005) *Foresight state of science review – experimental psychology*. London: Department of Trade and Industry.

Sakai, J.T., Hall, S.K., Mikulich-Gilbertson, S.K., and Crowley, T.J. (2004) Inhalant use, abuse, and dependence among adolescent patients: commonly comorbid problems. *J Am Acad Child Adolesc Psychiatry* 43(9): 1080–1088.

Sanchez, V., O'Shea, E., Saadat, K.S., Elliott, J.M., Colado, M.I., and Green, A.R. (2004) Effect of repeated ('binge') dosing of MDMA to rats housed at normal and high temperature on neurotoxic damage to cerebral 5-HT and dopamine neurones. *J Psychopharmacol* 18(3): 412–416.

Schifano, F., Oyefeso, A., Webb, L., Pollar, M., Corkery, J., and Ghodse, A.H. (2003) Review of deaths related to taking ecstasy, England and Wales, 1997–2000. *BMJ* 326: 80–81.

Schroeder, J.P., Iller, K.A., and Hodge, C.W. (2003) Neuropeptide-Y Y5 receptors modulate the onset and maintenance of operant ethanol self-administration. *Alcohol Clin Exp Res* 27(12): 1912–1920.

Schultz, W. (2001) Reward signaling by dopamine neurons. *Neuroscience* 7: 293–302.

Sheffler, D.J. and Roth, B.L. (2003) Salvinorin A: the 'magic mint' hallucinogen finds a molecular target in the kappa opioid receptor. *Trends Pharm Sci* 24: 107–109.

Shepard, J.D., Bossert, J.M., Liu, S.Y., and Shaham, Y. (2004) The anxiogenic drug yohimbine reinstates methamphetamine seeking in a rat model of drug relapse. *Biol Psychiatry* 55(11): 1082–1089.

Shoptaw, S., Yang, X., Rotheram-Fuller, E.J., *et al.* (2003) Randomized placebo-controlled trial of baclofen for cocaine dependence: preliminary effects for individuals with chronic patterns of cocaine use. *J Clin Psychiatry* 64(12): 1440–1448.

Shpilenya, L.S., Muzychenko, A.P., Gasbarrini, G., and Addolorato, G. (2002) Metadoxine in acute alcohol intoxication; a double-blind, randomized, placebo-controlled study. *Alcohol Clin Exp Res* 26: 340–346.

Shulgin, S. (2004) *Studying consciousness.* Exploring Consciousness conference, Bath, UK. June.

Shulgin, S. and Shulgin, A. (1991) *PIHKAL: a chemical love story.* Berkeley, California: Transform Press.

Shulgin, S. and Shulgin, A. (1997) *TIHKAL: the continuation.* Berkeley, California: Transform Press.

Simantov, R. (2004) Multiple molecular and neuropharmacological effects of MDMA (Ecstasy). *Life Sciences* 24: 803–814.

Sinha, R., Talih, M., Malison, R., Cooney, N., Anderson, G.M., and Kreek, M.J. (2003) Hypothalamic-pituitary-adrenal axis and sympatho-adreno-medullary responses during stress-induced and drug cue-induced cocaine craving states. *Psychopharmacology* 170(1): 62–72. Epub 4 July.

Smit, F., Bolier, L., and Cuijpers, P. (2004) Cannabis use and the risk of later schizophrenia: a review. *Addiction* 99: 425–430.

Snyder, S. (2002) Forty years of neurotransmitters: a personal account. *Arch Gen Psych* 59: 983–994.

Sobel, B.F., Sigmon, S.C., Walsh, S.L., *et al.* (2004) Open-label trial of an injection depot formulation of buprenorphine in opioid detoxification. *Drug Alcohol Depend* 73(1): 11–22.

Solinas, M., Panlilio, L.V., Antoniou, K., Pappas, L.A., and Goldberg, S.R. (2003) The cannabinoid CB1 antagonist N-piperidinyl-5- (4-chlorophenyl)-1-(2,4-dichlorophenyl) -4-methylpyrazole-3-carboxamide (SR-141716A) differentially alters the reinforcing effects of heroin under continuous reinforcement, fixed ratio, and progressive ratio schedules of drug self-administration in rats. *J Pharmacol Exp Ther* 306(1): 93–102. Epub 26 March.

Soyka, M. and Chick, J. (2003) Use of acamprosate and opioid antagonists in the treatment of alcohol dependence: a European perspective. *Am J Addict* 12(Suppl 1): S69–80.

Stinus, L., Cador, M., Zorrilla, E.P., and Koob, G.F. (2004) Buprenorphine and a CRF(1) antagonist block the acquisition of opiate withdrawal-induced conditioned place aversion in rats. *Neuropsychopharmacology* 12 May. Epub ahead of print.

Stromberg, M.F., Mackler, S.A., Volpicelli, J.R., O'Brien, C.P., and Dewey, S.L. (2001) The effect of gamma-vinyl-GABA on the consumption of concurrently available oral cocaine and ethanol in the rat. *Pharmacol Biochem Behav* 68(2): 291–299.

Sumnall, H.R., Wagstaff, G.F., and Cole, J.C. (2004) Self-reported psychopathology in poly-drug users. *J Psychopharmacol* 18(1): 75–82.

Swift, W., Hall, W., and Teesson, M. (2001) Characteristics of DSM-IV and ICD-10 cannabis dependence among Australian adults: results from the National Survey of Mental Health and Wellbeing. *Drug Alcohol Depend* 63(2): 147–153.

Szekeres, H.J., Atack, J.R., Chambers, M.S., *et al.* (2004) 3,4-Dihydronaphthalen-1(2H)-ones: novel ligands for the benzodiazepine site of a5-containing GABAA receptors. *Bioorganic Med Chem Lett* 14: 2871–2875.

Tomar, S.L., Connolly, G.N., Wilkenfeld, J., and Henningfield, J.E. (2003) Declining smoking in Sweden: is Swedish Match getting the credit for Swedish tobacco control's efforts? *Tob Control* 12: 368–371.

Twigg, L., Moon, G., and Walker, S. (2004) *The smoking epidemic in England.* London: Health Development Agency.

Valdez, G.R., Sabino, V., and Koob, G.F. (2004) Increased anxiety-like behavior and ethanol self-administration in dependent rats: reversal via corticotropin-releasing factor-2 receptor activation. *Alcohol Clin Exp Res* 28(6): 865–872.

Valdez, G.R., Zorrilla, E.P., Roberts, A.J., and Koob, G.F. (2003) Antagonism of corticotropin-releasing factor attenuates the enhanced responsiveness to stress observed during protracted ethanol abstinence. *Alcohol* 29(2): 55–60.

van der Stelt, M. and Di Marzo, V. (2003) The endocannabinoid system in the basal ganglia and in the mesolimbic reward system: implications for neurological and psychiatric disorders. *Eur J Pharmacol* 480(1–3): 133–150.

Verdoux, H. and Tournier, M. (2004) Cannabis use and risk of psychosis: an etiological link? *Epidemiol Psychiatr Soc* 13(2): 113–119.

Vetulani, J. (2001) Drug addiction. Part III: Pharmacotherapy of addiction. *Pol J Pharmacol* 53: 415–434.

Volkow, N.D., Fowler, J.S., and Wang, G.J. (1999) Imaging studies on the role of dopamine in cocaine reinforcement and addiction in humans. *J Psychopharmacol* 13: 337–345.

Vollenweider, F.X. and Liechti, M.E. (2000) Acute psychological and physiological effects of MDMA ('Ecstasy') after haloperidol pretreatment in healthy humans. *Eur Neuropsychopharmacol* 10: 289–295.

Vorel, S.R., Ashby C.R., Jr., Paul, M., *et al.* (2002) Dopamine D3 receptor antagonism inhibits cocaine-seeking and cocaine-enhanced brain reward in rats. *J Neurosci* 22(21): 9595–9603.

Walker, D.L., Ressler, K.J., Lu, K.T., and Davis, M. (2002) Facilitation of conditioned fear extinction by systemic administration or intra-amygdala infusions of D-cycloserine as assessed with fear-potentiated startle in rats. *J Neurosci* 22(6): 2343–2351.

Walker, D.D., Venner, K., Hill, D.E., Meyers, R.J., and Miller, W.R. (2004) A comparison of alcohol and drug disorders: is there evidence for a developmental sequence of drug abuse? *Addict Behav* 29(4): 817–823.

Waszkielewicz, A. and Bojarski, J. (2004) γ-hydroxybutyric acid (GHB) and its chemical modifications: a review of the GHBergic system. *Pol J Pharmacol* 56: 43–49.

Weiss, F., Ciccocioppo, R., Parsons, L.H., Katner, S., Liu, X., Zorrilla, E.P., Valdez, G.R., Ben-Shahar O., Angeletti, S., and Richter, R.R. (2001) Compulsive drug-seeking behavior and relapse. Neuroadaptation, stress, and conditioning factors. *Ann NY Acad Sci* 937: 1–26.

Wichniak, A., Brunner, H., Ising, M., Pedrosa Gil, F., Holsboer, F., and Friess, E. (2004) Impaired hypothalamic-pituitary-adrenocortical (HPA) system is related to severity of benzodiazepine withdrawal in patients with depression. *Psychoneuroendocrinology* 29(9): 1101–1108.

Wilens, T.E. (2001) Attention-deficit/hyperactivity disorder and the substance use disorders: the nature of the relationship, who is at risk, and treatment issues. *Primary Psychiatry* 11(7): 63–70.

Williams, K., Wu, T., Colangelo, C., and Nairn, A.C. (2004) Recent advances in neuro-proteomics and potential application to studies of drug addiction. *Neuropharmacol* 47: 148–166.

Wilson, R.I. and Nicoll, R.A. (2002) Endocannabinoid signaling in the brain. *Science* 296: 678–682.

Wingerchuck, G. (2004) Cannabis for medical purposes: cultivating science, weeding out the fiction. *Lancet* 264: 315–316.

Wlaz, P. (1998) Anti-convulsant and adverse effects of the glycineB receptor ligands, D-cycloserine and L-701,324: comparison with competitive and non-competitive N-methyl-D-aspartate receptor antagonists. *Brain Res Bull* Aug, 46(6): 535–540.

Wolf, M.E. (1998) The role of excitatory amino acids in behavioral sensitization to psychomotor stimulants. *Prog Neurobiol* 54(6): 679–720.

Wong, C.G.T., Gibson, K.M., and Snead III, O.C. (2004) From the street to the brain: neurobiology of the recreational drug γ-hydroxybutyric acid. *Trends Pharm Sci* 25(1): 29–34.

World Health Organization (1992) *International classification of diseases*, 10th edition. Geneva: WHO.

Xu, M. and Zhang, J. (2004) Molecular genetic probing of dopamine receptors in drug addiction. *Curr Opin Drug Discov Devel* 7(5): 703–708.

Xu, G.P., Van Bockstaele, E., Reyes, B., Bethea, T., and Valentino, R.J. (2004) Chronic morphine sensitizes the brain norepinephrine system to corticotropin-releasing factor and stress. *J Neurosci* 24(38): 8193–8197.

Zachariou, V., Brunzell, D.H., Hawes, J., *et al.* (2003) The neuropeptide galanin modulates behavioral and neurochemical signs of opiate withdrawal. *Proc Natl Acad Sci USA* 100(15): 9028–9033. Epub 9 July.

Zacny, J., Bigelow, G., Compton, P., Foley, K., Iguchi, M., and Sannerud, C. (2003) College on Problems of Drug Dependence taskforce on prescription opioid non-medical use and abuse: position statement. *Drug Alcohol Depend* 69: 215–232.

Zarrindast, M.R., Faraji, N., Rostami, P., Sahraei, H., and Ghoshouni, H. (2003) Cross-tolerance between morphine- and nicotine-induced conditioned place preference in mice. *Pharmacol Biochem Behav* 74(2): 363–369.

Zhu, H., Jenab, S., Jones, K.L., and Inturrisi, C.E. (2003) The clinically available NMDA receptor antagonist dextromethorphan attenuates acute morphine withdrawal in the neonatal rat. *Brain Res Dev Brain Res* 142(2): 209–213.

General Resources

No recommendation is given on the reliability or accuracy of these sources.

Miller, R.L. (2002) *The encyclopedia of addictive drugs*. Westport: Greenwood Press.

www.bap.org.uk/
www.drinkanddrugs.net/
www.drugscope.org.uk/
www.erowid.org/
www.forbes.com/
www.phrma.org/
www.statistics.gov.uk/
www.wired.com/

10 APPENDIX: ACRONYMS

ADHD	attention-deficit hyperactivity disorder
AMPA	α-amino-3-hydroxy-5-methyl-4-isoxazoleproprionic acid
BAP	British Association for Psychopharmacology
BDNF	brain-derived neurotrophic factor
2CT7	2,5-dimethoxy-4-(*n*)-propylthiophenethylamine
CREB	cyclic-AMP response element binding protein
CREST	Clinical Research Efficacy Screening Trial
CRF	corticotrophin-releasing factor
DMT	N,N-dimethyltryptamine
EAA	excitatory amino-acids
FDA	US Food and Drug Administration
GABA	gamma-aminobutyric acid
GHB	gamma-hydroxybutyrate
HIV	human immunodeficiency virus
IV	intravenous
LAAM	levo-alpha-acetyl methadol
LSD	D-lysergic acid diethylamide
MDA	3,4-methylenedioxyamphetamine
MDEA	3,4-methylenedioxy-N-ethylamphetamine
MDMA	3,4-methylenedioxy-N-methylamphetamine
NIDA	US National Institute on Drug Abuse
NMDA	N-methyl-D-aspartate
PCP	phencyclidine
PMA	4-methoxyamphetamine
SSRI	selective serotonin reuptake inhibitor
THC	delta-9-tetrahydrocannabinol

Psychological Treatments of Substance Misuse and Dependence

Val Curran and Colin Drummond

1 EXECUTIVE SUMMARY

This review summarises what is known about psychological treatments for addictions, examines gaps in the evidence base, and looks to the future at treatment and research in relation to new drugs, new opportunities and new priorities.

A wide range of psychological interventions have been developed based on existing psychological theories of addictive behaviour. These include conditioning and cognitive theories. The evidence base for the effectiveness of psychological interventions in treating addictive behaviour is strong, particularly in relation to alcohol, stimulant, cannabis and opiate dependence. In the latter, psychological intervention is an effective adjunct to methadone maintenance treatment. In alcohol, stimulant and cannabis dependence, psychological treatments are the main intervention approach.

Brief psychological interventions are particularly effective in the context of opportunistic screening and in medical settings for people not seeking alcohol treatment. However, there is a need for more pragmatic research into cost effectiveness and implementation, particularly in the UK treatment setting. There is a need for research on psychological interventions in polydrug misuse and in people with psychiatric comorbidity, which are becoming increasingly prevalent. More research is needed on intensive and longer term interventions for people with more severe addiction problems. These will require more innovative research methods than the typical one-year follow-up randomised controlled trials used to date.

Future research on psychological interventions needs to identify the key 'active ingredients' which lead to a successful treatment outcome for particular groups of substance misuser, as well as treatment 'matching' effects in more typical treatment settings. Care co-ordination and integrated care pathways are increasingly advocated by health commissioners but require more systematic research to assess cost effectiveness and optimal implementation strategies.

The development of new mood altering and 'lifestyle' drugs may lead to new forms of drug dependence and this will present new challenges for clinical psychology and psychological treatment research. Future psychological treatments will need to be based on more comprehensive evidence which details the key elements of therapies that work most effectively for particular individuals and classes of drugs.

This should build on three main areas of development: neuroscience and experimental psychology, new technology, and pharmacological treatments. Neuroscience and experimental psychology have begun to increase our understanding of the mechanisms of drug dependence such as the effect of exposure to drug-related cues, attentional bias and the impact of the client's cognitive function on information processing, all of which have implications for the use of psychological interventions. New technologies such as mobile phones could provide a useful adjunct in the real-world environment to more office-based psychological interventions. The Internet has the potential to deliver health information and addiction interventions to a much wider population, with a potential public health impact. Psychological interventions have the potential to enhance compliance and improve outcomes with pharmacological interventions.

Overall we conclude that psychological interventions applied to particular forms of addiction are highly cost effective. The potential of future more effective treatments delivered to a wider range of substance misusers is considerable. We need to develop the UK evidence base for effectiveness of psychological interventions.

2 INTRODUCTION

Addiction problems have increased in the UK in the last 20 years. The misuse of drugs is at its highest level ever and alcohol misuse at its highest point in

50 years. There are over 8 million adults in Britain drinking above the Government's safe weekly levels (Prime Minister's Strategy Unit, 2003). Alcohol misuse is associated with 150 000 hospital admissions and 22 000 premature deaths per annum. Smoking leads to 150 000 premature deaths per annum (Prime Minister's Strategy Unit, 2003). This rise in drug use has been accompanied by enormous costs to society. One estimate puts the cost of drug misuse at £12 billion per annum (Godfrey *et al.*, 2002). The Prime Minister's Strategy Unit has highlighted the large and growing problems caused by alcohol (Prime Minister's Strategy Unit, 2003). It is estimated that alcohol misuse costs the country £20 billion per annum. Gambling addiction remains a significant problem and may increase with deregulation and the further availability of gambling opportunities. All of this points to the need to find effective intervention strategies to combat both chemical and behavioural addictions.

There have been several recent comprehensive reviews of the research base of addiction treatment, and further reviews are in progress. Substance misuse treatment research was reviewed in a task force review (Department of Health, 1996) and there have been systematic reviews of treatments for opiate dependency (Amato *et al.*, 2004; Mayet *et al.*, 2004) and for substance-using people with severe mental illness (Jeffery *et al.*, 2000). The British Association for Psychopharmacology guidelines on substance misuse treatment include a review of treatment research (Lingford-Hughes *et al.*, 2004). Miller *et al.* (1995) have produced a comprehensive systematic review of the evidence for the effectiveness of treatment for alcohol problems. The National Institute for Health and Clinical Excellence (NICE) is developing guidance on evidence-based interventions for substance misuse. The National Treatment Agency for Substance Misuse has commissioned a review of the evidence base for treating alcohol misuse and dependence as part of the development of the National Alcohol Harm Reduction

Strategy. It is not our aim to provide a further review of this literature. Instead we summarise what we know about which psychological treatments work and examine the gaps in the existing evidence base. We then look to the future for psychological treatments and research – to new drugs, new opportunities and new priorities.

2.1 What is the Basis of Psychological Treatment?

Clinical psychology applies psychological principles to assessing and preventing substance abuse and treating people with substance-use problems. Psychological treatments encompass a wide range of interventions which are based on different theories of substance dependence. The main treatment approaches used are shown in Table 7.1. Although these are labelled separately, in practice there is a lot of overlap. Many treatments raid the theoretical cupboard to combine aspects of cognitive, behavioural and social interventions.

The roots of psychological treatments are embedded in behavioural and cognitive theories. Behavioural theories see substance misuse as a set of learned or 'conditioned' behaviours. There are two major types of conditioning. 'Classical conditioning' was based on Ivan Pavlov's classic experiment on dogs. Pavlov's dogs would salivate naturally when given food. However, if he rang a bell a few minutes before he gave them food, they soon began to salivate at the bell. They had become conditioned to respond (salivate) to the conditioned stimulus (the bell). Likewise, a person's use of heroin may be paired with particular objects (e.g. syringes), places (dealer's flat), people (heroin-using friends) or feelings (e.g. being bored or lonely). Because of the frequent pairings of these with the drug in the past, syringes, drug-using friends and so on become conditioned stimuli. Figure 7.1 illustrates Drummond *et al.*'s (1990) conditioning model for craving alcohol, where conditioned stimuli are those associated

TABLE 7.1   A brief summary of the main psychological therapies used in treating substance misuse

BEHAVIOURAL THERAPY (BT)

A structured therapy focusing on changing behaviour and the environmental factors that trigger maladaptive behaviour. Includes:

Cue exposure treatment (CET)

A structured treatment involving exposure to drug-related cues that have been associated with past drug use without consumption of the drug. This is intended to lead to a reduction (or habituation) of reactivity to drug cues and hence to a reduced likelihood of relapse.

Community reinforcement approach (CRA)

A behavioural approach that focuses on what the client finds rewarding in his or her social, occupational and recreational life. It aims to help him or her change their lifestyle and social environment to support long-term changes in behaviour whereby using substances is less rewarding that not using them.

Contingency management (CM)

Also known as voucher-based therapy, this aims to encourage adaptive behaviour by rewarding the client for attaining agreed goals (e.g. no use of illicit drugs as checked by urine screens) and not rewarding them when these goals are unmet (e.g. illicit drug use). Vouchers can usually be exchanged for consumer goods.

Cognitive therapy (CT)

A structured therapy using cognitive techniques (e.g. challenging a person's negative thoughts) and behavioural techniques (e.g. behavioural experiments; activity planning) to change maladaptive thoughts and beliefs.

Cognitive behavioural therapy (CBT)

A combination of both cognitive and behavioural therapies.

Relapse prevention (RP)

Uses several CBT strategies to enhance the client's self-control and prevent relapse. It highlights problems that the client may face and develops strategies that he or she can use to deal with high-risk situations.

Motivational interviewing (MI)

A focused approach aiming to enhance motivation for changing substance use by exploring and resolving the individual's ambivalence about change.

Motivational enhancement therapy (MET)

A brief intervention based on MI which also incorporates a 'check-up' assessment and feedback.

TWELVE-STEP APPROACHES

Interventions used by self-help organisations like Alcoholics Anonymous. They are based on a philosophy that adopts an illness model and sees substance use as stemming from an innate vulnerability. An individual must acknowledge their addiction and the harm it has caused to themselves and others; they must also accept their lack of control over use and thus the only acceptable goal is abstinence.

OTHER APPROACHES

The involvement of partners and family through marital and family therapy builds on the known social context of substance use. There are also various forms of counselling, group therapy and milieu therapy.

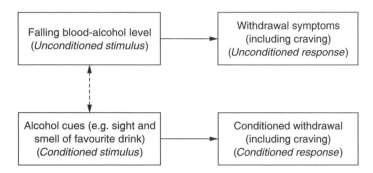

FIGURE 7.1   Drummond *et al.*'s (1990) conditioning model of alcohol craving.

with drinking. One behavioural treatment that builds on this theory is cue exposure. A person dependent on alcohol, for example, would be taken into a pub and, rather than following his or her automatic conditioned response of buying alcohol, would be helped to respond differently, perhaps by buying a non-alcoholic drink. Overtime, the conditioned response would reduce and eventually disappear (be 'extinguished').

A second behavioural theory is called 'operant conditioning'. This builds on the fact that an action that leads to a reward is more likely to be repeated than one that leads to no reward or to a punishment. A drug can be a very strong reward, activating the brain's natural pleasure pathways. Treatments based on this theory aim to reduce the value of the reward (the drug) while increasing the value of other, preferable, rewards. Thus, contingency management provides rewards (vouchers for consumer goods) when a client has not used drugs, while community reinforcement aims to build on what the client finds personally rewarding in their social, occupational and leisure activities and so increase the reward value of those activities while decreasing the reward value of drug use.

People also learn behaviours by watching or imitating other people and this is the basis of 'social learning theory'. Many treatments for substance abuse emphasise how being with other substance users can make it difficult to avoid use. They may also include social skills training and the enhancement of positive social support for the client, for example, through partners.

Cognitive theories stress how our 'cognitions' – thoughts and beliefs – can shape our behaviour and emotions. In a sense, we acquire 'thought habits' just like we have behavioural habits. A widely used cognitive model is that of Beck *et al.* (1993) which is shown in Figure 7.2. Here, cues – which can be either internal (such as feelings and body symptoms) or external (stimuli associated with drug use) – activate the person's beliefs ('I'm a hopeless addict'). These in turn lead to automatic thoughts ('I can't deal with X unless I've used') which produce cravings for the drug. To deal with cravings, other thoughts ('I deserve a break') are used to permit the person to use the drug and then to focus on strategies to obtain the drug. Cognitive treatments focus on changing dysfunctional beliefs and maladaptive thoughts through the therapist working collaboratively with the person to challenge those cognitions and through the client self-monitoring their thoughts, feelings and behaviours in daily life.

Other models focus on motivation. One motivational model emphasises that there are 'stages' for the user on the journey to changing their drug behaviour (Prochaska and DiClemente, 1983). In the 'precontemplation' stage, the person does not perceive a problem with their drug use; in the 'contemplation' stage, he or she may be

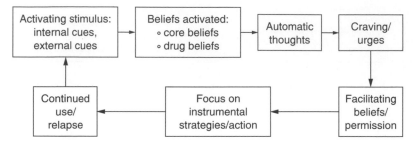

FIGURE 7.2   Beck *et al.*'s (1993) cognitive model of substance misuse.

worried about their drug use but does not want to change it; in the 'determination' stage, a commitment is made to change in the near future followed by 'action' where behaviour is changed, and followed in turn by 'maintenance' – trying to stick to it. Motivational treatments focus on the client's ambivalence about changing their behaviour, identify which stage they are at and facilitate progress towards action and maintenance.

Many treatments combine elements of behavioural, cognitive and motivational approaches. For example, relapse prevention combines cognitive and behavioural treatments to help those who have stopped using drugs to remain drug-free and cope with situations where they might relapse.

2.2 How do We Judge Whether a Treatment Works?

An intervention that works – an 'effective therapy' – is primarily judged to be one that results in abstinence or a significant reduction in substance use. Because substance misuse is a complex disorder involving psychological, biological and social factors, it often impacts on several areas of a person's life such as employment, relationships, criminality, physical health and health risks of HIV and hepatitis. These are often regarded as secondary 'outcome' measures.

3 WHERE ARE WE NOW? THE CURRENT EVIDENCE BASE ON PSYCHOLOGICAL TREATMENTS

It is well established that psychological therapies are effective in the treatment of substance misuse. For cocaine, crack, amphetamines, cannabis and alcohol, psychological interventions are the effective interventions. As yet, there are no effective pharmacological treatments. For other substances, such as heroin, psychological care and social help are as important as substitute prescribing.

Some psychological interventions (notably those focusing on motivation for change and those aiming to help prevent relapse) appear to be effective across a wide range of substances, whereas others are more substance-specific. While pharmacological treatment is focused mainly on replacing, blocking or sensitising the individual to the drug, (see Chapter 6, Pharmacology and Treatments), psychological treatments often take a broader focus. Substance misuse is rarely an isolated problem and clients usually have other psychological and social difficulties. It may be – and we don't yet know – that many advantages of psychological treatment are revealed at a later stage of treatment when drug-dependency issues are less prominent and individuals can focus on their broader psychological problems (Roth and Fonagy, 2005).

Brief treatments are often as effective as longer ones. However, for individuals who are more severely dependent, longer or more intensive treatments may be more helpful. It is useful to distinguish between extensiveness and intensiveness. A few sessions spread over a longer period can often be as effective as many more sessions given within a shorter period. Because of the difficulty in retaining many clients in treatment, methods that are effective over fewer sessions may sometimes be more practical.

The best outcomes are generally found when the focus of treatment is a direct change in drug use and drug-related behaviour and when there are higher levels of social support (Miller *et al.*, 1999). A person's willingness to engage in treatment and their initial response to it are also associated with better outcomes. Outcomes are often disappointing, and relapse rates high. However, this is to be expected because, like diabetes or hypertension, substance dependency is a chronic relapsing condition. Many individuals will need multiple treatments before they change their substance use. This means it is important to take a long-term perspective of the effectiveness of interventions.

The bulk of treatment studies are North American, with comparatively few based in the UK. Although many interventions take place in Britain, other methods such as community reinforcement, contingency management and family interventions are backed by good North American evidence but are not yet widely used in the UK (Wanigaratne *et al.*, 2005).

While most treatment trials are with clients selected for one primary substance of abuse, many clients seen in clinics regularly use several drugs, often taking one drug to prolong the effects or counteract the 'come down' of another. Further, clinical trials often exclude individuals who have serious co-morbidity such as personality disorder or medical problems (Humphreys and Weisner, 2000).

In the next section we briefly summarise the evidence for which psychological therapies are effective with which main substances of dependence. More detailed

accounts are given by Lingford-Hughes *et al.* (2004) and Roth and Fonagy (2005). As pharmacological treatments are reviewed in detail by Nutt in Chapter 6, we discuss them here only in the context of whether they can enhance the effectiveness of psychological therapies.

3.1 Alcohol

There is strong evidence for the effectiveness of motivational enhancement therapy (MET) (Dunn *et al.*, 2001; Miller and Willbourne, 2002; Burke *et al.*, 2003; Slattery *et al.*, 2003). The largest treatment trial to date – Project Match – involved 1726 clients across the US and compared MET with two other therapies: cognitive behavioural therapy (CBT) and Twelve-Step Facilitation (TSF) therapy (Project Match Research Group, 1997). The main outcome measures were the percentage of days per month that the client did not drink and the number of drinks they had in each drinking session. Results showed four sessions of MET to be as effective as 12 of either CBT or TSF. All treatments led to significant reductions in drinking after therapy and at 1- and 3-year follow-ups. Although a main aim of Project Match was to see which clients benefited from which therapy, few client 'matches' emerged. This suggests that the brief therapy (MET) was as effective as longer therapies regardless of the severity of alcohol dependence. What is probably more important than 'matching' treatments to clients is the relationship between therapist and client. MET is briefer than the other therapies, costs less and is as effective as them (Cisler *et al.*, 1998). This suggests that MET should replace these other therapies.

Building on this suggestion, the recent, rigorous multicentre UK Alcohol Treatment Trial (UKATT), with 742 clients, compared three sessions of MET with eight sessions of social behaviour and network therapy (SBNT) (UKATT research team, in press). SBNT was developed specifically for the trial on the basis of evidence that overcoming alcohol problems is helped when there is support from family and friends (Miller and Willbourne, 2002). SBNT contains elements of family therapy, community reinforcement, relapse prevention and social skills training. UKATT showed that SBNT was as effective as MET in reducing alcohol consumption, dependence and problems. Both treatments also improved clients' health-related quality of life. Although SBNT cost more per client (£170) than MET (£115), there was no significant difference in overall cost-effectiveness and both approaches saved six times as much as they cost in terms of health, social and criminal justice services.

There is also good US evidence for at least the short-term effectiveness of community reinforcement approaches. These usually combine a spectrum of interventions (social skills training, behaviour contracting, stress management and behavioural marital therapy) (Azrin *et al.*, 1982; Mattick and Jarvis, 1993). General counselling about alcohol is better than no treatment at all but not as effective as CBT, MET or TSF. Similarly, behavioural marital therapy is effective in the short term but there is little evidence of any long-term impact (Mattick and Jarvis, 1993; O'Farrell *et al.*, 1993). Social skills training is also effective, although less so with individuals who have neuropsychological impairment (Smith and McCrady, 1991).

Relapse prevention is effective and can be enhanced by adding pharmacological treatments (Irvin *et al.*, 1999). There is good evidence that abstinence rates can be improved when psychosocial treatments (notably relapse prevention, CBT and MET) are combined with acamprosate (Feeney *et al.*, 2002) and naltrexone (O'Malley *et al.*, 1992). Not all patients respond to these drug treatments and there is no known basis for predicting this (Lingford-Hughes *et al.*, 2004).

Another behavioural approach which has shown some promising results is cue-exposure treatment (Drummond *et al.*, 1990; Monti *et al.*, 1993; Drummond and Glautier, 1994). In this approach, alcohol-dependent individuals are exposed to cues such as the sight and smell of a favourite drink, without actually consuming alcohol. Exposure can involve recalling the memory of cues, or actual exposure to them. This is similar to cue-exposure treatment in phobic or obsessive compulsive disorders. Cue exposure has also included exposure to a priming dose of alcohol and resisting the temptation to consume further alcohol (Rankin *et al.*, 1982). There is clear evidence of reactivity to alcohol cues, including alcohol craving, which is related to the severity of alcohol dependence (Drummond, 2000). Small-scale clinical efficacy trials have shown some positive benefits of this approach in reducing relapse to drinking. However, to date, no large-scale clinical or cost-effectiveness trials have been conducted. Cue exposure has become the main treatment approach in phobic and obsessive compulsive disorder and these disorders have known resemblances to addictions.

Brief interventions are generally opportunistic and occur in non-specialist settings such as primary care or accident and emergency (A&E). They do not work with dependent drinkers who are seeking help for alcohol problems (Moyer *et al.*, 2002). Instead, they are targeted at people who drink heavily and aim to reduce the amount they drink. There is a substantial body of evidence showing their effectiveness (e.g. Fleming *et al.*, 2002; Ockene *et al.*, 1999) and this is true in both primary care (e.g. Miller and Willbourne, 2002; Moyer *et al.*, 2002) and A&E (e.g. Crawford *et al.*, 2004). They generally result in a 20–30% reduction in excessive drinking. Brief interventions are also highly cost-effective, suggesting that screening for alcohol and drug use should become routine in primary care and A&E. There is some evidence for the efficacy of brief intervention in psychiatric populations (e.g. Baker *et al.*, 2002; Hulse and Tait, 2002, 2003).

3.2 Benzodiazepines

There are two very different populations of benzodiazepine users. One population has taken standard, prescribed doses of these drugs over months or years. Although some find it relatively easy to stop following advice from their doctor, others are more dependent and may need support to gradually reduce their dose over time. For these users, it is not clear whether additional psychological treatments are helpful or not. It may depend on what problem (e.g. anxiety, sleep problems) led to the prescription in the first place. About 14 per cent of older adults in the UK take benzodiazepine sleeping pills each night. Curran *et al.* (2003) found that 80 per cent of older adults who had taken these every night for an average of 17 years successfully stopped taking them following a gradual reduction in dose and information about sleep hygiene. Compared with a group who kept taking their sleeping pills, the withdrawers showed subtle improvements in cognitive function. At the same time, this gradual reduction in dose did not produce withdrawal symptoms, or changes in sleep. It is not clear yet whether similar issues of dependency will arise with the newer drugs used to treat sleep problems, called the 'Z drugs' (zopiclone, zolpidem, zaleplon). They act in the brain in a very similar way to benzodiazepines and there have been reports of transient memory problems associated with Z-drugs (Terzano *et al.*, 2003).

The second population uses benzodiazepine, often at very high doses, alongside other drugs. Benzodiazepines may be used to reduce the come-down from crack or to prolong the effects of heroin (Lingford-Hughes *et al.*, 2004). We know very little about treating illicit benzodiazepine use by polydrug users. There is a significant concern about seizures if someone stops benzodiazepines abruptly after using large doses. It is important to see a person's benzodiazepine use within the broader picture of their crack, heroin or alcohol use.

3.3 Opiates

The vast majority of treatment programmes for heroin users involve a two-pronged approach of substitute prescribing alongside substantial, and very variable, psychosocial therapies. Perhaps because pharmacological treatment, especially methadone maintenance, is so widespread, there has been less research on psychological treatments for opiate dependence than for alcohol or cocaine dependence. Most studies have therefore evaluated psychosocial treatments in the context of methadone maintenance, whose goal is the reduction of illicit drug use and its associated harms and risks (Mattick *et al.*, 2003a,b).

There is robust evidence from US studies of the effectiveness of contingency management (CM) (Griffith *et al.*, 2000) and community reinforcement approaches (CRAs) (Gruber *et al.*, 2000). Motivational interviewing is also effective (Saunders *et al.*, 1995). There is some evidence that family treatment can produce additional benefits to individual treatment, especially in terms of adherence and of retention in treatment (Fals-Stewart and O'Farrell, 2003).

Although most psychological interventions are in the context of maintenance rather than abstinence as a treatment goal, several studies of withdrawal from opiates have contrasted various pharmacological regimes and these invariably have psychosocial adjuncts. There is some evidence that CM can reduce dropout rates from withdrawal programmes (Lingford-Hughes *et al.*, 2004). However, over 40 years of research has shown that after opiate withdrawal, a majority of clients relapse to heroin use, so maintenance is a more realistic aim.

Cue-exposure treatment has been studied in opiate dependence (Dawe *et al.*, 1993). Small-scale clinical studies have shown robust reactivity to opiate drug cues (e.g. the sight of injecting equipment, or video tapes of people injecting opiates). No positive clinical effects of cue-exposure treatment have been found so far.

There is more recent recognition that a minority of people who have been prescribed opiates like morphine or oxycodone for pain may become dependent (e.g. Zacny and Gutierrez, 2003). This area has recently been reviewed by the Pain Society (2004).

Little is known about the best psychological treatment for dependence on normal-dose opiate analgesics.

3.4 Stimulant Drugs

Psychosocial interventions are the mainstay in treating dependence on stimulant drugs, cocaine, crack and amphetamines (mainly methamphetamine). At present, there is no evidence that any pharmacological treatments can enhance outcome (Lingford-Hughes et al., 2004).

Behavioural therapies, especially CM approaches, are effective. When the effectiveness of CM alone and combined with an intensive behavioural therapy were compared, the combined therapy was more effective (Higgins et al., 2003). Roozen et al.'s (2004) systematic review found that community reinforcement approaches plus incentives were effective in treating cocaine addiction. Cognitive therapy is also effective (Carroll et al., 1994), even with cocaine addicts who are also opiate dependent and receiving methadone maintenance (Condelli et al., 1991). For cocaine-dependent clients in methadone maintenance programmes, both cognitive therapy and CM are effective but the combination of the two is no more effective than either alone (Rawson et al., 2002).

The National Institute of Drug Abuse (NIDA) collaborative cocaine study (Crits-Christoph et al., 1999), with nearly 500 patients, compared four treatments. All four groups received drug group counselling (DGC) which incorporated the TSF philosophy. It was given either alone or in combination with one of three other therapies: individual drug counselling, cognitive therapy, and supportive expressive therapy, over a 6-month period. At 3 months, about half had dropped out and only 28 per cent completed the treatment. All treatments led to decreased drug use but the most effective in reducing cocaine use was individual drug counselling combined with DGC. Crits-Christoph et al. (1999) suggest this may be because it specifically focused on stopping current drug use. On a wide range of other outcome measures, there were no differences between treatments. Relapse prevention is also effective in promoting abstinence from stimulant drugs over longer periods (Carroll et al., 1994).

3.5 Nicotine

There have been a large number of clinical trials, mainly centred on the effectiveness of nicotine replacement treatments (NRT, including gums, lozenges, patches and inhalers) rather than psychosocial interventions. Silagy et al. (2003) reviewed 96 high-quality trials and showed that NRT improves abstinence at 6 months, regardless of the type of NRT used. These authors also concluded that additional behavioural support improved success. Although bupropion is also an effective pharmacological treatment for nicotine dependency (Hughes et al., 2004), there is not enough evidence about which psychosocial treatments may be used in combination with it to enhance overall effectiveness.

Around 80 per cent of people who misuse alcohol and/or illicit drugs also smoke cigarettes, and this is three times the rate for the general population (Richter et al., 2002; Romberger and Grant, 2004). Lingford-Hughes et al. (2004) conclude that although there is a lack of randomised control trials of smoking cessation in people being treated for the use of other substances, there is some evidence that combining behavioural therapies with NRT may be effective in increasing smoking cessation rates.

3.6 Other Substances

A wide range of substances is associated mainly with intermittent or 'recreational' use. Users of these drugs are virtually never seen in specialist clinics, where the focus is on dependence. Many of the drugs mentioned above are used both intermittently and dependently. The use of alcohol in this way is considered normal in many countries and intermittent use of cannabis or cocaine is considered 'subculturally normal' by many young people. Other 'recreational' substances include Ecstasy, ketamine, gamma-hydroxybutyrate (GHB) and lysergic acid diethylamide (LSD).

3.6.1 Cannabis

After nicotine and alcohol, cannabis (marijuana) is the most widely used mood-altering drug (World Health Organisation, 2003). Although the majority of cannabis users would be seen as recreational users who do not have a serious drug problem, there may be a subset who develop a dependent pattern of use. There has been very little research on how to treat this. Most relevant are two randomised controlled trials by Stephens et al. (1994, 2000), the first of which showed that a psychosocial group intervention and a social support group were equally effective in reducing cannabis use. The second showed that motivational interviewing and relapse prevention were equally effective. Dennis et al. (2004) have reported that motivational enhancement therapy combined with CBT is the most cost-effective of psychosocial interventions with adolescent cannabis users, with some evidence in favour of the community reinforcement approach.

3.6.2 Ketamine

Ketamine ('Special K') use appears to be increasing among young people, especially club-goers (Mixmag, 2004). However, there have been only a few sporadic cases of ketamine addiction (e.g. Hurt and Ritchie, 1994). Although there is little evidence of dependence, there is concern about the psychological consequences of using such drugs frequently. Both controlled laboratory studies and studies with recreational ketamine users have shown that it induces transient schizophrenia-like symptoms. It also produces marked impairments of memory and cognitive function (Krystal et al., 1994; Curran and Morgan, 2000; Morgan et al.,

2004a). One concern is whether it produces long-term effects. A recent longitudinal study suggests that users may have persisting memory impairments even after they cease or substantially reduce their use of ketamine (Morgan et al., 2004b).

3.6.3 Ecstasy

Similarly, the concerns about ecstasy use are possible long-term psychological effects rather than dependence. Weekend ecstasy use is associated with low mood a few days later that, in a minority of users, may approach clinical levels of depression (Curran and Travill, 1997; Verheyden et al., 2003). Although mood generally returns to normal after a week (Curran et al., 2004), there is evidence that some users will show low mood and subtle memory decrements even a year or more after they have stopped using ecstasy (Curran and Verheyden, 2003; Thomasius et al., 2003). A central issue here is the extent to which these decrements predated drug use or were a consequence of it.

Recreational use by young people often involves a variety of drugs so that it is difficult to tease apart which drug or drug combination is contributing to which psychological effect. Further, certain combinations become fashionable cocktails, for example 'Calvin Klein' or 'CK' is a cocaine/ketamine mix. A major concern is the recent drop in price of many drugs. Ecstasy cost about £8 a tablet in 2001 but £2 in 2004. This has increased its availability to young teenagers who may be more vulnerable to adverse drug effects.

3.7 The Evidence Base on Psychological Interventions in Addictions

Psychological interventions are effective in reducing, or maintaining abstinence from, most forms of substance misuse, either alone or in combination with pharmacological interventions. Psychological interventions also have effects on multiple domains of substance-related problems including drug use itself and psychological functioning. In many cases, the effects of psychological and pharmacological intervention are additive. Overall, psychological intervention is most likely to be effective when it is conducted in a structured, standardised way, by appropriately trained and competent therapists. Therapist factors are important in determining the effectiveness of psychological interventions. However, overall, the evidence of efficacy of psychological interventions across substances is relatively robust, with clinically significant effects. The evidence base on cost-effectiveness and effectiveness in the typical clinical setting is less robust, and larger-scale clinical effectiveness studies are required. There is also a limited evidence base from the UK clinical setting. Most of the research is conducted in North America.

Across psychological interventions and substances, mechanisms of effect are not yet clearly identified and it is possible that different treatment approaches have different mechanisms. There may also be unidentified common mechanisms of effect of different psychological approaches. Client factors such as social stability, motivation, psychiatric comorbidity and personality disorder are also important in determining the engagement with and outcome of psychological interventions.

Where directly compared, intervention approaches based on motivational, cognitive behavioural, psychodynamic and TSF principles all show similar evidence of effectiveness, with no clear leading approach. This may suggest common mechanisms, or that therapist factors may be more influential than the differences between psychological approaches. Individualised, conjoint and group approaches show similar effectiveness, as do psychological interventions conducted in both inpatient and community settings. There has been no robust demonstration of matching effects, where specific treatments are preferentially effective for particular types of individual

(but see Section 3.8, Limitations of the existing treatment research evidence base, below).

Brief interventions have been tested extensively in alcohol dependence and show robust evidence of efficacy and some evidence of effectiveness, particularly in those with less severe alcohol dependence. It is important to note that cost effectiveness has rarely been studied in brief interventions or in fact most psychological interventions. So a lack of evidence does not necessarily indicate that psychological interventions are not cost effective. However, given the existing evidence base, brief interventions are the first line of psychological treatment in substance misuse, with other more intensive interventions reserved for those who do not respond to less-intensive approaches. Until there is more robust evidence of treatment matching, a stepped approach to intervention is indicated (e.g. Sobell and Sobell, 2000).

Surprisingly, brief interventions have been less often studied in other forms of substance misuse. In nicotine dependence, there is clear evidence that brief interventions are less effective than more intensive approaches in regular smokers (Lingford-Hughes *et al.*, 2004). There is also some limited evidence of efficacy of brief intervention for sedative dependence. However, it will be important to study the effectiveness of brief interventions with other forms of substance misuse, particularly in those with less-severe dependence.

Cue exposure treatment shows some promising effects in alcohol, but no evidence of efficacy in nicotine or opiate dependence. So far, clinical cue-exposure treatment studies have been small-scale. But, given the promising effects, larger clinical trials, particularly in alcohol dependence, are indicated.

Considering the similarities in efficacy of a range of psychological interventions, based on different theoretical models across a range of substances, further research on the common effective ingredients of psychological treatment is required. It would also be of interest to study why psychological treatments sometimes and with certain individuals do not succeed. Promising areas here include failures of client engagement and of therapeutic alliance between client and therapist. Again, this might help to point out common effective and ineffective ingredients of treatments.

3.8 Limitations of the Existing Treatment Research Evidence Base

There are several limitations to the existing treatment research evidence base. They are due to the selection of study populations, the range and nature of the substances studied, assumptions about the nature of addiction and treatment, lack of attention to the context of treatment, lack of comparability of outcome measures, and an overall lack of research, specifically in the UK treatment setting. This points to limitations in the generalisability of the existing evidence base to the typical treatment setting. This presents difficulties for clinicians and policy makers in deciding on the appropriateness of specific treatments for particular individuals and populations.

3.8.1 Selection of Study Populations

The 'gold standard' for the evaluation of addiction treatments is the randomised controlled trial (RCT), believed to provide the most compelling evidence for treatment effectiveness because it aims to minimise bias and protect internal validity. The predominant RCT in the addiction field is the efficacy trial, which further aims to protect internal validity by conducting studies in 'ideal' conditions, typically in single-site teaching hospitals or research-active clinical settings. Subject populations recruited in these settings may not be representative of the wider population of patients. A further selection bias exists in typically excluding groups that might compromise the internal validity of a trial or may prove difficult to follow up.

Patients with serious physical or psychiatric comorbidity, the elderly, the homeless and polydrug misusers are often excluded from RCTs. Patient groups that might present particular problems in the research design or where consent may be difficult are also typically excluded, for example, those with psychiatric disorders, learning disabilities or literacy problems, pregnant women, children and young people. Minority populations and populations in which substance misuse is less prevalent are often under-represented, partly through difficulties in recruiting sufficient numbers to make clear conclusions about the effectiveness of a treatment in that population. This can include women and ethnic-minority groups.

Some trial designs may inherently bias the selection of subjects. Intake assessment procedures or the choice of interventions may put off some groups from agreeing to participate. It is well documented that RCTs of screening and brief intervention for alcohol problems favour the recruitment of older males. Further, RCTs that involve a significant change from current practice in a clinic in order to evaluate a new treatment introduce a selection bias towards patients who are willing to accept randomisation, rather than having a particular preference as to what treatment they want, especially when major change is involved, for example, methadone detoxification versus methadone maintenance. There is a need for addiction treatment research to be more inclusive and for study samples to be more representative of the treatment-seeking population. This will require an appreciation by research funding bodies that more inclusivity may increase the cost of research. For example, we need more research on interventions for alcohol misuse in pregnancy, which will involve considerably greater screening costs because of the low prevalence of alcohol misuse in this group. We also need to be clearer about the limitations of attempting to generalise research findings to populations under-represented in, or completely excluded from, RCTs.

3.8.2 The Range of Substances Studied

Another inherent problem with RCTs of treatment efficacy in drug misuse and dependence is the drive to have a relatively homogeneous study population. Typically, studies of alcohol dependence will exclude polydrug misusers and those dependent on Class A (and often Class B) drugs, but include nicotine and cannabis use and dependence. Studies of Class A drug misusers are typically less exclusive, but often involve treatments aimed at altering behaviour with specific substances rather than examining an individual's substance misuse in the round. There has been hardly any research on interventions for alcohol misuse among opiate-dependent patients, even though nearly 30 per cent of opiate-dependent patients presenting to treatment also misuse alcohol. The findings of such trials are often not generalisable to the more typical treatment-seeking substance misuser.

There is also a bias towards studying alcohol and Class A drug dependence. This has partly been shaped by political priorities rather than issues of prevalence or presenting clinical need. The result has been a paucity of research on treatment for recreational drug misuse (including cannabis and club drugs) and a bias towards studying older age groups of drug misusers. The misuse of prescription drugs (including steroids, benzodiazepines and opiates) is a large problem clinically, but there is hardly any treatment research to guide clinical practice.

3.8.3 Assumptions about Addictions and Treatments in Treatment Research

RCTs are the most appropriate research design to evaluate treatments for acute medical conditions, particularly pharmacological interventions. However, evaluating treatments for addictions, and in particular psychosocial interventions, poses several challenges. While there remains an important place for RCTs in the evaluation of addiction treatment, further consideration needs to be given to the design of such research.

Many addictions are chronic, relapsing disorders. A large proportion of addicted patients will relapse after a period of abstinence, achieved with or without treatment. Factors such as social support, social stability, and physical illnesses can often be more influential in determining the outcome of addictions than treatment itself. Interventions often take place over many months or years, and their outcome may be determined by the cumulative effect of multiple episodes of treatment, interacting with non-treatment factors. Some addicts may progress from one addiction to another through substitution, for example, cannabis dependence giving way to opiate dependence, followed by alcohol dependence, or prescription-drug dependence.

Treatment evaluation research in addiction typically studies the impact of two or more treatment approaches, or interventions, of differing intensity over a period of 12 months. Studies that include longer follow-up often find that promising effects at 12 months are subsequently lost. The interpretation of this research is further complicated by patients obtaining non-scheduled interventions during the follow-up period, as they would do in the more typical clinical setting.

These difficulties have led some researchers to call for less emphasis on the intensity of interventions and more on the 'extensity' of treatment over an extended period of time. It has also been suggested that addictions would be better served by a more chronic-care approach to treatment evaluation, which is increasingly common in diseases such as diabetes and hypertension. Studies of a stepped-care approach to addiction intervention have also been suggested. Stepped care includes a significant component of longer-term monitoring and adjustment of treatment interventions to response. However, it appears that both researchers and research funding bodies are wary of a significant departure from the standard RCT design, which is more suited to acute care.

Psychosocial interventions present particular practical problems for treatment evaluation research. These include assuring the fidelity of treatment, treatment adherence, patient and assessor blinding, and therapist factors. None of these problems is insurmountable and there are good examples of optimal research designs to evaluate psychosocial treatments. Project Match is the largest and probably most rigorous RCT of psychosocial intervention ever conducted. However, the rigour of an RCT of psychosocial intervention comes at the cost of external validity. The rigour of a trial such as Project Match would be difficult to replicate in the typical clinical addiction setting.

3.8.4 The Context of Treatment

The clinical context in which a treatment approach is studied may have a large impact on its effectiveness. Several studies have been conducted of the relative efficacy of inpatient versus outpatient treatment, generally with little evidence of differences in outcome between the two. However, such research has several limitations, including limited statistical power, narrow subject selection, and the lack of a clear specification of the components of interventions. More recent research is beginning to point to potential differences, particularly cohort studies rather than RCTs (e.g. Project Match). While this may be related to sampling bias, it is possible that cohort studies exclude less of the more severe cases and more typically reflect actual treatment, and provide greater information of relevance to clinical and policy decision making.

Increasingly, addiction treatment is being conducted in the context of coercion through criminal justice agencies including prison, arrest referral and court orders. Assumptions are often made that treatments, particularly psychosocial treatments, conducted under coercion will perform in the same way as when patients are actively seeking help.

Since patient motivation is likely to be an important mediating variable in outcome, it cannot be assumed that coercive treatments are equivalent to voluntary ones.

Current policies often seek to extend the role of substance misuse interventions into clinical settings in which they have seldom or never been evaluated. Thus the UK Department of Health's Alcohol Harm Reduction Strategy (Prime Minister's Strategy Unit, 2004) emphasises the importance of alcohol intervention in mental health populations, despite its poor research base. Most of the brief alcohol intervention research has been conducted in primary care, often excluding patients with serious psychiatric co-morbidity. More systematic research is needed to evaluate the performance of treatment interventions in different clinical contexts. This is another area in which stepped care might offer opportunities for research.

3.8.5 Outcome Measures

One of the difficulties in comparing outcomes across research studies has been the lack of comparability of the measures of outcomes used. In some studies, particularly older research, the outcome measures are of unknown validity. Recent developments in research methodology, notably in Project Match, have identified research instruments and outcome evaluation methods that are valid and reliable. The methods used to measure alcohol consumption, often the main outcome of interest, have a large impact on the validity of the data.

Overall, there is a lack of economic analysis in treatment outcome research into addictions. The cost effectiveness of treatments is of major concern to policy makers and it would be of assistance to include health economic measures in treatment studies. This should take account of current methodologies in health economic research. Further, such research often requires larger sample sizes and longer follow-up to obtain meaningful data.

3.8.6 *Treatment Research in the UK*

Much of the world's treatment research takes place in the United States. There has been a lack of investment in clinical addiction research in the UK, more so in the past decade than in the preceding two. There is only one MRC-funded clinical research programme on addiction and there have been a handful of clinical addiction research projects funded by the MRC in the last decade. The Department of Health, NHS Research and Development and the Alcohol Education and Research Council have funded a few small-scale clinical trials in addiction, but there has been no sustained programme of clinical research. The clinical studies that have been funded have tended to be short term, and too statistically underpowered to form clear conclusions. This lack of investment contrasts with the considerable, and increasing, level of spending on clinical addiction services provision by the NHS and the Home Office. The Home Office has not been funding clinical trials in the addiction field, but has introduced pilot methodologies to establish the feasibility rather than the effectiveness of addiction interventions in the criminal justice system.

This means that the evidence base for the effectiveness of treatment in the UK is largely reliant on overseas research, principally from the US. Our research shows that this may not easily translate to the NHS setting or to the cultural context of the UK. Many of the new initiatives to develop addiction treatment services in the UK, costing several millions of pounds, have not been evaluated in the UK. The risk is that these treatment developments may be ineffective or not cost-effective, and therefore have minimal impact on the problem of addiction. There is a lack of infrastructure for clinical addiction research in the UK, including a lack of career opportunities for clinical addiction scientists. When funding is occasionally available to conduct clinical addiction research, it is difficult to find research-active professionals to do it.

Further, because there has been no UK national strategy for clinical addiction research, addiction tends to compete poorly for funding and is often not rated as highly as some other disciplines. All of this points to the need for a national clinical addiction research strategy, a specific funding stream for clinical addiction research, a national clinical addiction research network, and investment in the research infrastructure for clinical addiction research.

4 PSYCHOLOGICAL TREATMENTS OF SUBSTANCE MISUSE AND DEPENDENCE: THE FUTURE?

4.1 Identifying the Most Effective Psychological Treatments

Most research on psychological interventions in drug dependence has been concerned with alcohol and there has been very limited psychological research on other forms of drug dependence. In opiate dependence, much of the focus has been on pharmacological interventions. There is some evidence of the efficacy of psychological interventions in opiate and cocaine dependence but there has been very little UK-based research on this to guide service development, with the exception of the UK CBT in Methadone Treatment Project (Drummond *et al.*, 2004) funded by the Department of Health. This showed that US research may not translate to the NHS setting. Similarly, psychological intervention is the mainstay of cocaine and cannabis treatment and deserves more research. And more research is needed on the cost-effectiveness of psychological treatments delivered in different contexts by different professionals, and in 'typical' rather than 'ideal' clinical settings.

4.2 Identifying Key 'Active Ingredients' of Treatment

While we know that psychological treatments are effective in treating addictive disorders, more research is needed to identify the key active ingredients of effective psychological treatments. There is some evidence that therapist factors such as skill, style and training are influential. There is also evidence that client factors such as readiness to change, gender, social support, severity of problems, and satisfaction with treatment are predictive of outcome (Connors *et al.*, 2000). In addition, there is evidence of interactions between client and therapist factors, including the importance of therapeutic alliance (Connors *et al.*, 2000; DiClemente and Scott, 1997). This is likely to involve complex interactions between a wide range of factors (Moos *et al.*, 1990). Efforts to identify 'matching' variables, interactions between individual client differences and treatment factors that predict better treatment outcomes, have had limited success so far (e.g. Project Match, 1997). This research needs to include more individuals with complex needs than it has hitherto, and would benefit from more observational and qualitative research designs rather than relying on RCT designs. Such research also needs to be more theory-driven (e.g. Beck *et al.*, 1993; Drummond *et al.*, 1990).

Many assumptions are made about what constitutes high-quality psychological treatment, by both service providers and commissioners. The general clinical psychology literature may have applications in the addiction field. But this area of research is at a relatively early stage and needs to be developed, particularly in the UK treatment setting. Again, observational, case control and qualitative methodologies are needed to generate and test research hypotheses.

4.3 Broadening the Contexts of Psychological Treatment

Most psychological treatment research has been conducted in specialised clinical settings, such as treatment centres with academic staff and highly trained therapists.

A notable exception to this is brief intervention. But, even here, there are limitations in studying the implementation and effectiveness of psychological interventions in the 'typical' clinical setting, which limit the generalisability of this research. Assumptions are often made about the applicability of psychological interventions in settings other than those in which they have been evaluated. For example, there has been limited research on the effectiveness of psychological interventions in coerced populations, and specifically in the criminal justice system. The UK has made a significant investment in expanding treatment (principally psychological interventions) in criminal justice settings without adequate research evidence of its effectiveness. There is an urgent need to commission quality research in this area.

Research is needed on effective methods of training and delivery of psychological treatments by non-addiction specialists, or those with limited addiction treatment experience, including GPs, practice nurses, social workers and probation officers. Again, many assumptions are made by policy makers about the training needs and effectiveness of interventions delivered by these groups. It may be that equipping generalists with more generic behavioural change skills is more effective than training to provide specific psychological interventions for particular types of addiction (Rollnick *et al.*, 1999).

Young people typically have a higher level of substance misuse than older people, but seldom access services equipped to provide appropriate interventions. New methods need to be found to increase young people's access to psychological interventions for substance misuse. The Internet and interactive computer programmes have potential in this regard and young people often use them to seek information about substance misuse.

4.4 Psychological Interventions for Comorbidity

Another treatment context that requires further research is psychiatric populations with comorbid substance misuse. We know that psychiatric patients have high levels of alcohol, tobacco, and both licit and illicit drug misuse, yet these co-occurring disorders are seldom identified or treated in psychiatric settings (Regier *et al.*, 1993; Barnaby *et al.*, 2003). Similarly, patients in specialist addiction treatment have a high prevalence of co-occurring psychiatric disorders, which are often poorly addressed. There is also a strong association between alcohol misuse and suicidality (Driessen *et al.*, 1998; Foster, 2001; McCloud *et al.*, 2004). Since comorbidity is associated with poor treatment outcome, this issue deserves more attention from research.

We could do with more specific research on which psychological and pharmacological interventions, delivered at which point in treatment, and by which professionals, are more likely to be effective. There is some research on the effectiveness of treatment for comorbidity delivered in specialised programmes (Jeffery *et al.*, 2000). But it is more likely that, in practice, the delivery of interventions for comorbidity will be through mainstream psychiatric services (Department of Health, 2002). So we need more research on brief and extended psychological interventions in mental health settings, similar to that already conducted in primary care. It is likely that the type of addiction interventions needed for this population will be different and perhaps more intensive than those applied in primary care.

4.5 Psychological Interventions Across the Lifespan

Most research on psychological interventions has been conducted in adults of working age. It is clear that different forms of substance misuse have different ages of onset and recovery (usually nicotine and alcohol beginning in mid-teens, drugs in later teens). Nicotine dependence tends to have a long history, while the prevalence of alcohol misuse and dependence declines stepwise with age, with its peak in the 18–24-year age band. Drug misuse also tends to decline with age

and is relatively rare after the forties. Drug misusers tend to present for treatment for the first time in their twenties, whereas in alcohol dependence this occurs commonly in the thirties and forties.

We also know that most substance misuse tends to recover without formal treatment intervention, so the group that presents for treatment may be importantly different from the wider population of substance misusers. It is also clear that the age of onset has an impact on the life course and severity of substance misuse, with earlier onset being associated with a more severe and chronic course. The life (including age) context in which substance misuse occurs may have an important bearing on its aetiology and the type of intervention that may be required (Andersen, 2004). Younger substance misusers do not tend to access the same general health and helping agencies as older people. Therefore in terms of screening and identification of substance misuse in younger people, consideration needs to be given to targeting identification and interventions in agencies more likely to be in contact with younger people (e.g. youth organisations, sexual health clinics, accident and emergency departments).

We noted earlier that there has been relatively little clinical research on psychological interventions in adolescents and the elderly. Further, it cannot be assumed that interventions suitable for adults of working age are applicable to other age groups.

4.6 The Role of Care Co-ordination, Managed Care and Integrated Care Pathways

It is generally accepted that co-ordinated care is more effective than interventions delivered in isolation (e.g. National Treatment Agency, 2002). There is also interest in the application of integrated care pathways (ICPs) to substance misuse treatment. ICPs have gained prominence in the management of several chronic or relapsing medical disorders (e.g. diabetes) and there is some research to support their effectiveness and cost effectiveness. Stepped-care interventions have been shown to provide a resource-efficient method of delivering medical services, as well as providing clinical algorithms for clinicians. This has so far had limited investigation in addictions and in the delivery of different intensities of psychological interventions (Sobell and Sobell, 2000).

There is also some evidence that co-ordination of care and active follow-up improve treatment outcomes in addictions (Miller *et al.*, 1999). However, there has been limited systematic research on this and the active ingredients of effective care coordination have yet to be identified.

'Assertive outreach' has gained prominence in the management of severe mental illness and has been researched in the management of schizophrenia (Burns *et al.*, 2002). It may also be applicable to the management of severe addictive disorders. However, even in the field of severe mental illness, it is unclear what aspects of outreach are most effective. Different psychological intervention approaches allied to care co-ordination need to be systematically researched.

4.7 Neglected Populations

There are many groups that are either under-represented or specifically excluded from addiction treatment research studies, including (e.g. adolescents, the elderly, women, ethnic-minority groups, the homeless, and those with severe mental illness and learning disabilities). Sometimes such exclusion is for good practical reasons and sometimes for no reason at all. The result, however, is that we have very little information on the effectiveness of treatments in these groups. It cannot be assumed that research evidence on the effectiveness of psychological interventions carried out in one population will be applicable to other populations.

There have been proposals to expand the delivery of psychological interventions to substance-misusing adolescents in the UK.

However, we have no research data on the effectiveness of interventions in this group. This points to the need for greater investment in research and development to guide rational spending on substance misuse treatment.

5 WHAT WILL BE THE DRUGS OF THE FUTURE?

5.1 New Synthetic Drugs and Rediscovered Plants

Given the human history of seeking new 'highs', it is a safe bet that a range of new synthetic drugs will emerge over the next few decades. Which of these become popular will depend not only on the drug but also on a host of sociocultural factors. Ecstasy was first synthesised in 1914 but had no impact until Alexander Shulgin re-synthesised it and gave it to some therapist friends who thought it could be a useful therapeutic tool to give to their patients. Its mass popularity, beginning in the 1980s, was intimately linked with the emergence of the rave scene. Ecstasy became the ultimate dance drug, providing the three 'Es': empathy, energy and euphoria. As well as totally new synthetics, there may be other drugs patented years ago that could be rediscovered to complement future forms of music, dance and social subcultures.

Recipes for making Ecstasy and related drugs can be found on the web and recipes for new synthetic drugs will doubtless find their way there too. Much will depend on how the web and web sales are monitored and curtailed. For dealers, synthetic drugs have an advantage over plant-derived drugs in that they can be made locally and avoid problems of transport across national boundaries. There will also be new 'designer cocktails' – combinations of drugs taken together.

Awareness of old, plant-based drugs which differing cultures have used for ritual or spiritual purposes will increase. Drug-users' websites already contain information about drugs such as ayahuasca and peyote. In the UK, there has been a recent rise in the use of psychoactive mushrooms (Mixmag, 2004) as some London market stalls now (legally) sell untreated fungi from various countries and postal ordering services are available countrywide.

New ways of getting high might also involve reformulations of such plants or of older substances to enhance or prolong their psychoactive hit. One could speculate that new developments might not even need a drug to be taken at all, for example, transcranial magnetic stimulation (TMS) targeted at pleasure pathways in the brain.

5.2 New Prescribed Drugs and Cosmetic Pharmacology?

The perfect drug ... Euphoric, narcotic, pleasantly hallucinant ... What you need is a gramme of soma. All the advantages of Christianity and alcohol; none of their defects ... Take a holiday from reality whenever you like and come back without so much as a headache or a mythology. (Huxley, 1932),

Seventy-odd years ago, Aldous Huxley imagined a 'brave new world' where the drug 'soma' would solve people's problems, or at least make them less aware of social inequalities. Analogies can perhaps be drawn with the use of alcohol and opium over history, and even with the extensive use of prescription drugs such as valium-type tranquillisers in the 1960s and 1970s and prozac-type antidepressants today.

There has always been a fuzzy line between the medical use of mood-altering drugs and their misuse. Opiates prescribed for pain, benzodiazepines for anxiety or sleep, sildenafil for sexual dysfunction, ketamine for anaesthesia and methylphenidate for attention-deficit hyperactivity disorder have all been used for non-medical purposes. This pattern is likely to be repeated. In addition, pharmaceutical companies seeking ever bigger markets are likely to produce drugs for treating cognitive impairment, perhaps targeted at individuals with normal age-associated memory decrement. If an ageing memory is seen to merit

medication, the line between 'illness' and health will also become increasingly fuzzy.

Some people have cosmetic surgery to change the shape of their nose or cosmetic dentistry to achieve those Hollywood-white teeth. Might there be a similar role for 'cosmetic' psychopharmacology? And what might we, as consumers, want of this? Drugs to decrease our appetite for high-calorie foods? Drugs to increase our happiness, or to forget upsetting experiences? Alcohol has long been used to increase 'confidence', caffeine to increase wakefulness and various drugs to improve performance in sport. In future, there will be many more drugs available for such purposes. The market for drugs to counteract age-related memory impairment or aid weight loss would be huge.

Such drugs may have adverse effects, including dependency, and will raise many ethical considerations. Will using them be seen as 'cheating' just as the use of performance enhancers in sport is today? Or, at the other extreme, will employers insist on workers using cognition-enhancing drugs to optimise their output? One can only speculate on how these new drugs might be regulated. A possibility may be a change in how 'illness' is perceived. For example, psychiatric classification used to diagnose discrete 'disorders' may change to encapsulate a continuum concept. This would have severe illness at one extreme and excellent health at the other, with varying shades of disorder in the middle. On this basis, perhaps there would be some logic in intensive drug treatment for severe disorders and less-intensive treatment for people with more minor complaints.

Government policy and public opinion will be important influences on all this. For example, an increasing number of countries are banning smoking in public places and placing more restrictions on advertising tobacco. If this (as early indications suggest) helps people to smoke less and so reduces the harm and medical costs of smoking, it is foreseeable that similar approaches will be taken to reduce excessive alcohol use along with the individual and social costs this incurs. It is also possible that the climate of opinion will change away from the prohibitionist present with its 'war on drugs' approach and towards acceptance of an individual's right to chemically change his or her consciousness as they please, as long as it does not adversely affect others. Current issues around cannabis – including both deregulation and medical use – will provide some fodder for this debate.

6 PSYCHOSOCIAL TREATMENTS OF THE FUTURE

Future treatments will need to be based on more comprehensive evidence which details the key elements of therapies that work most effectively for particular individuals. For this, we need to carry out systematic research on a range of psychosocial treatments across a range of UK settings (e.g. specialist clinics, mainstream medical services). But future treatments will build on three main areas: the rapid developments in neuroscience and experimental psychology that have taken place in the last decade; new technology; and developments in pharmacological treatments.

6.1 How will Future Treatments Build on Developments in Neuroscience and Experimental Psychology?

There have been major developments over the last decade in our understanding of the brain correlates of drug dependence. This has been particularly spearheaded by brain-imaging studies. There has also been progress in understanding the psychological consequences of drug dependency both in terms of how drugs may affect an individual's cognitive ability and their sensitivity to differing rewards (see Chapter 5, Experimental Psychology and Research into Brain Science, Addiction and Drugs). Further, many additional advances have been made by combining brain-imaging methods with psychological techniques to determine how the brain responds to rewards such as

drug-related cues or how it is activated in different decision-making tasks.

Increasingly, research has shown that alcohol- and drug-dependent clients have significant neurocognitive impairment, particularly of the so-called 'executive' processes mediated by the prefrontal cortex. These processes are involved in inhibitory control of behaviour (the brain's brakes), in decision-making and planning. For example, about 75 per cent of people across a range of substance-use disorders are significantly impaired on an experimental decision-making task (Bechara, 2003). In particular, their decision making seems to be abnormally influenced by short-term rather than long-term outcomes (Bechara *et al.*, 2001). This, as well as poor inhibitory control and planning, probably reflects dysfunction of the dopaminergic pathways, which have been widely implicated in addictive behaviour, but other systems are likely to be involved as well [especially glutamate but also gamma-aminobutyric acid (GABA)].

As yet, it remains unclear how far these disturbances are a consequence of drug use, or predate and serve as vulnerability factors for it. Block *et al.* (2002) traced back school achievement records of people in treatment for substance dependence and found they were significantly impaired compared with controls on cognitive tests when aged 12, and before they started using drugs. However, even allowing for these early differences, there were still additional impairments in their current functioning. This suggests that pre-existing deficits are confounded by impairments subsequent to using drugs. Such cognitive impairments may impact negatively on progress in treatments and increase relapse rates. This suggests that cognitive rehabilitation – which is widely used with patients who have brain damage – may be a useful addition to treatment packages for substance-use disorders. As yet, this has not been researched as an area of treatment.

In their Incentive Sensitisation model of addiction, Robinson and Berridge (2000) argue that repeated drug use sensitises (enhances the reactivity of) the brain's reward system so that drug-related stimuli elicit stronger reactions, 'grabbing the individual's attention' and becoming increasingly salient. In effect, drugs hijack the brain's natural reward system. This leads to heightened 'cravings' which, compounded with poor response inhibition, lead to increasingly compulsive substance use (Jentsch and Taylor, 1999).

Building on these ideas, and integrating evidence from their own elegant brain-imaging studies, Volkow *et al.* (2003) have put forward a model of drug dependency (Figure 7.3). This model views dependence as a state arising initially from the reward provided by a drug. This reward value triggers a series of adaptations in four brain circuits. The four circuits (and the main, but not exclusive, brain areas implicated) are those involved in control (prefrontal cortex and cingulate gyrus); memory (hippocampus, amygdala), motivation and drive (orbitofrontal cortex and subcallosal cortex) and reward or saliency (nucleus accumbens and ventral pallidum). These four circuits work together, and change with experience. When an individual becomes drug dependent, the interaction between these four circuits changes so that the greater value of the

drug in three of the circuits (reward, drive and memory) overcomes the inhibitory control circuit. This loss of inhibitory control, combined with the positive feedback following drug consumption, strengthens links between the memory, reward and drive circuits and thereby perpetuates drug use.

As Volkow *et al.* (2003) point out, their model supports treatments that address multiple aspects of drug dependence. Specifically, they suggest four main strategies for intervention:

- decreasing the rewarding effects of the drug,
- increasing the value of other reinforcers,
- weakening learned drug responses,
- strengthening inhibitory control.

They give examples of how, in the first instance, the rewarding effects of the drug can be reduced by pharmacological treatments that either block the reinforcing effects of the drug or make its effects unpleasant. For the other three strategies they give examples of behavioural and cognitive treatments.

Many psychosocial approaches in current use broadly address multiple components within Volkow *et al.*'s model. Motivational treatments centre on the drive and reward components. Contingency management and

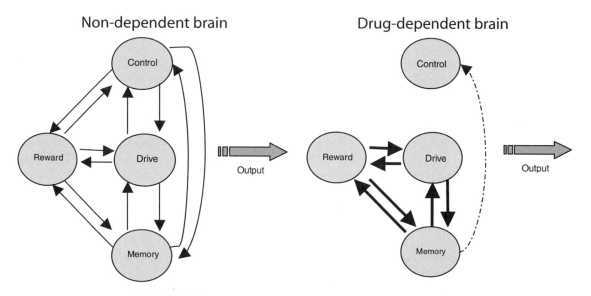

FIGURE 7.3   Volkow *et al.*'s (2003) model of drug dependency.

community reinforcement also involve drive and reward in aiming to increase the salience of non-drug reinforcers. Other behavioural treatments such as response prevention and cue exposure focus on control. Although no treatments currently focus on memory, successful interventions may eventually lead to a reduction in learned associations as drug-use behaviours are extinguished and new rewarded behaviours learned.

Developments in neuroscience have only begun to impact on the treatment of drug dependence. This is partly because, as yet, we do not know the effects of different treatments on the brain's response to drugs. It makes sense that successful treatments should enhance control mechanisms and reduce the brain's response to substance-related cues. The time course of brain changes following abstention from drugs may be protracted. For example, in a study with detoxified methamphetamine users, Wang et al. (2004) found some evidence that protracted abstinence (for months) from drug use was associated with a reversal of some methamphetamine changes in brain function but not others.

One impact that developments in neuroscience may well have in the future is to provide quantitative outcome measures such as changes in brain response to drug-related cues during functional imaging, or even changes in dopamine D2 receptor availability. The idea would be to assess clients when they start treatment and reassess at various stages afterwards. Conceivably such measures could eventually be used on an individual basis, potentially providing correlates of what stage of change a client had reached. A less resource-intensive outcome measure could be based on changes in how much of the individual's attention is grabbed by drug-related cues. Experimental studies have shown that substance users find drug-related stimuli more attention-grabbing than other types of stimuli (e.g. Bradley et al., 2003; Field et al., 2004; Townshend and Duka, 2001; Weinstein et al., 1998). A small-scale study by Cox et al. (2002) looked at attentional bias towards alcohol-related stimuli at the

beginning and end of a four week alcohol-detoxification programme. An increase in bias towards alcohol over the four weeks was found in those people who had relapsed back to drinking three months later. Those who had managed to stay abstinent showed a slight decrease in bias. There are very few studies of changes in cognitive bias over treatment but these may prove to be fruitful ways of assessing an individual's progress or even predicting outcome in treatment.

Similarly, based on the impairment of executive function associated with chronic drug use, other outcome measures which would be worth exploring could be change in performance on executive function tasks such as in Bechara et al.'s (2001) or Roger et al.'s (1999) gambling tasks.

Many current therapies place a load on the client's cognitive abilities and involve new learning. Assessing clients' cognitive function when they enter treatment may have additional use in allowing researchers to explore whether this may be one factor that helps to predict who benefits most from which types of 'evidence-based' psychological therapies.

6.2 How will Psychosocial Treatments Build on New Technologies?

A major aim of therapy is to develop an individual's motivation, skills and support to cope with not using substances in daily life. An important aspect is to help the individual generalise from the therapeutic situation to his or her real world. Although various ways to facilitate this are already in use, rapid advances in mobile phone technology offer a potentially powerful therapeutic aid for the future. This technology could replace current homework sheets and allow input to be given in difficult circumstances. Communication could be set up so that particularly high ratings could trigger a signal at a clinic help centre. Links with a therapist could be made in high-risk situations and previously agreed strategies reinforced to help the individual cope. As relapse often occurs as an impulsive response to cravings triggered by conditioned cues, mobiles may contribute positively to prevent relapse, especially in more motivated clients. Agreed timetables for input could provide a more detailed record of the client's difficulties and this could enhance the effectiveness of therapy sessions themselves. New communications technology could facilitate a more online form of therapy reaching beyond service contexts and into the individual's own world.

This approach might also enhance the effectiveness of brief interventions for heavy drinkers. Further, it may be a useful alternative to penal sentences for some substance users in the criminal justice system, perhaps in combination with electronic monitoring devices.

The Internet is already widely used as a source of information, and some drug-users' sites are reliable in the information they put out. There is scope for such sites to be used more interactively, and potentially for online therapy. One of the advantages of this approach could be for the many people with substance-use problems who never seek treatment. A more anonymous therapy may appeal to those who want help but without the stigma often associated with substance-use problems. Early intervention online could be widely accessible to people with excessive alcohol or drug use, and could be a first step in the treatment of those identified as being at risk. It would also offer significant advantages in terms of cost effectiveness.

6.3 How will Innovations in Pharmacological Treatment Impact on Psychosocial Treatments?

Because substance dependence is a complex disorder involving psychological, social and biological factors, we will not get far by treating the biological aspect in isolation. However, advances in pharmacological treatments may enhance psychosocial treatments. Theoretically, a psychological and a pharmacological intervention could combine positively, negatively or show no interaction. A positive interaction is seen with replacement opiates for heroin dependency where, without the suppression of craving by methadone, it is unlikely that a client could focus on talking with a therapist. Similarly, psychological interventions can be used to enhance adherence with pharmacological treatments. On the other hand, effective pharmacological treatment may reduce motivation for more personally effortful therapies. Taking a substitute drug such as methadone only involves swallowing, and if this is seen to be the main help, a client may have little motivation to engage in therapy, let alone to carry out 'homework' tasks which are part of most cognitive behavioural approaches. It is also possible that a pharmacological treatment that interferes with memory could impact negatively on progress in learning-based therapies. For example, benzodiazepines dose-dependently impair episodic memory (Curran, 1991) and methadone can also cause transient memory impairment around the time peak brain drug concentrations are achieved (Curran *et al.*, 2001). Finally, there is the issue of the clients' attributions. Do they see improvements in their drug use as being due to the pharmacological treatment rather than their own self-efficacy? Research on the mechanisms by which psychosocial and pharmacological treatment interact would help clarify these issues. For example, Littleton (1995) argues that the drug acamprosate may act by suppressing the normal conditioned responses (e.g. physiological response, craving) to alcohol-related cues (e.g. going into a pub).

There will soon be new ways of delivering pharmacological treatments for opiate dependence. For example, in the next few years a 'depot' formulation of buprenorphine will become available (Sobel *et al.*, 2004). Once injected, this will suppress opiate withdrawal symptoms and block the effects of self-administered opiates for about a month. This could have advantages for psychosocial treatments. A depot formulation should suppress cravings more continuously over time than a dose of methadone given daily (the latter also having all the psychological effects of more frequent use). By reducing cravings triggered by cues, this could widen the opportunity for therapists to improve the client's psychosocial skills and work on relapse prevention (Kleber, 2004).

Further, buprenorphine can be given outside the clinic in a mainstream medical centre and psychosocial treatments could also be given alongside it. There may be advantages in treating individuals away from a clinic population of other drug users. An implantable buprenorphine will soon be undergoing clinical trials (Kleber, 2004). This involves implanting small impregnated rods under the skin, and these may be pharmacologically effective for a period of years. These new treatments may be helpful for a subgroup of drug-dependent people who are relatively stable and who have jobs and effective social networks. They also extend the medical tool-chest, giving more options that may be useful at different stages of an individual's change in drug use. Depot injections or implants of buprenorphine may help suppress cravings but, without concurrent psychosocial input, it is highly unlikely that the individual will remain in treatment.

As Sobel et al. (2004) point out, what we crucially need are studies of which psychological therapies are optimised by these new pharmacological treatments.

There are no existing pharmacological treatments targeted at stimulant misuse. Their future development may enhance psychosocial interventions. Further, drug dependency is a form of learning, albeit maladaptive learning. Is it conceivable that future pharmacological agents may be able to influence learning and memory – to 'forget' old associations between drugs and related cues or enhance new learning of more adaptive behaviours? In the longer term, there is a possibility of delivering 'pleasure' not with drugs but with TMS. One could speculate that this may aid the treatment of drug dependency, although repeated TMS will incur its own costs. Finally, there is the question of how people will obtain drug treatments. Although the current focus

for opiate misuse is mainly on specialist treatment centres, there are already a range of alternatives (e.g. local pharmacy, supervised injection rooms, general practice) and it is possible that there may be advantages to extending prescription rights to other health workers.

6.4 Early Intervention in the Future?

The effectiveness of brief motivational interventions for excessive alcohol use has been clearly demonstrated (Burke et al., 2003). Recently, Bernstein et al. (2005) showed in a US RCT that a similar intervention was effective for heroin and cocaine use. They took hair samples from nearly 24 000 people attending a hospital drop-in clinic and from these identified over 1000 drug users. A 20-minute motivational interview was carried out by a trained 'peer' – an outreach worker who had themselves previously had problematic drug use. This significantly reduced the numbers using heroin and cocaine at a 6-month follow-up assessment which again screened hair samples. If this kind of intervention were made routinely available across A&E settings, it could have a significant impact in reducing the numbers of people who go on to need specialist treatment. Some would argue that we should extend drug testing of individuals to schools and the workplace and so allow for more widespread early intervention. There are clearly many ethical issues here.

7 PREVENTION STRATEGIES IN THE FUTURE?

One question which still puzzles scientists is why only a minority of people exposed to drugs go on to become dependent. Recent developments in neuroscience have begun to suggest some of the answers. People who are dependent on cocaine, alcohol or heroin show decreased densities of the dopamine D2 receptor (Volkow et al., 1999, 2002). Further, people who did not abuse drugs but had naturally low levels of D2 receptors found the effects of a stimulant (methylphenidate) more enjoyable than did people with high levels of these receptors (Volkow *et al.*, 1999). So, one of the many variables influencing vulnerability to substance-use disorders may be the inherited availability of D2 receptors. Genetics (as well as a multitude of developmental and environmental factors) is known to play a role in alcoholism. Relatives of alcoholics have a larger endorphin response to alcohol, and lower plasma endorphin levels, than non-relatives (Gianoulakis *et al.*, 1996). Further, relatives of alcoholics given ketamine reported it to be less unpleasant and somewhat more euphoric than people unrelated to alcoholics (Petrakis *et al.*, 2004).

The mapping of the human genome means we will in future be able to inform people of risk for substance-use disorders. This will not be simple given the complexity of gene–gene as well as gene–environment interactions. Genetic counselling of individuals identified as being at risk for addiction will probably have no major impact on the treatment of those who already have substance dependence, but may help with prevention. Vaccines to prevent drug abuse are already in development and we will need to determine their up- and downsides. Again, their use will involve a myriad ethical issues.

8 CONCLUSIONS

A range of psychological therapies have already been shown to be effective in treating substance misuse and dependency. Future treatments will build on developments in neuroscience, technology and pharmacology. They will broaden both the settings and the accessibility of treatment, and will increasingly be used earlier in an individual's development of substance-use problems. Economic analysis suggests that treatments are cost-effective. For example, the National Institute of Drug Abuse

(NIDA; 2004) in the United States concludes that every \$1 spent in treatment of drug abuse saves \$4–7 in reduced legal, social, community and health costs; in Britain, UKATT (2005) estimates that £1 saves £6 in similar costs. The potential of future, more effective, treatments for the wide range of people with problematic substance use is exciting. What we need now is rigorous research on these innovative approaches to provide a strong UK evidence base for future clinical practice.

References

Amato, L., Davoli, M., Ferri, M., Gowing, L., and Perruci, C. (2004) Effectiveness of interventions on opiate withdrawal treatment: an overview of systematic reviews. *Drug Alcohol Depend* 73: 219–226.

Andersen, A. (2004) The life-course approach to research on heavy alcohol drinking. *Addiction* 99: 1489.

Azrin, N.H., Sisson, R.W., Meyers, R., and Godley, M. (1982) Alcoholism treatment by disulfiram and community reinforcement therapy. *Behav Ther Exp Psychiatry* 13: 105–112.

Baker, A., Lewin, T., Reichler, H., Clancy, R., Carr, V., Garrett, R., Sly, K., Devir, H., and Terry, M. (2002) Motivational interviewing among psychiatric in-patients with substance use disorders. *Acta Psychiatr Scand* 106: 233–240.

Barnaby, B., Drummond, C., McCloud, A., Burns, T., and Omu, N. (2003) Substance misuse in psychiatric inpatients: comparison of a screening questionnaire survey with case notes. *BMJ* 327: 783–784.

Bechara, A. (2003) Risky business: emotion, decision-making, and addiction. *J Gambl Stud* 19: 23–51.

Bechara, A., Dolan, S., Denburg, N., Hindes, A., Anderson, S.W., and Nathan, P.E. (2001) Decision-making deficits, linked to a dysfunctional ventromedial prefrontal cortex, revealed in alcohol and stimulant abusers. *Neuropsychologia* 39: 376–389.

Beck, A.T., Wright, F.D., Newman, C.F., and Liese, B.S. (1993) *Cognitive therapy of substance abuse.* New York: Guilford.

Bernstein, J., Bernstein, E., Tassiopoulos, K., Heeren, T., Levenson, S., and Hingson, R. (2005) Brief motivational intervention at a clinic visit reduces cocaine and heroin use. *Drug Alcohol Depend* 77: 49–59.

Block, R.I., Erwin, W.J., and Ghoneim, M.M. (2002) Chronic drug use and cognitive impairments. *Pharmacol Biochem Behav* 73: 491–504.

Bradley, B.P., Mogg, K., Wright, T., and Field, M. (2003) Attentional bias in drug dependence: vigilance for cigarette-related cues in smokers. *Psychol Addict Behav* 17: 66–72.

Burke, B.L., Arkowitz, H., and Menchola, M. (2003) The efficacy of motivational interviewing: a meta-analysis of controlled clinical trials. *J Consult Clin Psychol* 71: 843–861.

Burns, T., White, I., Byford, S., Fiander, M., Creed, F., and Fahy, T. (2002) Exposure to case management: relationships to patient characteristics and outcome. Report from the UK700 trial. *Br J Psychiatry* 181: 236–241.

Carroll, K.M., Rounsaville, B.J., Nich, C., Gordon, L.T., Wirtz, P.W., and Gawin, F. (1994) One-year follow-up of psychotherapy and pharmacotherapy for cocaine dependence: delayed emergence of psychotherapy effects. *Arch Gen Psychiatry* 51: 989–997.

Cisler, R., Holder, H.D., Longabaugh, R., Stout, R.L., and Zweben, A. (1998) Actual and estimated replication costs for alcohol treatment modalities: case study from Project Match. *J Stud Alcohol* 59: 503–512.

Condelli, W.S., Fairbank, J.A., Dennis, M.L., and Rachal, J.V. (1991) Cocaine use by clients in methadone programs: significance, scope, and behavioural interventions. *J Subst Abuse Treat* 8: 203–212.

Connors, G.J., DiClemente, C.C., Dermen, K.H., Kadden, R., Carroll, K.M., and Frone, M.R. (2000) Predicting the therapeutic alliance in alcoholism treatment. *J Stud Alcohol* 61: 139–149.

Cox, W.M., Hogan, L.M., Kristian, M.R., and Race, J.H. (2002) Alcohol attentional bias as a predictor of alcohol abusers' treatment outcome. *Drug Alcohol Depend* 68: 237–243.

Crawford, M.J., Patton R., Touquet, R., Drummond, C., Byford, S., Barrett, B., Reece, B., Brown, A., and Henry, J.A. (2004) Screening and referral for brief intervention of alcohol-misusing patients in an emergency department: a pragmatic randomised controlled trial. *Lancet* 364(9442): 1334–1339.

Crits-Christoph, P., Siqueland, L., Blaine, J., Frank, A., Luborsky, L., Onken, L.S., Muenz, L.R., Thase, M.E., Weiss, R.D., Gastfriend, D.R., Woody, G.E., Barber, J.P., Butler, S.F., Daley, D., Salloum, I., Bishop, S., Najavits, L.M., Lis, J., Mercer, D., Griffin, M.L., Moras, K., and Beck, A.T. (1999) Psychosocial treatments for cocaine dependence: National Institute on Drug Abuse Collaborative Cocaine Treatment Study. *Arch Gen Psychiatry* 56: 493–502.

Curran, H.V. (1991) Benzodiazepines, memory and mood: a review. *Psychopharmacology* 105: 1–8.

Curran, H.V. and Morgan, C. (2000) Cognitive, dissociative and psychotogenic effects of ketamine in recreational users on the night of drug use and three days later. *Addiction* 95: 575–590.

Curran, H.V. and Travill, R.A. (1997) Mood and cognitive effects of ± 3,4 methylene-dioxymethamphetamine (MDMA, 'ecstasy'): week-end 'high' followed by mid-week 'low'. *Addiction* 92: 821–831.

Curran, H.V. and Verheyden, S.L. (2003) Altered response to tryptophan supplementation after long-term abstention from MDMA ('Ecstasy') is highly correlated with human memory function. *Psychopharmacology* 169: 91–103.

Curran, H.V., Kleckham, J., Bearn, J., Strang, J., and Wanigaratne, S. (2001) Effects of methadone on cognition, mood and craving in detoxifying opiate addicts: a dose-response study. *Psychopharmacology* 154: 153–160.

Curran, H.V., Collins, R., Fletcher, S., Yuen Kee, S.C., Woods, R.T., and Iliffe, S. (2003) Older adults and withdrawal from benzodiazepine hypnotics in general practice: effects on cognitive function, sleep, mood and quality of life. *Psychol Med* 33: 1223–1237.

Curran, H.V., Rees, H., Hoare, T., Hoshi, R., and Bond, A. (2004) Empathy and aggression: two faces of ecstasy? A study of interpretive cognitive bias and mood changes in ecstasy users. *Psychopharmacology* 173: 425–433.

Dawe, S., Powell, J., Richards, D., Gossop, M., Marks, I., Strang, J., and Gray, J.A. (1993) Does post-withdrawal cue exposure improve outcome in opiate addiction? A controlled trial. *Addiction* 88: 1233–1245.

Dennis, M., Godley, S.H., Diamond, G., Tims, F.M., Babor, T., Donaldson, J., Liddle, H., Titus, J.C., Kaminer, Y., Webb, C., Hamilton, N., and Funk, R. (2004) The Cannabis Youth Treatment (CYT) Study: Main findings from two randomized trials. *J Subst Abuse Treat* 27: 197–213.

Department of Health (1996) *Report of an independent review of drug treatment services in England: the task force to review services for drug misusers.* www.dh.gov.uk/PublicationsAndStatistics/Publications/PublicationsStatistics/PublicationsStatisticsArticle/fs/en?CONTENT_ID=400758&chk=uzpyfS

Department of Health (2002) *Mental health policy implementation guide: dual diagnosis good practice guide.* London: Department of Health.

DiClemente, C.C. and Scott, W. (1997) Stages of change: interactions with treatment compliance and involvement. *NIDA Research Monographs* 165: 131–156.

Driessen, M., Veltrup, C., Weber, J., John, U., Wetterling, T., and Dilling, H. (1998) Psychiatric co-morbidity, suicidal behaviour and suicidal ideation in alcoholics seeking treatment. *Addiction* 93: 889–894.

Drummond, D.C. (2000) What does cue-reactivity have to offer clinical research? *Addiction* 95, Suppl 2: S129–144.

Drummond, D.C. and Glautier, S. (1994) A controlled trial of cue exposure treatment in alcohol dependence. *J Consult Clin Psychology* 62: 809–817.

Drummond, D.C., Cooper, T., and Glautier, S.P. (1990) Conditioned learning in alcohol dependence: implications for cue exposure treatment. *Br J Addict* 85: 725–743.

Drummond, D.C., Kouimtsidis, C., Reynolds, M., Russell, I., Godfrey, C., McCusker, M., Coulton, S., Parrott, S., Davis, P., Tarrier, N., Turkington, D., Sell, L., Williams, H., Abou-Saleh, M., Ghodse, H., and Porter, S. (2004) *The effectiveness and cost-effectiveness of cognitive behaviour therapy for opiate misusers in methadone maintenance treatment: a multicentre randomised controlled trial (UKCBTMM[UK CBT in methadone maintenance treatment project]).* Final report to the Department of Health Research and Development Directorate. February 2004.

Dunn, C., Deroo, L., and Rivara, F. (2001) The use of brief interventions adapted from motivational interviewing across behavioural domains: a systematic review. *Addiction* 96: 1725–1742.

Fals-Stewart, W. and O'Farrell, T.J. (2003) Behavioural family counselling and naltrexone for opioid-dependent patients. *J Consult Clin Psychol* 71: 432–442.

Feeney, G., Young, R., Connor, J., Tucker, J., and McPherson, A. (2002) Cognitive behaviour therapy combined with the relapse-prevention medication acamprosate: are short-term treatment outcomes for alcohol dependence improved? *Austr NZ J Psychiatry* 36: 622–628.

Field, M., Mogg, K., and Bradley, B.P. (2004) Cognitive bias and drug craving in recreational cannabis users. *Drug Alcohol Depend* 74: 105–111.

Fleming, M.F., Mundt, M.P., French, M.T., Manwell, L.B., Stauffacher, E.A., and Barry, K.L. (2002) Brief physician advice for problem drinkers: long-term efficacy and benefit-cost analysis. *Alcohol Clin Exp Res* 26: 36–43.

Foster, T. (2001) Dying for a drink. Global suicide prevention should focus more on alcohol use disorders. *BMJ* 323(7317): 817–818.

Gianoulakis, C., Krishnan, B., and Thavundayil, J. (1996) Enhanced sensitivity of pituitary beta-endorphin to ethanol in subjects at high risk of alcoholism. *Arch Gen Psychiatry* 53: 250–257.

Godfrey, C., Eaton, G., McDougall, C., and Culyer, A. (2002) *The economic and social costs of Class A drug use in England and Wales, 2000.* Home Office Research Study 249. www.homeoffice.gov.uk/rds/pdfs2/hors249.pdf

Griffith, J.D., Rowan-Szal, G.A., Roark, R.R., and Simpson, D.D. (2000) Contingency management in outpatient methadone treatment: a meta-analysis. *Drug Alcohol Depend* 58: 55–66.

Gruber, K., Chutuape, M.A., and Stitzer, M.L. (2000) Reinforcement-based intensive outpatient treatment for inner city opiate abusers: a short-term evaluation. *Drug Alcohol Depend* 57: 211–223.

Higgins, S.T., Sigmon, S.C., Wong, C.J., Heil, S.H., Badger, G.J., Donham, R., Dantona, R.L., and Anthony, S. (2003) Community reinforcement therapy for cocaine-dependent outpatients. *Arch Gen Psychiatry* 60: 1043–1052.

Hughes, J., Stead, L., and Lancaster, T. (2004) Antidepressants for smoking cessation. *The Cochrane Database of Systematic Reviews.* Issue 4; doi: 10.1002/14651858.CD000031.pub2.

Hulse, G.K. and Tait, R.J. (2002) Six-month outcomes associated with a brief alcohol intervention for adult in-patients with psychiatric disorders. *Drug Alcohol Rev* 21: 105–112.

Hulse, G.K. and Tait, R.J. (2003) Five-year outcomes of a brief alcohol intervention for adult in-patients with psychiatric disorders. *Addiction* 98: 1061–1068.

Humphreys, K. and Weisner, C. (2000) Use of exclusion criteria in selecting research subjects and its effect on the generalizability of alcohol treatment outcome studies. *Am J Psychiatry* 57: 588–594.

Hurt, P.H. and Ritchie, E.C. (1994) A case of ketamine dependence. *Am J Psychiatry* 151: 779.

Huxley, A. (1932) *A brave new world.* London: Perennial Classics.

Irvin, J.E., Bowers, C.A., Dunn, M.E., and Wang, M.C. (1999) Efficacy of relapse prevention: a meta-analytic review. *J Consult Clin Psychol* 67: 563–570.

Jeffery, D.P., Ley, A., McLaren, S., and Siegfried, N. (2000) Psychosocial treatment programmes for people with both severe mental illness and substance misuse. *The Cochrane Database of Systematic Reviews.* Issue 2. doi: 10.1002/14651858.CD001088.

Jentsch, J.D. and Taylor, J.R. (1999) Impulsivity resulting from frontostriatal dysfunction in drug abuse: implications for the control of behavior by reward-related stimuli. *Psychopharmacology (Berl)* 146: 373–390.

Kleber, H.D. (2004) Treatment of drug dependence enters a new high technological era. *Addiction* 99: 1476–1477.

Krystal, J.H., Karper, L.P., Seibyl, J.P., Freeman, G.K., Delaney, R., Bremner, J.D., Heninger, G.R., Bowers, M.B. Jr, and Charney, D.S. (1994) Subanesthetic effects of the non-competitive NMDA-antagonist, ketamine, in humans. *Arch Gen Psych* 51: 199–214.

Lingford-Hughes, A.R., Welch, S., and Nutt, D.J. (2004) Evidence-based guidelines for the pharmacological management of substance misuse, addiction and comorbidity: recommendations from the British Association for Psychopharmacology. *J Psychopharmacol* 18: 293–335.

Littleton, J. (1995) Acamprosate in alcohol dependence: how does it work? *Addiction* 90: 1179–1188.

Mattick, R. and Jarvis, T. (1993) *An outline for the management of alcohol problems: Quality Assurance Project.* Sydney: National Drug and Alcohol Research Centre.

Mattick, R., Breen, C., Kimber, J., and Davoli, M. (2003a) Methadone maintenance therapy versus no opioid dependence. *The Cochrane Database of Systematic Reviews.* Issue 2. doi: 10.1002/14651858.CD002209.

Mattick, R., Kimber, J., Breen, C., and Davoli, M. (2003b) Buprenorphine maintenance versus placebo or methadone maintenance for opioid dependence. *The Cochrane*

Database of Systematic Reviews. Issue 2. doi: 10.1002/14651858.CD002207.pub2.

Mayet S., Farrell M., Ferri M., Amato, L. and Davoli, M. (2004) Psychosocial treatment for opiate abuse and dependence. *The Cochrane Database of Systematic Reviews.* Issue 4. Art. No: CD004330. doi: 10.1002/14651858.CD004330.pub2.

McCloud, A., Barnaby, B., Omu, N., Drummond, C., and Aboud, A. (2004) Relationship between alcohol use disorders and suicidality in a psychiatric population: in-patient prevalence study. *Br J Psychiatry* 184: 439–445.

Miller, W.R. and Willbourne, P.L. (2002) Mesa Grande: a methodological analysis of clinical trials of treatments for alcohol use disorders. *Addiction* 97: 265–277.

Miller, J.M., Brown, T.L., Simpson, N.S., Handmaker, T.H., Bien, L.F., Luckie, H.A., Montgomery, R.K., Hester, J.S., and Tonigan, S. (1995) What works? A methodological analysis of the alcohol treatment outcome literature. In: R.K. Hester and W.R. Miller (eds), *Handbook of alcoholism treatment approaches.* Needham Heights: Allyn and Bacon: 12–44.

Miller, W.R., Baker, C., Blackburn, I.M., James, I., and Reichelt, K. (1999) Effectiveness of cognitive therapy training. *J Behav Ther Exp Psychiatry* 30: 81–92.

Mixmag (2004) A nation of caners – what state are you in? *Mixmag* 33–45. London: UK, Emap.

Monti, P.M., Rohsenow, D.J., Rubonis, A.V., Niaura, R.S., Sirota, A.D., Colby, S.M., Goddard, P., and Abrams, D.B. (1993) Cue exposure with coping skills treatment for male alcoholics: a preliminary investigation. *J Consult Clin Psychol* 61: 1011–1019.

Moos, R., Finney, J., and Cronkite, R. (1990) *Alcoholism treatment: context, process, and outcome.* New York: Oxford University Press.

Morgan, C.J.A., Mofeez, A., Bradner, B., Bromley, L., and Curran, H.V. (2004a) Acute effects of ketamine on memory systems and psychotic symptoms in healthy volunteers. *Neuropsychopharmacology* 29: 208–218.

Morgan, C.J.A., Riccelli, M., Maitland, C.H., and Curran, H.V. (2004b) Long-term effects of ketamine abuse: evidence of persisting impairment of source memory in recreational users. *Drug and Alcohol Depend* 75: 301–308.

Moyer, A., Finney, J.W., Swearingen, C.E., and Vergun, P. (2002) Brief interventions for alcohol problems: a meta-analytic review of controlled investigations in treatment-seeking and non-treatment-seeking populations. *Addiction* 97: 279–292.

National Institute of Drug Abuse (2004) Measuring and improving costs, cost-effectiveness, and cost–benefit for substance-abuse treatment programs www.nida.nih.gov/IMPCOST/IMPCOSTIndex.html

National Treatment Agency (2002) *Models of care for the treatment of adult drug misusers.* London: National Treatment Agency.

Ockene, J.K., Adams, A., Hurley, T.G., Wheeler, E.V., and Herbert, J.R. (1999) Brief physician- and nurse-practitioner-delivered counselling for high-risk drinkers: does it work? *Arch Intern Med* 159: 2198–2205.

O'Farrell, T.J., Choquette, K.A., Cutter, H.S.G., Brown, E.D., and McCourt, W.F. (1993) Behavioral marital therapy with and without additional couples relapse prevention sessions for alcoholics and their wives. *J Stud Alcohol* 54: 652–666.

O'Malley, S.S., Jaffe, A.J., Chang, G., Schottenfeld, R.S., Meyer, R., and Rounsaville, B. (1992) Naltrexone and coping skills therapy for alcohol dependence. *Arch Gen Psychiatry* 49: 881–887.

Pain Society (2004) *Recommendations for the appropriate use of opioids for persistent non-cancer pain.* The Pain Society, London, March 2004.

Petrakis, I.L., Limoncelli, D., Gueorguieva, R., Jatlow, P., Boutros, N.N., Trevisan, L., Gelernter, J., and Krystal, J.H. (2004) Altered NMDA glutamate receptor antagonist response in individuals with a family vulnerability to alcoholism. *Am J Psychiatry* 161: 1776–1782.

Prime Minister's Strategy Unit (2003) *Alcohol Harm Reduction Project: interim analytical report.* www.strategy.gov.uk/work_areas/alcohol_Misuse/interim.asp

Prime Minister's Strategy Unit (2004) Alcohol harm reduction strategy for England. www.strategy.gov.uk/downloads/su/alcohol/pdf/CabOffce%20AlcoholHar.pdf

Prochaska, J.O. and DiClemente, C.C. (1983) Stages and processes of self-change of smoking: toward an integrative model of change. *J Consult Clin Psychol* 51: 390–395.

Project Match Research Group (1997) Matching alcoholism treatments to client heterogeneity: Project Match post-treatment drinking outcomes. *J Stud Alcohol* 58: 7–29.

Rankin, H., Hodgson, R., and Stockwell, T. (1982) Cue exposure and response prevention with alcoholics: a controlled trial. *Behav Res Ther* 21: 435–446.

Rawson, R.A., Huber, A., McCann, M., Shoptaw, S., Farabee, D., Reiber, C., and Ling, W. (2002) A comparison of contingency management and cognitive-behavioral approaches during methadone maintenance treatment for cocaine dependence. *Arch Gen Psychiatry* 59: 817–824.

Regier, D.A., Farmer, M.E., Rae, D.S., Locke, B.Z., Keith, S.J., Judd, L.L., and Goodwin, F.K. (1993) Comorbidity of mental disorders with alcohol and other drug abuse: results from the epidemiologic catchment area (ECA) study. *J Am Med Associ* 264: 2511–2518.

Richter, K.P., McCool, R.M., Okuyemi, K.S., Mayo, M.S., and Ahluwalia, J.S. (2002) Patients' views on smoking cessation and tobacco harm reduction during drug treatment. *Nicotine Tob Res* 4, Suppl 2: S175–S182.

Robinson, T.E. and Berridge, K.C. (2000) The psychology and neurobiology of addiction: an incentive-sensitization view. *Addiction* 95: S91–S117.

Rogers, R.D., Everitt, B.J., Baldacchino, A., Blackshaw, A.J., Swainson, R., Wynne, K., Baker, N.B., Hunter, J., Carthy, T., Booker, E., London, M., Deakin, J.F., Sahakian, B.J., and Robbins, T.W. (1999) Dissociable deficits in the decision-making cognition of chronic amphetamine abusers, opiate abusers, patients with focal damage to prefrontal cortex, and tryptophan-depleted normal volunteers: evidence for monoaminergic mechanisms. *Neuropsychopharmacology* 20: 322–339.

Rollnick, S., Mason, P., and Butler, C. (1999) *Behaviour change: a guide for healthcare professionals.* London: Churchill Livingstone.

Romberger, D.J. and Grant, K. (2004) Alcohol consumption and smoking status: the role of smoking cessation. *Biomed Pharmacother* 58: 77–83.

Roozen, H., Boulogne, J., Tulder, M., van den Brink, W., De Jong, C.A., and Kerkhof, A.J. (2004) A systematic review of the effectiveness of the community reinforcement approach in alcohol, cocaine and opioid addiction. *Drug Alcohol Depend* 74: 1–13.

Roth, A.D. and Fonagy, P. (2005) *What works for whom? A critical review of psychotherapy research.* New York: The Guilford Press.

Saunders, B., Wilkinson, C., and Phillips, M. (1995) The impact of brief motivational intervention with opiate users attending a methadone programme. *Addiction* 90: 415–424.

Silagy, C., Lancaster, T., Stead, L., Mant, D., and Fowler, G. (2003) Nicotine replacement therapy for smoking cessation. *The Cochrane Database of Systematic Reviews.* Issue 3. doi: 10.1002/14651858.CD000146.pub2.

Slattery, J., Chick, J., Cochrane, M., Godfrey, C., Kohli, H., Macpherson, K., Parott, S., Quinn, S., Single, A., Tochel, C., and Watson, H. (2003) *Prevention of relapse in alcohol dependence.* Health Technology Assessment Report 3. Glasgow: Health Technology Board for Scotland.

Smith, D.E. and McCrady, B.S. (1991) Cognitive impairment among alcoholics: impact on drink refusal skills acquisition and treatment outcome. *Addict Behav* 16: 265–274.

Sobel, B.F., Sigmon, S.C., Walsh, S.L., Johnson, R.E., Liebson, I.A., Nuwayser, E.S., Kerrigan, J.H., and Bigelow, G.E. (2004) Open-label trial of an injection depot formulation of buprenorphine in opioid detoxification. *Drug Alcohol Depend* 73: 11–22.

Sobell, M.B. and Sobell, L.C. (2000) Stepped care as a heuristic approach to the treatment of alcohol problems. *J Consult Clin Psychol* 68: 573–579.

Stephens, R.S., Roffman, R., and Simpson, E.E. (1994) Treating adult marijuana dependence: a test of the relapse prevention model. *J Consult Clin Psychol* 62: 92–99.

Stephens, R.S., Roffman, R.A., and Cutin, L. (2000) Comparison of extended versus brief treatments for marijuana use. *J Consult Clin Psychol* 68: 898–908.

Terzano, M.G., Rossi, M., Palomba, V., Smerieri, A., and Parrino, L. (2003) New drugs for insomnia: comparative tolerability of zopiclone, zolpidem and zaleplon. *Drug Safety* 26: 261–282.

Thomasius, R., Petersen, K., Buchert, R., Andresen, B., Zapletalova, P., Wartberg, L., and Nebeling, B. (2003) Mood, cognition and serotonin transporter availability in current and former ecstasy (MDMA) users. *Psychopharmacology* 167: 85–96.

Townshend, J.M. and Duka, T. (2001) Attentional bias associated with alcohol cues: differences between heavy and occasional social drinkers. *Psychopharmacology* 157: 67–74.

UKATT research team (2005) Effectiveness and cost-effectiveness of treatment for alcohol problems: findings of the randomised United Kingdom Alcohol Treatment Trial (UKATT). *BMJ* 331: 541, 544.

Verheyden S., Henry, J., and Curran H.V. (2003) Acute, sub-acute and long-term subjective consequences of ecstasy (MDMA) consumption in 430 regular users. *Human Psychopharmacol* 18: 1–11.

Volkow, N.D., Wang, G.J., Fowler, J.S., Hitzemann, R., Angrist, B., Gatley, S.J., Logan, J., Ding, Y.S., and Pappas, N. (1999) Association of methylphenidate-induced craving with changes in right striato-orbitofrontal metabolism in cocaine abusers: implications in addiction. *Am J Psychiatry* 156: 19–26.

Volkow, N.D., Wang, G.J., Fowler, J.S., Thanos, P.P., Logan, J., Gatley, S.J., Gifford, A., Ding, Y.S., Wong, C., and Pappas, N. (2002) Brain DA D2 receptors predict reinforcing effects of stimulants in humans: replication study. *Synapse* 46: 79–82.

Volkow, N.D., Fowler, J.S., and Wang, G.J. (2003) The addicted human brain: insight from imaging studies. *J Clin Invest* 111: 1444–1451.

Wang, G.J., Volkow, N.D., Chang, L., Miller, E., Sedler, M., Hitzemann, R., Zhu, W., Logan, J., Ma, Y., and Fowler, J.S. (2004) Partial recovery of brain metabolism in methamphetamine abusers after protracted abstinence. *Am J Psychiatry* 161: 242–248.

Wanigaratne, S., Davis, P., Pryce, K., and Brotchie, J. (2005) *The effectiveness of psychological therapies on drug misusing clients.* A briefing paper of the National Treatment Agency. London: Department of Health.

Weinstein, A., Lingford-Hughes, A., Martinez-Raga, J., and Marshall, J. (1998) What makes alcohol-dependent individuals early in abstinence crave for alcohol: exposure to the drink, images of drinking, or remembrance of drinks past? *Alcohol Clin Exp Res* 22: 1376–1381.

World Health Organisation (2003) Expert Committee on Drug Dependence. *World Health Organ Tech Rep Ser* 915, i–v, 1–26.

Zacny, J.P. and Gutierrez, S. (2003) Characterizing the subjective, psychomotor, physiological effects of oral oxycodone in non-drug-abusing volunteers *Psychopharmacology* 170: 242–254.

CHAPTER

8

Cognition Enhancers

Roy Jones, Kelly Morris and David Nutt

1 EXECUTIVE SUMMARY

The search for treatments for dementia, alongside other scientific and societal changes, has prompted the development of symptomatic treatments and disease-modifying drugs for people with degenerative brain diseases, mild cognitive impairment, and psychiatric diseases that involve cognition impairment. The enhancement of aspects of cognition, such as learning and memory, now seems possible for people with normal age-related decline and in healthy people, although so far the effects of these cognition enhancers are modest. The next two decades are likely to bring deeper knowledge of the mechanisms of learning, memory, and forgetting, together with an understanding of the relationship between changes in molecules, cells and brain circuits, and changes in cognition. Already, research efforts by the pharmaceutical industry are poised to deliver many more disease modifiers and putative cognition enhancers, though limitations exist in translating laboratory findings into effective interventions for human use.

If effective interventions become available, their general use will bring health, social, ethical and regulatory issues. The widespread use of cognition enhancers for healthy people could have substantial impact and potentially become problematic as a minority may have abuse liability. Mechanisms do not exist currently to regulate cognition enhancers for non-medical purposes, though social changes together with commercial pressures mean that their use for enhancement is likely to be increasingly required, desired and accepted. Their use for disease-related impairments seems unlikely to cause concerns if cost-effective treatments are used to enhance function and quality of life. New challenges will include the development of biomarkers to allow early intervention and the targeting of therapies for the best effect on the individual.

2 DEFINITIONS AND SCOPE OF REVIEW

'Cognition enhancement' is the use of various strategies to boost cognitive functions – ie mental states that underpin information-processing tasks such as attention, memory, and selective forgetting. The term was originally used for the treatment of disease-associated cognitive impairment, such as in dementia and schizophrenia. Subsequently, the term expanded to encompass the use of interventions for mild cognitive impairment (MCI), currently defined as cognitive deficits that do not overtly impair function. MCI has a greater risk of progression to dementia than for age-related cognitive decline, which is probably synonymous with normal ageing (Figure 8.1). Now 'cognition enhancement' is applied to the use of interventions for normal ageing and in well people for non-medical purposes. Many agents are marketed to UK consumers as cognition enhancers or nootropics. This term describes substances thought to enhance mental functions, and is interchangeable with 'smart drugs' or 'smart pills'. Definitions of pharmacological terms are given elsewhere (see Chapter 6, Pharmacology and Treatments).

This review is not a comprehensive account of dementia treatment or of all agents with cognition-enhancing properties. The pace of change is such that new developments are likely to be announced almost as soon as this review is published. Instead, we offer a representative account of the underlying science, current and potential agents, and strategies for drug development, plus forward-looking predictions of the field. A particular target of cognition enhancers is the augmentation of learning and memory, and these are the focus of this review. However, our review and predictions apply to other functions, such as attention and selective or useful forgetting, as well as to traditionally non-cognitive aspects of subjective experience such as mood and empathy.

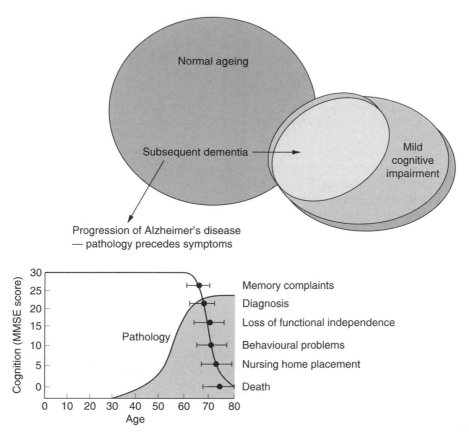

FIGURE 8.1 Progression to dementia in normal ageing versus mild cognitive impairment – the latter might be linked with early pathology.

3 BACKGROUND

Advances in our understanding of central nervous system functioning in health and disease have brought with them the potential for altering that functioning with psychoactive substances. The search for interventions that might halt cognitive decline was initiated within dementia research, and then applied to Parkinson's disease (PD) and other neurodegenerative and neurodevelopmental conditions such as schizophrenia and epilepsy.

Alongside the development of such disease-modifying drugs, changes in society and attitudes have occurred. People in the UK and similar nations are living longer. The current generation aged over 55 is also the richest in history, and aspires to an active retirement free from illness. However, age-related memory impairment begins to accelerate from 55 years, and the likelihood of having Alzheimer's disease (AD) or a related dementia rises substantially in old age, with 20 per cent of those aged over 80 affected. Now the most common reason for nursing home admission is not physical but cognitive impairment.

Within the past few decades, the preprogrammed decline in body systems that occurs with ageing has become a target for intervention, in addition to the prevention of age-related diseases such as AD. Increasing public interest in technologies for enhancement beyond therapy or prevention has encompassed the possibility of cognitive improvement in healthy people. Notably, the Cochrane Dementia and Cognitive Impairment Group, registered in August, 1995, altered its name and scope in 2000 to the Cochrane Dementia and Cognitive *Improvement* Group (CDCIG).

By 2010, the market for AD therapy alone is expected to grow from 16 million patients to 21 million in the seven major pharmaceutical markets, while AD drug sales could exceed $8 billion (£4.4 billion; www.leaddiscovery.co.uk/reports/vg010.html). Substantial numbers of people already have other neurodegenerative conditions (eg PD), MCI, or cognitive decline due to psychiatric disease. This group may be additionally important because depressed elderly people, like those with MCI, may have an increased risk of progression to dementia (Lyketsos *et al.*, 2004). Added to these trends is the over-the-counter and Internet availability of cognition-enhancing agents, while consumers are more informed about psychoactive substances, and more likely to take a preventative approach to future cognitive decline. Already, early intervention in neurodegenerative and related diseases is a public priority.

Research on cognition, neuroscience, and ageing has provided a multidisciplinary platform to inform development of disease-modifying drugs and, more recently, potential cognition enhancers. Key developments include: animal models, including transgenic animals with added or deleted genes to help indicate potential cognitive mechanisms (see Chapter 4, Genomics), imaging techniques to investigate brain structure and functional activity (see Chapter 9, Neuroimaging), and increasingly sophisticated neuropsychological testing of cognitive functions (see Chapter 5, Experimental Psychology and Research). Although the correspondence between these various strands of evidence remains unclear, for example, how neuropsychological deficits relate to changes in brain structure and functioning – the emerging field of cognitive neuroscience has begun to relate them and apply the findings to normal ageing and disease states (Cabeza, 2004; Cabeza *et al.*, 2004).

4 BASIS OF LEARNING AND MEMORY

Much has been discovered about the cellular and molecular basis of learning and memory in several species, although we still do not know comprehensively how new information is perceived, stored, consolidated, and retrieved or forgotten over timescales that vary from seconds to decades. The next 20 years are likely to bring much greater understanding of learning and memory, and our ability to manipulate these pathways will undoubtedly increase.

The central mechanism thought to underpin memory is synaptic plasticity (Silva, 2003) – changes in the strength and size of synapses that increase or decrease efficiency of transmission. Roles in learning, memory and forgetting are also attributed to new synapse formation (synaptogenesis) and loss, the proliferation and survival of new neurons (neurogenesis), and neuronal cell death (neurotoxicity and apoptosis). Each process provides possible targets for cognition enhancement and selective forgetting in healthy people, while processes important in disease-associated cognitive decline are important targets for early therapeutic intervention. Figure 8.2 shows the dramatic brain atrophy seen in AD compared with a healthy person.

4.1 Long-term Potentiation

The fundamental model of synaptic plasticity is long-term potentiation (LTP) – an increase in synaptic signalling after the synchronised stimulation of connected neurons. One classic example of LTP involves binding of the neurotransmitter glutamate to NMDA (N-methyl-D-aspartate) receptors. Glutamate binding opens a channel in the receptor, allowing charged atoms (ions) to

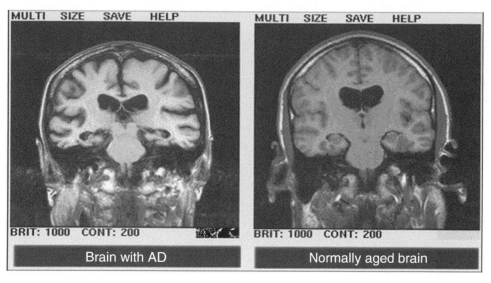

FIGURE 8.2 Gross differences in brain structure between Alzheimer's disease and normal ageing.

flow into the cell. At rest, the NMDA receptor channel is plugged by magnesium ions, so glutamate binding opens the channel but ions cannot flow through. When the membrane gains positive charge due to the transmission of an electrical signal, the magnesium ions leave the channel. When NMDA receptors open, calcium ions flow in to trigger a cascade of molecular events (Lisman, 2003), in addition to the flow of sodium ions that can result in onward transmission of the electrical signal.

Potentiation arises because short-term calcium-triggered events increase the sensitivity of the cell to further signals, so when a particular event is repeated, persistent and increasing activation of that circuit results in learning. The calcium influx acts to increase the sensitivity and number of a second glutamate receptor – AMPA (α-amino-3-hydroxy-5-methyl-4-isoxazoleproprionic acid; Lisman, 2003), which increases the amount of sodium ions allowed into the cell with each stimulation, further increasing the strength of synaptic signalling.

More permanent changes that could underlie longer-term memory require the synthesis of new proteins (Bradshaw *et al.*, 2003), in both presynaptic and postsynaptic neurons (Lisman, 2003). In humans, CREB (cyclic-AMP response element binding protein) is one factor that facilitates protein production (Josselyn *et al.*, 2001). Inward calcium flow indirectly activates CREB, which induces gene expression. Increased gene expression can lead to production of more receptors, as well as structural proteins that 'cement' the synaptic connection between two repeatedly communicating neurons. Presynaptic strengthening may also involve the addition of new receptors, and thus synapse size is increased on each side. Another important process is the production of neurotrophic factors that stimulate nerve growth and increase the complexity of neural connections, such as nerve growth factor (NGF) and brain-derived neurotrophic factor (BDNF). Roles in other short-term and longer-term more complex changes in brain and behaviour are beginning to be assigned to neurotrophic factors (Russo-Neustadt, 2003).

The formation and storage of very long-term memories is not well understood but some authors propose self-perpetuating reactions, such as those involving protein kinases and CREB, as one ongoing mechanism (Robertson and Sweatt, 1999).

The state of activation or depression in individual neural circuits may need reinstatement by repeated activation or depression, while synaptic weakening may be important to remove unnecessary connections. These two processes may occur particularly during sleep (Abraham, 2003; Walker and Stickgold, 2004).

Synaptic plasticity occurs in several brain structures. For example, the hippocampus has been implicated in encoding memories, in short-term or working memory, and in contextual learning or sequential memory (such as travel routes), while the neocortex is implicated in long-term memory storage and recall (Lisman, 2003; Hedou and Mansuy, 2003). The cerebellum has been implicated in learning direct and especially timed actions, such as riding a bicycle (Okano et al., 2000), while the amygdala seems key to emotion-related memory (Blair et al., 2001).

4.2 Effects of Attention, Emotion and Stress

Several factors affect the success of LTP and its inverse state, long-term depression (LTD). Neurotransmitters like acetylcholine, dopamine, serotonin, and CRF (corticotrophin-releasing factor) can alter the strength of LTP and LTD. The counterpart in the whole organism is likely to be effects of attention, stress and emotion on cognition.

Acetylcholine may play a key part in focusing learning and memory, and the loss of cholinergic projections is a classic feature of dementia. Activation of these projections can enhance LTP, at least in the hippocampus (Colgin et al., 2003; Ovsepian et al., 2004). Serotonin has been shown to both promote and inhibit learning (Barbas et al., 2003; Meneses, 2003), while dopamine acts to potentiate both LTP and LTD, depending on interactions between receptors (Centonze et al., 2001). Other neurotransmitters implicated in enhancing LTP include neuropeptides, such as somatostatin (Roozendaal, 2002).

The effects of stress on memory are complex, and depend on the type and phase of memory, the stressor involved, and its timing and duration. Glucocorticoids (steroid stress hormones) interact with noradrenaline, dopamine, and perhaps acetylcholine to generate appropriate learning responses for acutely stressful situations. High glucocorticoid levels impair memory retrieval but improve memory consolidation in fearful situations, but not in simply novel, arousing situations (Roozendaal, 2002; Woodson et al., 2003). Thus, fearful situations may produce strong new memories that 'overwrite' old memories, leading to amnesia for previous related knowledge (Diamond et al., 2004a). In such situations, the amygdala may generate new emotion-related memory while simultaneously the hippocampal-prefrontal cortex circuit is impaired (Diamond et al., 2004b).

In the long term, high glucocorticoids impair several learning-related processes (Erickson et al., 2003). Other inhibitory states, including those with high levels of GABA (gamma-aminobutyric acid) (Kalueff and Nutt, 1996/7), cannabinoids (Hill et al., 2004), and inflammatory immune chemicals (Barrientos et al., 2003) may impair both new memory and the retrieval of old learning. Endogenous cannabinoid signalling appears to be important in extinguishing aversive memories (Marsicano et al., 2002).

4.3 Ageing, MCI and Disease

Any process that leads to cognitive impairment, including normal ageing, may impact on common structures and processes, including LTP and LTD, neural connectivity, cellular calcium regulation, protein formation and destruction (proteolysis), neurotransmitter and hormone levels, and cerebral blood flow (Barnes, 2003; Wu et al., 2002; Jones, 2004; McNaught, 2004; Toescu et al., 2004; Prickaerts et al., 2004). Neural connectivity involves the formation, survival, and loss of synapses and neurons and effects on dendrites (nerve filaments) and dendritic spines where synapses form. Many of these processes are inter-related. Calcium regulation also seems important for dendritic changes, while abnormal protein formation can induce neurotoxicity. Finally, the balance between disruptive and compensatory mechanisms, such as the ability to recruit new brain regions to perform specific tasks, is thought to be crucial in determining clinical cognitive impairment (Cabeza *et al.*, 2004).

Normal ageing, MCI and early disease thus share similarities, although some of the changes seen during normal ageing seem distinct from established disease pathology. For example, normal ageing shares some similarities with AD, such as the presence of β-amyloid plaques, reduced blood flow, neuropeptide changes, and reduced cholinergic function, but not others such as neurofibrillary tangles and neuritic plaques. Whether normal ageing, MCI and AD represent a spectrum of outcomes or different entities is debated – more likely, a subset of people with MCI have early AD (Cabeza *et al.*, 2004; Ferris, 2004). But while the relationships between normal ageing, MCI and various disease processes await full definition, the study of what seem to be individual entities may inform understanding of others, such as the loss of neural connectivity in ageing, AD and schizophrenia (Jones, 2004) or the disruptions in proteolysis that underlie different neurodegenerative diseases (McNaught, 2004).

Notably, disease processes start several years earlier than clinical problems. Some of those affected will be categorised with MCI, while up to 60 per cent of people with MCI show such pathology. A far higher proportion of people with MCI will develop dementia than those with normal age-related deficits, so genetic, neurochemical and imaging tests are in development to distinguish potential signs of early disease (Ferris, 2004; DeKosky and Marek, 2003). Development of such biomarkers could allow early intervention with disease-modifying drugs. Since some early disease changes may be shared by those with normal ageing, the distinction between disease modification and cognition enhancement might be somewhat artificial.

However, this distinction allows us to consider cognition-enhancing agents separately.

5 CURRENT COGNITION ENHANCERS

Many different strategies are proposed to enhance cognition. Most interventions target either disease pathologies or the processes underlying normal cognition, particularly synaptic plasticity. Many act via more than one pathway or target. Strategies and treatments for cognition enhancement include:

- general measures such as exercise and environmental enrichment
- correction of underlying factors such as hypertension
- nutrients
- herbal medicines
- pharmaceuticals
- psychological and learning strategies (see Chapter 5, Experimental Psychology and Research)
- electromagnetic interventions, eg transcranial magnetic stimulation, brain-computer interfaces (see Chapter 3, Neuroscience of Drugs and Addiction).

5.1 General Measures

Environmental enrichment alters the structure of rodent brains and improves learning and memory, apparently by changes in gene expression related to neuron structure, synaptic plasticity, and transmission (Rampon *et al.*, 2000). Such changes might be prompted via neurotrophin expression (eg BDNF; Russo-Neustadt, 2003). Parallel findings in elderly people are that leisure activities and physical exercise are linked with lower risks of dementia and cognitive decline respectively (Verghese *et al.*, 2003; Yaffe *et al.*, 2001).

5.2 Correction of Underlying Factors

Cognitive impairment has been linked with hypertension, high cholesterol levels, diabetes and possibly the menopause. Early correction of some of these might slow cognitive decline.

Several randomised controlled trials (RCTs) have investigated the effects of lowering blood pressure on risk of dementia, although a Cochrane review is awaited (McGuiness *et al.*, 2005). One large trial (Syst-Eur) found that nitrendipine, a calcium-channel blocker, plus add-on medications was associated with a 50 per cent reduction in dementia, compared with a placebo (Forette *et al.*, 1998), which increased with longer follow-up (Forette *et al.*, 2002). However, this finding could be related to other effects of calcium-channel blockers (see below). Further, a recent study found that use of brain-penetrating angiotensin-converting enzyme inhibitors (but not non-brain-penetrating agents nor calcium-channel blockers) slowed progression of AD (Ohrui *et al.*, 2004).

A Cochrane review on diabetes management and cognitive impairment reviewed five trials, but none were of sufficient quality (Areosa Sastre and Grimley Evans, 2005). A Cochrane review on statins for AD found a similar lack of available trials (Scott and Laake, 2005). Other evidence on the effect of statins is contradictory (Shepherd *et al.*, 2002; Sparks *et al.*, 2002) so the possibility of an additional benefit on cognitive impairment remains open.

The Cochrane review on hormone-replacement therapy (HRT) for menopausal symptoms found five small trials, none of which provided convincing evidence of delay in the progression of dementia (Hogervorst *et al.*, 2005a). A similar conclusion was drawn over nine trials on protection from cognitive impairment (Hogervorst *et al.*, 2005b). The US Women's Health Initiative Memory Study indicated more than doubling of dementia risk in women on HRT and aged 65 years or more (Shumaker *et al.*, 2003). These and unrelated concerns have led to cautions against the use of HRT in older women, especially those with dementia. Soya extract, which contains oestrogen-like compounds, was given to postmenopausal women in an RCT that reported some

benefits on cognition after 12 weeks (Duffy *et al.*, 2003). The long-term consequences of a high soya diet continue to be debated.

5.3 Nutrients and 'Nutraceuticals'

Many dietary supplements are recommended by various sources to improve cognition, including 'nutraceuticals' – dietary components or similar that act like drugs. These agents are widely available in UK retail outlets. Such agents are usually well tolerated and no abuse potential is known for those listed.

Table 8.1 summarises all specific dietary supplements reviewed by the CDCIG that are regulated in the UK under the Food Safety Act 1990.

5.3.1 Vitamin E +/– Other Antioxidant Vitamins

Free radicals such as toxic oxygen products are linked with neuronal damage in AD and might be important in normal ageing. A recent review of dietary factors in AD (Luchsinger and Mayeux, 2004) included seven cohort studies that related vitamin E intake (including supplements) to the risk of cognitive impairment, including dementia. All studies considered dietary sources with and without vitamin C supplements, and three also investigated carotenoid intake. One study found no relation between antioxidant intake and AD, while three found an inverse relationship between dietary intake of vitamin E and dementia. The other three studies explored use of supplements. All found some benefit of vitamins E and C supplementation, one reported a reduced risk of vascular dementia (but not AD), one a reduced risk of AD, and one increased global cognition scores.

The 2002 Cochrane review included only one randomised trial of vitamin E, selegiline, both or placebo in AD (Tabet *et al.*, 2005. Although vitamin E was linked with a greater effect than selegiline or combined

TABLE 8.1 Potential cognition enhancers available as dietary supplements in the UK – summary of Cochrane reviews.

Name	Proposed mechanism	Evidence	Conclusion	Comments
Vitamin E	Antioxidant-scavenging of free radicals	Cochrane review (update 2002) in AD (Tabet et al., 2005)	Insufficient evidence of efficacy	Included only one RCT of vitamin E, selegiline or both
Vitamin B6	Treatment of undetected deficiency and reduction in homocysteine levels	Cochrane review (update 2003) for cognition (Malouf and Grimley Evans, 2005)	No evidence for short-term benefit in healthy people but more RCTs needed	Included two trials in healthy people only. Both papers report memory benefits
Vitamin B12	As for B6	Cochrane review (update 2003) for cognitive impairment (Malouf and Areosa Sastre, 2005)	Insufficient evidence of efficacy	Included two trials of people with dementia and low B12
Folate	As for B6	Cochrane review (update 2003) for people with cognitive impairment or healthy elderly (Malouf et al., 2005)	No significant benefit of folate supplementation with or without B12 – important issue that needs further RCTs	Four RCTs were included, one in healthy elderly people. One studied combined B12/folate supplements
Thiamine	Previous evidence for benefit of thiamine in AD	Cochrane review (update 2003) for AD (Rodriguez-Martin et al., 2005)	Not possible to draw any conclusions	Included three studies that amounted to less than 50 participants overall
Thiamine	Alcohol misuse results in thiamine deficiency, which can lead to cognitive impairment as part of Wernicke–Korsakoff syndrome	Cochrane review (update 2003) for people with or at risk of Wernicke–Korsakoff syndrome due to alcohol misuse (Day et al., 2005)	Insufficient evidence to guide prescribing for prophylaxis or treatment	Included one trial only, which reported benefit with high dose intramuscular thiamine (200 mg/day) after 2 days
Lecithin (phosphatidyl-choline)	A cell membrane component and the major dietary source of choline needed to synthesise acetylcholine	Cochrane review (update 2003) for cognitive impairment including dementia (Higgins and Flicker, 2005)	Available evidence does not support use for dementia, although a moderate effect cannot be excluded	Included 12 RCTs – only one trial, of subjective memory problems, reported dramatic effects

continued

TABLE 8.1—Continued

Name	Proposed mechanism	Evidence	Conclusion	Comments
DHEA and DHEA sulphate	Neurosteroids that enhance glutamate effects and inhibit GABA effects. Antiglucocorticoid action may lead to neuroprotective and immune-enhancing effects	Cochrane review (update 2004) for cognitive function (Huppert and Van Niekerk, 2005)	No support for an improvement of memory or other cognitive functions	Three studies of healthy older people, and one in perimenopausal women with decreased well-being
Alpha-lipoic acid	Several mechanisms, including enhanced mitochondrial function and antioxidant properties	Cochrane review (update 2004) for dementia (Sauer et al., 2005)	No RCTs included, thus use cannot be recommended	Benefit proposed from non-randomised trials and preclinical research only
Acetyl-L-carnitine	Similar roles to alpha lipoic acid	Cochrane review (update 2003) for dementia (Hudson and Tabet, 2005)	Evidence for benefit on clinical global impression only, thus no evidence to recommend routine use	11 RCTs included, all in people with AD
Ginkgo biloba	Multiple actions, including vaso-dilatation, anticoagulation, antioxidant actions, and effects on neurotransmitters	Cochrane review (update 2002) for cognitive impairment and dementia (Birks and Grimley Evans, 2005)	Highly variable trial quality and inconsistent results even among better trials	Large, high-quality long-term trial needed, given inconsistent effects and good safety

treatment, falls were increased in the vitamin E arm. For cognitive impairment in healthy elderly people, one good-sized trial found little effect of antioxidant vitamins for up to 12 months (Smith et al., 1999).

5.3.2 Vitamins B6, B12, and Folate

Deficiencies of vitamins B6, B12, and folate reduce the conversion of homocysteine to methionine or cysteine, while raised homocysteine has been linked with cerebrovascular disease and neuronal toxicity. Some evidence exists from epidemiological and non-randomised studies that reduced homocysteine levels or increased B6, B12, and/or folate can reduce dementia risk or improve cognition, although not all studies found positive findings (Luchsinger and Mayeux, 2004).

Deficiency of vitamin B6 is linked to various neuropsychiatric disorders and the rationale for its use is to treat undetected deficiency. A Cochrane review found no significant differences with treatment (Malouf and Grimley Evans, 2005), although individual papers have reported significant improvements in aspects of memory performance.

B12 deficiency affects more than 10 per cent of older people, and is associated with neuropsychiatric disorders. Folate deficiency has been linked to cerebral cortical atrophy at autopsy. One Cochrane review included two small randomised trials in demented people with low B12, and found no significant benefit on cognitive impairment (Malouf and Areosa Sastre, 2005). A second Cochrane review included four RCTs of folic acid with or without B12 for healthy people, or individuals with cognitive impairment or dementia (Malouf et al., 2005). All trials found no significant benefits.

5.3.3 Thiamine and Alcohol

Thiamine has been the treatment of choice for Wernicke–Korsakoff syndrome for 50 years. This syndrome, caused by thiamine deficiency, is most commonly due to heavy alcohol intake. Thiamine replacement can reverse early cognitive changes and is commonly prescribed (Lingford-Hughes et al., 2004), although evidence to guide prescribing is virtually non-existent (Day et al., 2005). High and no alcohol intake in middle age is linked with later cognitive impairment (Anttila et al., 2004) while moderate alcohol intake may be protective against dementia (Luchsinger and Mayeux, 2004), except in those with the APOE epsilon-4 allele (Anttila et al., 2004). Whether a link exists between cognitive impairment and thiamine deficiency cannot be determined from current evidence (Rodriguez-Martin et al., 2005).

5.3.4 Choline Precursors and Membrane Components

Various choline precursors such as the major dietary phospholipid lecithin (phosphatidylcholine) have been used in an attempt to accelerate acetylcholine synthesis. Lecithin is also a key component of neuronal cell membranes, which are degraded during cerebral ischaemia to free fatty acids and free radicals. A Cochrane review (Higgins and Flicker, 2005) of 12 trials of lecithin, involving 265 people with AD, 21 people with PD, and 90 people with subjective memory problems, did not find any substantial effects, except

in the study on memory problems. The authors conclude that a moderate effect cannot be excluded but a large RCT is not a priority. Some beneficial effects have been reported for the related phosphatidylserine (Kidd, 1999) although overall the evidence is inconclusive.

Marine-derived omega-3 fatty acids, especially docosahexaenoic acid, are purported to improve cell-membrane fluidity and cause less damage on membrane degradation than omega-6 fatty acids. Five cohort studies have explored the link between fats, fish intake, and risk of dementia or AD (Luchsinger and Mayeux, 2004). Overall, these studies suggest that high fish intake, unsaturated fats, and omega-3 fatty acids may be protective. Few trials have been done on marine-derived fatty acids for cognitive impairment, except for those trials done in preterm infants. One RCT reported abnormal levels of essential fatty acids in 36 patients with AD, and found a significant benefit of supplementation (Corrigan et al., 1991).

5.3.5 Neurosteroids and Melatonin

Dehydroepiandrosterone (DHEA) and its sulphate DHEAS are neurosteroids that enhance glutamate signalling and reduce GABA inhibition. Their antiglucocorticoid action may have neuroprotective and immune-enhancing effects. Some, but not all, studies have found lower levels of DHEA/S in people with dementia. However, a Cochrane review of four trials in people without cognitive impairment found few significant findings (Huppert and Van Niekerk, 2005). The authors suggest that benefit may be evident only in large, longer trials.

Melatonin is a hormone with clock-setting properties that is secreted at night from the pineal gland, at levels that decrease with ageing. Positive effects of melatonin have been reported on sleep and cognition in elderly people (Zhdanova et al., 2001) and in people with dementia (Asayama et al., 2003) although other trials have been negative. A Cochrane review is planned (Rusak-Maguire and Forbes, 2005).

TABLE 8.2   Some putative cognition-enhancing herbs.

Acorus calamas	*Embelia ribes*	*Nicotiana tabacum*
Angelica archangelica	*Emblica officinalis*	*Paeonia emodi*
Asparagus racemosus	*Eugenia caryophyllus*	*Panax ginseng*
Bacopa monniera	*Evodia rutaecarpa*	*Piper longum*
Biota orientalis	*Galanthus nivalis*	*Polygala tenuifolia*
Boerhavia diffusa	*Ginkgo biloba*	*Polygonum multiflorum*
Celastrus paniculatus	*Glycyrrhiza glabra*	*Pongamia pinnata*
Centella asiatica	*Huperzia serrata*	*Rosmarinus officinalis*
Clitoria ternatea	*Hydrocotyl asiatica*	*Salvia lavandulifolia*
Codonopsis pilosula	*Lawsonia inermis*	*Salvia miltiorrhiza*
Convolvulus pluricaulis	*Lycoris radiata*	*Schizandra chinensis*
Coptis chinensis	*Magnolia officinalis*	*Terminalia chebula*
Crocus sativus	*Melissa officinalis*	*Tinospora cordifolia*
Curcuma longa	*Nardostachys jatamansi*	*Withania somnifera*

5.3.6 *Other Endogenous Antioxidants*

Two endogenous antioxidants – alpha-lipoic acid and acetyl-L-carnitine – have been studied in people with dementia. Both are important in energy metabolism and might protect against oxidative damage to brain genetic material, thus improving memory (Liu *et al.*, 2002). However, a Cochrane review found no suitable RCTs of alpha-lipoic acid, and benefit in two small non-randomised studies (Sauer *et al.*, 2005). A reasonable body of evidence exists for global benefits with short- to medium-term use of acetyl-L-carnitine in AD, but without apparent benefit in most other measures (Hudson and Tabet, 2005). Thus global benefits may be due to chance.

5.4 Herbal Medicines

The use of herbs for cognitive improvement occurs in many traditions, including Chinese, Ayurvedic, and European herbalism. Usually herbal preparations are well tolerated but they can have harmful side-effects, including interactions with pharmaceuticals (de Smet, 2002; Barnes *et al.*, 2003). The only herb that has been reviewed by the CDCIG is *Ginkgo biloba* (Birks and Grimley Evans, 2005), commonly used for memory disorders and often also taken with ginseng (eg *Panax ginseng*) (Howes and Houghton, 2003;

Vohora and Mishra, 2004). Some herbs with evidence of cognition-enhancing action are listed in Table 8.2 (Howes and Houghton, 2003; Vohora and Mishra, 2004; Kennedy *et al.*, 2003; Kennedy *et al.*, 2004; Perry *et al.*, 2003).

The European Commission adopted a Directive on Traditional Herbal Medicinal Products (30 April 2004), prompted by concerns over public protection from the sale of ineffective or potentially harmful products. At the time of writing, the UK had until October 2005 to implement the Directive, although herbs legally available on 30 April 2004 receive transitional protection until April 2011.

5.4.1 Ginkgo Biloba *and* Ginseng

Extracts of *Ginkgo biloba* leaves are prescribed in Germany and France for cerebral insufficiency, memory and concentration problems. A recent Cochrane review found that the quality of trials is highly variable. Moreover, trials with superior methodology have inconsistent results (Birks and Grimley Evans, 2005). Nevertheless, most studies report at least some improvement in the overall functioning, cognition and activities of daily living in people with dementia. The authors advise that a large, high-quality trial is needed. A large trial is now underway (2005) in London. A potentially hazardous interaction could occur with anticoagulant drugs such as warfarin and aspirin (de Smet, 2002).

Many studies have been done in healthy people to assess whether ginkgo has positive effects. A review of nine trials found mixed results, which could be explained by dose variations (Canter and Ernst, 2002; Kennedy et al., 2000). A Cochrane review of the effect of ginkgo on cognition in healthy populations is planned (Lee and Birks, 2005).

Ginkgo is thought to act in several ways (Birks and Grimley Evans, 2005; Gold et al., 2002) including vasodilatation, anticoagulant effects, antioxidant actions, neuroprotection, and neurotransmitter changes. Ginkgo is often taken together with ginseng (eg Panax ginseng) as the two are traditionally said to be synergistic (Howes and Houghton, 2003; Vohora and Mishra, 2004). Panax ginseng is reported to have multiple effects, including neuroprotection (Howes and Houghton, 2003; Vohora and Mishra, 2004). The few studies differ on whether ginseng has cognition-enhancing properties in healthy people (Kennedy et al., 2002; Wesnes et al., 2000). Ginseng is reported to have a greater effect on brain electrical activity than ginkgo (Kennedy et al., 2003).

5.5 Pharmaceuticals

Several processes are targets for current agents aimed to improve cognition, although effect sizes are modest. Table 8.3 summarises the evidence from the CDCIG for licensed medicines. Most of these are prescription-only medicines in the UK or elsewhere (British Medical Association, Royal Pharmaceutical Society, 2004). Few have abuse potential.

5.5.1 Acetylcholine

Cholinesterase Inhibitors

Three agents that inhibit the breakdown of acetylcholine by blocking acetylcholinesterase are licensed for treatment of mild-to-moderate AD (British Medical Association, Royal Pharmaceutical Society,

2004) – donepezil, galantamine and rivastigmine. Galantamine, found in *Galanthus nivalis* and other plants, may also act via nicotinic receptors while rivastigmine also inhibits butyrylcholinesterase, which may be important in later-stage AD. The CDCIG has found beneficial effects on cognition, functioning, and behaviour for:

- donepezil in AD treated for up to a year (Birks and Harvey, 2005) and vascular dementia treated for up to 6 months (Malouf and Birks, 2005)
- galantamine for AD treated for up to 6 months (Olin and Schneider, 2005)
- rivastigmine for AD treated for 6 months (Birks et al., 2005); one trial of rivastigmine found some efficacy for dementia with Lewy bodies (Wild et al., 2005).

Efficacy trials comparing the three agents have been criticised over their methodology and reporting (Hogan et al., 2004). Cognition-enhancing effects have been reported in healthy people. Although one study of donepezil found a slight worsening on some measures (Beglinger et al., 2004), another found some improvement (Yesavage et al., 2002). Tolerability is generally similar for the three drugs.

Nicotine

Nicotine stimulates nicotinic cholinergic receptors and also releases acetylcholine, while the metabolite cotinine might be neuroprotective. Little RCT evidence of the effects of nicotine exists in AD (Lopez-Arrieta and Sanz, 2005) and while some studies have documented improvements in attention (Sahakian et al., 1989; Jones et al., 1992; White and Levin, 1999) in such patients, others have not (Lopez-Arrieta and Sanz, 2005). Some evidence exists of cognition-enhancing effects in healthy elderly people (Min et al., 2001) and improvements in attention for elderly people with memory impairment (White and Levin, 2004). Improvements in psychomotor performance in healthy volunteers are larger in smokers than in non-smokers, probably due to the offsetting of

TABLE 8.3   UK pharmaceutical drugs that act on cognition – summary of Cochrane reviews.

Name	Proposed mechanism	Evidence	Conclusion	Comments
Donepezil	Acetyl-cholinesterase inhibitor	Cochrane review (update 2003) in AD (Birks and Harvey, 2005)	Efficacy in all stages of disease, for up to a year's treatment	Cost-effectiveness data awaited for AD treatment
		Cochrane review (update 2003) in vascular cognitive impairment (Malouf and Birks, 2005)	Benefits for probable and possible mild-to-moderate disease for 6 months	Extension of studies and better diagnostic criteria are desirable
Galantamine	Acetyl-cholinesterase inhibitor; also possible cholinergic agonist	Cochrane review (update 2004) in AD (Olin and Schneider, 2005)	Consistent positive benefits in mild-to-moderate disease with 3–6 months' treatment	Daily dose of 16 mg titrated over 4 weeks offered best tolerability
Rivastigmine	Acetyl-cholinesterase and butyryl-cholinesterase inhibitor	Cochrane review (update 2000) in AD (Birks et al., 2005)	Benefits on various markers in mild-to-moderate AD after 26 weeks of 6–12 mg	Further study needed on optimum dosage to minimise side-effects
		Cochrane review (update 2003) in Lewy body dementia (Wild et al., 2005)	Benefits in some markers only if observed cases analysed	Evidence for efficacy is weak
Nicotine	Acetylcholine agonist and releaser	Cochrane review (update 2002) in AD (Lopez-Arrieta and Sanz, 2005)	Unable to find evidence for or against benefit	One trial found, but did not present results suitable for inclusion
D-cycloserine	Partial NMDA agonist – enhances glutamate signalling	Cochrane review (update 2002) in AD (Jones et al., 2005)	No place for this agent in treatment of AD	Lack of positive effects in well-powered controlled trials
Memantine	Moderate NMDA antagonist – may protect from excitatory cell death	Cochrane review (update 2004) in dementia (Areosa Sastre and Sheriff, 2005)	Clinically noticeable reduction in deterioration at 28 weeks	Benefit discernible in moderate-to-severe disease only, but early benefits seen, and well tolerated
Nimodipine	Calcium-channel blocker – might reduce neuronal death due to excess calcium influx	Cochrane review (update 2002) in various dementias (Lopez-Arrieta and Birks, 2005)	Some short-term benefits in dementia due to unclassified or mixed disease, Alzheimer's, or vascular dementia	Further evaluation of unavailable trial data is desirable, and new research must focus on longer-term outcomes

continued

TABLE 8.3—Continued

Name	Proposed mechanism	Evidence	Conclusion	Comments
Propentofylline	Adenosine uptake and phosphodiesterase inhibitor – also anti-inflammatory effects	Cochrane review (update 2002) in dementia (Frampton *et al.*, 2005)	Limited evidence of benefits in AD, vascular dementia, or mixed disease	Review limited by unavailable data on 1200 patients not released
Selegiline	Monoamine oxidase-A inhibitor – promotes dopamine signalling	Cochrane review (update 2002) in AD (Birks and Flicker, 2005)	No evidence of clinically meaningful benefit	Further trials in AD are not justified
Piracetam	Metabolic enhancement, antithrombotic, and neuropro-tectant	Cochrane review (update 2001) in dementia or cognitive impairment (Flicker and Grimley Evans, 2005)	Does not support use	Further evaluation warranted both on available data and as new studies
Hydergine	Increased cerebral blood flow, effects on neurotransmitters	Cochrane review (update 2000) in dementia (Olin *et al.*, 2005)	Significant treatment effects on generic scales	Selection criteria for trials is outdated so benefit remains uncertain
Nicergoline	As above, plus antioxidant and neuroprotectant properties	Cochrane review (update 2002) in dementia and other age-related cognitive impairment (Fioravanti and Flicker, 2005)	Some positive benefits on cognition and behaviour in older patients with mild-to-moderate impairment	Studies have differing outcomes; also, newer diagnostic criteria not used so not clear who might benefit
Vinpocetine	Metabolic and blood-flow enhancement, antithrombotic, neuroprotectant, phosphodiesterase inhibitor	Cochrane review (update 2002) in cognitive impairment and dementia (Szatmari and Whitehouse, 2005)	Evidence does not support clinical use	Large trials in well-defined populations are needed to evaluate efficacy
CDP-choline	Precursor of phosphatidyl-choline	Cochrane review (update 2003) for chronic cerebral disorders in the elderly (Fioravanti and Yanagi, 2005)	Some evidence of positive benefits on memory and behavioural disturbances (up to 3 months)	Longer trials warranted with current diagnostic criteria

withdrawal effects (Tucha and Lange, 2004). The abuse potential of pharmaceutical nicotine is thought to be low (see Chapter 6, Pharmacology and Treatments).

5.5.2 Excitatory Amino-acids

D-cycloserine and Glycine

The antituberculosis antibiotic (British Medical Association, Royal Pharmaceutical Society, 2004) D-cycloserine acts as a partial agonist at the glycine-binding site on NMDA receptors to enhance glutamate signalling. A Cochrane review of two of the four studies of D-cycloserine for AD found no benefits (Jones *et al.*, 2005). Only one other small trial reported benefits (Tsai *et al.*, 1999a). The authors attribute this short-term finding to the use of higher doses (100 mg/day) than in other trials.

Research on D-cycloserine includes the finding that 15 mg can reverse scopolamine-induced amnesia in healthy people (Jones *et al.*, 1991). Subsequently, a trial of biologically available glycine found improvements in episodic memory in young students and middle-aged men. The latter group also sustained benefits to attention (File *et al.*, 1999). These findings may provide the rationale for the unproven suggestion that trimethylglycine is a cognition enhancer.

Related agents have also been investigated for cognitive decline in schizophrenia, together with newer generations of antipsychotics (so-called 'atypical' antipsychotics) (Heresco-Levy *et al.*, 2002, 2004; Tsai *et al.*, 1999b, 2004; Evins *et al.*, 2000). It is suggested that atypical antipsychotics act on NMDA receptors in addition to monoamines, which could explain why these agents might preserve cognition more than classic antipsychotics that antagonise dopamine. However, the extent to which these agents preserve cognition is debated (Harvey and Keefe, 2001; Harvey *et al.*, 2003). Atypical antipsychotics increase the risk of stroke in people with dementia, although this risk may be small (Herrmann *et al.*, 2004; Gill *et al.*, 2005).

Memantine

This moderate-affinity NMDA antagonist may prevent neurotoxicity due to over-activity of excitatory amino-acids such as glutamate, and thus enhance learning and memory. A Cochrane review of memantine for dementia found significant broad benefits in moderate-to-severe AD, vascular dementia and combined or non-specified dementia, though some effects were modest (Areosa Sastre and Sheriff, 2005). Adverse effects were low, and the authors conclude that more studies are needed. Subsequently, an RCT has found memantine beneficial when added to donepezil (Tariot *et al.*, 2004). Memantine is licensed in the UK for moderate-to-severe AD and is usually well tolerated (British Medical Association, Royal Pharmaceutical Society, 2004), although hallucinations are occasionally reported.

Little evidence exists for the effects of memantine on cognition in healthy volunteers, although the drug can impair conditioned behaviours in humans and animals (Schugens *et al.*, 1997; Hart *et al.*, 2002; Popik *et al.*, 2003), suggesting potential for use in addiction. However, one report suggests that the drug may have mild subjective stimulant effects (Hart *et al.*, 2002).

5.5.3 Calcium Channels

Calcium-channel Blockers

Calcium influx into neurons occurs via both NMDA channels and voltage-dependent calcium channels – excessive calcium influx can cause neurotoxicity. Thus, calcium-channel blockers have been investigated for effects on cognition, effects on blood flow and also on voltage-dependent calcium channels, which assume greater importance with ageing (McNaught, 2004). A Cochrane review of nimodipine in dementia reviewed nine of 14 possible trials (Lopez-Arrieta and Birks, 2005). Pooled data indicated benefit on various scales including cognition but not on functioning. Nimodipine and related drugs, but not nitrendipine

(Forette *et al.*, 1998), are licensed in the UK for hypertension treatment (British Medical Association, Royal Pharmaceutical Society). Preclinical and animal research also indicate benefits from nimodipine and nivaldipine.

5.5.4 Adenosine and Phosphodiesterase

Cell signalling by cyclic AMP (cAMP) is important in various types of LTP. Inhibition of phosphodiesterase particularly type 4, which breaks down cAMP, can increase cAMP signalling, while antagonism at adenosine receptors acts indirectly to inhibit phosphodiesterase. AD pathology may in part depend on blocking cAMP signalling (Vitolo *et al.*, 2002). Thus, cognition is potentially enhanced by adenosine antagonists such as caffeine, and by phosphodiesterase inhibitors, both non-specific (eg papaverine and propentofylline) and specific (eg rolipram).

Caffeine

The role of the world's most popular drug as a cognition enhancer is a longstanding controversy. Experimental data indicate that caffeine can enhance the turnover of central noradrenaline in low arousal states, and may have cholinergic actions (Smith *et al.*, 2003). However, recent data suggest that caffeine only enhances cognition in caffeine-dependent people in withdrawal, eg after a 6–8-hour sleep (Rogers *et al.*, 2003; Heatherley *et al.*, 2005). High doses can cause side-effects in vulnerable people while caffeine withdrawal involves headaches and tiredness.

Propentofylline

This phosphodiesterase inhibitor also blocks adenosine uptake, and has other actions including NGF secretion. Nine RCTs have been conducted in people with various types of dementia but five ($n = 1200$) remain unpublished (Frampton *et al.*, 2005). Thus, a Cochrane review considered only four RCTs but did find limited evidence of benefit on cognition and functioning (Frampton *et al.*, 2005). However, the application for European licensing for this agent was unsuccessful.

Rolipram

This selective type-4 phosphodiesterase inhibitor enhances long-term retention of contextual learning (Barad *et al.*, 1998). In addition, it corrected learning deficits in a mouse model of a congenital syndrome associated with impaired cognition (Bourtchouladze *et al.*, 2003). Rolipram is licensed in some European countries and Japan, though not the UK, as an antidepressant.

5.5.5 Monoamines

The monoamine neurotransmitters – dopamine, serotonin, and noradrenaline – have substantial and complex effects on cognition. The interaction of dopamine and glutamate can promote LTP and LTD in various brain regions (Centonze *et al.*, 2001). Dopamine neurotransmission, which is important for motor function and cognition, declines with age and these age-related decreases may contribute to impaired attention and mental flexibility plus other deficits (Volkow *et al.*, 1998). Dopamine D2 receptors appear important for verbal learning and executive function (Mozley *et al.*, 2001), while D1 receptors are implicated in spatial working memory (Muller *et al.*, 1998).

Serotonergic projections modulate various aspects of learning and memory (Ovsepian *et al.*, 2004; Barbas *et al.*, 2003; Harvey, 2003). However, the contribution of the 14 receptor types (Barbas *et al.*, 2003) plus indirect effects due to cortical modulation of other monoamines is complex (Millan *et al.*, 2000). Serotonin appears to modulate the impact of dopamine upon spatial working memory (Luciana *et al.*, 1998; Harrison *et al.*, 2004b) and attention (Matrenza *et al.*, 2004), while serotonin alone appears to modulate declarative memory (Harrison *et al.*, 2004a).

Drugs that act via noradrenaline can have cognition-impairing or enhancing effects (Middleton *et al.*, 1999; Berridge and Waterhouse, 2003), perhaps due to the complex cortical interaction between noradrenaline and dopamine (Arnsten, 2001). Some agents that enhance noradrenergic function might act as stimulants directly, or indirectly by increasing cortical dopamine. States that involve increased noradrenergic activity have been linked with enhanced emotional memory formation (eg posttraumatic stress disorder) and impaired working memory (Berridge and Waterhouse, 2003).

Methylphenidate

Methylphenidate (see Chapter 6, Pharmacology and Treatments) is the cognition enhancer with the best evidence base, improving various aspects of cognition in children and adults with ADHD (Kutcher *et al.*, 2004; Biederman and Spencer, 2004). The short- and long-acting preparations licensed for ADHD (British Medical Association, Royal Pharmaceutical Society, 2004) work by reducing dopamine uptake into neurons via the dopamine transporter. Guidance from the UK's National Institute for Health and Clinical Excellence recommends that such treatments be used after remedial measures have been tried (National Institute for Clinical Excellence, 2000). However, large RCTs report little benefit from such support, whether alone or in addition to medication (MTA Cooperative Group, 1999, 2004). One concern over long-term psychostimulant treatment is the potential to mildly restrict growth, perhaps due to appetite suppression (MTA Cooperative Group, 2004).

In people with ADHD, the abuse potential of this psychostimulant is low (Kollins *et al.*, 2001; Kollins, 2003). Indeed, appropriate treatment in childhood is linked with reduced substance misuse later (Wilens, 2001). However, methylphenidate can be abused if it is administered via routes that provide rapid increases in blood levels (Volkow and Swanson, 2003). New formulations are designed to prevent such abuse.

A trend has developed for healthy students and others to take methylphenidate as a cognition enhancer, particularly for situations like exams. Studies have reported improvements in working memory in young adults, which have been linked with changes in cerebral blood flow (Mehta *et al.*, 2000; Elliott *et al.*, 1997). However, other evidence suggests a lack of effect in elderly men and young sleep-deprived volunteers (Turner *et al.*, 2003a; Bray *et al.*, 2004). Its use has been explored in pilot studies for HIV-associated cognitive slowing, post-stroke recovery, and traumatic brain injury.

Amphetamines

Amphetamines, including dexamphetamine sulphate and mixed amphetamines, are psychostimulants with efficacy in ADHD (British Medical Association, Royal Pharmaceutical Society, 2004; Kutcher *et al.*, 2004; Biederman and Spencer, 2004). In addition, amphetamines are reported to enhance several cognition measures in healthy volunteers, including response speed (Kumari *et al.*, 1997) and retention and recall of verbal memory (Soetens *et al.*, 1995), with variable effects on accuracy of responding. Amphetamines act indirectly to prompt release of dopamine, are linked with synaptic plasticity (Butefisch *et al.*, 2002), and thus may help with cognitive decline. Such agents have been used by various armed forces for years. However, a major problem with rapid-acting dopamine agonists is the potential for abuse. Outside certain contexts, amphetamines can lead to dependency, and may cause neurodegeneration and psychosis (see Chapter 6, Pharmacology and Treatments).

Other Dopaminergic Agents, Including Antipsychotics

In general, dopamine antagonists such as the classic antipsychotics (eg haloperidol (Kumari *et al.*, 1997)) act to impair working memory and other aspects of cognitive function, while agents that promote dopaminergic actions, especially at D1 receptors

(Muller *et al.*, 1998; Castner *et al.*, 2000), act to enhance working memory. D1 agonist effects may be particularly important to reverse cognitive deficits in schizophrenia (Castner *et al.*, 2000). Agents with dopamine agonism include buproprion and the selective D2 agonist bromocriptine. D2 receptors are thought to be involved in executive functions, such as planning, which explains some reported effects of bromocriptine (McDowell *et al.*, 1998). However, studies in healthy volunteers found that the drug impaired some aspects of executive function but improved spatial memory (Mehta *et al.*, 2001). Another study found effects on working memory were inversely related to baseline function (Kimberg *et al.*, 1997), a frequent finding with psychostimulants.

Selegiline inhibits the breakdown of dopamine by monoamine oxidase A and has been studied in PD and AD. A Cochrane review found some benefit of selegiline in AD plus good tolerability. However, benefits seemed unlikely to be clinically meaningful (Birks and Flicker, 2005). Use in PD together with levodopa has been linked with increased mortality and falls (Ben-Shlomo *et al.*, 1998). Selegiline might be useful for HIV-associated cognitive decline (Sacktor *et al.*, 2000).

Atomoxetine

Atomoxetine is a novel treatment for ADHD (British Medical Association, Royal Pharmaceutical Society, 2004) that acts as a noradrenaline reuptake inhibitor to indirectly enhance cortical dopamine levels. It is generally well tolerated in children and adults. Abuse potential has not been reported, and monkeys do not reliably self-administer the drug, unlike methylphenidate (Wee and Woolverton, 2004). Reboxetine is a similar agent that is licensed for depression (British Medical Association, Royal Pharmaceutical Society, 2004).

Antidepressants and Anxiolytics

Treatment with selective serotonin-reuptake inhibitors (SSRIs) has been linked with performance enhancement, with vigilance impairment, and with no effect on cognition (Hasbroucq *et al.*, 1997; Riedel *et al.*, 2005; Siepmann *et al.*, 2003). These discrepancies may be explained by differing SSRI actions on neurotransmitters other than serotonin (5HT). For example, sertraline, which has additional dopaminergic activity, causes no vigilance impairment, in contrast to citalopram, which has the greatest serotonergic activity (Riedel *et al.*, 2005). These drugs and similar agents that work additionally or exclusively via noradrenaline may also enhance mood-congruent memory recall (Harmer *et al.*, 2004) Reports from animal studies that 5HT3 antagonists, such as ondansetron, might enhance cognition have not been validated in humans (Broocks *et al.*, 1998).

In people with schizophrenia, agents like tandospirone that activate 5HT1A receptors are linked with improved memory (Sumiyoshi *et al.*, 2001). However, the fact that 5HT1A binding releases dopamine in the prefrontal cortex has led some authors to suggest that 5HT1A-binding drugs, including atypical antipsychotics, act to enhance cognition via dopaminergic mechanisms (Bantick *et al.*, 2001), particularly the latest agents, aripiprazole, a dopamine partial agonist, and ziprasidone, a D2 antagonist.

Other Noradrenergic Agents

Brain adrenoreceptors are implicated in arousal and attention, and the impact these have on sensory processing and memory, especially emotional and working memory (Middleton *et al.*, 1999; Berridge and Waterhouse, 2003). Thus, α_2-receptor agonists (eg clonidine, guanfacine) improve, whereas α_1-agonists impair, working memory, perhaps in a similar fashion to high noradrenergic states like stress. Further, α_1-agonists and β-receptor antagonists impair formation of emotional memory, particularly during memory review, which has led to the hope of using agents such as β-blockers for selective forgetting of traumatic memories.

5.5.6 Other Stimulant Pathways

Modafinil

Modafinil is a novel wakefulness-promoting agent of unknown mechanism. It is licensed in the UK to treat excessive daytime sleepiness associated with narcolepsy, sleep apnoea, and other conditions such as shift work (British Medical Association, Royal Pharmaceutical Society, 2004), and has good reported tolerability. Anecdotal reports suggest off-label use of the agent by students, pilots and military personnel, among others. Small studies suggest that modafinil has benefits for ADHD in children (Rugino and Samstock, 2003) and adults (Turner *et al.*, 2004a), and in schizophrenia ((Turner *et al.*, 2004b). Most reports (Turner *et al.*, 2003b; Wesensten *et al.*, 2002), but not all (Randall *et al.*, 2003) suggest that modafinil moderately enhances cognition in healthy volunteers, in addition to effects on alertness. Various lines of evidence suggest low potential for abuse (Myrick *et al.*, 2004). Adrafinil is a little-studied related compound.

5.5.7 Cerebral Metabolism and Blood Flow

Modern brain-imaging techniques (Chapter 9, Neuroimaging) demonstrate that conscious effort is underpinned by increases in cerebral metabolism and blood flow. Vasodilator agents like naftidrofuryl have been proposed to enhance cognition. Vascular dementia was thought to be the main condition that might respond to cerebral vasodilators, but impaired blood flow may occur in other disorders. Several other cognition enhancers have at least partial actions on these diffuse processes, including phosphodiesterase inhibitors and calcium-channel blockers. Other agents include the pyrrolidinones (racetams), ergot alkaloids, and vinpocetine, although these have additional mechanisms.

Naftidrofuryl

Naftidrofuryl is licensed in the UK as a peripheral vasodilator (British Medical Association, Royal Pharmaceutical Society, 2004), and is prescribed for dementia in several other countries. Even as an oral medication, side-effects, including hepatitis and liver failure, may limit its use. A Cochrane review of its use for cognition enhancement is planned (Smith *et al.*, 2005).

Pyrrolidinones

Many pyrrolidinone derivatives are available worldwide, including piracetam, oxiracetam, aniracetam, nefiracetam and levetiracetam. Piracetam was the first reported nootropic agent. Since then, racetams have been studied in and used for several disorders, including dementia, post-concussion syndrome, post-surgical neuroprotection, alcohol-related cognitive impairment, and dyslexia. Piracetam is currently prescribed in several European countries for cognitive impairment, including dementia, and is approved in the UK for adjunctive treatment of myoclonus (British Medical Association, Royal Pharmaceutical Society, 2004). Levetiracetam has recently been approved in the UK for adjunctive treatment of partial epilepsy (British Medical Association, Royal Pharmaceutical Society, 2004). Nefiracetam is in clinical trials for dementia and post-stroke treatment.

Many trials have been done of piracetam, although a Cochrane review of piracetam for dementia or cognitive impairment excluded several of these on methodological grounds (Flicker and Grimley Evans, 2005). The remainder had inconsistent results, although overall, piracetam carried around threefold odds of improvement compared with a placebo. Levetiracetam has potent anti-seizure activity so this agent may preserve cognition in people with epilepsy (Cramer *et al.*, 2003). The racetams are reported to have good tolerability.

Actions of piracetam include enhancement of brain metabolism and neuroprotection (Flicker and Grimley Evans, 2005). At higher doses, the agent may be antithrombotic. Nefiracetam binds to GABA-A, and potentiates activity at NMDA and acetylcholine nicotinic receptors, and aniracetam acts via acetylcholine and glutamate.

Ergot Derivatives

Derivatives of natural ergot alkaloids such as hydergine (co-dergocrine – a mixture of four ergoloid mesylates) and nicergoline have been used for decades in dementia and age-related cognitive impairment, as well as for arterial hypertension and insufficiency (Olin et al., 2005; Fioravanti and Flicker, 2005). Hydergine is approved in the UK as an adjunct in elderly patients with mild-to-moderate dementia (British Medical Association, Royal Pharmaceutical Society, 2004) and is licensed in the USA for idiopathic mental decline (Olin et al., 2005). Nicergoline is available in some 50 countries, but not the UK, for treatment of vascular disorders, including cerebrovascular disease (Fioravanti and Flicker, 2005).

An updated Cochrane review with a meta-analysis of 12 trials found an overall significant benefit of hydergine for dementia symptoms (Olin et al., 2005). Some inconsistencies between trials may be due to the dose and the duration of therapy. Benefit may be evident mainly for younger patients and those with vascular dementia. Some evidence exists for limited benefit in people with mild memory impairment and healthy elderly. Tolerability is generally good.

A Cochrane review of 14 trials of nicergoline found generally consistent results in its favour, although the benefits were not always statistically or clinically significant (Fioravanti and Flicker, 2005). In one trial with electroencephalogram (EEG) outcomes, nicergoline was found beneficial for both multi-infarct and Alzheimer-type dementia, and resulted in EEG indicators of enhanced vigilance and increased cognitive processing. The drug has also been found useful in elderly hypertensive patients with white-matter changes on brain scanning but no dementia (Bes et al., 1999).

Ergot alkaloids have marked effects on blood flow, which were originally thought to be the main mechanism of action.

However, more complex actions, including neurotransmitter changes, are reported (Olin et al., 2005). Nicergoline might also have antioxidant and neurotrophic actions (Fioravanti and Flicker, 2005).

Vinpocetine

Vinpocetine was synthesised from apovincamine, an alkaloid in Vinca minor. Clinical studies report selective enhancement of cerebral blood flow and metabolism, including enhanced glucose uptake, which may protect against the effects of hypoxia and ischaemia (Vas et al., 2002; Bonoczk et al., 2002). Non-clinical studies also suggest raised intracellular energy storage, neuroprotectant and anticonvulsant activity, phosphodiesterase inhibitor action and reduced platelet aggregation (Szatmari and Whitehouse, 2005).

These promising studies have not been supported by good-quality RCTs. A Cochrane review identified only three studies totalling 583 people, which showed some benefits. However, few patients were treated for more than six months, hence the conclusion that the evidence does not support clinical use (Szatmari and Whitehouse, 2005). Vinpocetine is not licensed in the UK. It is probably well tolerated.

5.5.8 Neuroprotection and Neural Growth

Several cognition enhancers are thought to work at least in part by protecting the brain from damage (Levi and Brimble, 2004), such as that due to oxidation, free radical damage or neurotoxicity. Agents that act through such mechanisms include memantine, melatonin, idebenone, cerebrolysin and potentially some endogenous neuropeptides and analogues. The secondary release of neurotrophic factors, such as NGF and BDNF, is a key action of phosphodiesterase inhibitors, among others.

Idebenone and Coenzyme Q10

Idebenone, a synthetic analogue of coenzyme Q10, is thought mainly to reduce oxidative damage, perhaps even in normal ageing. In particular, idebenone protects cell membranes and mitochondria and the latter also helps preserve energy storage (Anonymous, 2001). It also promotes release of NGF, together with other proposed actions (Zs-Nagy, 1990) including effects on monoamine turnover (Yamazaki *et al.*, 1989; Kawakami and Itoh, 1989). A Cochrane review of idebenone was planned but is withdrawn currently. Several RCTs and two open studies have been reported in various populations, including mixed disease. Most are small and of limited duration, and findings are contradictory. This agent is not licensed in the UK. Tolerability is thought to be good. Coenzyme Q10 is available as a dietary supplement but has not been studied for efficacy in humans.

Cerebrolysin

Cere (cerebrolysin) is a mixture of peptides and amino-acids derived from purified pig brain proteins. This intravenous preparation has been evaluated in various RCTs, mainly for AD, which show persistence of cognition improvement beyond the treatment period (Bae *et al.*, 2000; Ruether *et al.*, 2000, 2001; Panisset *et al.*, 2002). These appear to confirm preclinical suggestions of neurotrophic action but a systematic review is awaited (Fragoso and Dantas, 2005).

Endogenous Neuropeptides and Analogues

Numerous small proteins are found in the brain. These neuropeptides have complex and multiple actions, and may act as hormones, neurotransmitters and local messengers. A role in cognition, including neuroprotective effects, has been proposed for vasopressin, somatostatin, growth hormone, insulin-like growth factor-1, neuropeptide Y, orexins, vasoactive intestinal polypeptide, glucagon-like peptides, galanin, nociceptin/orphanin FQ, pro-opiomelanocortin derivatives, TRH (thyrotropin-releasing hormone), and others. Thus far, inconclusive clinical research has been mostly limited to studies on vasopressin and analogues (eg desmopressin). Long-term vasopressin treatment did exert a modest effect on attention in healthy elderly (Perras *et al.*, 1997), while short-term memory improvement is reported in children taking desmopressin for bedwetting (Muller *et al.*, 2001).

5.5.9 Miscellaneous Agents

The antidepressant tianeptine prevents and reverses the adverse effects of glucocorticoids and stress on dendritic changes and synaptic plasticity, brain morphology, and memory (Diamond *et al.*, 2004a; McEwen *et al.*, 2002). Although a serotonergic action was assumed, tianeptine might act to protect neurons from excessive actions of excitatory amino-acids.

The putative cognition enhancer Gerovital H3 contains procaine, a local anaesthetic related to the psychostimulant cocaine (see Chapter 6, Pharmacology and Treatments), and other ingredients that produce para-amino-benzoic acid and diethylaminoethanol in the body. One reported action is increased production of choline, though many other actions, including monoamine-oxidase inhibition, are claimed. The related dimethylaminoethanol (DMAE) is marketed as a dietary supplement.

CDP-choline (citicholine) is thought to accelerate resynthesis of membranes and suppress damaging release of free fatty acids. CDP-choline is licensed as a drug in several European countries, but not the UK. The Cochrane review of CDP-choline suggests positive effects on memory and behaviour in populations with mixed cerebral disorders, such as cerebrovascular disease (Fioravanti and Yanagi, 2005). The authors suggest that further research needs to focus on longer-term studies in populations with well-defined disorders.

6 COGNITION ENHANCERS IN DEVELOPMENT

The following overview of developmental drug leads includes drugs at clinical trial stage (www.phrma.org) and some that have shown promise in preclinical tests and animal models, although the latter information is not comprehensive due to variations between companies in their publishing practices. Findings in animal models and pre-clinical studies do not reliably translate to effects in humans, and the likelihood is that most of these agents will be abandoned due to inefficacy or intolerable side-effects. However, the approaches detailed seem likely to be pursued.

6.1 Glutamate

Many companies are developing agents that act on glutamate via NMDA and AMPA receptors. Effects are thought to encompass increased synaptic plasticity, compensation for loss of glutamate signalling in disease and normal ageing, and increased production of neurotrophic factors such as BDNF. Compounds that alter glutamate signalling are under investigation for PD, dependency and addiction, anxiety, schizophrenia, and pain.

Ampakines (eg Ampalex) and related agents potentiate the action of AMPA receptors to increase LTP. They might also be neuroprotective. Results in rodent models and in early clinical trials have been generally positive. Ampalex is currently in a phase-II clinical trial for AD and has completed phase-II studies for MCI (www.costexpharm.com). Other AMPA-targeted agents are in development (Scapecchi et al., 2004; Manetti et al., 2003). Several NMDA antagonists have been developed. CP101606 is in phase II trials for head injury and NPS1506 is in phase I trials for prevention of ischaemic damage due to head injury and stroke.

Other potential targets to influence glutamate signalling are metabotropic receptors, which act in a different manner from other glutamate receptors (van Dam et al., 2004; Singer, 2004). One concern over this and other glutamatergic targets is the possibility that excess stimulation could cause neurotoxicity, seizures or hallucinations. A large clinical trial of a potential anti-anxiety agent targeted at metabotropic glutamate receptors was halted after rodents developed seizures on the drug (Singer, 2004).

6.2 Calcium Channels

Various calcium channels are implicated in synaptic plasticity, particularly with ageing, while excessive calcium flow into neurons leads to neurotoxicity. MEM1003, which modulates calcium flow into cells, began phase I testing in healthy volunteers in 2003 (www.memorypharma.com), while final data could be available before 2008 if the drug reaches phase III testing for dementia and MCI (Hall, 2003).

6.3 Maxi-K Channels

Opening of maxi-K channels (potassium M-channels) controls the excitability of neurons due to excess calcium (Gribkoff et al., 2001). Agents that open these channels have potential for neuroprotection and treatment of epilepsy (eg retigabine). Despite promising results from phase I and II trials, BMS204352 failed to demonstrate superior efficacy over placebo in a phase III trial for acute stroke. Other agents have been identified that show promise in preclinical studies (Gribkoff et al., 2001).

6.4 CREB and Phosphodiesterase

The protein CREB responds to increasing levels of cAMP in the cell to promote events involved in LTP (Tully et al., 2003), and may act as a switch to turn newly acquired knowledge into long-term memory (Scott et al., 2002). At least two companies are working on type-4 phosphodiesterase inhibitors, which increase levels of cAMP and thus indirectly enhance the action of CREB. MEM1414 (www.memorypharma.com) has started phase I clinical trials while HT0712 (www.helicontherapeutics.com) has been extensively tested in animal models. A future target might also be the suppression or antagonism of the CREB repressor protein.

6.5 Acetylcholine

Many new compounds in development target acetylcholine. The cholinesterase inhibitor phenserine, which also may reduce toxic β-amyloid (Shaw *et al.*, 2001), is in human trials, as is the combined cholinesterase inhibitor and monoamine oxidase inhibitor ladostigil, which may have neuroprotectant, antidepressant, and cognition-enhancing properties (Weinstock *et al.*, 2003; Buccafusco *et al.*, 2003). Other approaches to increasing cholinergic neurotransmission include choline uptake enhancers (eg MKC231) and cholinergic agonists, which stimulate nicotinic and muscarinic receptors. MKC231 represents a new class of agent thought to reverse cholinergic deficits. It also offers protection against calcium-induced neurotoxicity (Akaike *et al.*, 1998). The agent showed some improvement in cognitive performance in early human trials, and is currently in phase IIb trials for AD (www.alz.org/resources/topicindex/MKC231.asp).

Several nicotinic agonists have been developed with the aim of increasing cognition-enhancing properties and reducing the side-effects of nicotine. ABT098 showed neuroprotectant and some cognitive-enhancing properties (Sullivan *et al.*, 1997; Decker *et al.*, 1997), but does not seem to have been developed further. GTS21 has shown promising results in animal models (Kem, 2000) and phase I clinical studies (Kitagawa *et al.*, 2003). Newer promising leads include TC1734, SIB1553A, and MEM3453. Another theoretical approach to increasing cholinergic transmission is the stimulation of muscarinic receptors, especially with M1 agonists, although evidence on agents such as talsaclidine (Weinrich *et al.*, 2001, 2002), xanomeline and sabcomeline suggests that this approach is not useful in humans.

6.6 Dopamine

Extensive research has led to various developmental drugs focused on altering dopaminergic neurotransmission, especially for cognition improvement in PD. Treatment of this low-dopamine state improves cognition and motor function, but also alters outcome-related learning (Frank *et al.*, 2004),

hence the importance of this neurotransmitter in drug dependence (see Chapter 6, Pharmacology and Therapeutics). The new monoamine-oxidase-B inhibitor rasagiline, which may also be neuroprotective, is in late clinical trials for AD and awaiting approval for PD (www.tevapharm.com). Another strategy involves inhibition of monoamine reuptake, for example by NS2330, an agent that increases levels of dopamine, noradrenaline and acetylcholine, which is in phase II trials for AD.

Stimulation of dopamine receptors might lead to long-term improvements in cognition, due to the phenomenon of sensitisation – an increase in sensitivity of the stimulated receptor (Castner and Goldman-Rakic, 2004). Full and partial dopamine agonists include piribedil, BP897, and ABT431 (Chapter 6, Pharmacology and Therapeutics), plus sumanirole, which is in phase II trials for PD. Drugs that rapidly enhance dopamine release may have abuse potential (see Chapter 6).

6.7 Serotonin

Binding to specific serotonin receptors might help improve cognition in neurodegenerative disease and in schizophrenia, possibly via changes in other neurotransmitters (Roth *et al.*, 2004). For example, 5HT6 antagonism can increase levels of acetylcholine, glutamate, dopamine and noradrenaline (Lacroix *et al.*, 2004). The 5HT6 antagonist SB742457 is in phase I trials for AD. Another drug, SL650155, a partial agonist at 5HT4 receptors, is in phase II trials for cognitive impairment and dementia (Bockaert *et al.*, 2004). 5HT1A agonists and 5HT2A antagonists might also impact on cognition. Xaliproden is a 5HT1A agonist that also mimics the action of NGF. It is in phase II trials for AD and neuropathy.

6.8 GABA

Several companies have agents in development that turn off GABA neurotransmission by partial inverse agonist action at the benzodiazepine receptor binding site. These agents are hoped to produce cognition-enhancing effects without adverse effects such as anxiety, eg PCALC36 (Lopes *et al.*, 2004). SB737552 (S8510) is in phase I trials for AD and vascular dementia. NS105 is a newer lead that appears to increase cholinergic neurotransmission and inhibits GABA-B receptor binding (Ogasawara *et al.*, 1999).

6.9 The Cannabinoid System

The extensive endocannabinoid system probably modulates learning by transmitting signals from post-synaptic neurons to cause presynaptic effects, such as synaptic weakening (Nicoll and Alger, 2004). Rimonabant (SR141716A) is currently under study for reduction in cravings (see Chapter 6, Pharmacology and Therapeutics) such as in smoking and to treat obseity. This and other cannabinoid-1 receptor antagonists have shown benefits in memory consolidation and might counteract the amnesic effect of β-amyloid in AD. However, the increased strength of memory formation might act as a source of interference when memory needs to change dynamically, indicating a trade-off in cognitive effects (Shiflett *et al.*, 2004). Dexanabinol, a synthetic cannabinoid, is in phase III trials for neuroprotection after traumatic injury, and phase II trials for neuroprotection during cardiac surgery. However, its main mechanism of action may be weak NMDA antagonism.

6.10 Histamine

Histamine-3 receptors inhibit release of several neurotransmitters involved in cognition. The histamine-3 antagonist A349821 increases histamine release and has shown cognition-enhancing properties in rodents (Esbenshade *et al.*, 2004).

6.11 Neurohormones and Neuropeptides

Interventions that promote or reduce activity of the multitude of hormones and peptides that act as neurotransmitters offer diverse potential strategies to enhance cognition, including receptor-binding agents, peptide releasers and synthetic peptides that mimic endogenous neuropeptide function or downstream targets. High, persistent circulating levels of glucocorticoids can impair memory functioning, so a current trial of mifepristone will determine whether antagonism of glucocorticoids can slow decline in AD (Belanoff *et al.*, 2002). Notably, inhibition of 11β-hydroxysteroid dehydrogenase with carbenoxelone improves cognition in healthy elderly and cognitively impaired people (Sandeep *et al.*, 2004).

NC1900 is an analogue of vasopressin that can enhance spatial memory, probably by acting on a specific receptor on cholinergic neurons (Mishima *et al.*, 2003). FK960 appears to enhance cerebral blood flow through release of somatostatin (Doggrell, 2004) but was not effective in humans. NAP, a peptide derived from a protein released by vasoactive intestinal polypeptide, has neuroprotectant properties (Gozes *et al.*, 2003). S17092 inhibits an enzyme that breaks down neuropeptides and showed promise in preclinical and clinical studies, but was abandoned after phase I studies (Morain *et al.*, 2002). Synthetic ligands have been developed including C3d, which binds to neural cell adhesion molecule (www.phoenixpeptide.com; Kiryushko *et al.*, 2003), and FG loop, which binds to fibroblast growth factor (FGF) receptor-1.

6.12 Other Molecular Targets

Several other strategies are under investigation, which mainly target disease processes associated with neurodegeneration. It is unclear whether any of these approaches will prove useful for cognition enhancement in other scenarios. However, those that target molecular messengers involved in cognitive processes inside neurons might prove useful in states other than neurodegeneration, such as agents acting on the protein kinase C that modulate effects of stress on working memory (Birnbaum *et al.*, 2004).

CEP1347 and AS601245 inhibit certain protein kinases – the latter neuroprotectant is in phase III trials for PD (www.cephalar.com). CPI1189 inhibits the potentially damaging immune chemical tumour necrosis factor-α and is in phase II trials for AD. One key strategy aims to mimic or enhance the activity of neurotrophic factors such as NGF, glial-cell-line-derived neurotrophic factor, and neuroimmunophilin ligands [eg GPI1485 (www.guilfordpharm. com) for PD; Mikol and Feldman, 1999]. One action of antidepressants is proposed to be neural growth due to release of neurotrophic factors like BDNF and FGF (Russo-Neustadt, 2003; Evans et al., 2004).

One example of agents that are probably selective for disease modification is in the development of several strategies to inhibit amyloid formation in AD, which depends on the breakdown of amyloid precursor protein by β- and γ-secretase enzymes. R-flurbiprofen lowers levels of β-amyloid, perhaps by altering secretase activity (Harrison et al., 2004), and is in phase II testing. This drug is of interest since it is one stereo-isomer (mirror-image) of the two found in the known drug flurbiprofen, in which R-flurbiprofen has markedly different properties from the anti-inflammatory L-flurbiprofen. Thus, any benefits of anti-inflammatory agents in dementia might at least partly be due to other mechanisms. Secretase inhibitors are under development but agents that target such ubiquitous substrates might be limited by systemic toxicity (Harrison et al., 2004b). Other agents that target β-amyloid in AD include Alzhemed, a glycosaminoglycan in phase III trials and AAB001, a monoclonal antibody in early human trials.

6.13 Genome and Stem Cells

The potential is immense for therapeutic strategies that target the genome, use cell replacement, or both (Tuszynski, 2002; Isacson, 2003; Rice and Scolding, 2004). In the next two decades, science in this area is likely to make major advances, although few successful therapies are expected given the poor success rate over the past decade or so. Two current approaches are in phase I trials of patients with AD, who are treated either with their own re-implanted skin cells engineered to carry the NGF gene, or with a virus to deliver the gene directly into the body (www.ceregene.com).

Various strategies are under study to use stem cells to replace dead neurons in neurodegenerative disease. Early clinical trials have been done for PD and traumatic brain injury, while therapy for stroke and other disorders is proven in animal models (Isacson, 2003; Björklund et al., 2003; Kelly et al., 2004; www.stemcellsinc.com). Difficulties with administration and unknown long-term effects mean that such strategies are unlikely to be employed for cognition enhancement for non-medical purposes, at least for a long time.

7 FUTURE COGNITION ENHANCERS

Several trends will impact on the future development and use of cognition enhancers.

7.1 Changes in Society

In the UK, moderately effective treatments for some neurodegenerative diseases are already available. These and other treatments are likely to impact on quality and length of life. The increased adoption of such strategies, and the development of new approaches to disease modification and cognition enhancement, will likely occur in the context of increasing longevity, which could further enhance the market for such interventions. In turn, drugs and other strategies that halt, prevent or reverse ageing processes, including cognitive impairment and age-related diseases, could perpetuate this cycle, in which a relatively healthy and wealthy elderly population seek to further lengthen lives lived in good health.

7.2 Increasing Knowledge

Scientific research is likely to continue to expand our knowledge of the mechanisms underlying cognition and their impairment in disease and normal ageing. Promising new avenues for disease-modifying drugs are being explored in the laboratory and in clinical trials. In addition, many people are conducting long-term self-experimentation by taking agents purported to be cognition enhancers. These trends will inform development of better agents and non-drug strategies that work via similar or novel mechanisms, though only modest effects are anticipated in the near future.

Comparative work may indicate an overlap between brain disorders and also with psychiatric diseases. Research on the mechanisms of disease-modifying and cognition-enhancing interventions could reveal agents that cross over for use in other conditions. For example, the MATRICS initiative to support development of drugs to treat cognitive deficits in schizophrenia (Marder and Fenton, 2004) may uncover drugs for use in other conditions, particularly those characterised by similar frontal cortical dysfunction. Strategies to screen known agents for novel properties might be similarly fruitful – recent highlights include potential effects of certain antibiotics for neuroprotection (Rothstein et al., 2005) and antiepileptics for longevity (Evason et al., 2005). Cognition enhancers for healthy people will be developed with the aim of targeting known and new substrates of normal cognition. There is also potential for interventions that act in more global ways. Possibilities include widely enhancing neural connectivity and facilitating the recruitment of other brain regions for specific functions.

Changes in pharmacological technologies, including high throughput screening for potential drug candidates, nanotechnology and rational drug design, may increase the pace and success rate of drug development. Genomic and proteomic techniques seek to identify large numbers of cellular changes in genetic 'messages' and protein products, respectively. They seem likely to provide insights into mechanisms of and variance in both pathology and drug actions (Morris and Wilson, 2004; Neuhold, 2004). Such knowledge is already starting to inform the development of biomarkers and drugs (Georganopoulou et al., 2005; Tully, 2004).

Advances in technologies to image the living brain and the combination of imaging techniques will expand our knowledge of cognitive processes, and could assist the targeting of therapies, at least in disease states (see Chapter 9, Neuroimaging). The nascent field of pharmacogenomics could allow treatments to be tailored to the genetic make-up of an individual, although an individual's future degree of cognitive impairment is likely to be much more difficult to predict (see Chapter 4, Genomics). Development of biomarkers for early brain changes in ageing and disease could allow early intervention and an emphasis on a preventative approach to cognitive decline.

7.3 Scientific Limitations

Years of research on learning and memory have not yet translated into highly effective disease-modifiers or cognition enhancers. One major impediment is the lack of good animal models and the consequent failure to translate findings in animals to efficacy in humans. Future developments seem likely to be more rapid for disease-modifying drugs than for mechanism-based cognition enhancers for healthy people. Already, transgenic animal models of AD have revealed potential pathways to new treatment strategies, although for other disorders, the genetic origins are much less clear and likely to be more complex. If similar animal models could be developed for other cognitively impairing neuropsychiatric diseases, progress could be markedly enhanced.

Strategies already exist for the rapid production and screening of transgenic animals for effects on cognition. Now robotic techniques have been developed to reduce the number of animals required and the screening times (Zhu *et al.*, 2004). Invertebrate models are an alternative strategy (Tully, 2004). In all cases, however, difficulties exist with the development of suitable tests to document the effect of gene mutations on cognition (Kas and Ree, 2004). Thus, the translation of such effects to humans remains an uncertain science. Commercial priorities mean that the extent of industry failures – compounds that enhanced learning and memory in animals but had no effect on humans, or had unacceptable side-effects – is not known, though some are reported.

In human studies, no biomarkers have yet been widely accepted even for AD, which raises the question of how to decide who should receive disease-modifying drugs. Moreover, we do not yet know how to accurately measure the full effects of drugs on cognition, nor do we know the most relevant indicators to predict desirable outcomes from therapies, such as maintaining independent living or reduced admission to nursing homes. The uncomfortable fact remains that despite huge research efforts, we do not yet know how to substantially enhance cognition in humans.

8 IMPLICATIONS

If effective cognition enhancers are developed, our capability to use them in the best way for individuals and society depends on several factors, mainly potential benefits and harms, plus ethical and social aspects of their use. The latter concepts have recently been reviewed (see Chapters 15, Ethical Aspects and 11 on Social Policy; Farah *et al.*, 2004; President's Council on Bioethics, 2003; Caplan and Elliott, 2004; Caplan, 2004). However, the social and ethical frameworks in which cognition enhancers could be used in the future will impact on

their benefits and harms, and so are briefly discussed here.

8.1 Potential Benefits and Harms

Cognition-enhancing technologies are likely to have three potential applications: disease states; MCI and normal ageing; and healthy cognition. In the cases of the first two applications, interventions may be useful for halting, preventing and reversing cognitive decline. The benefits to society of reductions in disease-related impairments and enhancements in human cognitive capabilities could potentially be enormous. Other benefits seem likely, including increased knowledge of human cognitive neuroscience and interventions that benefit other conditions.

However, for people with brain disease, treatments that halt cognitive decline and lengthen life without improving its quality might be undesirable. Likewise, the prospect of halting normal ageing and the subsequent prolongation of life, if it turns out to be possible, raises dilemmas if an individual's life is of poor quality. Impacts on health and social costs plus societal effects related to an ageing population also seem likely.

One possibility is that pharmaceutical companies will not be able to deliver effective cognition enhancers within the next 20 years (Rose, undated), while research already suggests that the effect of cognition enhancers might be unpredictable, or vary according to baseline function, genetic make-up, gender, and other variables. Some aspects of cognition may be easier to enhance than others. If increasing memory is possible but not improved selective forgetting, cognition enhancement could lead to remembering of excess clutter and would be a liability during distressing events. Trade-offs between enhancement of one function and impairment of another seem likely, and are already noted in normal brain functioning, for example, when attention on work is distracted by a need to attend to other stimuli. With cognition enhancement, one example is seen with the 'Doogie mouse' engineered to have excess NMDA receptor function, which shows increased learning ability (Tang *et al.*, 1999) but might have enhanced sensitivity to pain (Wei *et al.*, 2001).

Current key concerns over harms are restricted to short-term adverse effects, although some compounds are likely to lead to dependence and have abuse potential. Few disease-modifying drugs seem likely to have abuse potential, especially if used to enhance a neurochemical deficit, eg children with ADHD who take amphetamines. Some cognition enhancers, especially stimulant-type drugs, might show an increasing trend for abuse. Already, modafinil and other drugs are available on what is effectively a black market, and some may be abused. For people who wish to enhance cognition for non-medical purposes, the risk–benefit ratio required of a drug should be lower than that for individuals with debilitating or terminal illnesses. However, the use of putative cognition enhancers that spans decades could lead to unanticipated long-term effects. This possibility necessitates costly long-term follow-up of research participants and post-marketing surveillance.

8.2 Health Economics

If cognition enhancers are available in the future, they are likely to have substantial economic impact. The provision of disease-modifying drugs for AD alone is likely to have a marked impact on health economics. Such treatments are usually prescribed for life, and the cost of provision of such agents will depend on the source of payment and the indication. NHS treatment of dementia to restore independent living could be more cost-effective than not providing such treatments, unless this results in an increasing population of cognitively astute but physically frail elderly. The provision of disease-modifying drugs and cognition enhancers could have cost implications for Government and society in other ways: the increasing care and pension costs of an ageing society; state provision of treatments or prophylaxis for MCI and age-related deficits in otherwise healthy elderly; the regulation

of over-the-counter medications; the provision of vigilance-promoting compounds for military and other state personnel; efforts to control the black market; treatment of individuals who develop dependency; and long-term monitoring of risk with extended use. Conversely, the development and marketing of effective disease modifiers and cognition enhancers is likely to represent a large growth industry, with associated economic impact (see Chapter 13, Economics of Addiction and Drugs.)

8.3 Regulation, Ethics, and Society

In the future, our regulatory capability will either encompass the current system of licensed prescription medicines, over-the-counter medicines, nutritional supplements and herbal medicines, or develop into new systems. Such systems could vary from regulation of all psychoactive substances to total deregulation. The former case could encompass several tiers of regulatory assessments according to likely efficacy, safety, source and availability. In the latter case, the regulatory authority could assume the role of providing independent assessment of and advice on agents, including safety alerts. MCI is a good example of how the creation of a disease label can pose diagnostic, regulatory and ethical issues (Whitehouse, 2004). (See also Kas and Ree, 2004; Chapter 15, Ethical Aspects.)

The widespread use of cognition enhancers could effect changes in individuals and across society. Use of such agents for purposes beyond therapy may pose ethical issues earlier than 2025 if their use becomes expected, mandated or coercive. Until recent legislation (www.cognitiveliberty.org/pdf/ccle_un-comments04.pdf), some US schools required children with ADHD to take medications as a condition of attendance (Farah *et al.*, 2004). In the longer term, these agents could alter inequity, but it remains an open question whether they will increase or decrease inequity, or both. The focus on aspects of ourselves as commodities is much discussed. It already happens, and the question is whether we want such trends to continue. The potential use of technologies to alter cognition in children and developing embryos presents additional technical and ethical issues.

With cognition enhancement, as with other scientific advances, a common pattern is the initial glorification of novel technology followed by demonisation as overuse ensues and adverse effects are discovered. The challenge over future cognition enhancers lies in gaining the appropriate balance in terms of individual benefits and harms, social effects, commercial prospects and public opinion.

9 CONCLUSIONS

Likelihood: Current research is likely to bring in-depth understanding of the mechanisms that underlie cognition, including learning, memory and selective forgetting. The effects of neurodegeneration and other disease states may differ overall from those in normal ageing but there may be an impact on similar processes. Diagnosis of disease states such as dementia is likely to become more accurate and be possible earlier in the disease course.

Future capability: Given the increasing elderly population, cognition enhancement is likely to be increasingly required, acceptable, and desirable, for therapeutic purposes, for MCI, and for normal ageing. At the same time, the trend for healthy people to use agents for cognition enhancement for non-medical purposes seems likely to accelerate. Agents that are developed to treat neurodegenerative disorders might prove useful in other conditions, including early disease states, but will not necessarily be effective for normal ageing or for cognition enhancement in healthy people.

Future applications: Industry efforts to develop cognition enhancers are likely to experience unprecedented growth over the next 20 years. Research may focus separately on the treatment and prevention of neurodegeneration; modification of normal ageing processes; and enhancement beyond therapy. Each of these groups represents a large potential market.

Likelihood: Most societies are likely to continue to experience an increase in the number and type of putative cognition enhancers over the next 20 years. Some understanding of markers to target treatments and to predict responses seems likely to develop.

Future capability: A greater range of options is likely to be available for modifying the course of cognition-impairing disorders, and probably for age-related changes. Less likely but possible are agents with large cognition-enhancing effects for use by all age groups beyond therapy. Targeting of treatments and prediction of individual responses might become possible, at least in some scenarios.

Future applications: More research is needed to ensure that disease-modifying drugs are used to maximise benefits and minimise harms, including research on markers to guide treatment choice. The future of cognition enhancers in healthy people is uncertain but diversion and off-label use seem likely to increase. Thus, mechanisms to license or otherwise regulate cognition enhancers marketed at healthy individuals are likely to be considered.

Likelihood: Agents that enhance cognition are likely to have both beneficial and harmful effects, including trade-offs when the enhancement of one faculty results in the impairment of another. Few agents are likely to be wholly safe, even when used by healthy people, except some dietary supplements. Few agents are anticipated to have abuse potential, although a minority, particularly stimulants, may lead to problematic use.

Future capability: The early effects of disease-modifying drugs and cognition enhancers are likely to be mainly predictable from their pharmacology, although a minority of immediate or early effects will be unexpected. Ongoing use of such agents could have consequences that take many decades to appear.

Future applications: Continued, long-term assessment after regulatory approval or other release into society of agents to enhance cognition will be important to detect later effects.

Likelihood: The widespread use of disease-modifying drugs and cognition enhancers is likely to have an impact on individuals and on wider society. The effects may not be restricted to enhancement of function but may also include selective impairment of functions.

Future capability: The increasing use of cognition enhancers for non-therapeutic purposes could impact on individual and societal concepts of intellect and intelligence, personality and personhood, although this is likely to become apparent only after effective agents have been available for several decades.

Future applications: The impact of cognition enhancement depends on its application. Few issues are anticipated with the treatment of disease, whereas the effects on society of widespread use of effective cognition enhancers or memory erasers could ultimately be substantial. Such effects could include situations in which cognitive manipulation becomes expected, mandatory or even coercive. Cognition enhancement could become another means by which inequities in society are increased or decreased.

Likelihood: If current mechanisms remain, non-therapeutic cognition enhancers are likely to be regulated as drugs available by prescription from medical practitioners, or as over-the-counter preparations that are widely available. Some agents could be considered as foods, nutrients or herbal medicines.

Future capability: Current mechanisms are inadequate to regulate and control the expected expansion of cognition enhancement by healthy individuals, particularly online purchasing. Industry and the public will look to Government to develop effective regulatory and safety measures.

Future applications: Updated mechanisms are likely to be required for the most rational assessment and control of cognition enhancement. The process might differ between agents, depending on their applications, for which different risk–benefit ratios will be acceptable. However, mechanisms to control sales via the Internet seem unlikely to be fully effective. Independent safety assessment and public education (for example, on risk–benefit management) might be means by which the authorities reduce potential harms.

References

Abraham, W.C. (2003) How long will long-term potentiation last? *Phil Trans R Soc Lond B* 358: 735–744.

Akaike, A., Maeda, T., Kaneko, S., and Tamura, Y. (1998) Protective effect of MKC-231, a novel high affinity choline uptake enhancer, on glutamate cytotoxicity in cultured cortical neurons. *Jpn J Pharmacol* 76(2): 219–222.

Anonymous (2001) Idebenone monograph. *Altern Med Rev* 6(1): 82–86.

Anttila, T., Helkala, E.-L., Viitanen, M., *et al.* (2004) Alcohol drinking in middle age and subsequent risk of mild cognitive impairment and dementia in old age: a prospective population-based study. *BMJ* 329: 539–544. Published online 10 August.

Areosa Sastre, A. and Grimley Evans, J. (2005) Effect of the treatment of type II diabetes mellitus on the development of cognitive impairment and dementia. In: *The Cochrane Library* Issue 1. Chichester, UK: John Wiley & Sons Ltd.

Areosa Sastre, A. and Sheriff, F. (2005) Memantine for dementia (Cochrane Review). In: *The Cochrane Library* Issue 1. Chichester, UK: John Wiley & Sons Ltd.

Arnsten, A.F. (2001) Modulation of prefrontal cortical–striatal circuits: relevance to therapeutic treatments for Tourette syndrome and attention-deficit hyperactivity disorder. *Adv Neurol* 85: 333–341.

Asayama, K., Yamadera, H., Ito, T., Suzuki, H., Kudo, Y., and Endo, S. (2003) Double blind study of melatonin effects on the sleep–wake rhythm, cognitive and non-cognitive functions in Alzheimer-type dementia. *J Nippon Med Sch* 70(4): 334–341.

Bae, C.Y., Cho, C.Y., Cho, K., *et al.* (2000) A double-blind, placebo-controlled, multicenter study of cerebrolysin for Alzheimer's disease. *J Am Geriatr Soc* 48(12): 1566–1571.

Bantick, R.A., Deakin, J.F.W., and Grasby, P.M. (2001) The 5-HT1A receptor in schizophrenia: a promising target for novel atypical neuroleptics? *J Psychopharmacol* 15(1): 37–46.

Barad, M., Bourtchouladze, R., Winder, D.G., Golan, H., and Kandel, E. (1998) Rolipram, a type IV-specific phosphodiesterase inhibitor, facilitates the establishment of long-lasting long-term potentiation and improves memory. *Proc Natl Acad Sci USA* 95: 15020–15025.

Barbas, D., DesGroseillers, L., Castellucci, V.F., Carew, T.J., and Marinesco, S. (2003) Multiple serotonergic mechanisms contributing to sensitization in aplysia: evidence of diverse serotonin receptor subtypes. *Learn Mem* 10(5): 373–386.

Barnes, C.A. (2003) Long-term potentiation and the ageing brain. *Phil Trans R Soc Lond B* 358: 765–777.

Barnes, J., Anderson, L.A., and Phillipson, J.D. (2003) Herbal therapeutics: herbal interactions. *Pharmaceutical J* 270: 118–121.

Barrientos, R.M., Sprunger, D.B., Campeau, S., et al. (2003) Brain-derived neurotrophic factor mRNA downregulation produced by social isolation is blocked by intrahippocampal interleukin-1 receptor antagonist. *Neurosci* 121: 847–853.

Beglinger, L.J., Gaydos, B.L., Kareken, D.A., Tangphao-Daniels, O., Siemers, E.R., and Mohs, R.C. (2004) Neuropsychological test performance in healthy volunteers before and after donepezil administration. *J Psychopharmacol* 18(1): 102–108.

Belanoff, J.K., Jurik, J., Schatzberg, L.D., DeBattista, C., and Schatzberg, A.F. (2002) Slowing the progression of cognitive decline in Alzheimer's disease using mifepristone. *J Mol Neurosci* 19(1–2): 201–206.

Ben-Shlomo, Y., Churchyard, A., Head, J., et al. (1998) Investigation by Parkinson's Disease Research Group of United Kingdom into excess mortality seen with combined levodopa and selegiline treatment in patients with early, mild Parkinson's disease: further results of randomised trial and confidential inquiry. *BMJ* 316: 1191–1196.

Berridge, C.W. and Waterhouse, B.D. (2003) The locus coeruleus-noradrenergic system: modulation of behavioral state and state-dependent cognitive processes. *Brain Res Rev* 42: 33–84.

Bes, A., Orgogozo, J.M., Poncet, M., Rancurel, G., Weber, M., Bertholom, N., Calvez, R., and Stehle, B. (1999) A 24-month, double-blind, placebo-controlled multicentre pilot study of the efficacy and safety of nicergoline 60 mg per day in elderly hypertensive patients with leukoaraiosis. *Eur J Neurol* 6(3): 313–322.

Biederman, J. and Spencer, T.J. (2004) Psychopharmacology of adults with attention-deficit/hyperactivity disorder. *Primary Psychiatry* 11(7): 57–62.

Birks, J. and Flicker, L. (2005) Selegiline for Alzheimer's disease (Cochrane Review). In: *The Cochrane Library* Issue 1. Chichester, UK: John Wiley & Sons, Ltd.

Birks, J. and Grimley Evans, J. (2005) Ginkgo biloba for cognitive impairment and dementia (Cochrane Review). In: *The Cochrane Library* Issue 1. Chichester, UK: John Wiley & Sons, Ltd.

Birks, J.S. and Harvey, R. (2005) Donepezil for dementia due to Alzheimer's disease (Cochrane Review). In: *The Cochrane Library* Issue 1. Chichester, UK: John Wiley & Sons Ltd.

Birks, J., Grimley Evans, J., Iakovidou, V., and Tsolaki, M. (2005) Rivastigmine for Alzheimer's disease (Cochrane Review). In: *The Cochrane Library* Issue 1. Chichester, UK: John Wiley & Sons Ltd.

Birnbaum, S.G., Yuan, P.X., Wang, M., et al. (2004) Protein kinase C overactivity impairs prefrontal cortical regulation of working memory. *Science* 306: 882–884.

Björklund, A., Dunnett, S.B., Brundin, P., et al. (2003) Neural transplantation for the treatment of Parkinson's disease. *Lancet Neurol* 2(7): 437–445.

Blair, H.T., Schafe, G.E., Bauer, E.P., Rodrigues, S.M., and LeDoux, J.E. (2001) Synaptic plasticity in the lateral amygdala: a cellular hypothesis of fear conditioning. *Learn Mem* 8: 229–242.

Bockaert, J., Claeysen, S., Compan, V., and Dumuis, A. (2004) 5-HT4 receptors. *Curr Drug Targets CNS Neurol Disord* 3(1): 39–51.

Bonoczk, P., Panczel, G., and Nagy, Z. (2002) Vinpocetine increases cerebral blood flow and oxygenation in stroke patients: a near infrared spectroscopy and transcranial doppler study. *Eur J Ultrasound* 15(1–2): 85–91.

Bourtchouladze, R., Lidge, R., Catapano, R., et al. (2003) A mouse model of Rubinstein–Taybi syndrome: defective long-term memory is ameliorated by inhibitors of phosphodiesterase 4. *Proc Natl Acad Sci USA* 100: 10518–10522.

Bradshaw, K.D., Emptage, N.J., and Bliss, T.V.P. (2003) A role for dendritic protein synthesis in hippocampal late LTP. *Eur J Neurosci* 18: 3150–3152.

Bray, C.L., Cahill, K.S., Oshier, J.T., *et al.* (2004) Methylphenidate does not improve cognitive function in healthy sleep-deprived young adults. *J Investig Med* 52(3): 192–201.

British Medical Association, Royal Pharmaceutical Society of Great Britain. (2004) *British National Formulary* Issue 48. September.

Broocks, A., Little, J.T., Martin, A., *et al.* (1998) The influence of ondansetron and M-chlorophenylpiperazine on scopolamine-induced cognitive, behavioral, and physiological responses in young healthy controls. *Biol Psychiatry* 43(6): 408–416.

Buccafusco, J.J., Terry, A.V. Jr, Goren, T., and Blaugrun, E. (2003) Potential cognitive actions of (n-propargly-(3r)-aminoindan-5-yl)-ethyl, methyl carbamate (tv3326), a novel neuroprotective agent, as assessed in old rhesus monkeys in their performance of versions of a delayed matching task. *Neurosci* 119(3): 669–678.

Butefisch, C.M., Davis, B.C., Sawaki, L., *et al.* (2002) Modulation of use-dependent plasticity by D-amphetamine. *Ann Neurol* 51(1): 59–68.

Cabeza, R. (2004) Neuroscience frontiers of cognitive aging: approaches to cognitive neuroscience of aging. In: R.A. Dixon, L. Bäckman, and L.-G. Nilsson (eds), *New frontiers in cognitive aging.* Oxford: Oxford University Press.

Cabeza, R., Nyberg, L., and Park, D. (eds). (2004) *Cognitive neuroscience of aging: linking cognitive and cerebral aging.* Oxford: Oxford University Press.

Canter, P.H. and Ernst, E. (2002) Ginkgo biloba: a smart drug? A systematic review of controlled trials of the cognitive effects of ginkgo biloba extracts in healthy people. *Psychopharmacol Bull* 36(3): 108–123.

Caplan, A.L. (2004) Straining their brains: why the case against enhancement is not persuasive. *Cerebrum* 6:14–18.

Caplan, A. and Elliott, C. (2004) Is it ethical to use enhancement technologies to make us better than well? *PLoS Medicine* 1(3): 169–172.

Castner, S.A. and Goldman-Rakic, P.S. (2004) Enhancement of working memory in aged monkeys by a sensitizing regimen of dopamine D1 receptor stimulation. *J Neurosci* 24(6): 1446–1450.

Castner, S.A., Williams, G.V., and Goldman-Rakic, P.S. (2000) Reversal of antipsychotic-induced working memory deficits by short-term dopamine D1 receptor stimulation. *Science* 287: 2020–2022.

Centonze, D., Picconi, B., Gubellini, P., Bernardi, G., and Calabresi, P. (2001) Dopaminergic control of synaptic plasticity in the dorsal striatum. *Eur J Neurosci* 13: 1071–1077.

Colgin, L.L., Kubota, D., and Lynch, G. (2003) Cholinergic plasticity in the hippocampus. *Proc Natl Acad Sci USA* 100(5): 2872–2877.

Corrigan, F.M., Van Rhijn, A., and Horrobin, D.F. (1991) Essential fatty acids in Alzheimer's disease. *Ann N Y Acad Sci* 640: 250–252.

Cramer, J.A., De Rue, K., Devinsky, O., Edrich, P., and Trimble, M.R. (2003) A systematic review of the behavioral effects of levetiracetam in adults with epilepsy, cognitive disorders, or an anxiety disorder during clinical trials. *Epilepsy Behav* 4(2): 124–132.

Day, E., Bentham, P., Callaghan, R., Kuruvilla, T., and George, S. (2005) Thiamine for Wernicke–Korsakoff syndrome in people at risk from alcohol abuse (Cochrane Review). In: *The Cochrane Library* Issue 1. Chichester, UK: John Wiley & Sons Ltd.

de Smet, P.A. (2002) Herbal remedies. *N Engl J Med* 347(25): 2046–2056.

Decker, M.W., Bannon, A.W., Curzon, P., *et al.* (1997) ABT-089 [2-methyl-3-(2-(S)-pyrrolidinylmethoxy)pyridine dihydrochloride]: II. A novel cholinergic channel modulator with effects on cognitive performance in rats and monkeys. *J Pharmacol Exp Ther* 283(1): 247–258.

DeKosky, S.T. and Marek, K. (2003) Looking backward to move forward: early detection of neurodegenerative disorders. *Science* 302: 830–835.

Diamond, D.M., Park, C.R., and Woodson, J.C. (2004a) Stress generates emotional memories and retrograde amnesia by inducing an endogenous form of hippocampal LTP. *Hippocampus* 14: 281–291.

Diamond, D.M., Campbell, A., Park, C.R., and Vouimba, R.-M. (2004b) Preclinical research on stress, memory, and the brain in the development of pharmacotherapy for depression. *Eur Neuropsychopharmacol* 14(Suppl 5): S491–494.

Doggrell, S.A. (2004) The potential of activation of somatostatinergic neurotransmission with FK960 in Alzheimer's disease. *Expert Opin Investig Drugs* 13(1): 69–72.

Duffy, R., Wiseman, H., and File, S.E. (2003) Improved cognitive function in post-menopausal women after 12 weeks of consumption of a soya extract containing isoflavones. *Pharmacol Biochem Behav* 75(3): 721–779.

Elliott, R., Sahakian, B.J., Matthews, K., Bannerjea, A., Rimmer, J., and Robbins, T.W. (1997) Effects of methylphenidate on spatial working memory and planning in healthy young adults. *Psychopharmacology* 131(2): 196–206.

Erickson, K., Drevets, W., and Schulkin, J. (2003) Glucocorticoid regulation of diverse cognitive functions in normal and pathological emotional states. *Neurosci Biobehav Rev* 27: 233–246.

Esbenshade, T.A., Fox, G.B., Krueger, K.M., *et al.* (2004) Pharmacological and behavioral properties of A-349821, a selective and potent human histamine H3 receptor antagonist. *Biochem Pharmacol* 68(5): 933–945.

Evans, S.J., Choudary, P.V., Neal, C.R., *et al.* (2004) Dysregulation of the fibroblast growth factor system in major depression. *Proc Natl Acad Sci USA* 101: 15506–15511. Early online edition, 11 October, doi: 10.1073 pnas.0406788101

Evason, K., Huang, C., Yamben, I., Covey, D.F., and Kornfeld, K. (2005) Anticonvulsant medications extend worm life-span. *Science* 307: 258–262.

Evins, A.E., Fitzgerald, S.M., Wine, L., Rosselli, R., and Goff, D.C. (2000) Placebo-controlled trial of glycine added to clozapine in schizophrenia. *Am J Psychiatry* 157(5): 826–828.

Farah, M.J., Illes, J., Cook-Deegan, R., *et al.* (2004) Neurocognitive enhancement: what can we do and what should we do? *Nat Rev Neurosci* 5: 421–446.

Ferris, S. (2004) Neuropsychological correlates of brain aging and early cognitive markers of MCI and AD. *Neuropsychopharmacology* Suppl 1 (ACNP annual meeting): S7.

File, S.E., Fluck, E., and Fernandes, C. (1999) Beneficial effects of glycine (bioglycin) on memory and attention in young and middle-aged adults. *J Clin Psychopharmacol* 19(6): 506–512.

Fioravanti, M. and Flicker, L. (2005) Nicergoline for dementia and other age-associated forms of cognitive impairment (Cochrane Review). In: *The Cochrane Library* Issue 1. Chichester, UK: John Wiley & Sons, Ltd.

Fioravanti, M. and Yanagi, M. (2005) Cytidinediphosphocholine (CDP choline) for cognitive and behavioural disturbances associated with chronic cerebral disorders in the elderly (Cochrane Review). In: *The Cochrane Library* Issue 1. Chichester, UK: John Wiley & Sons Ltd.

Flicker, L. and Grimley Evans, J. (2005) Piracetam for dementia or cognitive impairment (Cochrane Review). In: *The Cochrane Library* Issue 1. Chichester, UK: John Wiley & Sons Ltd.

Forette, F., Seux, M.L., Staessen, J.A., *et al.* (1998) Prevention of dementia in randomised double-blind placebo-controlled Systolic Hypertension in Europe (Syst-Eur) Trial. *Lancet* 352: 1347–1351.

Forette, F., Seux, M.L., Staessen, J.A., *et al.* (2002) Systolic Hypertension in Europe Investigators. The prevention of dementia with antihypertensive treatment: new evidence from the Systolic Hypertension in Europe (Syst-Eur) study. *Arch Intern Med* 162(18): 2046–2052.

Fragoso, Y. and Dantas, D.C. (2005) Cerebrolysin for Alzheimer's disease (Protocol for a Cochrane Review). In: *The Cochrane Library* Issue 1. Chichester, UK: John Wiley & Sons Ltd.

Frampton, M., Harvey, R.J., and Kirchner, V. (2005) Propentofylline for dementia (Cochrane Review). In: *The Cochrane Library* Issue 1. Chichester, UK: John Wiley & Sons Ltd.

Frank, M.J., Seeberger, L.C. and O'Reilly, R.C. (2004) By carrot or by stick: cognitive reinforcement learning in Parkinsonism. *Science* 306: 1940–1943.

Georganopoulou, D.G., Chang, L., Nam, J.M., *et al.* (2005) Nanoparticle-based detection in cerebral spinal fluid of a soluble pathogenic biomarker for Alzheimer's disease. *Proc Natl Acad Sci USA* 102(7): 2273–2276. Epub 4 February.

Gill, S.S., Rochon, P.A., Herrmann, N., *et al.* (2005) Atypical antipsychotic drugs and risk of ischaemic stroke: population-based retrospective cohort study. *BMJ* 24 January. Epub ahead of print.

Gold, P.E., Cahill, L., and Wenk, G.L. (2002) Ginkgo biloba: a cognitive enhancer? *Psych Sci Public Interest* 3(1): 2–11.

Gozes, I., Divinsky, I., Pilzer, I., Fridkin, M., Brenneman, D.E., and Spier, A.D. (2003) From vasoactive intestinal peptide (VIP) through activity-dependent neuroprotective protein (ADNP) to NAP: a view of neuroprotection and cell division. *J Mol Neurosci* 20(3): 315–322.

Gribkoff, V.K., Starrett, J.E., and Dworetzky, S.I. (2001) Maxi-K potassium channels: form, function, and modulation of a class of endogenous regulators of intracellular calcium. *Neuroscientist* 7(2): 166–177.

Hall, S.S. (2003) The quest for a smart pill. *Sci Am* 289: 54–57, 60–65.

Harmer, C.J., Shelley, N.C., Cowen, P.J., and Goodwin, G.M. (2004) Increased positive versus negative affective perception and memory in healthy volunteers following selective serotonin and norepinephrine reuptake inhibition. *Am J Psychiatry* 161(7): 1256–1263.

Harrison, B.J., Olver, J.S., Norman, T.R., Burrows, G.D., Wesnes, K.A., and Nathan, P.J. (2004a) Selective effects of acute serotonin and catecholamine depletion on memory in healthy women. *J Psychopharmacol* 18(1): 32–40.

Harrison, T., Churcher, I., and Beher, D. (2004b) Gamma-secretase as a target for drug intervention in Alzheimer's disease. *Curr Opin Drug Discov Devel* 7(5): 709–719.

Hart, C.L., Haney, M., Foltin, R.W., and Fischman, M.W. (2002) Effects of the NMDA antagonist memantine on human methamphetamine discrimination. *Psychopharmacology* 164(4): 376–384. Epub 5 October.

Harvey, J.A. (2003) Role of the serotonin 5-HT(2A) receptor in learning. *Learn Mem* 10(5): 355–362.

Harvey, P.D. and Keefe, R.S. (2001) Studies of cognitive change in patients with schizophrenia following novel antipsychotic treatment. *Am J Psychiatry* 158(2): 176–184.

Harvey, P.D., Green, M.F., McGurk, S.R., and Meltzer, H.Y. (2003) Changes in cognitive functioning with risperidone and olanzapine treatment: a large-scale, double-blind, randomized study. *Psychopharmacology* 169(3-4): 404–411. Epub 18 February.

Hasbroucq, T., Rihet, P., Blin, O., and Possamai, C.A. (1997) Serotonin and human information processing: fluvoxamine can improve reaction time performance. *Neurosci Lett* 229(3): 204–208.

Heatherley, S.V., Hayward, R.C., Seers, H.E., and Rogers, P.J. (2005) Cognitive and psychomotor performance, mood, and pressor effects of caffeine after 4, 6 and 8 hours' caffeine abstinence. *Psychopharmacology* 5 February. Epub ahead of print.

Hedou, G. and Mansuy, I.M. (2003) Inducible molecular switches for the study of long-term potentiation. *Phil Trans R Soc Lond B* 358: 797–804.

Heresco-Levy, U., Ermilov, M., Shimoni, J., Shapira, B., Silipo, G., and Javitt, D.C. (2002) Placebo-controlled trial of D-cycloserine added to conventional neuroleptics, olanzapine, or risperidone in schizophrenia. *Am J Psychiatry* 159(3): 480–482.

Heresco-Levy, U., Ermilov, M., Lichtenberg, P., Bar, G., and Javitt, D.C. (2004) High-dose glycine added to olanzapine and risperidone for the treatment of schizophrenia. *Biol Psychiatry* 55(2): 165–171.

Herrmann, N., Mamdani, M., and Lanctot, K.L. (2004) Atypical antipsychotics and risk of cerebrovascular accidents. *Am J Psychiatry* 161(6): 1113–1115.

Higgins, J.P.T. and Flicker, L. (2005) Lecithin for dementia and cognitive impairment (Cochrane Review). In: *The Cochrane Library* Issue 1. Chichester, UK: John Wiley & Sons Ltd.

Hill, M.N., Froc, D.J., Fox, C.J., Gorzalka, B.B., and Christie, B.R. (2004) Prolonged cannabinoid treatment results in spatial working memory deficits and impaired long-term potentiation in the CA1 region of the hippocampus in vivo. *Eur J Neurosci* 20: 859–863.

Hogan, D.B., Goldlist, B., Naglie, G., and Patterson, C. (2004) Comparison studies of cholinesterase inhibitors for Alzheimer's disease. *Lancet Neurol* 3: 622–626.

Hogervorst, E., Yaffe, K., Richards, M., and Huppert, F. (2005a) Hormone replacement therapy to maintain cognitive function in women with dementia. In: *The Cochrane Library* Issue 1. Chichester, UK: John Wiley & Sons Ltd.

Hogervorst, E., Yaffe, K., Richards, M., and Huppert, F. (2005b) Hormone replacement therapy for cognitive function in postmenopausal women. In: *The Cochrane Library* Issue 1. Chichester, UK: John Wiley & Sons Ltd.

Howes, M.-J.R. and Houghton, P. (2003) Plants used in Chinese and Indian traditional medicine for improvement of memory and cognitive function. *Pharm Biochem Behav* 75: 513–527.

Hudson, S. and Tabet, N. (2005) Acetyl-L-carnitine for dementia (Cochrane Review). In: *The Cochrane Library* Issue 1. Chichester, UK: John Wiley & Sons Ltd.

Huppert, F.A. and Van Niekerk, J.K. (2005) Dehydroepiandrosterone (DHEA) supplementation for cognitive function (Cochrane Review). In: *The Cochrane Library* Issue 1. Chichester, UK: John Wiley & Sons Ltd.

Isacson, O. (2003) The production and use of cells as therapeutic agents in neurodegenerative diseases. *Lancet Neurol* 2(7): 417–424.

Jones, L.B. (2004) Loss of spines and neuropil. In: J. Smythies (ed.) Disorders of synaptic plasticity and schizophrenia. *Int Rev Neurobiol* 59: 1–18.

Jones, R.W., Wesnes, K.A., and Kirby, J. (1991) Effects of NMDA modulation in scopolamine dementia. *Ann N Y Acad Sci* 640: 241–244.

Jones, G.M., Sahakian, B.J., Levy, R., Warburton, D.M., and Gray, J.A. (1992) Effects of acute subcutaneous nicotine on attention, information processing and short-term memory in Alzheimer's disease. *Psychopharmacology* 108(4): 485–494.

Jones, R., Laake, K., and Oeksengaard, A.R. (2005) D-cycloserine for Alzheimer's disease (Cochrane Review). In: *The Cochrane Library* Issue 1. Chichester, UK: John Wiley & Sons Ltd.

Josselyn, S.A,. Shi, C., Carlezon, W.A., Neve, R.L., Nestler, E.J., and Davis, M. (2001) Long-term memory is facilitated by cAMP response element-binding protein overexpression in the amygdala. *J Neurosci* 21(7): 2404–2412.

Kalueff, A. and Nutt, D.J. (1996/7) Role of GABA in memory and anxiety. *Depression Anxiety* 4: 100–110.

Kas, M.J.H. and Ree, J.M.V. (2004) Dissecting complex behaviours in the post-genomic era. *Trends Neurosci* 27(7): 366–369.

Kawakami, M. and Itoh, T. (1989) Effects of idebenone on monoamine metabolites in cerebrospinal fluid of patients with cerebrovascular dementia. *Arch Gerontol Geriatr* 8(3): 343–353.

Kelly, S., Bliss, T.M., Shah, A.K., *et al.* (2004) Transplanted human fetal neural stem cells survive, migrate, and differentiate in ischemic rat cerebral cortex. *Proc Natl Acad Sci USA* 101(32): 11839–11844. Epub 27 July.

Kem, W.R. (2000) The brain alpha7 nicotinic receptor may be an important therapeutic target for the treatment of Alzheimer's disease: studies with DMXBA (GTS-21). *Behav Brain Res* 113(1–2): 169–181.

Kennedy, D.O., Scholey, A.B., and Wesnes, K.A. (2000) The dose-dependent cognitive effects of acute administration of ginkgo biloba to healthy young volunteers. *Psychopharmacology* 151(4): 416–423.

Kennedy, D.O., Scholey, A.B., and Wesnes, K.A. (2002) Modulation of cognition and mood following administration of single doses of ginkgo biloba, ginseng, and a ginkgo/ginseng combination to healthy young adults. *Physiol Behav* 75(5): 739–751.

Kennedy, D.O., Scholey, A.B., Drewery, L., Marsh, V.R., Moore, B., and Ashton, H. (2003) Electroencephalograph effects of single doses of ginkgo biloba and panax ginseng in healthy young volunteers. *Pharmacol Biochem Behav* 75: 701–709.

Kennedy, D.O., Little, W., and Scholey, A.B. (2004) Attenuation of laboratory-induced stress in humans after acute administration of *Melissa officinalis* (lemon balm). *Psychosom Med* 66: 607–613.

Kidd, P.M. (1999) A review of nutrients and botanicals in the integrative management of cognitive dysfunction. *Altern Med Rev* 4(3): 144–161.

Kimberg, D.Y., D'Esposito, M., and Farah, M.J. (1997) Effects of bromocriptine on human subjects depend on working memory capacity. *Neuroreport* 8: 3581–3585.

Kiryushko, D., Kofoed, T., Skladchikova, G., Holm, A., Berezin, V., and Bock, E. (2003) A synthetic peptide ligand of neural cell adhesion molecule (NCAM), C3d, promotes neuritogenesis and synaptogenesis and modulates presynaptic function in primary cultures of rat hippocampal neurons. *J Biol Chem* 278(14): 12325–12334. Epub 26 December 2002.

Kitagawa, H., Takenouchi, T., Azuma, R., *et al.* (2003) Safety, pharmacokinetics, and effects on cognitive function of multiple doses of GTS-21 in healthy, male volunteers. *Neuropsychopharmacology* 28(3): 542–551.

Kollins, S.H. (2003) Comparing the abuse potential of methylphenidate versus other stimulants: a review of available evidence and relevance to the ADHD patient. *J Clin Psych* 64(Suppl II): 14–18.

Kollins, S.H., MacDonald, E.K., and Rush, C.R. (2001) Assessing the abuse potential of methylphenidate in nonhuman and human subjects: a review. *Pharmacol Biochem Behav* 68: 611–627.

Kumari, V., Corr, P.J., Mulligan, O.F., Cotter, P.A., Checkley, S.A., and Gray, J.A. (1997) Effects of acute administration of D-amphetamine and haloperidol on procedural learning in man. *Psychopharmacology* 129(3): 271–276.

Kutcher, S., Aman, M., Brooks, S.J., *et al.* (2004) International Consensus Statement on Attention-Deficit/Hyperactivity Disorder (ADHD) and Disruptive Behaviour Disorders (DBDs): clinical implications and treatment practice suggestions. *Eur Neuropsychopharmacol* 14(1): 11–28.

Lacroix, L.P., Dawson, L.A., Hagan, J.J., and Heidbreder, C.A. (2004) 5-HT6 receptor antagonist SB-271046 enhances extracellular levels of monoamines in the rat medial prefrontal cortex. *Synapse* 51(2): 158–164.

Lee, H. and Birks, J. (2005) Ginkgo biloba for cognitive improvement in healthy individuals (Protocol for a Cochrane Review). In: *The Cochrane Library* Issue 1. Chichester, UK: John Wiley & Sons, Ltd.

Levi, M.S. and Brimble, M.A. (2004) A review of neuroprotective agents. *Curr Med Chem* 11(18): 2383–2397.

Lingford-Hughes, A.R., Welch, S., and Nutt, D.J.; British Association for Psychopharmacology. (2004) Evidence-based guidelines for the pharmacological management of substance misuse, addiction and comorbidity: recommendations from the British Association for Psychopharmacology. *J Psychopharmacol* 18(3): 293–335.

Lisman, J. (2003) Long-term potentiation: outstanding questions and attempted synthesis. *Phil Trans R Soc Lond B* 358: 829–842.

Liu, J., Head, E., Gharib, A.M., *et al.* (2002) Memory loss in old rats is associated with brain mitochondrial decay and RNA/DNA oxidation: partial reversal by feeding acetyl-L-carnitine and/or R-alpha-lipoic acid. *Proc Natl Acad Sci USA* 99(4): 2356–2361.

Lopes, D.V.S., Caruso, R.R.B., Castro, N.G., Costa, P.R.R., da Silva, A.J.M., and Noel, F. (2004) Characterization of a new synthetic isoflavonoid with inverse agonist activity at the central benzodiazepine receptor. *Eur J Pharmacol* 495: 87–96.

Lopez-Arrieta, J.L.A., and Birks, J. (2005) Nimodipine for primary degenerative, mixed and vascular dementia. In: *The Cochrane Library* Issue 1. Chichester, UK: John Wiley & Sons Ltd.

Lopez-Arrieta, J.L.A. and Sanz, F.J. (2005) Nicotine for Alzheimer's disease (Cochrane Review). In: *The Cochrane Library* Issue 1. Chichester, UK: John Wiley & Sons Ltd.

Luchsinger, J.A. and Mayeux, R. (2004) Dietary factors and Alzheimer's disease. *Lancet Neurol* 3: 579–587.

Luciana, M., Collins, P.F., and Depue, R.A. (1998) Opposing roles for dopamine and serotonin in the modulation of human spatial working memory functions. *Cerebral Cortex* 8: 218–226.

Lyketsos, C., Sheppard, J.M., Tschanz, J., Norton, M., Fitzpatrick, A., and Breitner, J.C. (2004) Epidemiology of depression in late life: relationship to cognitive disorders. *Neuropsychopharmacology* Suppl 1 (ACNP annual meeting): S53.

Malouf, R. and Areosa Sastre, A. (2005) Vitamin B12 for cognition (Cochrane Review). In: *The Cochrane Library* Issue 1. Chichester, UK: John Wiley & Sons Ltd.

Malouf, R. and Birks, J. (2005) Donepezil for vascular cognitive impairment (Cochrane Review). In: *The Cochrane Library* Issue 1. Chichester, UK: John Wiley & Sons Ltd.

Malouf, R. and Grimley Evans, J. (2005) Vitamin B6 for cognition (Cochrane Review). In: *The Cochrane Library* Issue 1. Chichester, UK: John Wiley & Sons Ltd.

Malouf, R., Grimley Evans, J., and Areosa Sastre, A. (2005) Folic acid with or without vitamin B12 for cognition and dementia (Cochrane Review). In: *The Cochrane Library* Issue 1. Chichester, UK: John Wiley & Sons Ltd.

Manetti, D., Martini, E., Ghelardini, C., *et al.* (2003) 4-Aminopiperidine derivatives as a new class of potent cognition enhancing drugs. *Bioorg Med Chem Lett* 13: 2303–2306.

Marder, S.R. and Fenton, W. (2004) Measurement and treatment research to improve cognition in schizophrenia: NIMH MATRICS initiative to support the development of agents for improving cognition in schizophrenia. *Schizophr Res* 72: 5–9.

Marsicano, G., Wotjak, C.T., Azad, S.C., *et al.* (2002) The endogenous cannabinoid system controls extinction of aversive memories. *Nature* 418: 530–534.

Matrenza, C., Hughes, J.M., Kemp, A.H., Wesnes, K.A., Harrison, B.J., and Nathan, P.J. (2004) Simultaneous depletion of serotonin and catecholamines impairs sustained attention in healthy female subjects without affecting learning and memory. *J Psychopharmacol* 18(1): 21–31.

McDowell, S., Whyte, J., and D'Esposito, M. (1998) Differential effect of a dopaminergic agonist on prefrontal function in traumatic brain injury patients. *Brain* 121(6): 1155–1564.

McEwen, B.S., Magarinos, A.M., and Reagan, L.P. (2002) Structural plasticity and tianeptine: cellular and molecular targets. *Eur Psychiatry* 17(Suppl 3): 318–330.

McGuiness, B., Todd, S., Passmore, P., and Bullock, R. (2005) The effects of blood pressure lowering on development of cognitive impairment and dementia in patients without apparent prior cerebrovascular disease (Protocol for a Cochrane Review). In: *The Cochrane Library* Issue 1. Chichester, UK: John Wiley & Sons Ltd.

McNaught, K.S.P. (2004) Proteolytic dysfunction in neurodegenerative disorders. In: Bradley, R.J., Harris, R.A. and Jenner, P. *Int Rev Neurobiol* 62: 95–120.

Mehta, M.A., Owen, A.M., Sahakian, B.J., Mavaddat, N., Pickard, J.D., and Robbins, T.W. (2000) Methylphenidate enhances working memory by modulating discrete frontal and parietal lobe regions in the human brain. *J Neurosci* 20: 1–6.

Mehta, M.A., Swainson, R., Ogilvie, A.D., Sahakian, J., and Robbins, T.W. (2001) Improved short-term spatial memory but impaired reversal learning following the dopamine D(2) agonist bromocriptine in human volunteers. *Psychopharmacology* 159(1): 10–20. Epub 11 September.

Meneses, A. (2003) A pharmacological analysis of an associative learning task: 5-HT(1) to 5-HT(7) receptor subtypes function on a pavlovian/instrumental autoshaped memory. *Learn Mem* 10(5): 363–372.

Middleton, H.C., Sharma, A., Agouzoul, D., Sahakian, B.J., and Robbins, T.W. (1999) Idazoxan potentiates rather than antagonizes some of the cognitive effects of clonidine. *Psychopharmacology* 145: 401–411.

Mikol, D.D. and Feldman, E.L. (1999) Neurophilins and the nervous system. *Muscle Nerve* 22: 1337–1340.

Millan, M.J., Lejeune, F., and Gobert, A. (2000) Reciprocal autoreceptor and heteroreceptor control of serotonergic, dopaminergic and noradrenergic transmission in the frontal cortex: relevance to the actions of

antidepressant agents. *J Psychopharmacol* 14(2): 114–138.

Min, S.K., Moon, I.W., Ko, R.W., and Shin, H.S. (2001) Effects of transdermal nicotine on attention and memory in healthy elderly nonsmokers. *Psychopharmacology* 159(1): 83–88. Epub 15 September.

Mishima, K., Tsukikawa, H., Miura, I., *et al.* (2003) Ameliorative effect of NC-1900, a new AVP4-9 analog, through vasopressin V1a receptor on scopolamine-induced impairments of spatial memory in the eight-arm radial maze. *Neuropharmacology* 44(4): 541–552.

Morain, P., Lestage, P., De Nanteuil, G., *et al.* (2002) S 17092: a prolyl endopeptidase inhibitor as a potential therapeutic drug for memory impairment. Preclinical and clinical studies. *CNS Drug Rev* 8(1): 31–52.

Morris, C.M. and Wilson, K.E. (2004) High-throughput approaches in neuroscience. *Int J Devl Neuroscience* 22: 515–522.

Mozley, L.H., Gur, R.C., Mozley, P.D., and Gur, R.E. (2001) Striatal dopamine transporters and cognitive functioning in healthy men and women. *Am J Psychiatry* 158(9): 1492–1499.

MTA Cooperative Group (1999) A 14-month randomized clinical trial of treatment strategies for attention-deficit/hyperactivity disorder. The MTA Cooperative Group. Multimodal Treatment Study of Children with ADHD. *Arch Gen Psychiatry* 56(12): 1073–1086.

MTA Cooperative Group (2004a) National Institute of Mental Health Multimodal Treatment Study of ADHD follow-up: 24-month outcomes of treatment strategies for attention-deficit/hyperactivity disorder. *Pediatrics* 113(4): 754–761.

MTA Cooperative Group (2004b) National Institute of Mental Health Multimodal Treatment Study of ADHD follow-up: changes in effectiveness and growth after the end of treatment. *Pediatrics* 113(4): 762–769.

Muller, U., von Cramon, D.Y., and Pollmann, S. (1998) D1- versus D2-receptor modulation of visuospatial working memory in humans. *J Neurosci* 18(7): 2720–2728.

Muller, D., Florkowski, H., Chavez-Kattau, K., Carlsson, G., and Eggert, P. (2001) The effect of desmopressin on short-term memory in children with primary nocturnal enuresis. *J Urol* 166(6): 2432–2434.

Myrick, H., Malcolm, R., Taylor, B., and Larowe, S. (2004) Modafinil: preclinical,

clinical, and post-marketing surveillance: a review of abuse liability issues. *Ann Clin Psych* 16: 101–109.

National Institute for Clinical Excellence. (2000) *Guidance on the use of methylphenidate (ritalin, equasym) for attention-deficit/hyperactivity disorder in childhood.* Technology Appraisal Guidance No 13. October.

Neuhold, L.A. (ed.) (2004) Human brain proteome. *Int Rev Neurobiol* 61.

Nicoll, R.A. and Alger, B.E. (2004) The brain's own marijuana. *Sci Am* Dec: 45–51.

Ogasawara, T., Itoh, Y., Tamura, M., *et al.* (1999) Involvement of cholinergic and GABAergic systems in the reversal of memory disruption by NS-105, a cognition enhancer. *Pharmacol Biochem Behav* 64(1): 41–52.

Ohrui, T., Tomita, N., Sato-Nakagawa, T., *et al.* (2004) Effects of brain-penetrating ACE inhibitors on Alzheimer disease progression. *Neurology* 63: 1324–1325.

Okano, H., Hirano, T., and Balaban, E. (2000) Learning and memory. *Proc Natl Acad Sci USA* 97(23): 12403–12404.

Olin, J. and Schneider, L. (2005) Galantamine for dementia due to Alzheimer's disease (Cochrane Review). In: *The Cochrane Library* Issue 1. Chichester, UK: John Wiley & Sons Ltd.

Olin, J., Schneider, L., Novit, A., and Luczak, S. (2005) Hydergine for dementia (Cochrane Review). In: *The Cochrane Library* Issue 1. Chichester, UK: John Wiley & Sons, Ltd.

Ovsepian, S.V., Anwyl, R., and Rowan, M.J. (2004) Endogenous acetylcholine lowers the threshold for long-term potentiation induction in the Ca1 area through muscarinic receptor activation. In vivo study. *Eur J Neurosci* 20: 1267–1275.

Panisset, M., Gauthier, S., Moessler, H., and Windisch, M.; Cerebrolysin Study Group. (2002) Cerebrolysin in Alzheimer's disease: a randomized, double-blind, placebo-controlled trial with a neurotrophic agent. *J Neural Transm* 109(7–8): 1089–1104.

Perras, B., Droste, C., Born, J., Fehm, H.L., and Pietrowsky, R. (1997) Verbal memory after three months of intranasal vasopressin in healthy old humans. *Psychoneuroendocrinology* 22(6): 387–396.

Perry, N.S.L., Bollen, C., Perry, E.K., and Ballard, C. (2003) Salvia for dementia therapy: review of pharmacological activity and pilot tolerability clinical trial. *Pharmacol Biochem Behav* 75: 651–659.

Persson, J., Bringlov, E., Nilsson, L.G., and Nyberg, L. (2004). The memory-enhancing effects of ginseng and ginkgo biloba in healthy volunteers. *Psychopharmacology* 172(4): 430–434. Epub 25 Nov (2003).

Popik, P., Wrobel, M., Rygula, R., Bisaga, A., and Bespalov, A.Y. (2003) Effects of memantine, an NMDA receptor antagonist, on place preference conditioned with drug and non-drug reinforcers in mice. *Behav Pharmacol* 14(3): 237–244.

President's Council on Bioethics. (2003) Beyond therapy: biotechnology and the pursuit of happiness. Washington, DC. October. www.bioethics.gov/reports/beyondtherapy/index.html

Prickaerts, J., Koopmans, G., Blokland, A., and Schoepens, A. (2004) Learning and adult neurogenesis: survival with or without proliferation. *Neurobiol Learn Mem* 81: 1–11.

Rampon, C., Jiang, C.H., Dong, H., *et al.* (2000) Effects of environmental enrichment on gene expression in the brain. *Proc Natl Acad Sci USA* 97(23): 12880–12884.

Randall, D.C., Shneerson, J.M., Plaha, K.K., and File, S.E. (2003) Modafinil affects mood, but not cognitive function, in healthy young volunteers. *Hum Psychopharmacol* 18(3): 163–73.

Rice, C.M. and Scolding, N.J. (2004) Adult stem cells-reprogramming neurological repair? *Lancet* 364(9429): 193–199.

Riedel, W.J., Eikmans, K., Heldens, A., and Schmitt, J.A.J. (2005) Specific serotonergic reuptake inhibition impairs vigilance performance acutely and after subchronic treatment. *J Psychopharmacol* 19: 12–20.

Robertson, E.D. and Sweatt, J.D. (1999) A biochemical blueprint for long-term memory. *Learn Mem* 6: 381–388.

Rodriguez-Martin, J.L., Qizilbash, N., and Lopez-Arrieta, J.M. (2005) Thiamine for Alzheimer's disease (Cochrane Review). In: *The Cochrane Library* Issue 1. Chichester, UK: John Wiley & Sons Ltd.

Rogers, P.J., Martin, J., Smith, C., Heatherley, S.V., and Smit, H.J. (2003) Absence of reinforcing, mood and psychomotor performance effects of caffeine in habitual non-consumers of caffeine. *Psychopharmacology* 167(1): 54–62.

Roozendaal, B. (2002) Stress and memory: opposing effects of glucocorticoids on memory consolidation and memory retrieval. *Neurobiol Learn Mem* 78: 578–595.

Rose, S. No way to treat the mind. http://nootropics.com/sceptic/

Roth, B.L., Hanizavareh, S.M., and Blum, A.E. (2004) Serotonin receptors represent highly favorable molecular targets for cognitive enhancement in schizophrenia and other disorders. *Psychopharmacology* 174(1): 17–24. Epub 2 December (2003).

Rothstein, J.D., Patel, S., Regan, M.R., *et al.* (2005) β-Lactam antibiotics offer neuroprotection by increasing glutamate transporter expression. *Nature* 433: 73–77.

Ruether, E., Husmann, R., Kinzler, E., *et al.* (2001) A 28-week, double-blind, placebo-controlled study with cerebrolysin in patients with mild to moderate Alzheimer's disease. *Int Clin Psychopharmacol* 16(5): 253–263.

Ruether, E., Ritter, R., Apecechea, M., Freytag, S., Gmeinbauer, R., and Windisch, M. (2000) Sustained improvements in patients with dementia of Alzheimer's type (DAT) 6 months after termination of cerebrolysin therapy. *J Neural Transm* 107(7): 815–829.

Rugino, T.A. and Samstock, T.C. (2003) Modafinil in children with attention-deficit hyperactivity disorder. *Pediatr Neurol* 29(2): 136–142.

Rusak-Maguire, A. and Forbes, D. (2005) Melatonin for cognitive impairment (Protocol for a Cochrane Review). In: *The Cochrane Library* Issue 1. Chichester, UK: John Wiley & Sons, Ltd.

Russo-Neustadt, A. (2003) Brain-derived neurotrophic factor, behavior, and new directions for the treatment of mental disorders. *Semin Clin Neuropsychiatry* 8(2): 109–118.

Sacktor, N., Schifitto, G., McDermott, M.P., Marder, K., McArthur, J.C., and Kieburtz, K. (2000) Transdermal selegiline in HIV-associated cognitive impairment: pilot, placebo-controlled study. *Neurology* 54(1): 233–235.

Sahakian, B., Jones, G., Levy, R., Gray, J., and Warburton, D. (1989) The effects of nicotine on attention, information processing, and short-term memory in patients with dementia of the Alzheimer type. *Br J Psychiatry* 154: 797–800.

Sandeep, T.C., Yau, J.L.W., MacLullich, A.M.H., *et al.* (2004) 11β-Hydroxysteroid dehydrogenase inhibition improves cognitive function in healthy elderly men and type 2 diabetics. *Proc Natl Acad Sci USA* 101(17): 6734–6739.

Sauer, J., Tabet, N., and Howard, R. (2005) Alpha lipoic acid for dementia (Cochrane Review). In: *The Cochrane Library* Issue 1. Chichester, UK: John Wiley & Sons Ltd.

Scapecchi, S., Martini, E., Manetti, D., *et al.* (2004) Structure-activity relationship studies on unifiram (DM232) and sunifiram (DM235), two novel and potent cognition enhancing drugs. *Bioorg Med Chem* 12(1): 71–85.

Schugens, M.M., Egerter, R., Daum, I., Schepelmann, K., Klockgether, T., and Loschmann, P.A. (1997) The NMDA antagonist memantine impairs classical eyeblink conditioning in humans. *Neurosci Lett* 224(1): 57–60.

Scott, H.D. and Laake, K. (2005) Statins for the prevention of Alzheimer's disease (Cochrane Review). In: *The Cochrane Library* Issue 1. Chichester, UK: John Wiley & Sons Ltd.

Scott, R., Bourtchouladze, R., Gossweiler, S., Dubnau, J., and Tully, T. (2002) CREB and the discovery of cognitive enhancers. *J Mol Neurosci* 19: 171–177.

Shaw, K.T.Y., Utsuki, T., Rogers, J., *et al.* (2001) Phenserine regulates translation of β-amyloid precursor protein mrna by a putative interleukin-1 responsive element: a target for drug development. *Proc Natl Acad Sci USA* 98(13): 7605–7610.

Shepherd, J., Blauw, G.J., Murphy, M.B., *et al.* On behalf of the PROSPER study group. (2002) Pravastatin in elderly individuals at risk of vascular disease (PROSPER): a randomised controlled trial. *Lancet* 360: 1623–1630.

Shiflett, M.W., Rankin, A.Z., Tomaszycki, M.L., and DeVoogd, T.J. (2004) Cannabinoid inhibition improves memory in food-storing birds, but with a cost. *Proc R Soc Lond B Biol Sci* 271(1552): 2043–2048.

Shumaker, S.A., Legault, C., Rapp, S.R., *et al.* (2003) WHIMS investigators. Estrogen plus progestin and the incidence of dementia and mild cognitive impairment in postmenopausal women: The Women's Health Initiative Memory Study: a randomized controlled trial. *JAMA* 289(20): 2651–2662.

Siepmann, M., Grossmann, J., Muck-Weymann, M., and Kirch, W. (2003) Effects of sertraline on autonomic and cognitive functions in healthy volunteers. *Psychopharmacology* 168(3): 293–298. Epub 12 April.

Silva, A.J. (2003) Molecular and cellular cognitive studies of the role of synaptic plasticity. *Memory J Neurobiol* 54: 224–237.

Singer, E. (2004) The master switch. *New Scientist* Mar 6: 35–37.

Smith, A.P., Clark, R., Nutt, D.J., Haller, J., Hayward, S., and Perry, K. (1999) Antioxidant vitamins and mental performance of the elderly. *Human Psychopharmacology* 14: 459–471.

Smith, A., Brice, C., Nash, J., Rich, N., and Nutt, D.J. (2003) Caffeine and central noradrenaline: effects on mood, cognitive performance, eye movements and cardiovascular function. *J Psychopharmacol* 17(3): 283–292.

Smith, P., Loy, C., and Wong, M. (2005) Naftidrofuryl for cognitive impairment (Protocol for a Cochrane Review). In: *The Cochrane Library* Issue 1. Chichester, UK: John Wiley & Sons, Ltd.

Soetens, E., Casaer, S., D'Hooge, R., and Hueting, J.E. (1995) Effect of amphetamine on long-term retention of verbal material. *Psychopharmacology* 119(2): 155–162.

Sparks, D.L., Connor, D.J., Browne, P.J., Lopez, J.E., and Sabbagh, M.N. (2002) HMG-CoA reductase inhibitors (statins) in the treatment of Alzheimer's disease and why it would be ill-advised to use one that crosses the blood-brain barrier. *J Nutr Health Aging* 6(5): 324–331.

Sullivan, J.P., Donnelly-Roberts, D., Briggs, C.A., *et al.* (1997) ABT-089 [2-methyl-3-(2-(S)-pyrrolidinylmethoxy)pyridine]: I. A potent and selective cholinergic channel modulator with neuroprotective properties. *J Pharmacol Exp Ther* 283(1): 235–246.

Sumiyoshi, T., Matsui, M., Yamashita, I., *et al.* (2001) The effect of tandospirone, a serotonin(1a) agonist, on memory function in schizophrenia. *Biol Psychiatry* 49(10): 861–868.

Szatmari, S.Z. and Whitehouse, P.J. (2005) Vinpocetine for cognitive impairment and dementia (Cochrane Review). In: *The Cochrane Library* Issue 1. Chichester, UK: John Wiley & Sons Ltd.

Tabet, N., Birks, J., Grimley Evans, J., Orrel, M., and Spector, A. (2005) Vitamin E for Alzheimer's disease (Cochrane Review). In: *The Cochrane Library* Issue 1. Chichester, UK: John Wiley & Sons Ltd.

Tang, Y.P., Shimizu, E., Dube, G.R., *et al.* (1999) Genetic enhancement of learning and memory in mice. *Nature* 401(6748): 63–69.

Tariot, P.N., Farlow, M.R., Grossberg, G.T., Graham, S.M., McDonald, S., and Gergel, I.; Memantine Study Group. (2004) Memantine treatment in patients with moderate to severe Alzheimer disease already receiving donepezil: a randomized controlled trial. *JAMA* 291(3): 317–324.

Toescu, E.C., Verkhratsky, A., and Landfield, P.W. (2004) Ca^{2+} regulation and gene expression in normal brain aging. *Trends Neurosci* 27(10): 614–620.

Tsai, G.E., Falk, W.E., Gunther, J., and Coyle, J.T. (1999a) Improved cognition in Alzheimer's disease with short-term D-cycloserine treatment. *Am J Psychiatry* 156(3): 467–469.

Tsai, G.E., Yang, P., Chung, L.-C., Tsai, I.-C., Tsai, C.-W., and Coyle, J.T. (1999b) D-serine added to clozapine for the treatment of schizophrenia. *Am J Psychiatry* 156: 1822–1825.

Tsai, G., Lane, H.Y., Yang, P., Chong, M.Y., and Lange, N. (2004) Glycine transporter I inhibitor, N-methylglycine (sarcosine), added to antipsychotics for the treatment of schizophrenia. *Biol Psychiatry* 55(5): 452–456.

Tucha, O. and Lange, K.W. (2004) Effects of nicotine chewing gum on a real-life motor task: a kinematic analysis of handwriting movements in smokers and non-smokers. *Psychopharmacology* 173(1–2): 49–56. Epub 11 December 2003.

Tully, T. (2004) From genes to drugs for cognitive dysfunction. *Neuropsychopharmacology* Suppl 1 (ACNP annual meeting): S33–34.

Tully, T., Bourtchouladze, R., Scott, R., and Tallman, J. (2003) Targeting the CREB pathway for memory enhancers. *Nat Rev Drug Discovery* 2: 267–277.

Turner, D.C., Robbins, T.W., Clark, L., Aron, A.R., Dowson, J., and Sahakian, B.J. (2003a) Relative lack of cognitive effects of methylphenidate in elderly male volunteers. *Psychopharmacology* 168(4): 455–464. Epub 7 May.

Turner, D.C., Robbins, T.W., Clark, L., Aron, A.R., Dowson, J., and Sahakian, B.J. (2003b) Cognitive enhancing effects of modafinil in healthy volunteers. *Psychopharmacology* 165(3): 260–269. Epub 1 November 2002.

Turner, D.C., Clark, L., Dowson, J., Robbins, T.W., and Sahakian, B.J. (2004a) Modafinil improves cognition and response inhibition in adult attention-deficit/hyperactivity disorder. *Biol Psychiatry* 55(10): 1031–1040.

Turner, D.C., Clark, L., Pomarol-Clotet, E., McKenna, P., Robbins, T.W., and Sahakian, B.J. (2004b) Modafinil improves cognition and attentional set shifting in patients with chronic schizophrenia. *Neuropsychopharmacology* 29(7): 1363–1373.

Tuszynski, M.H. (2002) Growth-factor gene therapy for neurodegenerative disorders. *Lancet Neurol* 1(1): 51–57.

van Dam, E.J.M., Kamal, A., Artola, A., de Graan, P.N.E., Gispen, W.H., and Ramakers, G.M.J. (2004) Group I metabotropic glutamate receptors regulate the frequency-response function of hippocampal Ca1 synapses for the induction of LTP and LTD. *Eur J Neurosci* 19: 112–118.

Vas, A., Gulyas, B., Szabo, Z., *et al.* (2002) Clinical and non-clinical investigations using positron emission tomography, near infrared spectroscopy and transcranial doppler methods on the neuroprotective drug vinpocetine: a summary of evidences. *J Neurol Sci* 203–204: 259–262.

Verghese, J., Lipton, R.B., Katz, M.J., *et al.* (2003) Leisure activities and the risk of dementia in the elderly. *N Engl J Med* 348: 2508–2516.

Vitolo, O.V., Sant'Angelo, A., Costanzo, V., Battaglia, F., Arancio, O., and Shelanski, M. (2002) Amyloid beta-peptide inhibition of the pka/creb pathway and long-term potentiation: reversibility by drugs that enhance cAMP signaling. *Proc Natl Acad Sci USA* 99(20): 13217–13221. Epub 20 September.

Vohora, D.S. and Mishra, L.C. (2004) Alzheimer's disease. In: Mishra, L.C. (ed.). *Scientific basis for ayurvedic therapies*. Florida: CRC Press.

Volkow, N.D. and Swanson, J.M. (2003) Variables that affect the clinical use and abuse of methylphenidate in the treatment of ADHD. *Am J Psychiatry* 160(11): 1909–1918.

Volkow, N.D., Gur, R.C., Wang, G.-J., *et al.* (1998) Association between decline in brain dopamine activity with age and cognitive and motor impairment in healthy individuals. *Am J Psychiatry* 155: 344–349.

Walker, M.P. and Stickgold, R. (2004) Sleep-dependent learning and memory consolidation. *Neuron* 44: 121–233.

Wee, S. and Woolverton, W.L. (2004) Evaluation of the reinforcing effects of atomoxetine in monkeys: comparison to methylphenidate and desipramine. *Drug Alcohol Depend* 75(3): 271–276.

Wei, F., Wang, G.D., Kerchner, G.A., *et al.* (2001) Genetic enhancement of inflammatory pain by forebrain NR2B overexpression. *Nat Neurosci* 4(2): 164–169.

Weinrich, M., Ceci, A., Ensinger, H.A., *et al.* (2002) Talsaclidine (WAL 2014 FU), a muscarinic M1 receptor agonist for the treatment of Alzheimer's disease. *Drug Dev Res* 56: 321–334.

Weinstock, M., Gorodetsky, E., Poltyrev, T., Gross, A., Sagi, Y., and Youdim, M. (2003) A novel cholinesterase and brain-selective monoamine oxidase inhibitor for the treatment of dementia comorbid with depression and Parkinson's disease. *Prog Neuropsychopharmacol Biol Psychiatry* 27(4): 555–561.

Wesensten, N.J., Belenky, G., Kautz, M.A., Thorne, D.R., Reichardt, R.M., and Balkin, T.J. (2002) Maintaining alertness and performance during sleep deprivation: modafinil versus caffeine. *Psychopharmacology* 159(3): 238–247. Epub 19 October 2001.

Wesnes, K.A., Ward, T., McGinty, A., and Petrini, O. (2000) The memory enhancing effects of a Ginkgo biloba/Panax ginseng combination in healthy middle-aged volunteers. *Psychopharmacology* 152(4): 353–361.

White, H.K. and Levin, E.D. (1999) Four-week nicotine skin patch treatment effects on cognitive performance in Alzheimer's disease. *Psychopharmacology* 143(2): 158–165.

White, H.K. and Levin, E.D. (2004) Chronic transdermal nicotine patch treatment effects on cognitive performance in age-associated memory impairment. *Psychopharmacology* 171(4): 465–471. Epub 8 October 2003.

Whitehouse, P.J. (2004) Regulatory aspects of mild cognitive impairment: towards a harmonized perspective. *Dialogues Clin Neurosci* 6(4): 409–414.

Wienrich, M., Meier, D., Ensinger, H.A., *et al.* (2001) Pharmacodynamic profile of the M1 agonist talsaclidine in animals and man. *Life Sci* 68(22–23): 2593–2600.

Wild, R., Pettit, T. and Burns, A. (2005) Cholinesterase inhibitors for dementia with Lewy bodies (Cochrane Review). In: *The Cochrane Library* Issue 1. Chichester, UK: John Wiley & Sons Ltd.

Wilens, T.E. (2001) Attention-deficit/hyperactivity disorder and the substance use disorders: the nature of the relationship, who is at risk, and treatment issues. *Primary Psychiatry* 11(7): 63–70.

Woodson, J.C., Macintosh, D., Fleshner, M., and Diamond, D.M. (2003) Emotion-induced amnesia in rats: working memory-specific impairment, corticosterone-memory correlation, and fear versus arousal effects on memory. *Learn Mem* 10: 326–336.

Wu, W.W., Oh, M.M., and Disterhoft, J.F. (2002) Age-related biophysical alterations of hippocampal pyramidal neurons: implications for learning and memory. *Ageing Res Rev* 1: 181–207.

Yaffe, K., Barnes, D., Nevitt, M., Lui, L.Y., and Covinsky, K. (2001) A prospective study of physical activity and cognitive decline in elderly women: women who walk. *Ann Int Med* 161(14): 703–708.

Yamazaki, N., Nomura, M., Nagaoka, A. and Nagawa, Y. (1989) Idebenone improves learning and memory impairment induced by cholinergic or serotonergic dysfunction in rats. *Arch Gerontol Geriatr* 8(3): 225–239.

Yesavage, J.A., Mumenthaler, M.S., Taylor, J.L., *et al.* (2002) Donepezil and flight simulator performance: effects on retention of complex skills. *Neurology* 59(1): 123–125.

Zhdanova, I.V., Wurtman, R.J., Regan, M.M., Taylor, J.A., Shi, J.P., and Leclair, O.U. (2001) Melatonin treatment for age-related insomnia. *J Clin Endocrinol Metab* 86(10): 4727–4730.

Zhu, Y., Kissinger, P.T., and Kissinger, C.B. (2004) Improving laboratory animal studies using robotics. *Pharmaceutical Discovery* 4(9): 34–41.

Zs-Nagy, I. (1990) Chemistry, toxicology, pharmacology and pharmacokinetics of idebenone: a review. *Arch Gerontol Geriatr* 11(3): 177–186.

Websites of Interest

No recommendation is given on the reliability of websites or the accuracy of their content.

www.acnp.org/
www.bap.org.uk/
www.bio.com/
www.ceri.com/index.shtml
www.drugdevelopment-technology.com/
www.erowid.org/smarts/smarts.shtml
www.jefallbright.net/taxonomy/page/or/191
www.leaddiscovery.co.uk/
www.nootropics.com/refs/index.html
www.pharmcast.com/
www.smart-publications.com/articles/articles.html

9

Neuroimaging

Hugh Garavan, Anne Lingford-Hughes, Terry Jones, Peter Morris,
John Rothwell and Steve Williams

1 EXECUTIVE SUMMARY

Functional neuroimaging techniques, particularly functional magnetic resonance imaging (fMRI), positron emission tomography (PET) and single photon emission tomography (SPET) are well suited to the study of drug addiction, including the mechanisms involved in its effects on the brain. These techniques have contributed much in the last decade or so to our understanding of this most challenging of social issues. But research effort in this area is not commensurate to the importance of the problem.

This report reviews the application of neuroimaging to the study of drug addiction, beginning with the defining pharmacology and studies of craving before considering the more cognitive aspects. The availability of small imaging systems, particularly for magnetic resonance imaging (MRI), but also increasingly for PET and SPET, and in a few cases for combined MRI/PET, enables non-invasive methodologies to be applied to animal models, examples of which are given in Section 4. The development of PET as a molecular imaging tool is considered in Section 5, and future developments in MRI, fMRI and their sister technique, magnetic resonance spectroscopy (MRS), in Section 6. Although not itself an imaging technique, transcranial magnetic stimulation (TMS) is increasingly being used in conjunction with neuroimaging techniques to explore the effects of inhibiting and modulating neural circuits. This approach is described in Section 7.

Although the vast majority of neuroimaging studies are based on fMRI, PET and SPET, these techniques lack temporal resolution. Where this is key, they are often supplemented by electroencephalography (EEG) or magnetoencephalography (MEG). A brief discussion of these is included in the final section.

2 FUNCTIONAL NEUROIMAGING IN THE STUDY OF DRUG ADDICTION: DEFINING PHARMACOLOGY AND CRAVING

2.1 Introduction

The use of functional neuroimaging in the field of substance misuse has grown considerably over the past decade, as understanding the neurobiology of addiction has become more of a clinical priority. There has been increased acceptance and development of drug treatments for addiction. In parallel an increasing range of imaging technologies applicable to studying hypotheses derived from a wealth of animal studies has emerged. This section focuses on the use of various imaging techniques to define the neural circuits involved in addiction and to measure changes in relevant parameters in the brain. The most common target for these studies has been cocaine addiction, but there is a growing literature about other stimulants such as ecstasy, methamphetamine, alcohol, opioids, nicotine and cannabis.

2.2 How the Drug is Delivered is Important

The effect of a drug depends on its pharmacology and on other complex interactions. For instance, is the substance of abuse given in the experiment as the users normally take it? The kinetics of drug use, its environment and other factors will all contribute to the measured effect of the drug.

2.2.1 Kinetics

The faster a drug gets into the brain, the greater the 'rush' and the potential for reinforcement. Volkow's group have used neuroimaging studies of methylphenidate, which blocks the dopamine transporter as cocaine does but is not as reinforcing, to show the significant contribution of drug kinetics to effect. The uptake of intravenous methylphenidate was very fast and was associated with subjective ratings of 'high' in healthy volunteers (Volkow et al., 1996a). This is similar to cocaine (Volkow et al., 1996b). In contrast, the clearance of methylphenidate was relatively slow compared with cocaine and it was still present in the brain after the subjective effects of methylphenidate had subsided. This prevented any further effects of subsequently administered methylphenidate, so reducing its reinforcing properties. Taking methylphenidate orally resulted in even slower accumulation in the brain, peaking at 60 minutes, and was not associated with pleasurable effects. This demonstrates why oral methylphenidate has low if any abuse liability.

2.2.2 How is the Drug Delivered?

In neuroimaging experiments, drugs have often been administered intravenously for practical reasons. But drugs are not always taken this way. Depending on what hypothesis is being tested, we must take account of the effect of the drug being given via a novel route. For example, it is likely that smoking a cigarette will have greater significance (salience) than intravenous nicotine administration, because it reproduces the way individuals usually receive nicotine. One study has shown that smoking a cigarette and intravenous nicotine both resulted in a similar pattern of increased regional cerebral blood flow (rCBF) in nicotine receptor regions of the brain such as the pons, midbrain and thalamus and also in the frontal cortex (Rose et al., 2003). However, smoking a cigarette resulted in a greater degree of regional brain activation than intravenous nicotine. Since nicotine levels were measured, we know that this was not a dose-related effect. It seems likely that the greater effect is due to the

superior salience of smoking compared with intravenous administration.

2.2.3 Anticipation

Since anticipation can enhance the effects of a drug, Volkow et al. (2003) studied the effects of methylphenidate in cocaine abusers when they expected to receive the drug and when they did not, i.e. when told they were getting a placebo. Expecting and receiving methylphenidate was associated with greater activation in the cerebellum and thalamus, whereas greater activation was seen in the orbitofrontal cortex if subjects were not expecting the drug. Increases in thalamic metabolism correlated with self-reports of 'high', which was 50 per cent greater when subjects expected it than when they did not. The thalamus receives dopaminergic projections and has reciprocal connections with the frontal cortex and striatum.

2.3 Pharmacology

2.3.1 Dopamine: Critical to All Substances of Abuse?

Over the last decade, many neuroimaging studies have investigated the dopamine system in addiction. Many studies have been performed in stimulant dependence, due to the direct effect of this class of drugs on dopamine neurotransmission, and possibly because problems of cocaine misuse receive high priority in the United States, where the majority of studies are performed.

Different aspects of dopaminergic function can be measured, including dopamine transporters (DAT), receptors and one of its metabolising enzymes, monoamine oxidase (MAO B). Striatal dopamine D2 receptor (DRD2) levels are commonly measured with ^{11}C-raclopride PET or ^{11}C-IBZM SPET. Tracers such as ^{11}C-FLB or epidepride labelled with C-11 for PET or I-123 for SPET can measure extra-striatal DRD2, but have not been applied to studying addiction. Various methods have been developed to distinguish anatomically between ventral and dorsal striatum to determine the status of DRD2 in these areas, which have different functions in relation to addiction (Martinez et al., 2004; Drevets et al., 1999).

Synaptic Markers: Dopamine Receptors

Reduced DRD2 levels have been found in all addictions studied in man, including cocaine, methamphetamine, opioid, and alcohol (see Volkow et al., 2002a, 2004). Thus, chronic use of a drug results in dopaminergic hypofunction which is thought to underlie dysphoria and irritability. These symptoms are particularly pronounced during substance withdrawal. Reduced DRD2 levels appear to persist for a long time. With cocaine addiction, little increase in DRD2 levels is seen after four months of abstinence. After a similar period of abstinence from alcohol, no increase has been observed. Reduced DRD2 levels in striatum have also been shown to be associated with reduced metabolism at rest in the orbitofrontal cortex (Volkow et al., 1993), a region known to be critical for impulse control and decision making.

Are reduced levels of DRD2 a consequence of substance misuse, or contributors to vulnerability? Volkow et al. (1999a, 2002b) reported that the level of striatal DRD2 was related to whether healthy volunteers liked or disliked methylphenidate (a stimulant that increases dopamine levels by blocking the dopamine transporter like cocaine). Individuals with high DRD2 levels described methylphenidate as unpleasant but those with low DRD2 levels experienced drug liking. In these individuals, such an increase is thought to compensate for dopaminergic hypofunction in their 'natural' pleasure–reward system, even among non-addicts, and therefore increases the risk of further use and misuse.

The important role of the dopamine system in addiction makes it important to understand what influences dopaminergic status. For instance, treatment often focuses on two things associated with dopaminergic hypofunction: coping with low mood and with lack of pleasure. One important modulator shown in monkeys is social hierarchy. After individual rearing, becoming a dominant monkey in social housing is associated with increased levels of DRD2, while subordinate animals show no changes in DRD2 levels (Morgan et al., 2002). Significantly, cocaine was less reinforcing in dominant animals than in subordinate monkeys. Therefore, in human and non-human primates, low DRD2 levels appears to be associated with drug liking (Volkow et al., 1999a; Morgan et al., 2002).

Synaptic Markers: Dopamine Transporters

Presynaptic DAT have been measured using various tracers with PET and SPET. Reduced DAT levels have been reported in stimulant users (McCann et al., 1998b; Volkow et al., 1997a). In alcoholism, both reduced and similar DAT levels have been found compared with control populations (Tiihonen et al., 1995; Volkow et al., 1996c; Repo et al., 1999). This discrepancy may be due to the type of alcohol-dependent patient studied. In those with a history of violence (similar to type 2 alcoholism, characterised by early age of onset, and antisocial, impulsive personality traits), DAT levels were similar to controls. In those without such a history (similar to type 1, characterised by late age of onset and anxiety) reduced levels were found. It is possible that neuroimaging may help in defining subtypes of alcoholism and other addictions by delineating their neurobiology.

Measuring Dopamine Levels

The tracers ^{11}C-raclopride and ^{123}I-IBZM have affinities similar to those of endogenous dopamine. This means that their binding is altered by changing levels of this neurotransmitter. This property has been widely exploited in addiction to test the fundamental hypothesis that the pleasure given by abused substances relates to their ability to increase dopamine levels. Both healthy volunteers and dependent patients have been studied.

In healthy volunteers stimulants such as methylphenidate and amphetamine were shown to reduce the binding of these radio-tracers, consistent with increased dopamine release (Laruelle et al., 1995; Volkow et al., 1997b), and the greater the reduction in tracer binding. The greater the release of dopamine, the greater was the high produced by the drug. Similarly in healthy volunteers, alcohol has been shown to release dopamine in the ventral striatum as it decreased ^{11}C-raclopride PET binding (Boileau et al., 2003). However, dopamine release was correlated with increased heart rate and a measure of 'impulsiveness' but not euphoria.

A few studies have been performed in dependent patients. In nicotine-dependent individuals, smoking a cigarette leads to reduced ^{11}C-raclopride binding in the left ventral striatum, and this is associated with reduced craving (Brody et al., 2004). In cocaine-dependent patients, Volkow et al. (1997b) found that methylphenidate produced less dopamine release than in control patients, supporting the hypothesis that dopamine hypofunction is present in dependence on stimulants. Schlaepfer et al. (1997) found that cocaine did increase dopamine levels in the striatum that related to its peak physiological and subjective effects, though less dopamine was released in more severely dependent patients.

2.3.2 Specific Substances of Abuse

No other neurotransmitter system has been as comprehensively studied as dopamine and therefore the remaining studies will be described by substance of abuse.

Ecstasy

Since Ecstasy increases serotonin (5HT) levels and preclinical experiments show it causes damage to the serotonergic system, imaging studies have focused on the 5HT system, primarily the 5HT transporter (5HTT). The SPET tracer, ^{123}I-β-CIT, labels both the 5HT and the DAT. However, in the striatum there are few 5HTT, and in the

raphe in the brainstem, there are few DAT. This anatomical separation allows ^{123}I-β-CIT to be used to label both transporters. The PET tracer, ^{11}C-McN5652, shows greater specificity for the 5HTT compared to DAT; however, its kinetics are complex.

Initial studies measuring the 5HTT with ^{11}C-McN5652 PET and ^{123}I-β-CIT SPET reported reduced levels throughout the brain (e.g. cortex, hippocampus) in ecstasy users and those abstinent for three weeks (McCann et al., 1998a; Semple et al., 1999). However, there has been debate about the limitations of these studies, concerning the individuals studied and the imaging protocols used. Nevertheless, more recent studies using the same tracers have reported reduced 5HTT levels in current ecstasy users throughout the brain, e.g. in the thalamus, caudate nucleus, midbrain (raphe), and medial temporal lobe (hippocampus; Thomasius et al., 2003; Buchert et al., 2004). 5HTT levels in ex-users were not significantly different from those in a control drug-naïve population. A specific effect of Ecstasy on 5HTT is likely since polydrug users who did not use Ecstasy had normal 5HTT levels.

Female Ecstasy users have been found to show greater 5HTT reductions than males (Reneman et al., 2001; Buchert et al., 2004). Why there is such gender difference is unknown, but this clearly has important implications for educating and advising the public about Ecstasy use.

Alcohol: GABA

The gamma-aminobutyric acid (GABA)-benzodiazepine receptor (GBzR) complex has been a focus of intense interests since many of the central effects of alcohol are mediated through its agonist action at the GBzR, and benzodiazepines alleviate alcohol withdrawal symptoms.

Using ^{11}C-flumazenil PET or ^{123}I-iomazenil SPECT, alcohol dependence has been shown to be associated with reduced levels of the GBzR, particularly in the frontal lobes (Gilman et al., 1996; Abi-Dargham et al., 1998; Lingford-Hughes et al., 1998). This reduction does not seem to be related to the length of abstinence, nor to grey-matter atrophy. These findings may reflect an alteration in the subunit profile of the GBzR as a means of reducing sensitivity to alcohol (i.e. tolerance). With regard to GBzR subtypes, both flumazenil and iomazenil appear non-selective, whereas ^{11}C-Ro15 4513 preferentially labels the alpha5 subtype (Lingford-Hughes *et al.*, 2002). However, we await new tracers to image other GBzR subtypes.

Alcohol: Serotonin

Serotonin (5HT) is implicated in many disorders that coexist with alcoholism, such as anxiety and depression, and also in controlling impulsive behaviour. Using ^{123}I-βCIT SPECT, Heinz *et al.* (1998) reported that alcohol dependence was associated with reduced levels of the 5HTT in the raphe nucleus in the brainstem (the only region which could be imaged), which correlated with ratings of depression and anxiety. Notably this reduction, but not alcoholism itself, was associated with a particular allelic variation *(ll)* of the 5HT transporter, suggesting that this polymorphism mediates susceptibility to the neurotoxic effects of alcohol (Heinz *et al.*, 2000).

2.3.3 Opioids

Neuroimaging has been used less often to investigate opioid dependence than for other drugs of dependence.

Opioid substitute drugs such as methadone and buprenorphine are widely used, but how much to prescribe relies on clinical assessment of illicit opioid use. However, it is not unusual for individuals to demand higher doses. Given the concerns about diversion and overdose, it would be valuable to know the relationship between dose and occupancy. It has been assumed that methadone and buprenorphine occupy opiate receptors, thus 'blocking' access to additional or 'on-top' illicit opioid use. Neuroimaging is well placed to investigate the relationship between dose, occupancy and effect to inform drug regimens, as with

the use of neuroimaging studies in antipsychotic prescribing in schizophrenia (Frankle and Laruelle, 2002).

Two PET studies using different tracers, ^{18}F-cyclofoxy (labels μ, κ opioid receptors) and ^{11}C-diprenorphine (labels μ, δ, κ opioid receptors), have investigated the dose–occupancy relationship in methadone-maintained addicts. Kling *et al.* (2000) measured available opioid receptors with ^{18}F-cyclofoxy and reported reduced labelling of opioid receptors in the thalamus, amygdala, caudate/putamen, and anterior cingulate cortex, compared with normal controls. Only in one region, the caudate/putamen, where ^{18}F-cyclofoxy binding was reduced by just 19 per cent to 32 per cent, was a correlation found between opiate receptor availability and plasma methadone levels. Melichar *et al.* (2004) did not find a reduction in ^{11}C-diprenorphine binding in a similar group of patients nor in animal studies, where much higher doses could be used, and instead hypothesised that methadone only occupies a small fraction of receptors, undetectable with ^{11}C-diprenorphine PET.

In contrast, using ^{11}C-carfentanil PET, the partial agonist buprenorphine has been clearly shown to dose-dependently occupy μ opioid receptors (Greenwald *et al.*, 2003). A relationship between occupancy and blocking the effects of an opioid agonist was also shown. Therefore it appears that methadone's efficacy may not depend on receptor blockade or reduction but probably on desensitising the receptor to opioids, whereas receptor blockade may contribute to buprenorphine's effectiveness.

Greenwald *et al.* (2003) noted that opioid-dependent patients had higher μ opioid receptor levels than healthy controls. It is noteworthy that increased opioid receptor levels have also been seen in cocaine (Zubieta *et al.*, 1996) and alcohol dependence (Lingford-Hughes *et al.*, unpublished) immediately after detoxification. Therefore a common neurobiological finding in dependence appears to be the increased availability of opioid receptors. This may be related to craving.

2.4 Studies of Changes in Blood Flow or Metabolism in Substance Misuse and Dependence

2.4.1 Mapping Neural Circuitry Associated with Craving

Exposure to salient cues often results in profound physiological and psychological responses, including increased pulse and craving. Cue exposure has therefore been used widely in neuroimaging studies of drug users to determine the neural networks associated with craving in order to define its underlying neurobiology and cognitive processes. Despite different patient populations, different substances abused and the use of different neuroimaging techniques, there is remarkable consistency in the brain regions whose activity is increased with cue exposure and craving. Areas such as the amygdala, anterior cingulate, dorsolateral prefrontal cortex and orbitofrontal cortex, which are involved in attention, emotional processing, goal-directed behaviour, associative learning, decision making, integration of information and response suppression, are commonly activated (see e.g. Grant et al., 1996; Childress et al., 1999; Garavan et al., 2000; Sell et al., 2000; Daglish et al., 2001; Wexler et al., 2001; Brody et al., 2002; Due et al., 2002; Myrick et al., 2004; Grusser et al., 2004). In particular, the changes seen in the orbitofrontal cortex have gained prominence due to its critical role in impulse control and decision making (Volkow and Fowler, 2000; London et al., 2000).

It is noteworthy that the relatively new 'connectivity' analysis that allows the determination of brain circuits involved in a brain process to be defined from functional neuroimaging studies has rarely been applied. Where it has, e.g. in two studies of opiate cue exposure and craving, interesting results have been found. Sell et al. (1999) reported activity in the anterior cingulate, left dorsolateral prefrontal cortices and the left extended amygdala correlated with the level of midbrain activation only during exposure to drug-related video. Daglish et al.

(2003) found activity in the anterior cingulate or orbitofrontal cortex covaried with activity in other brain regions involved in memory (hippocampus), attention (middle temporal gyrus) and sensory processing (auditory cortex, striate cortex). Together these data support the view that the brain regions involved in these fundamental brain processes are 'hijacked' by drugs of addiction (Figure 9.1).

While the considerable consistency between studies is notable, there are some discrepancies that are likely to be due to different cue-exposure paradigms, subjects studied, availability of the drug during or after the experiment, mood and degree of physiological arousal. Another important variable, often overlooked, is whether subjects are in treatment and, if so, with what aim, for example, abstinence or controlled use. In their review, Wilson et al. (2004) draw attention to the fact that cue exposure generally results in activation of the dorsolateral prefrontal and orbitofrontal cortices in non-treatment-seeking individuals but not in those in treatment. They suggest that activation of the dorsolateral prefrontal cortex reflects generation and maintenance of behavioural goals aimed at obtaining a reward and that activation of the orbitofrontal cortex reflects anticipation of getting the drug. Therefore 'craving' may have a different neurobiology depending on whether the individual is intending to use the drug again.

2.5 Conclusions

- Neuroimaging studies have contributed significantly to our understanding of the effects of substance misuse on the brain and illustrate the broad range of brain regions involved.
- Key to future applications are:
  - increased availability of functional neuroimaging centres, particularly those offering dedicated research availability of SPET and PET,
  - technological advances to provide improved resolution, shorter acquisition

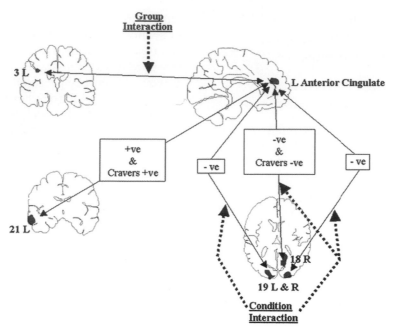

FIGURE 9.1   Brain regions (Brodmann areas) associated with the left anterior cingulate region. Solid lines with labels indicate a direct relationship between brain regions, with the label specifying the analyses when this relationship was demonstrated. Dotted lines denote a modulation of the relationship by scan condition or subject group. *Source:* Daglish *et al.*, 2003. (Reprinted from *Neuroimage*, 20, Daglish *et al.*, 'Functional connectivity analysis...', pp. 1964–1970, copyright 2003, with permission from Elsevier.)

times and development of PET/SPECT tracers that:

- can label neurotransmitter systems of interest, e.g. glutamate,
- are sensitive to neurotransmitters.

The use of these techniques to understand the interplay between environment and genes in addiction is still in its infancy.

3 FUNCTIONAL NEUROIMAGING IN THE STUDY OF DRUG ADDICTION

3.1 Introduction

Substance dependence is characterised by a loss of control over behaviour. Despite their best efforts and expressed preferences, drug-dependent individuals often appear incapable of exerting sufficient control over their drug urges and their drug-seeking and drug-taking behaviours. This suggests that cognitive processes involved in controlling human behaviour may be compromised in dependent individuals and that such processes should be investigated if we are to understand, treat and prevent drug abuse. While much research attests to compromised cognitive abilities in drug abusers, relatively little research has been conducted into the functional neuroanatomy that underlies these impairments. Another feature of much of the extant literature is the use of complex tasks that engage many distinct cognitive processes. As a consequence, it is difficult to infer from compromised performance on such tasks what specific cognitive process or processes are affected and what specific cortical areas may be altered. Functional neuroimaging studies that focus on distinct, well-characterised cognitive processes that are guided by current theory thus afford us the best chance to understand the behavioural control processes of drug abusers. It is these studies that are the subject of this report.

3.2 Drug Abuse and Impaired Learning from Feedback

A large body of research suggests that drug-abusers are compromised in how they process feedback and incorporate it into their performance (Bechara *et al.*, 2002; Bolla *et al.*, 2002; Finn *et al.*, 2002; Grant *et al.*, 2000; Lyvers and Yakimoff, 2003; Mazas *et al.*, 2000; Monterosso *et al.*, 2001; Petry *et al.*, 1998; Stout *et al.*, 2005; Whitlow *et al.*, 2004; Yechiam *et al.*, 2005). For example, Finn and colleagues (2002) employed a GO/NOGO task in which subjects were required to learn through feedback (small monetary gains or losses or mild shock) which were the GO stimuli to which they should respond, and which were the NOGO stimuli to which they should withhold responding. Alcoholics with a history of conduct disorder were impaired in learning these response contingencies. Drug-abuse-related impairment in learning from feedback is also apparent on a standard neuropsychological test of frontal lobe function, the Wisconsin Card Sorting Test (WCST). In this task, stimuli presented on individual cards vary in shape, colour and number (e.g. a typical card may contain two red triangles) and subjects must sort the cards according to one of these dimensions. They must infer the appropriate sorting rule from feedback and must be able to adjust their behaviour responsively as the experimenter occasionally changes the sorting rule. Chronic marijuana users have shown increased errors (Bolla *et al.*, 2002), while alcohol and stimulant abusers (Bechara *et al.*, 2002) and heroin abusers (Lyvers and Yakimioff, 2003), tested after 15 or more days of abstinence, demonstrated abnormal persistence in making selections which, as they were repeatedly told, were incorrect.

Much research into the decision making of drug users has employed the Iowa Gambling Task (IGT), a task which captures important aspects of decision making, most notably the ability to learn from feedback. In this task, subjects make selections from four decks of cards, with each selection yielding a monetary loss or gain. Some decks are more advantageous than others as they are associated with greater overall winnings. However, it is often not immediately apparent which decks are better, so subjects must learn from their selections, a task that is made challenging as decks that are worse overall often yield large rewards on individual selections. Thus, the IGT involves aspects of decision making that may be particularly germane to drug abuse, such as learning from feedback, delaying gratification, and downplaying immediate large rewards relative to slower incremental gains. Notably, compared to their control groups, drug abusers are more persistent in making disadvantageous choices on this task, despite repeatedly receiving feedback that they are losing (Bartzokis *et al.*, 2000; Bechara *et al.*, 2002; Bolla *et al.*, 2002; Finn *et al.*, 2002; Grant *et al.*, 2000; Mazas *et al.*, 2000; Monterosso *et al.*, 2001; Petry *et al.*, 1998; Stout *et al.*, 2005; Whitlow *et al.*, in press; Yechiam *et al.*, 2005).

3.2.1 Neuroimaging of Altered Sensitivity to Feedback

Imaging studies suggest that the IGT engages a distributed set of neural regions (Ernst *et al.*, 2002, 2003) associated with coding the motivational significance of stimuli (orbitofrontal and ventromedial frontal cortex), the formation of new memories (hippocampus), action monitoring (anterior cingulate cortex), and working memory (dorsolateral prefrontal cortex). In parallel to appreciating the number of distinct cortical areas engaged by the task, cognitive investigations have attempted to identify which particular aspect of the IGT decision-making process is impaired in drug abusers. Experimental manipulations of the task, such as displaying the win/loss probabilities of each deck (Stout *et al.*, 2005) or revealing the top card from each deck before the selection is made (Yechiam *et al.*, 2005), and cognitive modelling of card-by-card selections (Busemeyer and Stout, 2002), point to a diminished response to losses in drug abusers. That is, drug abusers appear to be less able to attend to loss information in the presence of information about wins, and, relative to comparison groups, their decision behaviour is under-influenced by their loss or, as has been observed in a proportion of substance abusers (Bechara *et al.*, 2002), overly influenced by their experiences of wins.

In agreement with the findings of the previous section, neuroimaging studies of drug abusers concur with this conclusion, with evidence of dysfunction in the anterior cingulate and in the ventral prefrontal cortex in users. As well as being implicated in performance of the IGT, these cortical areas appear to serve critical roles in monitoring behaviour and guiding decisions and thus are likely to be key brain centres underpinning a cognitive contribution to addiction. A role for prefrontal cortex in drug abuse would be expected from existing evidence of differences between drug users and controls in brain metabolism, brain morphology, and brain functional activation (Bolla *et al.*, 2004; Liu *et al.*, 1998; Matochik *et al.*, 2003; Stapleton *et al.*, 1995; Volkow *et al.*, 1992). For example, the functioning of the anterior cingulate cortex (ACC), which has previously been implicated in addiction and its

cognitive sequelae (Goldstein and Volkow, 2002; Peoples, 2002; Volkow *et al.*, 2002a), has been observed to be hypoactive in drug users relative to drug-naïve controls in attention switching (Kubler *et al.*, 2005), Stroop (Bolla *et al.*, 2004; Eldreth *et al.*, 2004), and inhibitory control (Hester and Garavan, 2004; Kaufman *et al.*, 2003) tasks. Evidence of ACC hypoactivity is also particularly pronounced in response to errors as revealed by an event-related fMRI investigation of commission errors on a GO/NOGO task (Kaufman *et al.*, 2003). In this investigation, cocaine users and controls performed a GO/NOGO task and brain activation in the ACC, which is typically found for performance errors (Hester *et al.*, 2004a), showed a diminished response in the users (see Figure 9.2). This finding on the neuroanatomical level matches well with the cognitive studies discussed above that revealed a blunted response to loses or negative feedback in drug abusers. Thus, the neuroimaging studies suggest a neuroanatomical substrate for the aberrant decision-making of drug abusers.

3.3 Addiction and the Anterior Cingulate Cortex

A diminished ACC response to errors has also been observed in opiate users (Forman *et al.*, 2004), on a Stroop task in

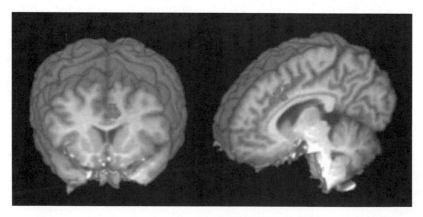

FIGURE 9.2   Reduced anterior cingulate activation observed in cocaine users relative to controls in response to commission errors on a GO/NOGO task. (This figure appears in the colour plate section.)

both cocaine (Bolla *et al.*, 2004) and marijuana users (Eldreth *et al.*, 2004), following alcohol administration (Ridderinkhoff *et al.*, 2003), and in other clinical groups such as schizophrenics and sufferers of attention-deficit hyperactivity disorder (ADHD) in whom monitoring abilities and behavioural control are compromised (Alain *et al.*, 2002; Fallgatter *et al.*, 2004). As seen in Section 2.1, many drugs of abuse are believed to exert their reinforcing effects by increasing dopamine (Volkow *et al.*, 2002a; Wise and Rompre, 1989). Evidence also points to a role for dopamine in error-related processing in the ACC, consistent with the concentration of dopamine receptors in this region (Volkow *et al.*, 1999b). Because of the relevance of dopamine to drug abuse and reward systems, this points to a neural system in drug abusers that might be responsible for deficient error processing. Indeed, Holroyd and Coles (2002) have proposed that the ACC error-related signal is driven by the same mesocorticolimbic dopamine system that generates ventral striatal responses related to expected and unexpected rewards and losses, as reported, for example, by Schultz (1997) and Schultz *et al.* (1997). Supporting this proposal, an increased error-related negativity (ERN, an electrophysiological component observed for errors) has been observed following amphetamine administration in non-dependent controls (de Bruijn *et al.*, 2003). As amphetamine increases synaptic levels of dopamine, and the ERN has been localised to the ACC (Dehaene *et al.*, 1994), this result is consistent with a role for ACC dopamine in error processes and, furthermore, with drugs of abuse being able to affect this process.

Direct support for this proposal comes from a recent study in which the infusion of cocaine in regular users led to more accurate performance in a GO/NOGO task, as well as increased error-related ACC activity (Kaufman *et al.*, under review). Thus, administering cocaine to chronic users appeared to correct the hypoactivity of the ACC to a level similar to those seen in drug-naïve controls. This 'normalisation' of a neurocognitive process through the administration of the abused drug is compelling evidence that cocaine can ameliorate abnormalities in the very neural systems that may have been altered by chronic use or that may have had a pre-existing abnormality that led to chronic use.

The functional integrity of error-related responses may be important for addiction because these, as well as other action monitoring processes, are thought to serve an essential monitoring function through initiating increased top-down, prefrontally-mediated attentional control and behavioural change (Botvinick *et al.*, 2004; Cohen *et al.*, 2000). For example, increased post-error slowing, indicative of a more attentive and cautious approach to a task, is associated with greater error-related ACC activation (Garavan *et al.*, 2002; Kerns *et al.*, 2004). Although the exact role of the ACC in monitoring performance is still debated (Botvinick *et al.*, 2004; Rushworth *et al.*, 2004), these results demonstrate drug-abuse-related differences in neural systems that are generally accepted as central to behavioural control.

3.4 Cognitive Neuroimaging of Addiction

Cognitive processes other than monitoring one's performance, and cortical areas other than the ACC, have been implicated in addiction. For example, structures such as the orbitofrontal cortex are important for performance of the IGT (Bechara *et al.*, 2000) and altered levels of activation in the orbitofrontal cortex have been observed in drug abusers (Bolla *et al.*, 2003; Goldstein *et al.*, 2001). The orbitofrontal cortex appears to play a critical role in assigning or adjusting valences to stimuli. Altered functioning of this structure may impact on the values assigned to the different decks in the IGT and, more importantly, may affect the emotional value given to drug use experiences despite knowledge of the adverse consequences of such use

(Bechara *et al.*, 2000). Hyperactivity in this region in cocaine users performing the IGT may reflect a hypersensitivity to reward (Bolla *et al.*, 2003), an interesting possibility given the ACC hypoactivity that has been suggested above to reflect a hyposensitivity to losses.

The compromised inhibitory control of drug users (Fillmore and Rush, 2002) may constitute another arena of drug-related executive dysfunction. Infusions of cocaine have been shown to improve inhibitory performance in cocaine users and to increase activation in right prefrontal regions that are considered critical for this function (Aron *et al.*, 2004; Garavan *et al.*, 1999). Although a full dose-response study has not been conducted, this result is consistent with a self-medication hypothesis in which cocaine may be cognitively reinforcing in a similar way to which it is understood to be affectively reinforcing (Khantzian, 1997). Such a result is also consistent with improvements in inhibitory control that have been observed with methylphenidate in patients with ADHD (Scheres *et al.*, 2003). In contrast, d-amphetamine administration has been observed to impair inhibitory control in amphetamine users (Fillmore *et al.*, 2003). While this effect appeared to be specific to certain contexts (the impairment was only observed if subjects were erroneously cued to expect a GO rather than a NOGO stimulus, thereby potentially including additional cognitive processes), it would seem that a thorough understanding of the specific circumstances and conditions in which drugs of abuse will help or hinder performance will require further investigation at both the cognitive and molecular levels (Koob and Le Moal, 1997).

3.5 Effects of Drug Craving on Cognition

The cognitive and neuroimaging data demonstrating deleterious interactions between working memory load and cognitive control functions (Bunge *et al.*, 2001;

Hester *et al.*, 2004b) may be of particular relevance to drug abuse. Abusers must try to control their behaviour (e.g. inhibit prepotent drug-seeking or drug-taking behaviours) while their working memories are occupied with drug-craving thoughts (Bonson *et al.*, 2002; Garavan *et al.*, 2000; Grant *et al.*, 1996). These interactions have recently been studied (Hester *et al.*, 2004a, 2004b, 2005) with tasks in which subjects were presented with memory sets of one, three or five items. Next, subjects were presented with a serial stream of letters, a minority of which were members of the memory set. Task instructions required a button press in response to all letters except memory set items. Thus, subjects had to combine a working memory demand (maintenance of a memory set) with a cognitive control demand (inhibiting a prepotent response to members of the memory set). The advantage of this dual-task design is that the maintenance of the memory set is integral to knowing when to inhibit. This prevents subjects from switching between the two task demands or arriving at other methods to circumvent the dual-task demand of the experiment. On accurate trials (i.e. successful inhibitions), ACC activity increased as a function of memory load in controls but did not change in users. Furthermore, this failure to activate the ACC was accompanied by reduced activity in the right prefrontal cortex, a cortical region which both functional imaging and lesion data suggest is critical for implementing inhibitory control (Aron *et al.*, 2004; Garavan *et al.*, 1999). Instead, it was the left cerebellum that showed increased inhibition-related activity as a function of memory load in the cocaine users. Exactly the opposite was found in controls, who performed better and had decreased load-dependent cerebellar activation.

A similar finding of increased cerebellar activity reported in alcoholics was interpreted as evidence that dysfunction of prefrontal circuits results in a dependence on cerebellar functions (Desmond *et al.*, 2003). A very similar pattern of activation change, reduced ACC and increased cerebellum, has recently been observed in marijuana users performing the IGT (Bolla *et al.*, 2005). Given the relationship between the ACC, action monitoring and the involvement of lateral prefrontal regions in performance when additional cognitive control is required, these results on cocaine, alcohol and marijuana users suggest that the compromised ACC functioning of users results in diminished prefrontal control over behaviour and, instead, given the poorer performance of the cocaine and marijuana users, reliance on suboptimal cerebellar structures.

These results suggest a number of future research directions. For example, are the neurocognitive deficits observed in drug users a cause or consequence of drug dependence? If these neurofunctional deficits are present prior to initial drug use, might they have predictive value for identifying individuals likely to become dependent on drugs? There is some evidence that this may be possible as measures of cognitive, affective and behavioural control in 10–12-year-olds have been shown to predict drug use at age 19 (Tarter *et al.*, 2003). Alternatively, if these deficits result from drug use, are they consequential for treatment outcome? For example, ACC hypoactivity in drug users has been shown to persist into abstinence (Bolla *et al.*, 2004; Eldreth *et al.*, 2004) and performance on cognitive tasks such as the Stroop that engage prefrontal areas are predictive of relapse in abstinent smokers (Waters *et al.*, 2003).

Whether neurofunctional alterations in drug abusers are a cause or consequence of drug use (or are a combination of both), the evidence that these alterations exist leads one to query whether it is possible to use behavioural or pharmacological treatments to improve the monitoring abilities of drug abusers for the amelioration of their behavioural problems. More research is required to determine if neurobiological mechanisms of altered functioning vary according to drug of choice or by the user's state, and whether these alterations are affected by a craving or withdrawal state.

4 FUNCTIONAL NEUROIMAGING IN PRECLINICAL MODELS OF ADDICTION

4.1 Introduction

The recent advent of non-invasive neuroimaging methods such as fMRI to complement more established PET methods will for the first time allow direct translation from preclinical laboratory experiments to the patient. These methods will yield new temporal information about both acute and long-term drug-induced structural and functional changes in the brain, as well as precise quantification and visualisation of the drug's distribution and elimination from the body. In addition, imaging has begun to reveal recovery of function and reappearance of neuronal markers in abstinent drug users. Furthermore, it has recently been mooted that brain imaging, in tandem with genetic and behavioural assessments, may help in identifying individuals predisposed to become addicts.

At present, there is too little neuroimaging research in preclinical models of addiction. More such studies are needed in these more ordered systems as they allow more controlled drug exposure and eliminate many of the potential confounds commonly observed in the clinic, such as poor compliance and multiple substance abuse. As we further establish and validate these novel neuroimaging methods, we envisage being able to more objectively assess the abuse potential of new drugs that penetrate the central nervous system as well as strengthening our critical evaluation of candidate pharmacotherapies for the treatment of drug addiction.

4.2 Heroin

One of the first preclinical, functional neuroimaging studies of addiction was performed by Stein and colleagues (Xu *et al.*, 2000). They showed that fMRI allows us to directly visualise the effects of acute, intravenous heroin administration at those central sites that are consistent with the distribution of opiate μ-receptors in the rat brain and which have previously been reported by *ex vivo* autoradiography. As the non-invasive nature of neuroimaging lends itself to serial investigations of the same subject, these researchers have built on these seminal observations with a more recent fMRI investigation to determine whether repeated self-administration (SA) of heroin produces tolerance or sensitisation in the rat brain. Under spontaneous respiration, acute heroin (0.1 mg/kg) administration induced a global decrease in blood-oxygen-level-dependent (BOLD) signal changes. Under artificial respiration, a region-specific increase in fMRI signal was identified in cortical regions, including the prefrontal cortex, cingulate, and olfactory cortex, which were significantly less in the pretreated, heroin-SA rats than in a matched group of saline control rats. These data suggest that repeated heroin-SA produces tolerance or desensitisation of opiate actions in the rat brain, which may in turn potentiate drug SA behaviour and drug intake (Xi *et al.*, 2004).

4.3 Models of Drug Withdrawal

fMRI can be used to examine drug dependence using a robust animal model of drug withdrawal. Two groups of rats chronically pretreated with increasing doses of morphine sulphate and then subjected to either placebo or precipitated withdrawal (using the opioid antagonist, naloxone) revealed statistically significant and localised changes in the brain signal intensity following administration of 1 mg/kg naloxone alone. The control group did not exhibit any statistically significant changes in behaviour, or brain fMRI signal intensity changes. Regional patterns of modulated activity included the retrosplenial, piriform, insular, entorhinal, cingulate, visual and auditory cortices, posterior fields of the hippocampus, and in particular the dentate gyrus (Lowe *et al.*, 2002).

4.4 Nicotine Dependence

fMRI has also been used to examine the neurobiological mechanisms through which nicotine produces dependence. Rats followed an established seven-day regime to induce physical dependence on nicotine and were then scanned before, during and after a mecamylamine (1mg/kg sc) or saline (1ml/kg) challenge. Mecamylamine, a nicotine antagonist, precipitated highly significant positive changes in the MRI signal contrast that were predominantly localised to the nucleus accumbens (NAc) of the nicotine-dependent rats (Figure 9.3). This observation is consistent with previous, more invasive, neurochemical investigations which have reported a decrease in dopamine in the NAc during nicotine withdrawal. This study further highlights the potential of this method to image the neurobiological events during nicotine dependence and withdrawal (Shoaib *et al.*, 2004).

4.5 Dopamine Circuits

It is well known from intracranial self-administration studies with specific dopamine receptor agonists that the shell of the NAc is a critical site of dopamine reward. We believe that the higher spatial resolution available with MRI will also allow us to image discrete subcomponents of this reward circuit (Figure 9.4). For example, using fMRI in combination with the selective dopamine agonist quinelorane (which at low doses acts specifically at D3 receptors but at higher concentrations acts at both D2 and D3 receptors), we can elicit selective activity of the core and shell of the NAc (Ireland *et al.*, 2005).

4.6 Effects of Anaesthetic

The neuroimaging data discussed above suffers from the potential confound of an interaction with the anaesthetic required to minimise subject movement. Furthermore, many of the anaesthetics of choice

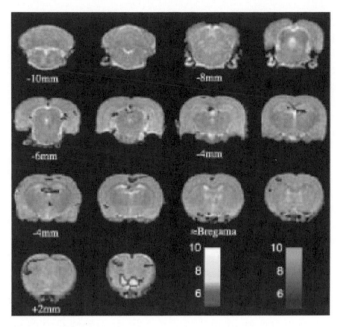

FIGURE 9.3 fMRI from the whole brain of a group of five nicotine-dependent rats following administration of the nicotine antagonist, mecamylamine, to precipitate drug withdrawal. The most significant changes are observed in the NAc, which plays a central role in the reward circuitry.

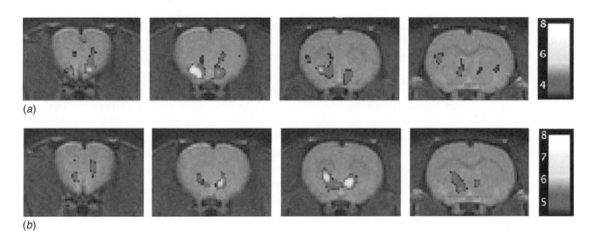

FIGURE 9.4 Group statistical parametric maps of the rat brain comparing statistically significant increases in BOLD contrast after administration of $3\,\mu g/kg$ quinelorane (*a*), or $30\,\mu g/kg$ quinelorane (*b*). At $3\,\mu g/kg$, quinelorane is associated with hypolocomotion and increases in BOLD are seen in the nucleus accumbens but at a dose associated with hyperlocomotion; at $30\,\mu g/kg$, additional BOLD increases are seen in the caudate-putamen and globus pallidus.

in addiction research (e.g. urethane and alpha-chloralose), while maintaining substantive central activity, do not allow subject recovery, thus defeating one of the main strengths of the imaging technique, which is repetition in the same animal. However, recent results from the Center for Comparative NeuroImaging at the University of Massachusetts Medical School have demonstrated the technical feasibility of studying psychostimulant-induced brain activity using MRI in fully conscious rats.

Methods were developed to image cocaine-induced changes in the BOLD signal prior to and following the intracerebroventricular injection of cocaine. Within five minutes of the injection, there was a significant increase in BOLD signal intensity in the substantia nigra, ventral tegmental area, NAc, dorsal striatum and prefrontal cortex, as compared with vehicle controls. No significant perturbations in normal cardiovascular and respiratory function were observed (Febo *et al.*, 2004). A follow-up study involving repeated cocaine administration reported lower BOLD responses in many of these brain regions, which again could not be attributed to variations in cerebrovascular reactivity between drug-naive rats and those repeatedly exposed to cocaine. Therefore, the lower metabolic activation in response to cocaine could reflect reduced neuronal or synaptic activity on repeated administration (Febo *et al.*, 2005).

5 MOLECULAR IMAGING AND THE ROLE OF PET

5.1 Role of Molecular Imaging

A key aim of this Foresight project is to 'provide challenging visions as to how scientific and technical advancement may impact on our understanding of addiction and drug use'. Here we address two major project questions relevant to molecular imaging. What are the effects of using psychoactive substances? What mechanisms do we have to manage the use of psychoactive substances?

To address these questions there are two general hypotheses:

- The introduction of psychoactive substances into the human body will produce chemical changes within brain tissue.
- The phenotypic profiles of humans at risk of addiction from psychoactive substances will be revealed as differences in neurochemistry within specific brain regions.

To answer these hypotheses in the context of the associated profiles of human behaviour, we need to measure selected aspects of the regional neurochemistry of the human brain in life. Molecular imaging offers a non-invasive means to provide the biomarkers needed to address these hypotheses. Unless such technology is used, within a broad portfolio addressing brain science and addiction, this area will remain in the scientific dark ages.

5.2 Developing the Future of PET-based Molecular Imaging for Addiction Research

5.2.1 New Radio-labelled PET Ligands for Addiction Research

From the examples shown, it will be clear that PET-based imaging is able to provide unique information on regional brain neurochemistry that is pertinent to addiction research and to showing the effects of psychoactive substances on the human brain. The underlying technology to derive relevant information is established, and it is justified to project forward and predict a unique future role for such studies. It is relevant to note that the key examples shown are based on the use of probes introduced some 20 years ago. These include ^{11}C-raclopride, a ligand for the D-2 receptor, ^{11}C-flumazenil, a ligand for the central benzodiazepine receptor, and ^{11}C-diprenorphine for the opiate receptor. The ligand for imaging the serotonin 5HT1A receptor, ^{11}C-Way 100063, was introduced some 10 years ago, while the tracer for imaging regional brain glucose metabolism, ^{18}FDG, was first introduced in man in 1976. Based on the exploitation record of such ligands in addiction research, there is a suggestion that, although there have been clear achievements, the field has not realised the full potential of the opportunities offered by PET.

The key future challenge is to provide imaging probes that are specific for the potentially wide spectrum of neuroreceptors and pathways that could be involved in the brain's response to psychoactive substances and the underlying addiction phenotype. In principle, it should be possible to make tracer equivalents of all new and old pharmaceutical products since their chemistry is fairly well worked out. There is a critical need for impetus and funding. Important neurotransmitter systems where we need tracers in addiction include GABA-A subtype receptors, glutamate receptor subtypes, and noradrenaline receptor subtypes. This needs to extend to optimising procedures to study the functional activation of these receptors and pathways in the addictive setting and in response to psychoactive substances.

5.3 Developing Collaborative Links with the Pharmaceutical Industry

The ligands that have been used successfully to date all stemmed from the pharmaceutical industry, which is the principal source of pharmacologically active molecules. Pipelines of more specific ligands and tracers for PET-based imaging research will need to be developed through partnerships between industry and academic medicine. This is needed to advance the understanding of addiction and the effects of psychoactive substances in the academic setting. Industry is turning to 'biomarkers' such as imaging to provide proofs-of-concept of the mechanisms and efficacy of new agents prior to the implementation of large and expensive clinical trials.

There has been a tendency to suggest that the pharmaceutical industry has been reluctant to play its partnership role with academia in advancing this field, with suggestions that it is developing a fortress approach to its own in-house developments. Since the field is in its infancy, with many high-risk areas to be developed, it remains an academic area where research has to be conducted within the setting of experimental medicine. Creating the environment for collaborations with industry, where the probes will be developed and exploited for

addiction research, calls for contributions from both academia and industry. To energise this partnership, which is vital for fully realising the future potential of molecular imaging for addiction research, it is worth itemising what academia needs to do to attract industry to channel its considerable resources into this area and share in the risks associated with such development.

5.4 Establishing Experimental Medicine-based Molecular Imaging Centres

Academia has to provide the experimental medicine infrastructure, centred on the high-technology facilities necessary for developing and applying PET methodology for clinical research. This requires the establishment of 'big science' research environments which address the major governance issues increasingly overlaid on clinical research. These issues include clinical accountability and legislation for the production and introduction of foreign substances into human volunteers, as well as the preclinical validation of new probes in such academic institutions. Such academic centres must be led by clinical science but remain committed to the discovery and development of new methodologies, especially the validation of new procedures in patients. These need to be followed by in-depth clinical research projects which give the platform for using such tools for both long-term studies in addiction and the proof-of-concept studies required by industry. Such environments need to be developed as science hotels. In the first instance, it will be imperative to attract individuals from the pharmaceutical industry to spend working periods in these institutes in order to foster symbiosis and to forge the conduits linking companies and universities. In addition, such 'hotels' need to be linked with UK networks of clinical research in order to undertake the most relevant and best-advised programmes of addiction research. This could be achieved by working within a UK consensus for future study as defined within the Foresight project. It would be difficult to develop such imaging research institutes solely for addiction research. They need to be shared by other areas of academic medicine that need PET-based molecular imaging. These include research into brain disorders in general as well as cancer. One such centre is currently being established at the University of Manchester.

5.5 Availability of PET/SPET Facilities

There are substantial benefits to UK society and the research community in having neuroimaging research centres that increase the availability of SPET and particularly PET. Usually this research cannot be commercially driven. The development of new PET cameras with computed tomography (CT) means that the radiation dosage has increased due to CT being used to produce the detailed anatomical images needed in oncology. This is likely to affect the research studies that are possible. The importance of clinical and commercial drivers, often concentrating on oncology, may also reduce the use of PET/SPET for understanding the neurobiology of mental health disorders, including addiction. Radionuclide imaging such as PET and SPET will never be wholly replaced by other neuroimaging techniques and needs to be nurtured in the UK as a critical tool to map the neuropharmacology of substance misuse and addiction.

5.6 The Importance to the Foresight Project of Utilising Molecular Imaging Centres

- Defining the most important addiction-related questions that can be answered by molecular imaging.
- Setting the scene for creating enduring networks for addiction research able to utilise and support national facilities within the UK.

6 ADVANCES IN MRI/S TECHNOLOGY

6.1 Ultra-high-field Strength Systems

6.1.1 Improvement in Sensitivity

Despite the undoubted success of fMRI, its interpretation and range of applications are limited by the low-activation contrast-to-noise ratio (CNR) of the BOLD effect, even at three tesla (3T). There is strong evidence that problems of sensitivity could be solved by working at higher magnetic fields, such as the seven tesla (7T) of planned future machines (see Figure 9.5).

6.1.2 Single-trial fMRI

This problem of low CNR is normally addressed by averaging over many trials of a standard block paradigm or a 'single event' study. However, this averaging, which is routine in EEG and MEG studies, assumes that the responses are consistent. Many mental phenomena of crucial importance in understanding brain injury or mental illness are fleeting in nature and might best be studied using a procedure that has sufficient sensitivity to detect the cerebral activity associated with single events. This might apply to transient mental symptoms such as auditory hallucinations, transient 'awareness' of sensation after damage to primary sensory brain regions, formal thought disorder, or obsessional ruminations; drug craving can also be similarly transient – to responses to external stimuli under circumstances where habituation is expected and to events in which subjects make erroneous responses to stimuli.

If the CNR in an fMRI study could be increased to the point that the analysis of an individual trial was possible, with reasonable spatial resolution, this would represent a 'quantum leap' in our ability to study brain function. The gain in going from a conventional high field of 1.5T is apparent. Events that can only be observed with 100 averages at 1.5T should be detected in a single shot at 7T.

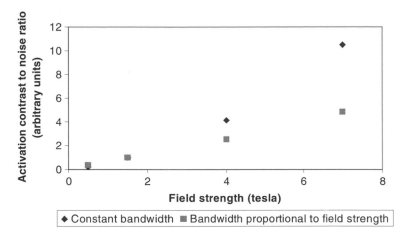

FIGURE 9.5 Variation in functional contrast-to-noise ratio with field strength. The upper line assumes that the signal-to-noise ratio increases linearly with field strength, whereas the lower line assumes that it increases only as the square root of field to accommodate the wider bandwidth necessary for the more rapid acquisition. This is a somewhat pessimistic view and represents a minimum bound. We expect the actual outcome to be closer to the upper curve.

Source: derived from Gati *et al.* (1997) for 0.5, 1.5 and 4T and from Hu *et al.* (2000) for 7T.

6.1.3 High-spatial-resolution fMRI

Functional domains are highly localised, and the increased CNR with higher fields can also be used to improve the resolution with which they can be mapped. Minimum voxel size is reduced by an order of magnitude at 7T relative to 1.5T. Working at 4T, Menon and Goodyear (1999) have mapped the ocular dominance columns in visual cortex at 1mm resolution. The spatial resolution is limited not only by the CNR, but also by the nature of the BOLD effect, in which contrast arises from dephasing the MR signal in and around capillaries and draining veins serving the activated area of cortex. This dephasing is a consequence of local inhomogeneity in the magnetic field related to the local concentration of deoxyhaemoglobin (dHb), and to the blood volume. There are sound theoretical reasons to expect, and good supporting evidence for thinking (Lee *et al.*, 1999), that the greatly reduced T2 of blood, relative to tissue, at higher fields (7T and above) effectively removes the intravascular component of the functional response [without the need for diffusion gradients (Duong *et al.*, 2000)], and limits the extravascular response to the smaller vessels

and capillaries, more intimately related to neural activity. The resulting improvement in localisation is expected to be highly significant. Other aspects of the haemodynamic response may offer improved functional resolution.

6.2 Magnetic Resonance Spectroscopy

6.2.1 ^{1}H MRS

^{1}H MRS is widely available on clinical MRI systems (it does not require additional hardware), but has enjoyed limited success in clinical diagnosis, mainly because of sensitivity limitations. Metabolites of interest typically are present in millimolar concentrations, thousands of times lower than the concentration of hydrogen in tissue water at 80M. In any case, relatively few metabolites can be reliably distinguished. However, it has had some impact in neurodegenerative disease, where the neuronal marker N-acetylaspartate (NAA), has provided a useful measure of the extent of degeneration. Other observable metabolites include creatine (and phosphocreatine), choline-containing compounds, inositol (a possible glial marker), and lactate. Of particular interest in the study of drug addiction, it is also possible to identify multiple resonances from GABA, glutamate and glutamine. The glutamate and glutamine peaks overlap at 1.5T, but as field strengths increases, so our ability to resolve them improves. It is possible that addiction may lead to changes in the levels of these and other neurotransmitters or in the ratio of glutamate to glutamine, reflecting altered recycling of glutamate via the glutamate–glutamine cycle.

6.2.2 ^{13}C MRS

In contrast to ^{1}H MRS, ^{13}C MRS enables metabolic rates to be determined. ^{13}C MRS was first applied to the human brain by Beckmann et al. in 1991. Their study was performed at 1.5T following [1-^{13}C]glucose administration. In 1994, Gruetter et al. achieved a time resolution of four minutes, enabling them to follow the incorporation of the labelled ^{13}C from [1-^{13}C]glucose into glutamate, glutamine and aspartate. There have been relatively few ^{13}C measurements of resting TCA cycle rate in the human brain, but there is good agreement between them, with a mean value of about 0.74 μmol/min/g. There is also reasonable agreement with the few measurements by PET of the cerebral metabolic rate for glucose (CMR_{glc}) which, if glucose is the sole substrate and is consumed aerobically, should be about half the TCA cycle rate since each glucose molecule generates two acetyl units. This agreement suggests that, under resting conditions, cerebral metabolism is essentially aerobic (Morris and Bachelard, 2003).

^{13}C MRS, both direct (Chhina et al., 2001) and indirect (^{1}H-{^{13}C}; Chen et al., 2001) has been used to study changes in TCA cycle rate in the human visual cortex on visual stimulation. Analysis of the MRS time-courses reveals increases in F_{TCA} of about 50% (Chhina et al., 2001), similar to the increases in CMR_{glc} reported in the PET studies, but strongly suggest, in contrast to these studies, that cerebral glucose is

metabolised oxidatively, even during intense visual stimulation. This is supported by the fact that neither under basal conditions nor during strong activation does the labelled isotope accumulate to any significant extent in lactate. It is also supported by the large increase in $CMRO_2$ seen in anaesthetised rats on forepaw stimulation (Hyder et al., 1996).

The same data used to determine F_{TCA} can be analysed to determine the rate of the glutamate/glutamine cycle, via which much of the neurotransmitter glutamate is recycled. Given the difficulty of such measurements, there is good agreement between them, with a mean rate of about 0.3 μmol/min/g (Morris and Bachelard, 2003). Sibson et al. (1998) have shown in rats that 80–90 per cent of the glutamine synthase flux can be attributed to glutamate–glutamine cycling, and that it is intimately related to the rate of oxidative glucose metabolism (the TCA cycle rate). The above discussion relates essentially to glutamate-mediated excitatory neurotransmission. Labelling from [1-^{13}C]glucose can also be seen in GABA, the principal inhibitory neurotransmitter, and there is increasing interest in this labelling pathway and its relation to inhibitory neurotransmission. Though inhibitory activity is believed to be energetically less costly, and there is as yet no established quantitative link between GABA labelling and inhibitory activity, it is likely that ^{13}C MRS will in the future also be able to furnish estimates of such activity.

Measurements of F_{TCA} and F_{cyc} are possible but difficult at current field strengths (3T). They will be substantially improved at higher fields (7T and up), but would really come of age in the context of drug addiction if they could be combined with hyperpolarised technologies. The rates of these reactions are such that instantaneous rate measurements would be possible if two orders of magnitude of sensitivity improvement could be achieved. Though this will not be easy to achieve, it is relatively modest on the scale of what is theoretically possible.

6.3 Hyperpolarised Technologies

Relative to most forms of spectroscopy, magnetic resonance is a very insensitive technique. The origin of this poor sensitivity lies in the small difference in energy between the nuclear Zeeman energy levels, and the resulting small difference in population of those energy levels, even in the highest magnetic fields currently available. At 3T, the field typically used for functional MRI studies, the proton polarisation is only about 1×10^{-5}. Put simply, the signal we detect at this field is only 0.001 per cent of what we would detect if the protons were fully polarised. Hyperpolarisation, a method for creating a highly non-equilibrium nuclear polarisation of selected chemical species, is ripe for development, and should lead to sensitivity improvements of up to 10 000, thereby creating exciting new opportunities for MRI and MRS. To date, most effort has been focused on noble gases (^{3}He and ^{129}Xe), in which polarisation levels in excess of 90 per cent have already been achieved.

6.3.1 Hyperpolarised Gases

Methods for Hyperpolarising Gases

Two optical pumping techniques, spin exchange (Ruth *et al.*, 1999) and metastable (Stoltz *et al.*, 1996) optical pumping (SEOP and MEOP), are used to produce hyperpolarised noble gases in sufficient quantity and level of polarisation for use with MRI. For ^{3}He, MEOP, where the gas is optically pumped at low pressure ($\sim$1 mbar) and then subsequently compressed to a pressure suitable for MRI (>1 bar), currently allows higher production rates (>10 bar litre/hour) and ultimate polarisation ($\sim$80%). The production stations are generally room-sized, complex and costly, but there is no inherent reason why they cannot be made much smaller, perhaps the size of a small fridge or ultimately a shoe box. For ^{129}Xe, SEOP techniques have been dramatically improved, with 70 per cent polarisation achieved at production rates of about 1 bar litre/hour.

Applications of Hyperpolarised Gases

These high levels of polarisation and good production rates, coupled with greatly improved storage times of up to 900 hours make ^{3}He an ideal candidate for lung ventilation studies. There is much research in this area, and the methodology is likely to receive approval by the US Food and Drug Administration for assessment of respiratory disorders in the very near term. The incorporation of ^{3}He (or ^{129}Xe) into microbubbles, which remain trapped in the vascular system, could be used to determine blood flow in a non-invasive manner, and may prove a useful alternative to standard fMRI. However, there is little ongoing work in this area.

^{129}Xe can likewise be used for lung ventilation studies in humans (Mugler *et al.*, 1997). However, it is also blood-soluble and lipophilic, and so penetrates into brain parenchyma; a 'dissolved phase' resonance can be observed which is a direct indicator of regional cerebral blood flow (rCBF). At present this application is limited by the anaesthetic properties of xenon. But this should be overcome by the considerably enhanced levels of hyperpolarisation now achievable. Potentially, this provides an attractive new method for the assessment of drug-induced changes in rCBF. The sensitivity of the chemical shift of the ^{129}Xe resonance to its environment can be used in an NMR analogue of fluorescence labelling, in which the fluorophore is replaced by a ^{129}Xe atom, caged in a clathrate. Binding to the target structure results in a shift in resonance frequency, allowing detection (Pietrass *et al.*, 1995). This technology remains at an early stage of development, but if successful would have very exciting implications for imaging in drug addiction.

6.3.2 Transfer of Polarisation

Hyperpolarised gases are limited in their application. However, if magnetisation could be transferred to other spin species, a whole new range of possibilities would open up. For transfer of magnetisation from ^{129}Xe, a solution of the target species in liquid xenon is producing promising results. ^{13}C, which can have a long T1 relaxation time and is a biologically versatile label, is a favoured recipient. ^{13}C NMR signals have been enhanced by between one and three orders of magnitude using the spin-polarisation-induced nuclear Overhauser effect (SPINOE) method at 1.5T (Navon *et al.*, 1996), and (more successfully) by thermal mixing at 5mT (Bowers *et al.*, 1993). These methods could be used to hyperpolarise ligands directly, or to hyperpolarise small, chemically reactive molecules, which can be used to mark larger molecules in the fashion of the synthesis of PET ligands.

6.3.3 *Other Approaches to Hyperpolarisation*

An interesting approach to hyperpolarisation is *para* hydrogen (*p*-H2) which is itself NMR silent, so that chemical reactions are required to generate observable ^{1}H hyperpolarisation. Signal amplification levels exceeding 10 000 have already been achieved by this approach. Semiconductor hyperpolarisation offers a further exciting possibility. However, the most promising approach is currently dynamic nuclear polarisation (DNP). This method relies on the fact that free electrons can be hyperpolarised relatively easily by the 'brute force' method, and the polarisation (of approaching 90 per cent) transferred to nuclear spins (usually ^{13}C) by microwave irradiation of the electron transition. ^{13}C polarisation of about 50 per cent has been achieved using this approach, and used as a vascular contrast agent in demonstrative MRI studies (Petersson, 2004). If suitable rapid synthesis and delivery systems could be produced, this would provide a method for instantaneous measurement of the regional cerebral metabolic rate for glucose – perhaps the most quantitative measure of brain activity currently envisaged. It could further open up exciting possibilities for measuring the activity of a range of neurotransmitter systems. Currently, this is an area of intense academic and commercial activity.

7 TRANSCRANIAL MAGNETIC STIMULATION

7.1 Relevance to Issues Addressed

TMS can address the Foresight project questions: What are the effects of using psychoactive substances? What mechanisms do we have to manage the use of psychoactive substances?

7.2 Scope of Technique

TMS is simply a non-invasive method of stimulating the brain. It achieves an effect similar to that seen in experiments where the skull is removed and an electrode is used to apply a direct electrical stimulus to the cortex. However, it is not as focused as the latter, usually activating an area of 1–2 cm^2. TMS does not spread deep into the brain and cannot activate thalamus or basal ganglia directly. However, it can stimulate areas on the surface that project to these structures and can therefore activate them indirectly:

TMS can address questions about brain function in four main ways.

7.2.1 *'Virtual Lesion' Effect*

Although we talk of 'stimulation' of an area, a TMS pulse actually has the effect of disrupting activity for about 100ms after each stimulus. This is termed a 'virtual lesion'. If we 'lesion' an area of cortex that is contributing to behaviour at the time the stimulus is given, behaviour will be disrupted. For example, a stimulus to the primary visual cortex produces a transient scotoma that can be detected if subjects are asked to detect the presence of briefly flashed visual stimuli in the 100ms period following the TMS pulse. The 'virtual lesion' method is commonly used in conjunction with fMRI/PET methods to verify that an activated area contributes to task performance (rather than being associated with it), and to provide an indication of when that activity is necessary.

7.2.2 Paired Pulse Methods

These can be used on motor cortex to test specific neural circuits. At present they can only be applied to motor cortex because of the way the effects are measured in terms of EMG potentials. They currently detect activity in GABAa, GABAb and cholinergic pathways and are sensitive to manipulations of these neurotransmitters by globally-acting central nervous system drugs.

7.2.3 TMS in Conjunction with Other Imaging Methods

TMS to one site activates both the input and output connections of that site, so that applying TMS in a functional imaging scanner can reveal connectivity of cortical areas. Moreover, the ease with which the connections are activated depends on their excitability at the time the stimulus is given, so active connections are highlighted above inactive ones. It is possible to test connectivity at rest and to compare how this changes during different tasks. At the present time, this procedure is being validated in the motor system. For example, stimulation of the primary motor cortex leads to changes in metabolic activity in premotor and supplementary motor cortex, thalamus and cerebellum. The method can potentially be applied to any part of the cortex.

A second application with imaging is to employ ligand imaging methods (Section 2) to show how stimulation of one area changes the release of neurotransmitters at the site of stimulation and sometimes at connected sites at a distance. So far, this method has demonstrated that the stimulation of frontal areas of cortex can lead to the release of dopamine in the basal ganglia. In the future, the method could be applied to other areas and other neurotransmitters depending on the ligands available.

7.2.4 Repetitive TMS

Repeated stimulation of cortex leads to after-effects that outlast the period of stimulation. These may be produced by processes analogous to long-term potentiation (LTP) or depression (LTD), which have been well-documented in animal experiments. It has been postulated that repeated applications of repetitive TMS (rTMS) could lead to very long-lasting effects on brain function that could have potential therapeutic value. This has led to trials of rTMS as a treatment for depression, obsessive compulsive disorder, migraine and several varieties of movement disorder. Currently, the results suggest that some positive effects may be obtained, but in no case have the effects been superior to conventional treatments. In the future, increased understanding of how rTMS works and what neural populations are targeted may help improve prospects.

7.3 Brain Science, Addiction and Drugs: Key Issues

7.3.1 Effects of Psychoactive Substances

TMS can explore these by comparing patterns of task-related brain activation in different populations of users. TMS in this case would be an adjunct to other methods of functional imaging. In addition, TMS can detect connectivity of brain areas, both at rest and during task performance, to test whether the use of psychoactive substances changes the organisation of brain areas. Finally, TMS can reveal how psychoactive substances can lead to changes in neurotransmitter release. In all cases, an important question will be whether the administration of such substances produces long-term effects on brain organisation that outlast the period of treatment.

7.3.2 Managing the Use of Psychoactive Substances

The main potential contribution here is to replace some treatments with rTMS-based methods, which are currently being tested in patients with depression. As noted above, present studies are suggestive of the possibility of weak effects. However, more studies need to be done to understand which of the infinite number of possible combinations of rTMS applications, in terms of duration of treatment, intensity of TMS pulse, frequency of rTMS, etc., are optimal and to determine the best sites of stimulation to apply the rTMS. The effects of TMS can be seen at connected sites at a distance from the stimulated area.

8 FURTHER DEVELOPMENTS

8.1 Magnetoencephalography

Functional MRI can provide useful information on the timing of neural activity, but there is a limit to the time resolution that can be achieved with techniques that are based on the haemodynamic response. In contrast, MEG is capable of high temporal resolution, but lacks the spatial resolution of fMRI. Recent developments, especially the increase in the number of channels, to 256, 512, or even more, have greatly improved resolution, and the ability to localise deep sources, but MEG is probably still used to greatest effect in combination with fMRI. Recently, the feasibility of combining fMRI and MEG has been established. In addition, a new GLM-beamformer method developed for processing MEG data enables changing patterns of activity to be mapped across all frequency ranges, including sustained fields (Brookes et al., 2004, 2005).

8.1.1 Availability of MEG in the UK

Until 2005, there was only one whole-head MEG system in the UK, located at Aston University. An indication of the growing interest in this technique is that by 2006 there are expected to be at least seven whole-head MEG systems installed in the UK.

8.2 Developmental Neuroscience

The use of PET/SPET in young people will probably never be possible due to the radiation exposure it involves. The use of structural MRI and fMRI and MEG to understand changes in young people is in its infancy but is growing. Neuroimaging will help us define brain regions involved in use, abuse and dependence in this population by repeating strategies already employed in adults and comparing the differences. It will also help us assess the impact on cognitive function and recovery, if any, if addicts stop drug abuse, and assess the impact of treatments. There is currently much less work in the UK in this area than the opportunity warrants. Some developmental neuroimaging centres are now being established, for example, the Brain and Body Centre at Nottingham.

References

Abi-Dargham, A., Krystal, J.H., Anjilvel, S., et al. (1998) Alterations of benzodiazepine receptors in type II alcoholic subjects measured with SPECT and [123I]iomazenil. Am J Psychiatry 155(11): 1550–1555.

Alain, C., et al. (2002) Neuropsychological evidence of error-monitoring deficits in patients with schizophrenia. Cereb Cortex 12: 840–846.

Aron, A.R., et al. (2004) Inhibition and the right inferior frontal cortex. Trends Cogn Sci 8: 170–177.

Bartzokis, G., et al. (2000) Abstinence from cocaine reduces high-risk responses on a gambling task. Neuropsychopharmacology 22: 102–103.

Bechara, A., et al. (2000) Emotion, decision making, and the orbitofrontal cortex. Cereb Cortex 10: 295–307.

Bechara, A., et al. (2002) Decision-making and addiction (part II): myopia for the future or hypersensitivity to reward? Neuropsychologia 40: 1690–1705.

Beckmann, N., Turkalji, I., Seelig, J., and Keller, U. (1991) ^{13}C NMR for the assessment of human brain glucose metabolism in vivo. Biochemistry 30: 6362–6366.

Boileau, I., Assaad, J.M., Pihl, R.O., Benkelfat, C., Leyton, M., Diksic, M., Tremblay, R.E., and Dagher, A. (2003) Alcohol promotes dopamine release in the human nucleus accumbens. *Synapse* 49: 226–231.

Bolla, K.I., *et al.* (2002) Dose-related neurocognitive effects of marijuana use. *Neurology* 59: 1337–1343.

Bolla, K.I., *et al.* (2003) Orbitofrontal cortex dysfunction in abstinent cocaine abusers performing a decision-making task. *Neuroimage* 19: 1085–1094.

Bolla, K.I., *et al.* (2004) Prefrontal cortical dysfunction in abstinent cocaine abusers. *J Neuropsychiatry Clin Neurosci* 16: 1–8.

Bolla, K.I., *et al.* (2005) Neural substrates of faulty decision-making in abstinent marijuana users. *Neuroimage* 26: 480–492.

Bonson, K.R., *et al.* (2002) Neural systems and cue-induced cocaine craving. *Neuropsychopharmacology* 26: 376–386.

Botvinick, M.M., *et al.* (2004) Conflict monitoring and anterior cingulate cortex: an update. *Trends Cogn Sci* 8: 539–546.

Bowers, C.R., Long, H.W., Pietrass, T., Gaede, H.C., and Pines, A. (1993) Cross polarization from laser-polarized solid xenon to $^{13}CO_2$ by low-field thermal mixing. *Chem Phys Lett* 205 (2–3): 168–170.

Brody, A.L., Mandelkern, M.A., London, E.D., Childress, A.R., Lee, G.S., Bota, R.G., Ho. M.L., Saxena, S., Baxter, L.R. Jr., Madsen, D., and Jarvik, M.E. (2002) Brain metabolic changes during cigarette craving. *Arch Gen Psychiatry* 59: 1162–1172.

Brody, A.L., Olmstead, R.E., London, E.D., Farahi, J., Meyer, J.H., Grossman, P., Lee, G.S., Huang, J., Hahn, E.L., and Mandelkern, M.A. (2004) Smoking-induced ventral striatum dopamine release. *Am J Psychiatry* 161: 1211–1218.

Brookes, M.J., Gibson, A.M., Hall, S.D., Furlong, P.L., Barnes, G.R., Hillebrand, A., Singh, K.D., Holliday, I.E., Francis, S.T., and Morris, P.G. (2004) A general linear model for MEG beamformer imaging. *Neuroimage* 23(3): 936–946.

Brookes, M.J., Gibson, A.M., Hall, S.D., Furlong, P.L., Barnes, G.R., Hillebrand, A., Singh, K.D., Holliday, I.E., Francis, S.T., and Morris, P.G. (2005) GLM-Beamformer method demonstrates stationary field, alpha ERD and gamma ERS co-localisation with fMRI BOLD response in visual cortex. *Neuroimage* 26: 302–308.

Buchert, R., Thomasius, R., Wilke, F., Petersen, K., Nebeling, B., Obrocki, J., Schulze, O., Schmidt, U., and Clausen, M. (2004) A voxel-based PET investigation of the long-term effects of 'Ecstasy' consumption on brain serotonin transporters. *Am J Psychiatry* 161: 1181–1189.

Bunge, S.A., *et al.* (2001) Prefrontal regions involved in keeping information in and out of mind. *Brain* 124: 2074–2086.

Busemeyer, J.R. and Stout, J.C. (2002) A contribution of cognitive decision models to clinical assessment: decomposing performance on the Bechara Gambling Task. *Psychol Assess* 14: 2523–2562.

Chen, W., Xiao-Hong, Z., Gruetter, R., Seaquist, E.R., Adriany, G., and Ugurbil, K. (2001) Study of tricarboxylic acid cycle flux changes in human visual cortex during hemifield visual stimulation using ^{1}H-[^{13}C] MRS and fMRI. *Magn Reson Med* 45: 349–355.

Chhina, N., Kuestermann, E., Halliday, J., Macdonald, I.A., Bachelard, H.S., and Morris, P.G. (2001) Measurement of human tricarboxylic acid cycle rates during visual activation by ^{13}C magnetic resonance spectroscopy *J Neurosci Res* 66: 737–746.

Childress, A.R., Mozley, P.D., McElgin, W., Fitzgerald, J., Reivich, M., and O'Brien, C.P. (1999) Limbic activation during cue-induced cocaine craving. *Am J Psychiatry* 156(1): 11–18.

Cohen, J.D., *et al.* (2000) Anterior cingulate and prefrontal cortex: who's in control? *Nature Neuroscience* 3: 421–423.

Daglish, M.R., Weinstein, A., Malizia, A.L., Wilson, S., Melichar, J.K., Britten, S., Brewer, C., Lingford-Hughes, A., Myles, J.S., Grasby, P., and Nutt, D.J. (2001) Changes in regional cerebral blood flow elicited by craving memories in abstinent opiate-dependent subjects. *Am J Psychiatry* 158: 1680–1686.

Daglish, M.R., Weinstein, A., Malizia, A.L., Wilson, S., Melichar, J.K., Lingford-Hughes, A., Myles, J.S., Grasby, P., and Nutt, D.J. (2003) Functional connectivity analysis of the neural circuits of opiate craving: 'more' rather than 'different'? *Neuroimage* 20: 1964–1970.

de Bruijn, E.R., *et al.* (2003) Action monitoring in motor control: ERPs following selection. *Psychophysiology* 40: 786–795.

Dehaene, S., *et al.* (1994) Localization of a neural system for error detection and compensation. *Psychol Sci* 5: 303–305.

Desmond, J.E., *et al.* (2003) Increased frontocerebellar activation in alcoholics during verbal working memory: an fMRI study. *Neuroimage* 19: 1510–1520.

Drevets, W.C., Price, J.C., Kupfer, D.J., Kinahan, P.E., Lopresti, B., Holt, D., and Mathis, C. (1999) PET measures of amphetamine-induced dopamine release in ventral versus dorsal striatum. *Neuropsychopharmacology* 21: 694–709.

Due, D.L., Huettel, S.A., Hall, W.G., and Rubin, D.C. (2002) Activation in mesolimbic and visuospatial neural circuits elicited by smoking cues: evidence from functional magnetic resonance imaging. *Am J Psychiatry* 159: 954–960.

Duong, T., Kim, D.S., and Kim, S.G. (2000) *Field dependence of the early negative and late positive BOLD response at 4.7 T and 9.4 T.* Proceedings of the 8th Annual Meeting of ISMRM, 994.

Eldreth, D.A., *et al.* (2004) Abnormal brain activity in prefrontal brain regions in abstinent marijuana users. *Neuroimage* 23: 914–920.

Ernst, M., *et al.* (2002) Decision-making in a risk-taking task: a PET study. *Neuropsychopharmacology* 26: 682–691.

Ernst, M., *et al.* (2003) Decision-making in adolescents with behavior disorders and adults with substance abuse. *Am J Psychiatry* 160: 33–40.

Fallgatter, A.J., *et al.* (2004) Altered response control and anterior cingulate function in attention-deficit/hyperactivity disorder boys. *Clin Neurophysiol* 115: 973–981.

Febo, M., Segarra, A.C., Nair, G., Schmidt, K., Duong, T.Q., and Ferris, C.F. (2005) The neural consequences of repeated cocaine exposure revealed by functional MRI in awake rats. *Neuropsychopharmacology* 30: 936–943.

Febo, M., Segarra, A.C., Tenney, J.R., Brevard, M.E., Duong, T.Q., and Ferris, C.F. (2004). Imaging cocaine-induced changes in the mesocorticolimbic dopaminergic system of conscious rats. *J Neurosci Methods* 139(2): 167–176.

Fillmore, M.T. and Rush, C.R. (2002) Impaired inhibitory control of behavior in chronic cocaine users. *Drug Alcohol Depend* 66: 265–273.

Fillmore, M.T., Rush, C.R., and Marczinski, C.A. (2003) *Drug Alcohol Depend* 71: 143.

Finn, P.R., *et al.* (2002) Early-onset alcoholism with conduct disorder: go/no go learning deficits, working memory capacity, and personality. *Alcohol Clin Exp Res* 26: 186–206.

Forman, S.D., *et al.* (2004) Opiate addicts lack error-dependent activation of rostral anterior cingulate. *Biol Psychiatry* 55: 531–537.

Frankle, W.G. and Laruelle, M. (2002) Neuroreceptor imaging in psychiatric disorders. *Ann Nucl Med* 16(7): 437–446.

Garavan, H., *et al.* (1999) Right hemispheric dominance of inhibitory control: an event-related fMRI study. *Proc Natl Acad Sci USA* 96: 8301–8306.

Garavan, H., Pankiewicz, J., Bloom, A., *et al.* (2000) Cue-induced cocaine craving: neuroanatomical specificity for drug users and drug stimuli. *Am J Psychiatry* 157(11): 1789–1798.

Garavan, H., *et al.* (2002) Dissociable executive functions in the dynamic control of behaviour: inhibition, error detection and correction. *Neuroimage* 17: 1820–1829.

Gati, J., Menon, R.S., Ugurbil, K., and Rutt, B.K. (1997) Experimental determination of the BOLD field strength dependence in vessels and tissues. *Magn Reson Med* 38: 296–302.

Gilman, S., Koeppe, R.A., Adams, K. *et al.* (1996) Positron emission tomographic studies of cerebral benzodiazepine-receptor binding in chronic alcoholics. *Ann Neurol* 40(2): 163–171.

Goldstein, R.Z. and Volkow, N.D. (2002) Drug addiction and its underlying neurobiological basis: neuroimaging evidence for the involvement of the frontal cortex. *Am J Psychiatry* 159: 1642–1652.

Goldstein, R.Z., *et al.* (2001) Addiction changes orbitofrontal gyrus function: involvement in response inhibition. *NeuroReport* 12: 2595–2599.

Grant, S., London, E.D., Newlin, D.B., *et al.* (1996) Activation of memory circuits during cue-elicited cocaine craving. *Proc Natl Acad Sci USA* 93: 12040–12045.

Grant, S., *et al.* (2000) Drug abusers show impaired performance in a laboratory test of decision making. *Neuropsychologia* 38: 1180–1187.

Greenwald, M.K., Johanson, C.E., Moody, D.E., Woods, J.H., Kilbourn, M.R., Koeppe, R.A., Schuster, C.R., and Zubieta, J.K. (2003) Effects of buprenorphine maintenance dose on mu-opioid receptor availability, plasma concentrations, and antagonist blockade in heroin-dependent volunteers. *Neuropsychopharmacology* 28: 2000–2009.

Gruetter, R., Novotny, E.J., Boulware, S.D., Mason, G.F., Rothman, D.L., Shulman, G.L., Prichard, J.W., and Whulman, R.G. (1994)

Localised ^{13}C NMR spectroscopy in the human brain of amino acid labelling from D-[1-^{13}C] glucose. *J Neurochem* 63: 1377–1385.

Grusser, S.M., Wrase, J., Klein, S., Hermann, D., Smolka, M.N., Ruf, M., Weber-Fahr, W., Flor, H., Mann, K., Braus, D.F., and Heinz, A. (2004) Cue-induced activation of the striatum and medial prefrontal cortex is associated with subsequent relapse in abstinent alcoholics. *Psychopharmacology (Berl)* 175: 296–302.

Heinz, A., Ragan, P., Jones, D.W., Hommer, D., Williams, W., Knable, M.B., Gorey, J.G., Doty, L., Geyer, C., Lee, K.S., Coppola, R., Weinberger, D.R., and Linnoila, M. (1998) Reduced central serotonin transporters in alcoholism. *Am J Psychiatry* 155: 1544–1549.

Heinz, A., Jones, D.W., Mazzanti, C., *et al.* (2000) A relationship between serotonin transporter genotype and in vivo protein expression and alcohol neurotoxicity. *Biol Psychiatry* 47(7): 643–649.

Hester, R. and Garavan, H. (2004) Executive dysfunction in cocaine addiction: Evidence for discordant frontal, cingulate and cerebellar activity. *J Neuroscience* 24: 11017–11022.

Hester, R., Fassbender, C., and Garavan, H. (2004a) Individual differences in error processing: a review and meta-analysis of three event-related fMRI studies using the GO/NOGO task. *Cereb Cortex* 14(9): 966–973.

Hester, R., *et al.* (2004b) Beyond common resources: the cortical basis for resolving task interference. *Neuroimage* 23: 202–212.

Hester, R. and Garavan, H. (2005) Neural correlates of error detection with and without awareness. *Memory and Cognition* 33: 221–223.

Holroyd, C.B. and Coles, M.G.H. (2002) The neural basis of human error processing: reinforcement learning, dopamine, and the error-related negativity. *Psychol Rev* 109: 679–709.

Hu, X., Yacoub, E., Andersen, P., Vaughan, T., Adriany, G., Merkle, H., and Ugurbil, K. (2000) *Initial experience with fMRI in humans at 7 Tesla.* Proceedings of the 8th Annual Meeting of ISMRM, Denver, 935.

Hyder, F., Chase, J.R., Behar, K.L., Mason, G.F., Siddeek, M., Rothman, D.L., and Shulman, R.G. (1996) Increased tricarboxylic acid cycle flux in rat brain during forepaw stimulation. *Proc Natl Acad Sci USA* 93: 7612–7617.

Ireland, M.D., Lowe, A.S., Reavill, C., James, M.F., Leslie, R.A., and Williams, S.C. (2005) Mapping

the effects of the selective dopamine d2/d3 receptor agonist quinelorane using pharmacological MRI. *Neuroscience* 133: 315–326.

Kaufman, J.N. and Garavan, H. Acute effects of cocaine on the functional neuroanatomy of cognitive control (11.2, Nov).

Kaufman, J.N. *et al.* (2003) Cingulate hypoactivity in cocaine users during a GO/NOGO task as revealed by event-related fMRI. *J Neuroscience* 23: 7839–7843.

Kerns, J.G., *et al.* (2004) Anterior cingulate conflict monitoring and adjustments in control. *Science* 303: 1023–1026.

Khantzian, E.J. (1997) The self-medication hypothesis of substance abuse disorders: a reconsideration and recent applications. *Harv Rev Psychiatry* 4: 231–244.

Kling, M.A., Carson, R.E., Borg, L., Zametkin, A., Matochik, J.A., Schluger, J., Herscovitch, P., Rice, K.C., Ho, A., Eckelman, W.C., and Kreek, M.J. (2000) Opioid receptor imaging with positron emission tomography and [(18)F]cyclofoxy in long-term, methadone-treated former heroin addicts. *J Pharmacol Exp Ther* 295: 1070–1076.

Koob, G.F. and Le Moal, M. (1997) Drug abuse: hedonistic homeostatic dysregulation. *Science* 278: 52–58.

Kubler, A., Murphy, K., and Garavan, H. (2005) Effects of cocaine use on attentional control within and between verbal and visuospatial working memory. *Eur J Neurosci* 21: 1984–1992.

Laruelle, M., Abi-Dargham, A., van Dyck, C.H., Rosenblatt, W., Zea-Ponce, Y., Zoghbi, S.S., Baldwin, R.M., Charney, D.S., Hoffer, P.B., Kung, H.F., *et al.* (1995) SPECT imaging of striatal dopamine release after amphetamine challenge. *J Nucl Med* 36: 1182–1190.

Lee, S., Silva, A.C., Urgurbil, K., and Kim, S.G. (1999) Diffusion weighted spin-echo fMRI at 9.4T: microvascular/tissue contribution to BOLD signal changes. *Magn Reson Med* 42(5): 919–928.

Lingford-Hughes, A.R., Acton, P.D., Gacinovic, S., *et al.* (1998) Reduced levels of GABA-benzodiazepine receptor in alcohol dependency in the absence of grey matter atrophy. *Br J Psychiatry* 173: 116–122.

Lingford-Hughes, A., Hume, S.P., Feeney, A., Hirani, E., Osman, S., Cunningham, V.J., Pike, V.W., Brooks, D.J., and Nutt, D.J. (2002) Imaging the GABA-benzodiazepine receptor subtype containing the alpha5-subunit in vivo with [11C]Ro 15 4513 positron emission tomography. *J Cereb Blood Flow Metab* 22: 878–889.

Liu, X., *et al.* (1998) Smaller volume of prefrontal lobe in polysubstance abusers: a magnetic resonance imaging study. *Neuropsychopharmacology* 18: 243–252.

London, E.D., Ernst, M., Grant, S., Bonson, K., and Weinstein, A. (2000) Orbitofrontal cortex and human drug abuse: functional imaging. *Cereb Cortex* 10: 334–42.

Lowe, A.S., Williams, S.C., Symms, M.R., Stolerman, I.P., and Shoaib, M. (2002) Functional magnetic resonance neuroimaging of drug dependence: naloxone-precipitated morphine withdrawal. *Neuroimage* 17(2): 902–910.

Lyvers, M. and Yakimoff, M. (2003) Neuropsychological correlates of opiod dependence and withdrawal. *Addict Behav* 28: 605–611.

Martinez, D., Broft, A., Foltin, R.W., Slifstein, M., Hwang, D.R., Huang, Y., Perez, A., Frankle, W.G., Cooper, T., Kleber, H.D., Fischman, M.W., Laruelle, M., and Frankle, W.G. (2004) Cocaine dependence and d2 receptor availability in the functional subdivisions of the striatum: relationship with cocaine-seeking behavior. *Neuropsychopharmacology* 29(6): 1190–1202.

Matochik, J.A., *et al.* (2003) Frontal cortical tissue composition in abstinent cocaine abusers: a magnetic resonance imaging study. *Neuroimage* 19: 1095–1102.

Mazas, C.A., *et al.* (2000) Decision-making biases, antisocial personality, and early-onset alcoholism. *Alcohol: Clin Exp Res* 24: 1036–1040.

McCann, U.D., Szabo, Z., Scheffel, U., Dannals, R.F., and Ricaurte, G.A. (1998a) Positron emission tomographic evidence of toxic effect of MDMA ('Ecstasy') on brain serotonin neurons in human beings. *Lancet* 352: 1433–1437.

McCann, U.D., Wong, D.F., Yokoi, F., Villemagne, V., Dannals, R.F., and Ricaurte, G.A. (1998b) Reduced striatal dopamine transporter density in abstinent methamphetamine and methcathinone users: evidence from positron emission tomography studies with [^{11}C]WIN-35,428. *J Neurosci* 18(20): 8417–8422.

Melichar, J.K., Hume, S.P., Williams, T.M., Daglish, M.R., Taylor, L.G., Ahmad, R., Malizia, A.L., Brooks, D.J., Myles, J.S., Lingford-Hughes, A., and Nutt, D.J. (2004) Using [^{11}C]-diprenorphine to image opioid receptor occupancy by methadone in opioid addiction: clinical and preclinical studies. *J Pharmacol Exp Ther.* doi: 10. 1124/pet.104. 072686.

Menon, R. and Goodyear, B.G. (1999) Submillimeter functional localization in human striate cortex using BOLD contrast at 4 Tesla: implications for the vascular point-spread function. *Magn Reson Med* 41(2): 230–235.

Monterosso, J., *et al.* (2001) Three decision-making tasks in cocaine-dependent patients: do they measure the same construct? *Addiction* 96: 1825–1837.

Moris, P., and Bachelard, H. (2003) Reflections on the application of 13C-MRS to research on brain metabolism. *NMR Biomed* 16: 303–312.

Morgan, D., Grant, K.A., Gage, H.D., Mach, R.H., Kaplan, J.R., Prioleau, O., Nader, S.H., Buchheimer, N., Ehrenkaufer, R.L., and Nader, M.A. (2002) Social dominance in monkeys: dopamine D2 receptors and cocaine self-administration. *Nat Neurosci* 5(2): 169–174.

Mugler, J.P. III, Driehuys, B., Brookeman, J.R., Cates, G.D., Berr, S.S., Bryant, R.G., Daniel, T.M., de Lange, E.E., Hunter Downs, J. II, Erickson, C.J., Happer, W., Hinton, D.P., Kassel, N.F., Maier, T., Phillips, C.D., Saam, B.T., Sauer, K.L., and Wagshul, M.E. (1997) MR imaging and spectroscopy using hyperpolarized ^{129}Xe gas: preliminary human results. *Magn Reson Med* 37: 809–815.

Myrick, H., Anton, R.F., Li, X., Henderson, S., Drobes, D., Voronin, K., and George, M.S. (2004) Differential brain activity in alcoholics and social drinkers to alcohol cues: relationship to craving. *Neuropsychopharmacology* 29: 393–402.

Navon, G., Song, Y.Q., Room, T., Appelt, S., Taylor, R.E., and Pines, A. (1996) Enhancement of solution NMR and MRI with laser-polarized xenon. *Science* 271(5257): 1848–1851.

Peoples, L.L. (2002) Will, anterior cingulate cortex, and addiction. *Science* 296: 1623–1624.

Petersson, J. (2004) Beyond relaxation contrast: agents for polarization enhancement in MRI. *Proc. 11th Ann. Meeting Int. Soc. Magn. Reson. Med*: 690.

Petry, N., *et al.* (1998) Shortened time horizons and insensitivity to future consequences in heroin addicts. *Addiction* 93: 729–738.

Pietrass, T., Gaede, H.C., Bifone, A., Pines, A., and Ripmeester, J.A. (1995) Monitoring xenon clathrate hydrate formation on ice surfaces with optically enhanced Xe-129 NMR. *J Am Chem Soc* 117(28): 7520–7525.

Reneman, L., Booij, J., de Bruin, K., Reitsma, J.B., de Wolff, F.A., Gunning, W.B., Den Heeten, G.J., and Van Den, B.W. (2001) Effects of dose, sex, and long-term abstention from use on toxic effects of MDMA (ecstasy) on brain serotonin neurons. *Lancet* 358: 1864–1869.

Repo, E., Kuikka, J.T., Bergstrom, K.A., Karhu, J., Hiltunen, J., and Tiihonen, J. (1999) Dopamine transporter and D2-receptor density in late-onset alcoholism. *Psychopharmacology (Berl)* 147: 314–318.

Ridderinkhof, K.R., *et al.* (2003) Alcohol consumption impairs detection of performance errors in mediofrontal cortex. *Science* 298: 2209–2211.

Rose, J.E., Behm, F.M., Westman, E.C., Mathew, R.J., London, E.D., Hawk, T.C., Turkington, T.G., and Coleman, R.E. (2003) PET studies of the influences of nicotine on neural systems in cigarette smokers. *Am J Psychiatry* 160: 323–333.

Rushworth, M.F.S., *et al.* (2004) Action sets and decisions in the medial frontal cortex. *Trends Cog Sci* 8: 410–417.

Ruth, U., Hof, T., Schmidt, J., Fick, D., and Jansch, H.J. (1999) Production of nitrogen-free, hyperpolarized Xe-129 gas. *Appl Phys B-Lasers and Optics* 68(1): 93–97.

Scheres, A., Oosterlaan, J., Swanson, J., Morein-Zamir, S., Meiran, N., Schut, H., Vlasveld, L., and Sergent, J.A. (2003) *J Ab Child Psychol* 31: 105.

Schlaepfer, T.E., Pearlson, G.D., Wong, D.F., Marenco, S., and Dannals, R.F. (1997) PET study of competition between intravenous cocaine and [^{11}C] raclopride at dopamine receptors in human subjects. *Am J Psychiatry* 154(9): 1209–1213.

Schultz, W., (1997) Dopamine neurons and their role in reward mechanisms. *Current Op Neurobiol* 7: 191–197.

Schultz, W. *et al.* (1997) A neural substrate of prediction and reward. *Science* 275: 1593–1599.

Sell, L.A., Morris, J., Bearn, J., Frackowiak, R.S., Friston, K.J., and Dolan, R.J. (1999) Activation of reward circuitry in human opiate addicts. *Eur J Neurosci* 11: 1042–1048.

Sell, L.A., Morris, J.S., Bearn, J., Frackowiak, R.S., Friston, K.J., and Dolan, R.J. (2000) Neural responses associated with cue-evoked

emotional states and heroin in opiate addicts. *Drug Alcohol Depend* 60: 207–216.

Semple, D.M., Ebmeier, K.P., Glabus, M.F., O'Carroll, R.E., and Johnstone, E.C. (1999) Reduced in vivo binding to the serotonin transporter in the cerebral cortex of MDMA ('ecstasy') users. *Br J Psychiatry* 175: 63–69.

Shoaib, M., Lowe, A.S., and Williams, S.C. (2004) Imaging localised dynamic changes in the nucleus accumbens following nicotine withdrawal in rats. *Neuroimage* 22(2): 847–854.

Sibson, N.R., Dhankhar, A., Mason, G.F., Rothman, D., Behar, K.L., and Shulman, R.G. (1998) Stoichiometric coupling of brain glucose metabolism and glutamatergic neuronal activity. *Proc Natl Acad Sci USA* 95: 316–321.

Stapleton, J.M., *et al.* (1995) Cerebral glucose utilization in polysubstance abuse. *Neuropsychopharmacology* 13: 21–31.

Stoltz, E., Villard, B., Meyerhoff, M., and Nacher, P.J. (1996) Polarization analysis of the light emitted by an optically pumped He-3 gas. *Appl Phys B-Lasers and Optics* 63(6): 635–640.

Stout, J.C., Rock, S.L., Campbell, M.C., Busemeyer, J.R., and Finn, P.R. (2005) Psychological processes underlying risky decisions in drug abusers. *Psychol Addict Behav* 19: 148–157.

Tarter, R.E., *et al.* (2003) Neurobehavioral disinhibition in childhood predicts early age at onset of substance use disorder. *Am J Psychiatry* 160: 1078–1085.

Thomasius, R., Petersen, K., Buchert, R., Andresen, B., Zapletalova, P., Wartberg, L., Nebeling, B., and Schmoldt, A. (2003) Mood, cognition and serotonin transporter availability in current and former ecstasy (MDMA) users. *Psychopharmacology (Berl)* 167: 85–96.

Tiihonen, J., Kuikka, J., Bergstrom, K., *et al.* (1995) Altered striatal dopamine re-uptake site densities in habitually violent and non-violent alcoholics. *Nat Med* 1(7): 654–657.

Volkow, N.D. and Fowler, J.S. (2000) Addiction, a disease of compulsion and drive: involvement of the orbitofrontal cortex. *Cereb Cortex* 10: 318–325.

Volkow, N.D., *et al.* (1992) Long-term frontal brain metabolic changes in cocaine abusers. *Synapse* 11: 184–190.

Volkow, N.D., Fowler, J.S., Wang, G.J., Hitzemann, R., Logan, J., Schyler, D.J.,

Dewey, S.L., and Wolf, A.P. (1993) Increased dopamine D2 receptor availability is associated with reduced frontal metabolism in cocaine users. *Synapse* 14: 169–177.

Volkow, N.D., Wang, G.J., Gatley, S.J., Fowler, J.S., Ding, Y.S., Logan, J., Hitzemann, R., Angrist, B., and Lieberman, J. (1996a) Temporal relationships between the pharmacokinetics of methylphenidate in the human brain and its behavioral and cardiovascular effects. *Psychopharmacology (Berl)* 123: 26–33.

Volkow, N.D., Wang, G.J., Fowler, J.S., Gatley, S.J., Ding, Y.S., Logan, J., Dewey, S.L., Hitzemann, R., and Lieberman, J. (1996b) Relationship between psychostimulant induced high and dopamine transporter occupancy. *Proc Natl Acad Sci USA* 93: 10388–10392.

Volkow, N.D., Wang, G.J., Fowler, J.S., et al. (1996c) Decreases in dopamine receptors but not in dopamine transporters in alcoholics. *Alcohol Clin Exp Res* 20(9): 1594–1598.

Volkow, N.D., Wang, G.J., Fischman, M.W., et al. (1997a) Relationship between subjective effects of cocaine and dopamine transporter occupancy. *Nature (Lond)* 386: 827–830.

Volkow, N.D., Wang, G.J., Fowler, J.S., Logan, J., Gatley, S.J., Hitzemann, R., Chen, A.D., Dewey, S.L., and Pappas, N. (1997b) Decreased striatal dopaminergic responsiveness in detoxified cocaine-dependent subjects. *Nature* 386: 830–833.

Volkow, N.D., Wang, G.J., Fowler, J.S., Logan, J., Gatley, S.J., Gifford, A., Hitzemann, R., Ding, Y.S., and Pappas, N. (1999a) Prediction of reinforcing responses to psychostimulants in humans by brain dopamine D2 receptor levels. *Am J Psychiatry* 156: 1440–1443.

Volkow, N.D., et al. (1999b) Imaging studies on the role of dopamine in cocaine reinforcement and addiction in humans. *J Psychopharmacology* 13: 337–345.

Volkow, N.D., Fowler, J.S., Wang, G.J., and Goldstein, R.Z. (2002a) Role of dopamine, the frontal cortex and memory circuits in drug addiction: insight from imaging studies. *Neurobiol Learn Mem* 78: 610–624.

Volkow, N.D., Wang, G.J., Fowler, J.S., Thanos, P.P., Logan, J., Gatley, S.J., Gifford, A., Ding, Y.S., Wong, C., Pappas, N., and Thanos, P. (2002b) Brain DA D2 receptors

predict reinforcing effects of stimulants in humans: replication study. *Synapse* 46: 79–82.

Volkow, N.D., Wang, G.J., Ma, Y., Fowler, J.S., Zhu, W., Maynard, L., Telang, F., Vaska, P., Ding, Y.S., Wong, C., and Swanson, J.M. (2003) Expectation enhances the regional brain metabolic and the reinforcing effects of stimulants in cocaine abusers. *J Neurosci* 23: 11461–11468.

Volkow, N.D., Fowler, J.S., and Wang, G.J. (2004) The addicted human brain viewed in the light of imaging studies: brain circuits and treatment strategies. *Neuropharmacology* 47: 3–13.

Waters, A.J., et al. (2003) Attentional bias predicts outcome in smoking cessation. *Health* 22: 378–387.

Wexler, B.E., Gottschalk, C.H., Fulbright, R.K., et al. (2001) Functional magnetic resonance imaging of cocaine craving. *Am J Psychiatry* 158(1): 86–95.

Whitlow, C., et al. (2004) Long-term heavy marijuana users make costly decisions on a gambling task. *Drug Alcohol Depend* 76: 107–111.

Whitlow, C., et al. (in press) Long-term heavy marijuana users choose high immediate gains despite higher future losses on a decision-making task. *Psychopharmacology*.

Wilson, S.J., Sayette, M.A., and Fiez, J.A. (2004) Prefrontal responses to drug cues: a neurocognitive analysis. *Nat Neurosci* 7: 211–214.

Wise, R.A. and Rompre, P.P. (1989) Brain dopamine and reward. *Ann Rev Psychology* 40: 191–225.

Xi, Z.X., Wu, G., Stein, E.A., and Li, S.J., (2004) Opiate tolerance by heroin self-administration: an fMRI study in rat. *Magn Reson Med* 52(1): 108–114.

Xu, H., Li, S.J., Bodurka, J., Zhao, X., Xi, Z.X., Stein, EA Xu, H., Li, S.J., Bodurka, J., Zhao, X., Xi, Z.X., and Stein, E.A. (2000) *Neuroreport* 11(5): 1085–1092.

Yechiam, E., et al. (2005) Individual differences in the response to forgone payoffs: an examination of high functioning drug abusers. *J Behav Decision Making* 18: 97–110.

Zubieta, J.K., Gorelick, D.A., Stauffer, R., Ravert, H.T., Dannals, R.F., and Frost, J.J. (1996) Increased mu opioid receptor binding detected by PET in cocaine-dependent men is associated with cocaine craving. *Nat Med* 2: 1225–1229.

CHAPTER

10

Drug Testing

David Cowan, David Osselton and Steven Robinson

1 EXECUTIVE SUMMARY

This review of drug testing outlines the methods available to analyse recreational, psychiatric, cognition-enhancing or mood-altering drugs. The review discusses the techniques currently used for the analysis of psychoactive drugs and attempts to fore-cast methods that are likely to find a place in drug analysis within the next few years and beyond. The review attempts to pre-dict how advances in analytical science, such as miniaturisation, linked with advances in electronics and increased instrumental sensitivity, might develop over the coming years.

Psychoactive drugs are chemically and structurally diverse and encompass a vast range of chemical entities. This review therefore considers drug testing on the basis of the analytical techniques employed rather than by the chemical or pharmacological classification of individual compounds. Examples are provided of the types of drug that may be tested for using different methods. The review includes a brief survey of inexpensive techniques that are suitable for near-patient monitoring, as well as those that require more complex laboratory analysis.

The principal interest of the commissioning body is the detection of drugs in living subjects rather than the dead, and we have confined discussion to biological specimens that may be easily collected from living persons.

The relative merits and limitations of various specimen types are discussed in relation to each analytical technique.

The three most likely significant advances will almost certainly be miniaturisation, enabling point-of-care analysis, high-throughput screening using an enhanced spectrophotometric detection of antibody binding of drugs of interest, and enhanced separation techniques for the discrimination of complex mixtures.

2 INTRODUCTION

The term 'psychoactive drug' is a loosely applied term used to describe substances that act on the central nervous system (CNS) to exert a psychological effect. There are many types of psychoactive drug which, for the purpose of this chapter, are considered to fall into two categories: those that are widely used for medicinal purposes and although they have some abuse potential are largely not abused, and those that have a significant abuse potential.

The purpose of drug testing is to determine whether an individual has used any particular substance that might have affected their well-being or behaviour. The most common scenarios where testing is undertaken to detect psychoactive drug use include workplace drug testing, forensic drug testing (e.g. with drugs and driving) and compliance with treatment. Most drug testing is restricted to these areas and is not widely applied to the analysis of psychoactive drugs used in medical practice unless they pose a threat to the safety of the individual. In workplace drug testing and treatment compliance testing, the objective of the procedure is to extend the window of detection to determine whether or not the subject had been taking drugs over a period of days or possibly months prior to specimen collection. In forensic drug testing, interest is focused more on whether an individual may have been affected by a drug substance at the time of a particular event such as driving a car or at the time of an assault. In order to obtain the most appropriate information, therefore, different types of samples may be used, depending on the reason for testing.

Testing for drugs of abuse evolved in the United States during the 1960s within the armed forces and was used extensively to monitor members of the armed forces on active duty in the 1970s. All early drug testing and most testing today is based on urine samples. As technology and our understanding of how drugs behave in the body have increased, screening tests have become available that may be used on a range of samples. The significant increase in the availability of psychoactive drugs in the mid- to late-1990s stimulated an increased interest in drug testing that resulted in the development of tests suitable for use within the workplace (point-of-care) as well as in the laboratory.

At the present time, testing for common drugs of abuse, whether in a clinical, forensic, sport or workplace setting, is usually undertaken as a two-step process. The first step normally involves a simple and inexpensive screening test followed by a more specific and definitive identification test (called a confirmatory analysis) that may also be quantitative. This review outlines the techniques currently in use for the screening and confirmation of commonly encountered psychoactive drugs and then considers how advances in technology and miniaturisation might be applied over the coming years. Discussion centres on the types of test available for the analysis of common drugs of abuse and medicinal drugs, as it is not possible to predict with any certainty what new psychoactive drugs will be introduced during the forthcoming 20 or more years. It might reasonably be predicted, however, that as advances are made in the miniaturisation of electronics and microfluidics (see Section 5), tests will be developed for near-patient use that will combine both screening and confirmation in a single test, and that the range of tests on offer will be extensive.

Most of the psychoactive drugs subject to misuse today have been used for centuries, including alcohol, opium derivatives, cannabis and cocaine, and it is envisaged that these, together with amphetamine and related compounds, will continue to be the most popular substances used for the foreseeable future. The most widely used psychoactive drugs (alcohol, heroin, morphine, cannabis and cocaine) are derived from natural sources or are easily synthesised from widely used industrial reagents in the case of synthetics such as amphetamines. These substances are easy to produce in large quantities at relatively low cost. Until supplies become limited there is little incentive for users to switch to alternatives. Although methods for the synthesis of numerous synthetic psychoactive amines have been published (Shulgin and Shulgin, 1991) few of these substances have attracted widespread use and few are regularly encountered other than amphetamine, methylamphetamine (MA), methylenedioxyamphetamine (MDA) and methylenedioxymethylamphetamine (MDMA, i.e. Ecstasy).

In addition to these common drugs of misuse, there are numerous psychoactive substances used medicinally that can affect performance, including the benzodiazepine anti-anxiety and sleep-inducing agents (e.g. diazepam, temazepam and flunitrazepam), hypnotics (e.g. zopiclone, zolpidem and zaleplon) and antipsychotics and antidepressants (e.g. fluoxetine and amitriptyline).

The analytical methods employed today in drug testing for psychoactive substances are determined by the chemistry of the individual substances. As our understanding increases about how and where different drugs act in the body, drug testing may turn towards the measurement of endogenous markers within the body, for example, the monitoring of neurotransmitters and neurotransmitter binding sites rather than the drugs themselves. But for the next 5–10 years at least, testing is likely to remain orientated towards the determination of the presence of psychoactive substances or their breakdown products. It is already possible to use electromagnetic scanning techniques to monitor changes to receptor binding in certain circumstances, but this technique is costly and therefore unlikely to be used routinely for drug-abuse screening.

The analytical techniques used for drug detection also depend on the chemical and physical properties of each substance or its breakdown products. Consequently, there is no universal test that can be applied to detect the presence of a drug and it is necessary to employ a range of different tests for different drugs.

3 TEST MATRICES

The chemistry of any particular drug and its biological breakdown products (metabolites) determines how it is distributed within the various body tissues and fluids, and therefore the time-window during which it may be detected in the various body secretions and excretions. Drugs that are lipid (fat) soluble, such as cannabinoids, tend to accumulate in the body's fat depots and may subsequently be released over a period of days or weeks into the general circulation of the body, whereas those that are more water-soluble can be eliminated within a few hours. The time spans over which drugs can be detected in different tissues may be influenced by a number of factors. These include the state of health of an individual, presence of disease, age, the properties of the drug and its distribution within the body, the quantity of drug taken, whether drug intake involved single or chronic dosing, and the sensitivity of the analytical methods used.

Historically, urine has been collected for drug testing as it is easy to collect, may be collected in large volumes and is easy to analyse. However, as a consequence of improvements in analytical technology, blood, oral fluid, sweat and hair are now being used with increasing frequency, depending on the rationale behind the test. Urine, oral fluid, sweat and hair are favoured for use in many drug testing applications because they can be collected non-invasively by suitably trained lay people. The collection of blood, however, is regarded as invasive and requires the use of more highly trained collectors such as doctors, nurses and phlebotomists.

3.1 Urine

Urine is the most widely used specimen employed for drug testing. Urine is produced in large quantities, is easy to collect and offers a wide window of detection, often facilitating the detection of drug use over a period of 2–4 days after the last dose was consumed. Table 10.1 summarises the approximate windows of detection for common drugs of abuse in urine. It should be noted that detection times can only be regarded as approximate since they are dependent on a number of factors, including the route by which the drug entered the body, the quantity taken, the frequency of use and the sensitivity and limits of detection of the assay.

The advantages and disadvantages associated with urine as a matrix (medium) for drug testing are summarised in Table 10.2. In many ways urine is an ideal matrix for drug testing since it is relatively easy to collect and analyse and, depending on the elapsed time between drug use and specimen collection, drugs may be present in much greater quantities than in other matrices. But because of the ease with which chemicals that may interfere with the analysis may be added to specimens during collection, observed collection may be necessary to prevent specimen adulteration. Observed collection is costly, unpleasant for both the donor and collector, and is regarded as a potential infringement of personal privacy.

TABLE 10.1 Approximate detection times for commonly used psychoactive drugs in urine (from Saunders and Barnes, 2002).

Drug	Approximate detection time in urine
Amphetamines	1–2 days
Benzodiazepines	0.5–7 days (depends on half-life)
Cannabinoids (single use)	Up to 3 days
Cannabinoids (moderate use – four times a week)	4 days
Cannabinoids (chronic use)	21 days or longer
Cocaine metabolites	2–3 days
Gamma-hydroxybutyrate (GHB)	0.5 day
Ketamine	2–4 days
Methadone	7–9 days (maintenance dosing)
Methamphetamine (single use)	1–3 days
Methamphetamine (heavy use)	3–5 days
Opiates	2 days
Phencyclidine (PCP)	8 days (approximately)

TABLE 10.2 Advantages and disadvantages of urine with respect to drug testing.

Advantages	Disadvantages
Easy to collect	Observed collection seen as infringement of privacy
Drugs present in high concentrations relative to other specimens	Results difficult to interpret – not ideal for forensic testing
Large volumes available	Often contains metabolites and little unchanged parent drug
Provides a history of recent drug use between 2 days and several weeks	Easy to adulterate unless collection is observed
A wide range of drug substances can be detected	
Easy to analyse	
Inexpensive to analyse	
Suitable for workplace and compliance testing	
Untreated urine can be screened directly without the need for sample pretreatment	
Point-of-care test kits are available for commonly abused drugs	

3.2 Blood

Blood is primarily used in forensic and some areas of clinical testing and is not commonly employed when screening for drugs of abuse. The advantage of blood analysis is that it provides information about how much of the drug is present in the circulating blood and can give an indication of whether the donor of the specimen is likely to be affected by the drug at the time of collection. But blood collection requires specially trained personnel and can be costly, its collection is regarded as invasive, and current analytical methods require extensive sample pretreatment prior to analysis, which is expensive.

The advantages and disadvantages of using blood for drug testing are summarised in Table 10.3. One of the potentially exciting consequences associated with the developments of miniaturisation combined with microfluidics is the possibility of being able

TABLE 10.3 Advantages and disadvantages of blood drug testing.

Advantages	Disadvantages
Provides indication of recent use	Requires specially trained personnel to collect specimens
Difficult for donor to adulterate	Low concentrations of drugs present, hence relatively short window of detection
Results can be interpreted	Analysis requires specialised laboratory facilities
	Analysis is complex, therefore tends to be costly
	Current technologies not developed for point-of-care testing

to analyse blood without the requirement for complex and expensive sample preparation procedures.

The use of blood for general non-clinical drug testing may not develop, owing to the issues surrounding its collection.

3.3 Oral Fluid

Recent advances in a technique known as lateral flow immunalysis (see Section 4.1) have resulted in the development of point-of-care drug tests for the analysis of oral fluid, a term that covers fluid collected from the mouth, including saliva and other secretions, together with cellular and food debris. It was originally believed that drugs secreted via saliva reflected the concentration of drug present in the circulating blood and that collection of this matrix would enable results to be interpreted. More recently, it has been demonstrated that the concentrations of some drugs in oral fluid (e.g. mono-acetylmorphine, morphine, codeine, cocaine and benzoylecgonine) may be exceptionally high and would not be representative of concentrations in the circulating blood. The most likely explanation for this phenomenon is buccal absorption following smoking or snorting (inhaling the drug in powder form), since the effect is particularly noticeable in association with drugs that are smoked or snorted, such as heroin, cocaine and crack cocaine.

Oral fluid is particularly attractive as a matrix for drug testing as it is inexpensive, easy and non-intrusive to collect, requires no special facilities, is difficult to adulterate and does not require complex sample preparation prior to confirmatory testing. It can be reasonably predicted that methods for oral-fluid drug screening will predominate during the next 5–10 years. The relative advantages and disadvantages associated with oral fluid as a matrix for drug testing are summarised in Table 10.4. An example of a hand-held point-of-care oral-fluid test device is shown in Figure 10.1.

3.4 Sweat

Many drugs are excreted in sweat and hence this matrix can be used as a source

TABLE 10.4 Advantages and disadvantages of oral-fluid drug testing.

Advantages	Disadvantages
Easy to collect	Sample size limited – could be overcome by miniaturisation
Can be collected and tested on site with no intrusion of privacy	Drug concentrations may be low and subsequently difficult to analyse
Difficult to adulterate	Interpretation complex
Can detect a wide range of drug substances	Confirmatory analysis requires sensitive analytical facilities
Suitable for workplace, compliance and forensic testing	Cannabis derivatives and benzodiazepines do not pass readily from blood into saliva, therefore potential sensitivity issues for general screening
Point-of care-test kits available for commonly abused drugs	
Indicates recent drug use for non-smoked drugs	
Nature of the matrix amenable for the development of new analytical techniques	

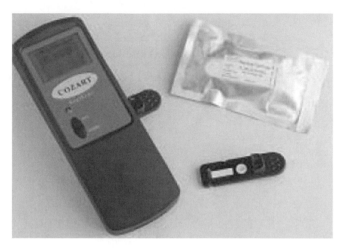

FIGURE 10.1   Hand-held point-of-care oral fluid test.

material for drug testing. Few manufacturers have devoted attention to the use of sweat as a routine specimen for drug testing, possibly because it is not easy to collect in large quantities for multiple drug screening and subsequent confirmatory analysis. Two types of test are currently available for testing drugs in sweat. One (see Figure 10.2) comprises a small absorbent pad that is wiped across an area of skin such as the forehead of an individual to collect a small quantity of sweat that can be subsequently analysed by lateral flow immunoassay. The other system comprises a small absorbent patch enclosed

within a tamper-evident adhesive cover that sticks to the skin rather like an Elastoplast dressing.

The patch is applied after cleaning the skin by swabbing and left in place for a number of days, during which excreted drugs are absorbed onto the pad prior to collection. The sweat patch is subsequently sent to the laboratory for analysis. The principal use of sweat patches is for the screening of prison inmates in the US.

The major disadvantages of sweat testing are that only very small amounts of sweat are collected, thus limiting the extent of analysis

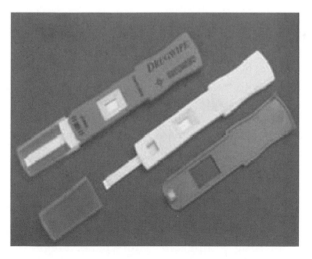

FIGURE 10.2   Point-of-care sweat testing device.

TABLE 10.5   Advantages and disadvantages of sweat drug testing.

Advantages	Disadvantages
Non-invasive – easy to collect	Not widely used – currently available tests are expensive if multidrug testing is required
Point-of-care tests available for common drugs of abuse	Small sample volumes collected – requires very sensitive and expensive analytical procedures
Sweat collection patches can be used to monitor drug-use history	High possibility of external contamination with simple point-of-care tests
	Interpretation difficult

with the present state of technology, and that skin can potentially become contaminated with drugs via environmental exposure prior to collection of the specimen. If a point-of-care device is used, prior swabbing of the skin to remove external contamination would also remove traces of drugs excreted in sweat. Although sweat testing is possible, these drawbacks have limited its take-up and we envisage that it will have only limited application in the future. The advantages and disadvantages associated with sweat testing are outlined in Table 10.5.

3.5 Hair

The introduction of methods for the analysis of drugs in hair has developed rapidly in recent years because hair theoretically offers a non-intrusive way to monitor an individual's drug-taking history over several months or even years. Drugs enter the hair during its formation within the scalp and also by diffusion into the hair from the outside environment or via sweat and sebaceous secretions. Since drugs can enter hair following environmental exposure it is desirable that testing is designed that can detect drug metabolites, since these can only be formed within the body and allow the analyst to distinguish between drug use and external contamination. The advantages and disadvantages of hair for drug testing are summarised in Table 10.6.

Hair may be used to back up disputed urine or oral fluid tests, particularly where an individual claims not to be a regular drug user and that, for example, his or her drink was spiked without their knowledge. In these circumstances, with hair analysis it may be possible to distinguish one-time from chronic drug use. Drug binding and subsequent retention in hair may be influenced by the types of melanin present (black or blond hair) and is thus subject to potential genetic and racial bias. Hair testing is currently confined to laboratory testing and is relatively expensive. The main uses of hair testing at the present time are in child custody dispute cases where one parent may be alleging the other to be unsuitable to have custody of a child because he or she is a drug user, or in cases where a urine drug test has been disputed.

4 ANALYTICAL METHODS

Drug detection techniques currently in use for the analysis of drugs in forensic, clinical, workplace and research environments are summarised in Table 10.7.

4.1 Routine Techniques in Use Today

Screening tests usually employ antibodies directed at a region of a test molecule, which is usually shared with other structurally

TABLE 10.6 Advantages and disadvantages of hair testing.

Advantages	Disadvantages
Provides history of drug use – several months – limited mainly by length of hair available for analysis	Prone to external contamination – essential to be able to show presence of drug metabolites to exclude allegations of external contamination
Specimens stable for years	Expensive to analyse – requires specialist laboratory facilities
Wide range of drugs can be detected in hair	Not suitable for point-of-care testing
Non-invasive to collect	Need to allow hair to grow for approximately 10 days after drug use prior to collection of specimens
Particularly useful if subject is required to be tested days or weeks after last drug use	Limited interpretation
Can be used in exhumed or mummified bodies to determine drug exposure prior to death	Results may be affected by cosmetic treatments such as dyeing and perming
	Some indication of racial or genetic bias
	Head hair can be shaved in an attempt to foil the test

related compounds. For example, the opiate drugs (heorin, morphine, codeine, dihydrocodeine) are structurally related to morphine, and an antibody raised against morphine will also react with codeine and heroin, among others. This is called cross-reactivity. A positive result in an opiate assay is therefore not specific enough to be of diagnostic value, but differentiates between someone who has taken an opiate and someone who has not. An immunoassay is a flexible technique that can provide a rapid, inexpensive and convenient method to screen large numbers of samples in a variety of matrices and allow the differentiation of negative from positive specimens, thus preventing the need for further, more complicated and expensive processing or investigation.

The reaction between antibody and drug molecule is measured by using a label which emits a detectable signal. Labels used in immunoassay include radioisotopes (RIA), enzymes, chemiluminescent molecules, particles such as colloidal gold, latex beads, rare earth metals, and fluorescent molecules. Immunoassay formats vary from systems designed for rapid point-of-care testing of a single sample through to fully automated systems that can process thousands of samples per day.

Enzyme immunoassay (EIA) and enzyme-linked immunosorbent assay (ELISA) are the most frequently used drug-screening techniques, and are often used interchangeably to describe non-radioisotopic assays. EIA and ELISA have largely replaced RIA as the assay system of choice because radioisotopes have more health and safety constraints on their use than enzyme-based reactions.

Immunoassay is the preferred screening technique in many areas, e.g. therapeutic drug monitoring, toxicological and workplace drug testing. The main difference between these applications is the degree of quantification required, and the selection of antibodies with the required

TABLE 10.7 Analytical techniques currently used for drug analysis in forensic, clinical and research applications in the UK.

Analytical technique[1]	Sensitivity	Scale of current use	Extent of likely future use	Matrix[2]	Suitable for point-of-care use	Applicable to a wide range of drugs
Immuno procedures	+++	++++	++++	BUHSOP	Yes	+++
General spectrophotometry (ultraviolet, infrared, fluorescence, visible)	+	+++	++	P	Yes	++++
Raman	+ → +++	+	+++	SOP	Not yet	++
Nuclear magnetic resonance	+ → ++	+	+++	BUP	No	+++
Gas chromatography–mass spectrometry	+++	++++	+++	All	Not yet	+++
Liquid chromatography–mass spectrometry	++++	+	++++	BUHSOP	Not yet	++++
Isotope ratio mass spectrometry	+	+	++	UP	No	++
Thin-layer chromatography	+	++	++	BUOP	No	++++
Gas chromatography–nitrogen phosphorous detector	++	++	+	BUSOP	No	++++
Gas chromatography–flame ionisation detector	+	+	+++	BBrUSOP	No	+++
Liquid chromatography–ultraviolet detector	+	++	+	BUP	No	++
Chemiluminescence	+++(+)	+	++	All	Not yet	++
Electrochemical detector	+++(+)	+	+	All	No	++
Capillary electrophoresis	+++(+)	+	+++	BUHSOP	Not yet	++++
Supercritical fluid chromatography	++	+	++	BUSOP	No	++
Time-of-flight mass spectrometry	+++	++	++++	P	Yes	++++

+ Low use/sensitivity; +++ High use/sensitivity. Matrix: B = blood; Br = breath; H = hair; O = oral fluid; S = sweat; U = urine; P = powders and solids.
[1] This is a generic table and does not differentiate between techniques that do or do not require sample preparation/purification.
[2] Applicability at concentrations less than 1 part per million.

cross-reactivity profiles. For example, drug-monitoring assays may require highly specific antibodies that are reactive only with a single chemical entity, whereas immunoassays used in toxicology or drug-abuse screening may be designed to be broadly cross-reactive with a whole drug group.

A further criterion for assay selection is whether the result is required immediately, or whether the collected sample can be sent to a laboratory for analysis. Most immunoassays are performed in the laboratory, either using plates with 96 or more reaction wells, allowing many samples to be analysed simultaneously, or on large autoanalysers (Figure 10.3) can process many hundreds of samples per hour. Homogeneous immunoassays do not require the separation of bound and free fractions, and as a result have been automated successfully in a number of different systems. Examples of such assays include enzyme multiplied immunoassay technique (EMIT), cloned enzyme donor immunoassay (CEDIA), fluorescence polarisation immunoassay (FPIA) and kinetic interaction of microparticles in solution (KIMS).

Point-of-care single-use cartridges are basically variants of a competitive ELISA assay run on a solid-phase strip rather than inside a well or tube. These tests employ a heterogeneous lateral flow mechanism using antibodies labelled with colloidal gold or other reactant particles which must be separated from the matrix before development of the result (Figures 10.4 and 10.5).

Figure 10.6 illustrates the process of 'lateral flow' screening for a single drug analyte. A drug-protein derivative is bound to a nitrocellulose membrane in a band at a

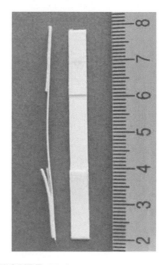

FIGURE 10.4 Lateral flow strip.

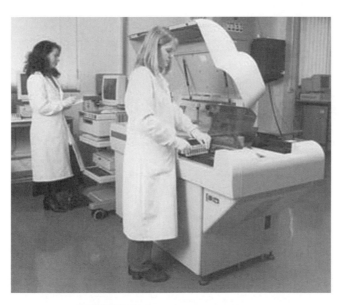

FIGURE 10.3 Laboratory analyser.

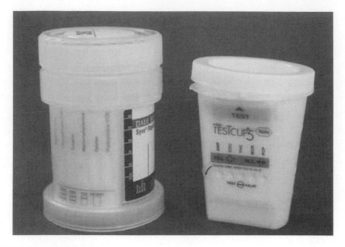

FIGURE 10.5   Lateral flow strip mounted on urine collection containers.

defined position on the strip (Figure 10.6). An antibody labelled with colloidal gold, coloured latex or an alternative visualisation probe is located in a pad that overlaps with the nitrocellulose membrane close to the point of the test strip where the sample is introduced. When urine, diluted oral fluid or some other liquid that might contain drugs is added to the pad, the labelled antibody migrates from the pad onto the cellulose

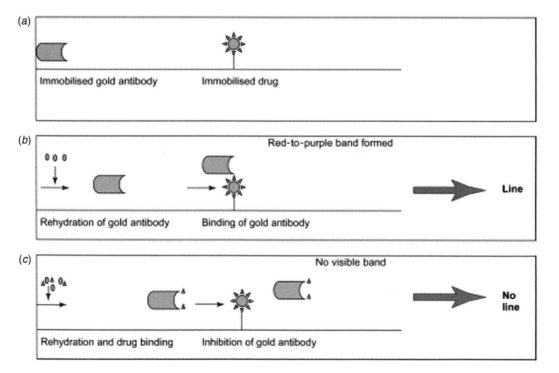

FIGURE 10.6   A competitive lateral flow immunoassay (Hand and Baldwin, 2004, reproduced with permission of the Royal Pharmaceutical Society).

membrane by capillary action. As the sample and rehydrated gold-labelled antibody flow along the membrane, any drug in the sample binds to the labelled antibody and inhibits it from binding to the immobilised drug on the membrane (Figure 10.6b and c). Separation of bound and free drug continues with the movement of liquid along the membrane strip. Where a specimen contains no drug, the antibody binds to the immobilised drug forming a visible line. In specimens containing drugs, the antibody binding sites are taken up by the drug in the specimen resulting in no antibody binding to the immobilised drugs on the membrane. A positive result is therefore indicated by no coloured band being formed on the strip, whereas a line will be observed if the donor's specimen does not contain drugs. It is possible to add a number of drug-derivative bands in different positions along the length of the nitrocellulose membrane together. With suitable matching labelled antibodies this allows the analysis of multiple drugs to be undertaken simultaneously in a single test cartridge.

Most commercially available test strips are interpreted visually by the test operator. However, the criticism has been offered that visual interpretation may be subjective. A number of point-of-care test strips are now being developed by the manufacturers to be read using small portable readers based on digital imaging to facilitate more accurate and consistent results (Figure 10.1).

Lateral-flow immunoassay test strips based on colloidal gold-labelled antibodies are currently limited to performing up to a maximum of around five or six tests per strip. This is usually sufficient for a drug-testing clinic, or for an employer who is mainly interested in determining whether a subject has used commonly available drugs of abuse. The upconverting phosphor system developed by OraSure Technologies, however, has the potential to offer up to 15 or more tests per strip. This could in theory offer clinicians much more information, perhaps including tests to determine whether individuals were infected with HIV, hepatitis and other drug-related diseases.

The future of immunoassay-based screening tests for drugs other than those currently subject to misuse is limited by the availability of suitable antibodies, and by market forces. The cost involved in the development and production of suitable antibodies is high and unless substantial commercial sales are predicted, companies involved with the production of test kits are reluctant to risk investment. The result is that there is always a significant time lag between a new drug being encountered and the availability of an immunoassay test for the new drug. Past experience has shown that drug test manufacturers have been reluctant to develop screening tests for the European market alone as this was perceived to be too small to be commercially viable. Given the assumption, however, that a suitable commercial market is available, the next predicted development in immunoassay screening is likely to involve the miniaturisation of tests so that 20 or more assays can be performed on a microchip platform. At least one company is currently developing an automated laboratory-based microchip system capable of offering the rapid screening of several hundred urine or oral-fluid samples per day for common drugs of abuse. Within a few years, such a system could be miniaturised to facilitate portability. The limitations associated with immunoassay testing might stimulate the development of drug testing based on different technologies in the future as miniaturisation is developed further.

4.2 The Fuel Cell

Fuel cell technology has been in use since the 1980s for measuring the amount of volatile substances, and in particular alcohol, in breath. Because fuel cells are small and relatively inexpensive, they are ideally suited for use in small portable or hand-held screening devices and have found widespread application for use by police officers at the roadside and also in workplace drug testing.

It is now possible to link alcohol-detecting fuel cells to electronic locks that can only be opened when an alcohol-free specimen of breath has been supplied. Such devices have been proposed to control entry onto the bridge of a ship or to prevent drivers from being able to start their car engines if they have more than a predetermined concentration of alcohol in their breath. In principle this offers a means of preventing an intoxicated person from driving while under the influence of alcohol, but is not totally secure and has not been widely implemented at the time of writing. The use of devices as a means of harm reduction is still rather limited. Fuel cell technology is particularly suitable for the analysis of volatile solvents and is unlikely to be applicable to the analysis of non-volatile substances or solid-dose formulations.

4.3 Mass Spectrometry (MS)

Any positive result from a screening test must be subjected to further, more specific, confirmatory analysis to identify and quantify the substance taken. The acknowledged 'gold standard' technique for drug identification is Mass Spectrometry (MS), coupled either to a gas chromatograph (GC–MS) or liquid chromatograph (LC–MS) to separate the compounds in a complex mixture. The mass spectrometer is a detector that produces a signal based on the structure of the analyte itself, and so is compound-specific. There are several types of mass spectrometer, but the most common for drug analysis use the quadrupole, ion trap and time-of-flight (TOF) mass analysers.

In some clinical and toxicological drug testing laboratories, LC–MS, or more specifically its powerful sibling technique LC–MS–MS, is being used to screen and confirm medicinal drugs and drugs of abuse. The cost of these systems can be prohibitive, but high-throughput applications make it more cost-effective. Mass spectrometry in its various configurations (e.g. GC–MS, or LC–MS, or TOF) is highly versatile and can be used to analyse common drugs of abuse and most drugs used in medical practice.

4.4 Liquid Chromatography–Mass Spectrometry (LC–MS)

This is one of many hyphenated techniques that combine the separation of components in complex mixtures such as biofluids with a sensitive means of detection and identification. In this case, the separation is facilitated by a flow of liquid under pressure through a short (10–20cm length, 2–5mm diameter) metal column packed with a silica-based medium. The components in the mixture will ideally interact with the medium to differing degrees and so will separate spatially. As the individual components leave the column, they pass into the mass spectrometer, where controlled fragmentation occurs. Measurement of the abundance and masses of the fragments produced gives a very specific 'mass spectrum' of the compound, which is then searchable against standard reference libraries of spectra to assist in obtaining an absolute identification of the compound.

The separation in this case is usually done at room temperature, making it ideally suited to the analysis of thermally sensitive compounds. It is also suited to the analysis of large molecules (e.g. small peptides), parent drugs and their conjugates (especially glucuronides and sulphates), which can provide information on the time since ingestion or administration. One example is the simultaneous measurement of free (non-conjugated) morphine and its more water-soluble glucuronide metabolites. A further benefit of this technique is that sample pretreatment and derivatisation are often unnecessary (unlike with GC–MS), which saves time and money. LC–MS is routinely used in toxicology, research and pharmaceutical laboratories, and many methods are available in the scientific literature for the separation, detection and quantification of many drugs and their metabolites.

An enhancement of this technique, LC–MS–MS, involves the addition of a second fragmentation facility and a second mass spectrometer. This can be used to generate structural information on individual fragments produced from the first fragmentation. These 'daughter' mass spectra provide additional discrimination where structurally similar compounds produce the same mass fragments. The use of MS–MS also improves sensitivity and is suitable for the analysis of a wide range of drug compounds that exert psychoactive effects. There are published methods which can screen a single sample extract for several compounds simultaneously using LC–MS–MS, demonstrating its analytical capability and value. It is likely that LC–MS–MS will soon replace GC–MS as the routine laboratory analytical tool for drug analysis. Modern LC columns are now being developed to provide greater resolution, or separating power, but require higher pressures to push the liquid through the columns. It is envisaged that these higher resolution systems will become routine in the next 10 years.

4.5 Gas Chromatography–Mass Spectrometry (GC–MS)

This is probably the most commonly used analytical technique in all fields of drug testing. Often referred to as the 'gold standard', this technique effects separation using the flow of a gas (usually helium) to carry the vaporised sample through a long (15–60m length, 0.2–0.5mm diameter) column whose inner surface is coated with a silica-based medium. The entire column is held in an oven, and heat is used to effect separation of the compounds from the medium. The sample must be soluble in a volatile organic solvent to allow vaporisation upon introduction into the gas flow, and must be thermally stable to withstand the high temperatures (up to 300°C) required to achieve separation.

In order to produce satisfactory separation and resolution, it is frequently necessary to perform sample clean-up (either liquid/liquid or solid-phase extraction) and

then derivatisation, the addition of a chemical 'cap' to cover up potentially active functional groups. This takes longer, but the result is better chromatographic separation than LC because the derivative has a higher mass and so produces more discriminatory mass spectra. The mass spectrometer is the same as that used in LC–MS, but there are very different methods of sample introduction to accommodate either a high pressure flow of liquid solvent, or helium gas.

Many toxicology laboratories will use a combination of LC– and GC–MS to enable the identification and quantification of any drug or metabolite known to have been ingested, or indicated from a preliminary screening test. Instrumentation is moderately expensive but, with automated sample introduction, large cost-effective batches can be processed unattended. As with LC–MS, it is possible to add further fragmentation capability to give GC–MS–MS, which has the same benefits of enhanced specificity and discrimination.

4.6 Nuclear Magnetic Resonance (NMR) Spectroscopy

This technique, like mass spectrometry, measures a physical characteristic of a molecule (or more precisely, the nuclei of its component atoms), producing specific information about the structure of the molecule. The property in question is 'spin', with an energy change due to the spin of an atomic nucleus being measurable in a strong magnetic field. It is especially useful for detecting molecules containing isotopes of carbon, hydrogen, nitrogen, fluorine, silicon and phosphorus, which covers the vast majority of therapeutic and abused drugs and their metabolites. There are functional groups that do not produce NMR spectra, and so this technique is sometimes used to complement other analyses such as MS.

It is possible to couple a liquid chromatograph to the NMR instrument, allowing spectra to be obtained from complex biofluids, although low sensitivity is a problem for trace analysis. NMR spectroscopy is commonly used on pure compounds, solid dosage forms or where a high concentration of analyte is present. This instrumentation is not routinely used in analytical laboratories, but is used in the pharmaceutical industry to provide structural information capable of distinguishing polymorphic forms of the same drug.

A development of NMR technology is used in the diagnosis of disease states *in vivo*, with the aid of magnetic resonance imaging (MRI) scanning instruments. This points towards the future possibility of non-invasive drug detection using the same or similar techniques. We predict that this technique will be increasingly applied to the analysis of psychoactive drugs and their metabolites at their site of action in the body (body scanning) and to study their interactions with receptors.

4.7 Capillary Electrophoresis (CE)

This is purely a separation technique and must be coupled to a suitable detector to produce a measurable response. Instead of using a flow of gas or liquid to transport the sample through a separation medium, the innate electrical charge on the drug molecule is used to separate it from other molecules of differing size and charge. In classic electrophoresis, the sample is introduced into a channel, usually in a gel, and a strong electric field is applied that effects separation based on size as well as charge, small molecules travelling further and faster than heavy ones. Traditionally, this technique has been used to separate high molecular weight molecules such as proteins and DNA fragments, but smaller molecules can also be separated in this way. In principle, any molecule which is naturally charged or can be made charged in a buffered solution can be analysed using CE. The discovery that the same principles could be applied to molecules travelling through a narrow silica capillary, and produce more focused results, has led to considerable interest in CE for drug analysis. CE offers the ability to analyse most types of psychoactive

drug and their metabolites including peptides, but suffers from the fact that it requires a very sensitive device to detect the small concentration of components submitted to this technique.

Capillary electrophoresis is seen as complementary to LC, but with the advantage of utilising smaller sample volumes ($\sim$10µl). More analytes are detectable than in LC because negatively charged anions, positively charged cations and non-charged neutrals can be detected simultaneously. Although it is less sensitive than LC, CE lends itself to miniaturisation, and the potential for portable (or even handheld) devices is evident. Instrument costs are similar to those for LC, but CE is much cheaper to run, with much lower solvent requirements.

Possible detectors include ultraviolet (UV) absorption, laser-induced fluorescence or even MS. CE as an analytical technique is becoming more popular, many drugs and their metabolites have been analysed by CE and the number of published methods is growing, but it has not become widespread or routine in many laboratories because of the popularity of LC.

4.8 Thin-layer Chromatography (TLC)

Thin-layer chromatography is probably the oldest analytical technique still in use today, although its use is very much diminished with the advent of GC and LC techniques.

Separation is effected by the flow of solvent up a silica-coated plate standing in the solvent (or mobile phase) causing the migration of components in the same direction; much like LC, only in one dimension. Once the solvent has reached the top of the plate, the run has finished and a visualisation reagent must be added to show up the position and quantity of the components. There are no general methods for drugs as a class, but there are a large number of methods for individual drugs defined by their therapeutic or chemical categories. Most use colour development as the detection method, while some rely on induced UV fluorescence, for example, for LSD and psilocin.

Thin-layer chromatography methods are most effective for the low-cost analysis of a large number of samples (e.g. drug screening in biological fluids and tissues, and in herbal preparations), for example, the Toxi-lab TLC system, which is widely used in clinical toxicology laboratories for qualitative screening of tissue and fluid samples.

4.9 Supercritical Fluid Chromatography (SFC)

This is another separation technique that must be coupled to an appropriate detector. It uses carbon dioxide at relatively high temperature and very high pressure, producing the supercritical fluid, and this is the carrier medium in the column. This technique is not widely used in drug testing or toxicology, although it offers the potential for analysing a wide range of psychoactive drugs.

4.10 Electrochemical Detection (ECD)

This is a very sensitive LC detector which measures the current produced by the electrolytic oxidation or reduction of analytes at the surface of an electrode. These detectors are quite sensitive (down to 10^{-15} mol) and also quite selective. Two types of detector are available. The coulometric detector has a large electrode surface at which the electrochemical reaction is taken to completion. The amperometric detector has a small electrode with a low degree of conversion. Despite the difference in conversion rate, in practice these two types have approximately the same sensitivity. Samples for ECD must be electrically conductive, and this is accomplished by the addition of inert electrolytes. These detectors are difficult to maintain, and so do not lend themselves to routine analyses and are not used in high-throughput drug testing laboratories.

5 EMERGING TECHNOLOGIES

5.1 Miniaturisation

It is likely that there will be a large increase in miniature instrumentation that does not require skilled operators available for use at point of care, by the roadside, or in the office (Tudos *et al.*, 2001). These systems rely on a variety of physico-chemical principles that are currently being refined. A recent example uses a disposable potentiometric sensor (Gracheva *et al.*, 2004). The speed of development and hence implementation of these systems will depend on the level of investment, which is relatively large since innovation in this field involves an interdisciplinary approach including physicists, analytical scientists and engineers. Commercial investment is limited because the market is insufficiently large. Typical examples of the emerging miniature devices are shown in Figures 10.7 and 10.8. The NanoChip microelectronic array (Figure 10.8) is the inner component of the NanoChip cartridge shown in Figure 10.7 and is a 100-site electronically powered microarray fluidic device for DNA and RNA

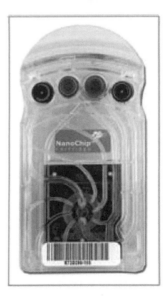

FIGURE 10.7 The NanoChip cartridge. (Sanchez-Felix, 2004. Reproduced with permission of the Royal Pharmaceutical Society.)

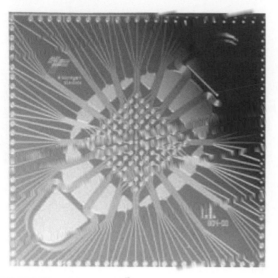

FIGURE 10.8 NanoChip microelectronic array. (Sanchez-Felix, 2004. Reproduced with permission of the Royal Pharmaceutical Society.)

analysis. Nanometre-sized low-dimensional semiconductors known as quantum dots (QDs) are also being investigated for use in drug and poison detection. One recent application of this technology has been in the development of a sensitive test for cyanide.

5.2 Time-of-flight (TOF) Mass Spectrometry

Time-of-flight mass spectrometry provides an example of where mass spectrometry is already beginning to be miniaturised to provide portable testing devices for the detection of solid-dosage forms of drugs (e.g. tablets, powders, and drugs on banknotes) and explosives. Advances in this field have received considerable attention as a response to the increase in drug trafficking (e.g. their use by Customs and Excise) and the potential threat from terrorism, as they can be used to screen for explosives at airports and sea terminals. TOF technology will play an increasing role in the laboratory for the analysis of a wide range of psychoactive drugs in biological fluids and tissues.

5.3 Isotope Ratio Mass Spectrometry (IRMS)

Although most psychoactive substances are foreign to the human body and their presence in body fluids is evidence of administration, some substances are virtually identical to those produced naturally in the body. Examples of these include testosterone, misused by sports competitors at least partly because of its behavioural effect, and gamma-hydroxybutyrate (GHB) allegedly used in drug-facilitated sexual assaults. Since the source of these administered 'pseudoendogenous' substances is different from the naturally produced endogenous material, a subtle difference in their natural isotope composition is often present. The IRMS technique has been used to detect sports cheats misusing testosterone, and work is underway to use the technique to provide evidence of GHB use. Unfortunately, the technique has relatively limited sensitivity at present, requiring about 20ng or more at the point of analysis, but is likely to improve by at least one order of magnitude over the next 10 years. The main use of this technique in the near future (2–8 years) will be to distinguish between endogenous and exogenous forms of the same substance in a biological specimen.

5.4 Coated Microsphere Technology

This technique is suitable for the quantitative measurement of up to 100 different analytes in each sample and generally relies on immunoprocedures. Thus, any substance for which suitable antibodies have been prepared should be amenable to analysis using this technique. The principle of operation is by the use of polystyrene microspheres (5.6 μm diameter in xMAP® technology; LuminexCorporation, 2001) that have been internally dyed with two spectrally distinct (red and infrared) fluorophores in appropriate precise proportions, enabling the production of up to 100 distinct sets of microspherical beads. Each of the bead sets may be coated with the appropriate antibodies to capture the analytes of interest, with a third fluorophore acting as a reporter of antibody binding. Multiple sets of the appropriately coated beads may be placed in 96-well microtitre plates and the samples of interest added to each well. The contents of each well may then be sampled with a suitable analyser (e.g. Luminex 100). Using a system of microfluidics, the beads in the sampled microtitre plate are sequentially excited via two different wavelength laser beams to identify each microsphere (in order to determine which antibody is present) and also to detect the presence of any reporter dye captured during the assay. With suitable automation such as using the Gilson 215 Multiprobe™ fluidics system, up to 32 000 wells per day have been analysed with, in theory, up to 320 000 different measurements of analytes. This technique has been proven for proteins and DNA. To date, it has not been fully explored for small molecule analysis but it has been used to measure the thyroid hormone T4 (Bellisario *et al.*, 2000a,b; Lukacs *et al.*, 2003; Pass, 2003).

5.5 Chemiluminescent Nitrogen Detector (CLND)

The chemiluminescent nitrogen detector (CLND) is specific for nitrogen-containing compounds, although it can also be set up to detect sulphur containing compounds. It is based on the chemiluminescent gas-phase reaction between ozone and nitric oxide which produces nitrogen dioxide formed in an electronically excited state. Relaxation of this excited state gives rise to light emission of 600–900nm. The intensity of the emission is proportional to the mass flow of the nitrogen dioxide through the detector. The technique has been successfully coupled with gas chromatography, liquid chromatography (Taylor *et al.*, 2002) and SFC (Shi *et al.*, 1997). The total nitrogen content can be determined quantitatively whatever the state of the nitrogen (except for diatomic nitrogen N_2) and most drugs of abuse contain at least one nitrogen atom. Sensitivity is of the order of 5pmol. Since SFC shows great promise for the separation of optical isomers of many substances, it is likely to be useful for the ready distinction of certain drugs of abuse, especially amphetamine, that are marketed legally in a single isomer (dexamphetamine), whereas much of the substance sold on the black market contains both forms of the molecule. Similarly, dextromethorphan is sold in cough mixtures and is not a controlled drug, whereas levorphanol is controlled under the Misuse of Drugs Act. Since levorphanol might need to be distinguished from dextrorphanol (the N-demethylated metabolite of dextromethorphan), SFC with CLND is likely to be a technique of the future.

5.6 Surface Plasmon Resonance (SPR; Turbadar, 1959; Kretschmann and Raether, 1968; Otto, 1968)

This is a detection technique that allows the quantitative estimation of one or more analytes concurrently within one assay, relying on the use of suitable immunoprocedures. Suitable antibodies are bound onto a thin metal (typically gold) surface that is coated onto a quartz prism. Total internal reflection occurs when light travelling in the quartz, which has a greater refractive index than at the interface, being in an aqueous solution, arrives at an angle of incidence above a critical angle. However, the light may be maximally coupled into the metal surface through the prism in such a way that, at the appropriate incident angle, the reflectivity is minimised. The incident light then feeds plasmons (the collective resonance of electrons near the surface of metal islands; Chalmers and Griffiths, 2002) in the metal and an enhanced evanescent wave is produced. Biospecific interactions occurring on the metal layer may be observed using this phenomenon since the interaction will change the solute concentration and hence its refractive index. Thus, suitable antibodies may be bound to the metal surface and the concentration of substance bound to the antibody quantified. No tagging or chemical derivatisation is required. A linear correlation between resonance angle shift and protein surface concentration has been shown (Stenberg *et al.*, 1991).

The technique is extremely sensitive (Kooyman *et al.*, 1988) and currently achieving quantitative sensitivities as low as 2×10^9 molecules, i.e. femtomoles of molecules of molecular weight of about 1000. At least one further order of magnitude of sensitivity is anticipated. The technique can readily be adapted for multi-sample parallel analysis, for example, by using a beam spreader to focus the beam of light on a line of samples and using a charge-coupled device to measure multiple reflectivity responses simultaneously. More than 100 parallel channels could be analysed simultaneously in the near future (Plant and Silin, 2004; www.cstl.nist.gov/biotech).

5.7 Surface-enhanced Resonance Raman Spectroscopy

Surface plasmons can also enhance Raman scattering. In contrast to surface-enhanced Raman spectroscopy, this allows the use of a smooth metal or single-crystal metal surface. Thus, in a similar manner to SPR, the interactions of biomolecules at the surface may be observed.

5.8 Total Internal Reflectance Fluorescence (TIRF)

Total internal reflection occurs when light travelling in a medium of higher refractive index such as quartz reaches an interface with a medium of lower refractive index such as an aqueous solution at an angle of incidence above a critical angle. Although the fully reflected light does not lose any net energy across the interface, an electrical field wave known as an evanescent field wave is produced that extends beyond the interface surface into the medium of lower refractive index, typically to a depth of about half of the wavelength of the light (Kroger *et al.*, 2002; Ruckstuhl *et al.*, 2003; Tedeschi

et al., 2003; Willard *et al.*, 2003; Jennissen and Zumbrink, 2004; Ohkawa *et al.*, 2004; Sapsford *et al.*, 2004).

The technique may be applied to fluorescent or fluorescently labelled compounds of interest. Only fluorophores adsorbed or otherwise in intimate contact with the interface will be excited and hence fluoresce, whereas those in bulk solution will not. The surface may be made biologically active, for example, with appropriate antibodies to substances of interest, so that fluorescently labelled compounds may be trapped at the surface. Since the excitation light is totally reflected away from the interface by total internal reflection, discrimination of the fluorescence signal from the excitation light is relatively effective, and so very good sensitivity and low limits of detection are achievable. The technique is non-destructive and rapid and more than 10 000 times more sensitive than other biosensor systems based on SPR.

6 THE FUTURE OF DRUG TESTING

It is predicted that new developments in analytical drug testing will be driven by commercial forces dictated by the potential market size. Although many of the technologies discussed above have the potential to be developed for drug testing, development will be dependent on market demand and manufacturers are unlikely to invest in the high cost of research and development without a clear indication of demand. So it is not possible to predict how fast, if at all, some of the techniques discussed in this review will be developed for drug testing. It is envisaged that emphasis will be directed towards producing more specific and reliable point-of-care tests to enable employers, those involved in law enforcement, and clinic-based practitioners to determine whether an individual may have used drugs.

Oral fluid offers many potential advantages over urine and is becoming a method of choice in certain areas. Technical advances should make a strong impact in developing the scope for screening drugs in oral fluid still further within the next 5–10 years.

The application of pharmacogenomics and our ability to prescribe drugs based on knowledge of an individual's genetic profile could well become a reality within five years, and some of this knowledge will have applicability to interpretative toxicology. Following the completion of the human genome project, microarray tests are currently being developed that will enable genetic variations between individuals to be determined. Such tests will, for example, enable physicians to analyse genes encoding drug-metabolising enzymes of the cytochrome P450 complex. Variations in these genes influence the metabolism of several drugs including antidepressants, psychotics, beta blockers, analgesics and some anticancer compounds. By enabling physicians to access information concerning an individual's genetic make-up, it should be possible to help prevent harmful drug interactions and to assure that drugs are used optimally. Near-patient testing should be developed in this area within the next 5–10 years. Detailed discussion of this is outside the scope of this review; see Chapter 4, Genomics.

Most drugs interact with specific sites (receptors) in the body, e.g. in the brain. Receptors may be isolated to provide the basis for drug assays depending on the specific interaction that occurs between drug and receptor. This use of receptor assays should be one of the most exciting innovations for the future. The use of DNA technology with yeast cells has enabled the production of specific receptors. For example, the use of glucocorticosteroid receptor assays has already been exploited. The significant benefit of this approach should be that it will be effective for most of the yet undiscovered psychoactive drugs. Other future techniques are likely to include the use of neural networks to deal with the complex analytical data produced by mass spectrometers and other instruments to simplify the detection of substances from a complex biological background. This approach is likely to become more important if metabolomics (the study of the small molecules, or metabolites, contained in a human cell, tissue or organ (including fluids) and involved in primary and intermediary metabolism) is used to indicate that a psychoactive substance has been used.

7 CONCLUSIONS

The three most likely significant advances will almost certainly be miniaturisation, enabling point-of-care analysis; high-throughput screening using enhanced spectrophotometric detection of antibody binding of drugs of interest; and enhanced separation techniques for the discrimination of complex mixtures.

The futuristic concept of a scenario where a simple probing device is placed on an area of the body may not, after all, be so far-fetched that it could not become a reality for the detection of common drugs within the next 25 years.

References

Bellisario, R., Colinas, R., *et al*. (2000a). Simultaneous quantitation of thyroxine (T4) and thyrotropin (TSH) from newborn dried blood-spot specimens with a multiplexed fluorescent immunoassay. *Am J Hum Genetics* 67(4): 1557.

Bellisario, R., Colinas, R.J. *et al*. (2000b) Simultaneous measurement of thyroxine and thyrotropin from newborn dried blood-spot specimens using a multiplexed fluorescent microsphere immunoassay. *Clin Chem* 46(9): 1422–1424.

Chalmers, J.M. and Griffiths, P.R. (eds) (2002) *Handbook of vibrational spectroscopy*. Chichester: John Wiley & Sons Ltd.

Gracheva, S., *et al*. (2004) Development of a disposable potentiometric sensor for the near patient testing of plasma thiol concentrations. *Anal Chem* 76(13): 3833–3836.

Hand, C. and Baldwin, D. (2004) Immunoassays. In: A.C. Moffat, M.D. Osselton, and B. Widdop (eds), *Clarke's analysis of drugs and poisons*. London: Pharmaceutical Press: 301–312.

Jennissen, H. P. and Zumbrink, T. (2004) A novel nanolayer biosensor principle. *Biosens Bioelectron* 19(9): 987–997.

Kooyman, R. P. H., Kolkman, H. *et al.* (1988) Surface-plasmon resonance immunosensors: sensitivity considerations. *Analytica Chimica Acta* 213(1–2): 35–45.

Kretschmann, E. and Raether, H. (1968) Radiative decay of non-radiative surface plasmons excited by light. *Z Naturforsch A: Phys Sci* A 23(12): 2135.

Kroger, K., Jung, A. *et al.* (2002) Versatile biosensor surface based on peptide nucleic acid with label free and total internal reflection fluorescence detection for quantification of endocrine disruptors. *Anal Chim Acta* 469(1): 37–48.

Lukacs, Z., Mordac, C. *et al.* (2003) Use of microsphere immunoassay for simplified multianalyte screening of thyrotropin and thyroxine in dried blood spots from newborns. *Clin Chem* 49(2): 335–336.

LuminexCorporation (2001) High-throughput screening on the Luminex 100™ System: rapid, efficient, accurate. *Technical Bulletin.* 2005: xMAP Technical Bulletins.

Ohkawa, J., Okuno, T. *et al.* (2004) Single-molecule observation under isotropic evanescent wave by advanced TIRF microscopy. *Biophys J* 86(1): 601A–601A.

Otto, A. (1968) A new method for exciting nonradiant plasma surface vibration. *Physica Status Solidi* 26(2): K99.

Pass, K.A. (2003) Commentary on: use of microsphere immunoassay for simplified multianalyte screening of thyrotropin and thyroxine in dried blood spots from newborns. *Clin Chem* 49(2): 336.

Plant, A.L. and Silin V. (2004) High-throughput screening of pharmaceuticals, NIST.

Ruckstuhl, T., Rankl, M. *et al.* (2003) Highly sensitive biosensing using a supercritical angle fluorescence (SAF) instrument. *Bios Bioelectron* 18(9): 1193–1199.

Sanchez-Felix, M. (2004) Emerging techniques. In: A.C. Moffat, M.D. Osselton, and B. Widdop (eds), *Clarke's analysis of drugs and poisons.* London: Pharmaceutical Press: 550–564.

Sapsford, K.E., Shubin, Y.S. *et al.* (2004) Fluorescence-based array biosensors for detection of biohazards. *J Appl Microbiol* 96(1): 47–58.

Saunders, J. and P. Barnes (2002) *Identification and treatment of pharmaceutical and illicit drug problems: a general practitioner's guide.* Brisbane, ADTRU: 44.

Shi, H., Taylor, L.T. *et al.* (1997) Chemiluminescence nitrogen detection for packed-column supercritical fluid chromatography with methanol modified carbon dioxide. *J Chromatogr A* 757(1–2): 183–191.

Shulgin, A. and A. Shulgin (1991) *Pihkal: a chemical loves story.* CA: Transform Press.

Spiehler, V. (2004) Drugs in saliva. In: A.C. Moffat, M.D. Osselton, and B. Widdop (eds), *Clarke's analysis of drugs and poisons* London: Pharmaceutical Press: 109–123.

Stenberg, E., Persson, B. *et al.* (1991) Quantitative-determination of surface concentration of protein with surface-plasmon resonance using radiolabeled proteins. *J Colloid Interface Sci* 143(2): 513–526.

Taylor, E.W., Jia, W.P. *et al.* (2002) Accelerating the drug optimization process: identification, structure elucidation, and quantification of in vivo metabolites using stable isotopes with LC/MSn and the chemi luminescent nitrogen detector. *Anal Chem* 74(13): 3232–3238.

Tedeschi, L., Domenici, C. *et al.* (2003) Antibody immobilisation on fibre optic TIRF sensors. *Biosen Bioelectron* 19(2): 85–93.

Tudos, A.J., Besselink, G.A.J. *et al.* (2001) Trends in miniaturized total analysis systems for point-of-care testing in clinical chemistry. *Lab on a Chip* 1(2): 83–95.

Turbadar, T. (1959) Complete absorption of light by thin metal films. *Proc Phys Soc London* 73(469): 40–44.

Willard, D., Proll, G. *et al.* (2003) New and versatile optical-immunoassay instrumentation for water monitoring. *Environ Sci Pollution Res* 10(3): 188–191.

Social Policy and Psychoactive Substances

Robin Room

1 EXECUTIVE SUMMARY

There are a number of strategies by which a society may seek to control psychoactive substances. One is control of availability, of which prohibition is the most extreme form. Others include education, public information and persuasion, environmental harm-reduction strategies, deterring behaviours connected with substance use, and the treatment of substance-use problems. It is possible to regulate the product, the provider or seller, the conditions of sale, or the buyer or consumer. There has been a wide diversity of rationales for governments seeking to control the supply and consumption of psychoactive substances.

Rankings of the risk or danger from different substances are reviewed. A ranking based on present levels of health harm puts tobacco and alcohol in the top two positions, but policy should take into account both present patterns of use and also the potential for harm under changed regimes.

Alcohol and tobacco are undercontrolled and cannabis is overcontrolled in terms of what the relative ratings for heavy use patterns would support.

Other factors besides the substance itself influence the harm with which it is associated, and should be taken into account in policies on substance use. They include the concentration of the substance, the mode of ingestion, and the location and circumstances of use.

The problems of substance use are felt most acutely at the local level, and there is a case for locating decisions on controls at local rather than universal levels. However, the globalisation of the current world puts limits on this approach.

In the context of western Europe, for alcohol, taxes (i.e., pushing up prices) are the most cost-effective strategy for reducing harm, followed by advertising bans, availability limits such as a weekend closing day, brief medical advice, and random traffic breath-tests. For tobacco, taxes (raising prices) are again the most cost-effective strategy, followed by an advertising ban, counter-advertising campaigns, bans on smoking in indoor public spaces, and nicotine replacement therapy.

Scenarios for the future include rethinking availability in terms of potential for harm. Obstacles to such recalibration include economic interests, international politics, and public attitudes. The coming into force of the Framework Convention on Tobacco Control can be expected to push forward the marginalisation of cigarette smoking. There is an urgent need for thinking and research on policies concerning alternative nicotine products, which offer substantial potential for reducing the harm related to nicotine use. Internationally, the same issues as for tobacco argue for the need for a Framework Convention on Alcohol Control. For cannabis, the long-term trend in Europe is towards a greater acceptance of recreational use.

Despite periodic fads and fashions, demand for psychoactive substances remains surprisingly conservative in terms of dominant substances. But developments can be expected in the area of performance enhancement.

Medications for addiction tend not to succeed, either because of problems of patient compliance or because of their ideological acceptability. Drug vaccines and depot formulations may short-circuit the issue of compliance, but they raise ethical, legal and social questions.

Growth in international transport and travel, and the rise of the Internet, are transforming the availability of psychoactive substances, nullifying national controls. Trade agreements and common markets also limit the scope of national controls on legal substances.

The weakening of market controls points towards a compensating increase in individual-level controls, whether through deterrence and punishment, or treatment. Despite the adverse side effects that accompany the singling-out of individuals, the tendency seems to be to broaden the net of social control with measures – such as the UK's anti-social behaviour orders (ASBOs) or random drug testing in various environments – applied to individual 'bad apples'.

2 OPTIONS FOR CONTROLLING PSYCHOACTIVE SUBSTANCES

From the beginning of recorded history, societies have sought to regulate psychoactive substances; the code of Hammurabi, from 3800 years ago, includes regulations on drink-shops (Hammurabi, 2000). But humans have been willing to go to extraordinary lengths to get psychoactive substances. The recognition that problems can accompany the pleasures of psychoactive substance use is also ancient. Many societies place a positive valuation on such substances. Regulations governing them have often been designed to guarantee an adequate supply of them for the elite.

A state's options for controlling the availability of psychoactive substances are limited. Modern states rarely opt for free availability in an open market. Instead, all substances taken into the body are controlled in some ways, for instance, for purity and accuracy of labelling. For caffeine, there are few special controls beyond the general rules on ingested substances. At the opposite extreme is total prohibition on production, sales, purchase and use. For a few psychoactive substances – heroin is an example in many countries, though not in the UK – this option is commonly exercised. In between are various options which involve a controlled market in the substance.

One common option is to raise prices by taxation. Another is controlling availability, for instance, by specifying the requirements for places of sale, limiting retail opening hours, or forbidding sale to particular classes of customers, for instance, of alcohol to those already drunk or below a certain age.

Other strategies include education, public information and persuasion, environmental harm-reduction strategies, deterring specific behaviours connected with substance use, and the treatment of substance-use problems.

2.1 Control Systems: the Existing Literature

Most discussions have revolved around two substances: alcohol and marijuana. For alcohol, comparative analysis has been invited by the many control systems that existed in the last century and before. Lemert (1962) put forward four 'models of social control' for alcohol: prohibitionary, educational, regulatory and the substitution of functional equivalents. Commenting on Lemert's analysis, Bruun (1971) proposed a tripartite division of control strategies, according to the aspect of substance use which they aimed to control: the 'phase of choice', i.e. decisions to use them; the 'phase of use', i.e. the amounts consumed; and

the 'phase of consequences', i.e. what we now term harm reduction. The US National Academy of Sciences report on *Alcohol and public policy* (Moore and Gerstein, 1981) adopted essentially the same tripartite division of strategies – distinguishing between 'regulating the supply of alcoholic beverages', 'shaping drinking practices directly', and 'reducing environmental risk' – reducing harm without necessarily affecting the drinking itself.

The special contribution of the literature on alcohol has been the recognition that a full public health control strategy must involve much more than prohibiting or regulating the availability of the substance.

For marijuana, the emphasis has been on prohibition and its alternatives. Kaplan's analysis (1970) discussed four alternatives: the 'vice model' of decriminalising possession and use; the 'medical model' of medical prescriptions for use; the 'licensing model', based on alcohol control; and the 'sugar candy model', where the substance is regulated only as a foodstuff would be.

An Australian tradition of discussion of alternative marijuana policies, initiated by a 1978 royal commission (South Australia, 1978), uses a similar typology of legislative options (McDonald *et al.*, 1994). The 'medical model' is dropped from consideration, and Kaplan's 'vice model' is divided into 'prohibition with civil penalties for minor offences' – as exists in South Australia and the Australian Capital Territory – and 'partial prohibition', legalising possession and cultivation for personal use, but retaining criminal penalties for growing or dealing in cannabis in commercial quantities.

Only recently has systematic discussion begun of alternative control systems for the whole range of psychoactive substances. The analysis by MacCoun *et al.* (1996; see also MacCoun and Reuter, 2001: 310–317, and Figure 11.1) places control regimes on a single dimension of restrictiveness, according to 'the extent of justification a user has to provide to obtain the drug'. But the authors recognise that a single-dimension

Proh	Pres	Reg	Model
■			**Pure prohibition**: Full prohibition, with no allowed use for any purpose whatever (e.g. heroin, marijuana)
■	■		**Prohibitory prescription**: Prohibited except for narrow therapeutic purposes unrelated to addiction; administered by a doctor or other health professional (e.g. cocaine)
■	■		**Maintenance**: Prescribed for relief of addiction; otherwise prohibited (e.g. methadone). Administered by an authorised agent or, for some patients, self-administered under tight supervision
	■	■	**Regulatory prescription**: Self-administered, under prescription, for relief of psychiatric problems (e.g. anxiety, depression). Otherwise prohibited (e.g. current US regime for Valium, Prozac)
	■	■	**Positive licence***: Available for any reason to any adult in possession of an appropriate licence, gained by demonstrated capacity for safe use (theoretical regime from Kleiman 1992)
		■	**Negative licence***: Available for any reason to any adult who has not forfeited the right by violating conditions of eligibility (theoretical regime from Kleiman 1992)
		■	**Adult market**: Available to any adult (e.g. alcohol)
		■	**Free market**: Available to any individual (e.g. caffeine)

Proh = prohibitory; **Pres** = prescription; **Reg** = regulatory
*Note added by RR: These regimes have actually existed for alcohol in various jurisdictions.

FIGURE 11.1   The spectrum of drug control regimes, in order of decreasing restrictiveness (according to MacCoun and Reuter, 2001: 311).

ranking has its limits when, as MacCoun *et al.* (1996) note, 'drug policy is inherently multi-dimensional'.

2.2 Classification of Regulation

An alternative way of classifying control regimes is in terms of who or what is being regulated or restricted. The object of control may be the product itself; the provider or seller; the conditions of sale or provision; and the buyer or consumer. National prohibition of alcohol in the United States involved few restrictions on the buyer or consumer, and provided for production and sale for religious and medical purposes. For marijuana in the Netherlands, the possession and sale of small quantities in limited circumstances is not penalised, but production and wholesaling are prohibited. Another example is doping in sports. It may not be illegal to distribute or possess the designated substances, but a sports participant who has the substance in their body is subject to penalties. Such contradictions are usually a sign of countervailing ideologies at work.

2.2.1 Regulation of the Product

Modern industrial societies typically regulate a large proportion of all marketed products, in terms of such factors as purity, safety, strength or size, and labelling and claims made for the product. Psychoactive substances tend to be subject to particularly stringent product controls. Controls on labelling, advertising and other promotional activities are also common. Price and other regulations may be used to favour more dilute or less harmful forms of the product.

Typically, regulation of the product is enforced primarily through the manufacturer or importer of the final form of the product. Manufacturing or importing often requires a licence, and the threat of losing it is an efficient and relatively inexpensive means of enforcement. Other parts of the chain of production and distribution may also be licensed.

2.2.2 Regulation of the Provider or Seller

A primary form of restriction of the market in psychoactive substances is to limit who can provide or sell the product. The state may itself operate all or part of the marketing chain. In 18 US states, all Canadian provinces, and four Nordic countries, the state operates the wholesale and/or retail levels of alcohol sales. Until recently, many countries operated tobacco monopolies, primarily to generate state revenue. In Sweden, the state operates the pharmacies for all prescription products.

Alternatively, the state may license producers and sellers. In the UK, licensing for public houses dates back to 1552 (Hunter, 2002), with *de facto* local licensing of sellers of alcoholic beverages existing considerably earlier (Bennett, 1996). In the case of internationally controlled psychoactive substances, states are obliged to license producers and sellers under international conventions. Again, the threat of losing the licence to produce, distribute or sell is an effective and inexpensive enforcement mechanism.

A special form of state licensing is the prescription system, in which doctors and chemists are given a licence, which may be removed for misconduct, to prescribe and provide or sell controlled medications. The prescription system is the primary means of regulation for most psychopharmaceuticals. Particularly for psychoactive medications, the licence to prescribe often comes with special restrictions. For instance, the most heavily controlled legally available psychoactive product in the US is methadone. Its provision is limited by prescription and to registered clinics or hospitals. Again, the primary enforcement mechanism is the threat of losing a licence to practise as a professional.

2.2.3 Regulation of the Conditions of Sale

Limits can also be put on the conditions of sale. In some US states, some alcoholic beverages must be sold in specific, dedicated shops. The number of shops may be limited. Dutch 'coffee shops' selling marijuana are another example of retailers that are heavily restricted by the state, in terms of the number of shops and their specialisation, and a limit on the amount that can be sold to a customer. In Canada, some pharmaceuticals that do not require prescription must nevertheless be sold in a pharmacy. Part of the alcohol control structure in many places is a set of controls on the hours of sale. For alcohol and now for tobacco products, there is a restriction that forbids selling to customers under a minimum age. It is now common to criminalise the attempt to purchase under the legal age. Historically, alcohol sales on credit were also often forbidden.

Other common regulations of the conditions of sale of alcoholic beverages apply, particularly to sale for on-premises consumption. They include specifications concerning design and layout, requirements on the availability of food, the prohibition of particular activities such as dancing, gambling or smoking, and a prohibition on serving someone who is already intoxicated. Again, the primary means of enforcement of conditions of sale has been the threat of cancellation of the licence of the provider or seller. Potential legal liability of the seller for harm resulting from prohibited sales has also become an important support for regulation of the conditions of sale, particularly in the US.

2.2.4 Regulation of the Buyer or Consumer

The state may prohibit or set limits on purchases by individual customers. Before 1955, Sweden had a rationing system in which civil servants decided the size of the ration of spirits that individuals could purchase each month (Frånberg, 1987), and alcohol rationing systems have been in effect elsewhere more recently (eg Schechter, 1986). In Nordic countries, individual-level controls also took the form of 'buyer surveillance' systems which attempted to reset dosage allowances in response to the individual's purchasing history (Järvinen, 1991). In some places, taverns were required to post and respect blacklists of drunkards who could not be served alcohol. Developing notions of privacy rights and of equality in treatment under the law have tended to make these kinds of restrictions on adults untenable in many places.

The primary regulation of the alcohol buyer or consumer these days is in terms of behaviour while or after drinking – particularly the offences of driving under the influence and of public drunkenness. Prohibitions on drinking at all in public places are also making a comeback in the UK and some other jurisdictions. In addition to these alcohol-specific offences, the intoxicated consumer is usually held responsible, with respect to the general criminal law, for the same standards of behaviour expected of the sober. This principle may conflict both with informal understandings that rules of behaviour are different under the influence of an intoxicant ('time-out', MacAndrew and Edgerton, 1969), and with judicial insistence that a guilty mind is necessary for conviction of a crime (Room, 1996). Changed attitudes to drink-driving show that it is possible to reduce problems from the use of psychoactive substances through deterring

the user. But it is inherently easier for the state to regulate the market by licensing those providing the psychoactive substances and thus threatening their commercial and professional interests.

2.3 Rationales for Controls on Psychoactive Substances

Governments have had many motives for controlling the supply and consumption of psychoactive substances, including:

- to raise revenue. Ideal commodities to tax are those with a controllable supply and low price elasticity, which psychoactive substances often are.
- to ensure purity or palatability. Modern European regulations on the purity or composition of alcoholic beverages date back in an unbroken tradition to medieval times (1266 in England; Hunter, 2002).
- as sumptuary or other symbolically discriminatory legislation. In many societies, access to psychoactive substances has been limited to categories defined by age, gender or social status. Often, use has been a prerogative of the powerful. In many village and tribal societies, the use of alcoholic beverages is forbidden for women. Now sumptuary prohibitions have retained their legitimacy only for children and special categories such as prisoners. Special taxes on luxury commodities, such as the special US federal tax rate for champagne and other sparkling wines, can be seen as a mild form of sumptuary control.
- to ensure fairness and equal opportunity. This applies mainly in sport. The *World anti-doping code* (World Anti-Doping Agency, 2003) states its fundamental purpose as being 'to protect the Athletes' fundamental right to participate in doping-free sport and thus promote health, fairness and equality for Athletes worldwide'.
- to favour or disfavour specific economic interests. Probably the most common

motivation for this sort of regulation has been to favour domestic over foreign producers. But this kind of regulation can cut many ways; eg between agricultural and manufactured products; between brand-name and generic pharmaceuticals; between products of a political ally and those of a rival or enemy.

- to enforce a religious principle or cultural value. Abstention from alcohol is a marker of an observant Muslim. Many Islamic countries that follow the *sharia* prohibit alcohol sales. In a European or North American context, it can be argued that regulations on psychoactive substances, particularly those seen as intoxicating, reflect a cultural bias against intoxication as a pleasure or recreation.

- to enforce or encourage work and family discipline. The earliest English alcohol control laws aimed to get 'sturdy beggars' out of the tavern and into the workforce at a time of labour scarcity. East German regulations in the 1970s forbade serving alcohol in the afternoon to someone in working clothes. The mid-afternoon closing hours for British pubs during most of the 20th century likewise removed a competitor for work and family time.

- to protect public order. Alcohol and other psychoactive drugs have often been associated with political subversion (Rorabaugh, 1981: 35), resulting in such measures as the repression of taverns in 1870s France (Barrows, 1991). The fact that coffeehouses and tobacco shops have also been seen as threats suggests that the perceived problem has been as much from congregating and sociability as from drug use. Alcohol has long been seen, with good reason (Room and Rossow, 2001), as a cause of violence both on the streets and in the family, and this view has played a major role in efforts at alcohol control (for present-day Britain, see Chatterton and Hollands, 2003; Hobbs *et al.*, 2003). For other drugs, an illegal status brings violence and public disorder (Fischer *et al.*, 1997), and there is sometimes a cultural association between some drugs and violence, but there is little evidence of a direct psychopharmacological effect on violence.

- to improve public health. This motive for regulation has come to the fore in recent years.

2.4 The Diversity of Aims and Targets within Public Health and Order

Many users of psychoactive substances argue that they are beneficial. They are used as anaesthetics and anodynes, and therapeutically for mental disorders. There can also be beneficial effects for physical health, for instance, alcohol's protective effect for heart disease, and the antinausea effects of cannabis. There is renewed discussion of potential beneficial effects of nicotine. Beneficial effects will undoubtedly continue to complicate the health message about psychoactive substances.

However, many psychoactive substances have severe and immediate adverse effects on the user (Fischer *et al.*, 1997). Often the risk of such consequences can be ameliorated by favouring dilute forms or safer modes of administration. Thus, death from overdose of alcohol is much less likely with beer than with spirits, and drinking coca tea is less likely to result in overdose than injecting cocaine.

Chronic consequences for the user are also an issue with many psychoactive substances. For some substances, such as alcohol, most of the chronic health risks are inherent in the main psychoactive ingredient. For others, such as tobacco and marijuana, this is not the case, and so regulations that affect the form and mode of administration are potentially important tools. There may also be chronic health consequences for those in the environment of the user. Smoke from cigarettes may harm those around the smoker, or a sexually transmitted disease may spread to the partner of an intravenous drug user who contracted the illness from sharing needles.

A third aspect of the consequences of substance use is in terms of effects on the user's thinking, judgement and behaviour.

Some of these effects are immediate. Alcohol or benzodiazepines, for instance, impair performance in complex tasks such as driving, causing risks both for the user and for others. At least in some cultures, drinking also seems to raise the risk of violent behaviour (Room and Rossow, 2001). Again, there is an extended range of potential interventions, and harm can be reduced by changing the physical or social environment of use, or by changing the response of others to the user, as well as by changing the user's behaviour.

Longer-lasting social consequences are usually related to a pattern of use over time. Particularly where there is repeated substance use to the point of intoxication, the result may be impairment of major social roles such as work performance or family participation. These consequences, too, are defined by the interaction of the user's behaviour with the reaction of others, and their occurrence and severity can be affected by changes in the reactions of others.

2.4.1 Addiction or Dependence per se

Addiction is a protean concept in the context of consequences of psychoactive substance use. Its core meaning in English-speaking cultures relates to the social consequences, and secondarily the health consequences, of recurrent use. The addict is the person who continues to use, despite having experienced the consequences (Room, 1973). More recently, definitions of addiction have diverged from this core meaning (Room, 1989) in two directions. One is a biologised concept focusing on the biological effects of drugs, particularly tolerance and withdrawal, which reinforce the continued use of the drug. The other direction has been towards a cognition- and feeling-oriented concept, focusing on the experiences of craving and impairment of control, often termed 'psychic' or 'psychological dependence'. In the 1961 Single convention on narcotic drugs (United Nations Office of Drug Control, 2004), 'addiction' as a 'serious evil for the individual' serves as

a main rationale for international controls. But, while invoking addiction may serve as a policy rationale, it plays little role in actual control policies (MacCoun, 2004).

2.5 Criteria for the Extent of Control of Psychoactive Substances

Some psychoactive substances are covered by international conventions controlling their production, distribution and use, while others are not. Alcohol is prominent among the substances not controlled internationally, and the controls on tobacco, through the Framework convention of tobacco control, are emergent and will initially be weak. At the other extreme, the regime with the tightest market controls (the Single convention of 1961) is applied to substances derived from three plants – the opium poppy, the coca bush and the cannabis plant. A generally less restrictive set of controls, the Convention on psychotropic substances of 1971, applies to synthesised substances such as LSD, amphetamines and diazepines.

Under the 1971 convention, a 'psychotropic substance' may be brought under international control if the World Health Organisation (WHO) finds that it has the capacity to produce a state of dependence and central-nervous-system stimulation or depression, resulting in hallucinations or disturbance in motor function or thinking or behaviour or perception or mood, and if there is sufficient evidence that the substance is likely to be abused so as to constitute a public health and social problem warranting the placing of the substance under international control (based on Article 2, Paragraph 4).

The official commentary on the 1971 convention (United Nations, 1976) notes that 'alcohol appears to be covered by' its wording but adds that the 'public health and social problem' that alcohol presents is not of such a nature as to warrant it being placed under 'international control'. Alcohol does not 'warrant' that type of control because it is not 'suitable' for the régime of the 1971 convention. The commentary then goes on to provide similar reasoning for why tobacco 'is not covered' by the paragraph.

2.5.1 Present Levels of Social and Health Harm

The WHO's estimates for the global burden of disease in 2000 suggest that tobacco accounts for 4.1 per cent of the total burden in disability-adjusted life years (DALYs) globally, alcohol for 4.0 per cent, and illicit drugs for 0.8 per cent. For developed societies such as the UK, the respective figures are 12.2 per cent, 9.2 per cent and 1.8 per cent (Ezzati et al., 2002). Another way of estimating harm is economic. One such estimate is for Canada for 1992: CAD9.6 billion for tobacco, $7.5 billion for alcohol, and $1.4 billion for illicit drugs (Single et al., 1998).

2.5.2 Potential for Harm

The most obvious objection to basing policy decisions on such estimates is that the present levels of social and health harm would alter if policies changed. One approach to estimating harm, adopted by a research team of which I was a member (Hall et al., 1999), was to compare the severity of effects for heavy users of different substances in their most harmful common form (see Table 11.1).

A limited measure of potential harm is the likelihood of an overdose from a substance. This is of significance for overdoses and for poison control, eg for labelling and child-proofing containers of the substance. The first column of figures in Table 11.2 shows partial results of a recent review of the literature by Gable (2004). The 'safety ratio' shown is the ratio between 'the usual effective dose for non-medical purposes' and the usual lethal dose, for the mode of administration specified.

Another dimension of danger is the level of intoxication produced by the substance, which 'increases the personal and social damage a substance may do' (Hilts, 1994). Obviously the level of intoxication produced by taking a substance is highly influenced by the dose taken, and the setting of the consumption. The second column of Table 11.2 shows rankings made by Jack Henningfield and Neal Benowitz on this (Hilts, 1994).

A more global approach to the problem was taken by a French committee chaired by Bernard Roques (Roques, 1999). The final two columns of Table 11.2 show the Roques committee's rankings on 'general toxicity' and 'social dangerousness'. As used in the report,

TABLE 11.1 A summary of adverse effects on health for heavy users of the most harmful common form of each of four drugs (according to Hall et al., 1999).

	Marijuana	Tobacco	Heroin	Alcohol
Traffic and other accidents	*		*	**
Violence and suicide				**
Overdose death			**	*
HIV and liver infections			**	*
Liver cirrhosis				**
Heart disease		**		*
Respiratory diseases	*	**		
Cancers	*	**		*
Mental illness	*			**
Dependence/addiction	**	**	**	**
Lasting effects on the foetus	*	*	*	**

* = less common or less well-established effect; ** = important effect.

TABLE 11.2   Ratings on dimensions of 'dangerousness'.

	Safety ratio (Gable, 2004)	Intoxicating effect (Hilts, 1994)	General toxicity (Roques, 1999)	Social dangerousness (Roques, 1999)
Marijuana	>1000 sm	4th highest	Very weak	Weak
Benzodiazepines (Valium)	nr	nr	Very weak	Weak (except when driving)
MDMA/Ecstasy	16 or	nr	Possibly very strong	Weak (?)
Stimulants	10 or	nr	Strong	Weak (possible exceptions)
Tobacco	nr	5th highest	Very strong	None
Alcohol	10 or	Highest	Strong	Strong
Cocaine	15 in	3rd highest	Strong	Very strong
Heroin	6 iv	2nd highest	Strong (except therapeutic use of opiates)	Very strong

nr = not rated; sm = smoked; or = oral; in = intranasal; iv = intravenous.
'Safety ratio = (usual effective dose for non-medical purposes)/(usual lethal dose).

'toxicity' includes long-term health effects such as cancer and liver disease, and infections and other consequences of mode of use, as well as acute effects.

The concept of 'social dangerousness' focuses on 'states of comportment which can generate very aggressive and uncontrolled conduct ... induced by the product or varied disorders (fights, robberies, crimes ...) in order to obtain it and risks for the user or others, for example in the case of driving a vehicle' [Roques, 1999: 296 (original in French)].

2.5.3 Dependence Dimensions

Ratings are also available of the dependence potential or addictiveness of different substances. For instance, Henningfield and Benowitz (Hilts, 1994) give comparative ratings of the different substances on withdrawal, tolerance, reinforcement and dependence, while the Roques committee report rates the substances on physical dependence and psychic dependence. On dependence, both Henningfield and Benowitz

rank the drugs in the following descending order: tobacco; heroin; cocaine; alcohol; caffeine; marijuana. The order implied by the ratings of the Roques committee on psychic dependence is: alcohol, heroin and tobacco; benzodiazepines and cocaine; stimulants; marijuana.

The overall message is that the present international system of classification and control of psychoactive substances can no longer be justified. Alcohol and tobacco are undercontrolled and cannabis is overcontrolled, in terms of relative harm. But there are substantial vested interests – material and ideological – at stake in maintaining the status quo. In particular, any comparison that looks across the licit–illicit boundary attracts controversy (Anonymous, 1998). ('Illicit' as used here means substances which are subject to international control when used non-medically.)

The relative danger or harmfulness of psychoactive substances cannot be escaped in any policy consideration with the overall aim of minimising health and social harm. But it should be recognised that the chemical substance itself, in its pure form, is only one among many factors in whether, and how much, harm occurs. Policies on substance use can considerably influence rates of harm by affecting such other factors. Here are some examples.

Concentration

Dilute forms of a substance often have less potential for harm than concentrated forms. It is not easy to die of an overdose of weak beer. But this is not always the case: low-nicotine, high-tar cigarettes are likely to cause more health harm than high-nicotine cigarettes. For licit substances, availability often varies substantially by concentration. In Sweden, beer containing less than 2.2 per cent alcohol is not counted as an alcoholic beverage, and is legally available to all ages. Beer containing up to 3.5 per cent alcohol is available in corner grocery stores (with beer containing less than 2.8 per cent alcohol having a price advantage from not being taxed for alcohol content). Stronger beer, along with other alcoholic beverages, is only available in a limited number of state-run stores (Hibell, 1984; Ramstedt, 2002).

There is mostly only anecdotal evidence of the effects of concentration for illicit substances. Less harm is presumed to result from chewing coca leaves or brewing coca tea than from snorting or injecting cocaine. On the other side of the debate, there is an argument that cannabis is much more potent now than it was previously and that, as a consequence, more harm will result (Manski *et al.*, 2001: 86), but in fact systematic information is not available on the implications of variations in potency for harm.

Mode of Ingestion

This is a dimension on which considerable information is available for some illicit substances. Health damage is less from smoking heroin than from injecting it, and probably less from eating marijuana than from smoking it. However, for some substances there is relatively little systematic knowledge of the effects on a population of measures designed to favour one mode of ingestion

over another. Often policies are made in the absence of systematic knowledge. For instance, the Swedish form of snuff known as *snus* is banned for sale in the European Union, except in Sweden, on the grounds that it is a health hazard. There are good public health arguments for promoting the use of *snus* as a less harmful alternative to smoking cigarettes (Gilljam and Rosaria Galanti, 2003), although there have also been counter-arguments. But at present the European legal system considers that it must make decisions on whether *snus* should remain banned on the basis of suppositions (Geelhoed, 2004).

Location of Use

Whether the substance is licit or illicit, policies can influence whether it is consumed in private or in public spaces. This can influence the harm from use. Again, there is a need to base such policy directions on careful studies. For instance, in the 1970s, Finnish alcohol policy was based on the presumption that drinking in a bar or restaurant would be more restrained than drinking at home. In fact, Partanen (1975) found that the empirical results in Helsinki were the opposite: 'people do not drink any more at home than in a restaurant, but they do it in a more leisurely manner, which seems to lead to a lower degree of intoxication'.

2.6 Universal or Local Controls?

Local regulation of psychoactive substance regulation entails abandoning a universal standard which applies the same level of control in all jurisdictions. This happened for alcohol control in the US and Canada after national prohibition. Local decision-making is consistent with the fact that the problems related to substance use are often most acutely felt at the local level (Room 1990; Room 2006). Such harm reduction strategies as needle exchanges and safe injection rooms (SIRs) for illicit substances have also most often been local initiatives. For drugs under international control, the local level can often act more flexibly, while national governments are more tightly bound by the rigidity of the international control system (van de Mheen and Gruter, 2004). But maintaining local controls on the marketing of legal substances is difficult in a globalised world. Consumer sovereignty also argues against rules which vary from place to place.

3 INSTRUMENTS AND MEANS OF GOVERNANCE AND CHANGE

Table 11.3 lists major strategies, other than market controls, for reducing substance use problems.

Even for licit substances, the police are potentially involved in setting the boundaries of behaviour, for instance, enforcing laws that forbid drinking in a park or ban smoking in public buildings. At least for illicit drugs and alcohol, treatment and counselling are also a part of most governments' response to substance-use problems. So is providing alternative activities – sports, leisure activities, etc. – which it is hoped will substitute for substance use. Reducing harm forms part of the treatment strategy for many illicit drugs. Particularly in the case of alcohol, such an approach – providing transportation after a party, providing water at raves, discouraging violence by the provision of trained bouncers, etc. – is widely recognised as a commonsense approach to 'living with drinking' or other drug use.

Effective planning in this area is inherently 'multisectoral', reaching across jurisdictional, professional and bureaucratic lines. For instance, Jha et al. (2000: 455) list between three and six agencies or ministries involved in each of eight typical activities of tobacco control programmes. The suppressed report of the Central Policy Review Staff on alcohol (Bruun, 1982) counted 16 government departments involved in alcohol policy in the UK in the late 1970s. The US National Drug Control Strategy for 1994 listed expenditures by 13 cabinet departments and a number of other government agencies (Office of National Drug Control Policy, 1994: 84–85). A review of US illicit-drug monitoring data identified 16 federal agencies involved in the collection of such data (Manski et al., 2001: 308–317).

4 POLICY IMPACT STUDIES

4.1 Alcohol Policy Impact Studies

There is a very substantial literature on the effects of alcohol-control policy changes on drinking amounts, patterns and problems (Babor et al., 2003). It generally excludes both the developing world (Room et al., 2002) and southern-European wine-based cultures. There is also an imperfect fit between what those involved in liquor licensing decisions

TABLE 11.3   Policy and prevention strategies, and institutions and professions involved.

Strategy	Institutions involved	Professions involved
Education	Schools, universities	Teachers
Persuasion	Media	Media professionals
Deterrence	Criminal justice	Police
Insulating use from harm	Pubs, nightclubs, public health agencies, others	Publicans, event promoters, health workers, others
Providing alternatives	(various)	(various)
Treatment and reintegration	Clinics, welfare offices, voluntary agencies	Doctors, nurses, social workers, experienced counsellors

may want to know and what is available in the literature on alcohol controls (Wagenaar and Toomey, 2000). The studies are sometimes done because a change was controversial in a particular jurisdiction, and funding an evaluation was a way of defusing the controversy. Other studies have been opportunistic, where a researcher seizes the chance to do a 'natural experiment' on some policy change but does not have a voice in the circumstances of the change. Often studies have made use of available data, such as per capita consumption data or mortality registers. Since research is usually a national government responsibility, its topical focus is not necessarily attuned to the concerns of local jurisdictions.

A new step forward, as part of the WHO-CHOICE programme (Choosing Interventions which are Cost-Effective; www.who. int/whosis/menu.cfm?path=evidence,cea& language=english) has been the comparison of the cost-effectiveness of different strategies and combinations of strategies to prevent alcohol-related problems (Chisholm et al., 2004) in terms of dollars per DALY saved. Table 11.4 shows some of the results from these analyses for the 'Europe-A' WHO subregion, roughly equal to the 25-member European Union. Since evidence was lacking for any effectiveness of mass media persuasion or school-based education (Foxcroft et al., 2003; Babor et al., 2003), these strategies were excluded from the analysis as having no apparent cost-effectiveness. In terms of cost-effectiveness per DALY saved, the most cost-effective strategy was raising taxes (and thus prices; this is even without counting the government revenue from taxes). In descending order, the other cost-effective strategies were a ban on advertising, limiting availability (the example used was Saturday closing for off-sales); random traffic breath-testing, and screening and brief medical advice.

4.2 Tobacco Policy Impact Studies

There are several synthetic reviews of the literature (eg Jha and Chaloupka, 1999; Jha et al., 2000; Rabin and Sugarman, 2001).

The literature is often aimed at assessing the impact of anti-smoking policy packages as a whole (eg Siegel and Biener, 1997; Pierce et al., 1998). There is a clear difference in emphasis between the literatures on alcohol and tobacco control. Raising the price through increased taxes looms even larger as a strategy for tobacco than it does for alcohol (see Chaloupka et al., 2001), followed by an advertising ban, counteradvertising campaigns, bans on smoking in indoor public places, and nicotine replacement therapy. Although a much greater proportion of the total harms from alcohol than from tobacco are to others, reducing harm from second-hand smoke has proved politically potent for tobacco control in a way that has not

TABLE 11.4   Comparative cost-effectiveness of alcohol interventions in 'Europe-A' (Chisholm et al., 2004).

	DALYs saved/million population	Average cost-effectiveness ratio
Tax: current	1365	333
Tax: current + 25%	1576	289
Tax: current + 50%	1764	258
Random traffic breathtests	247	2467
Saturday closing for off-sales	251	1087
Advertising ban	459	594
Brief medical advice	1889	2351

been true in alcohol policy except for drink-driving. A strong emphasis in the tobacco literature has been put on contextual prohibitions – bans on smoking at work and in public places – which are largely taken for granted for alcohol.

The two policy impact literatures have also reached substantially different conclusions about the effects of counteradvertising campaigns. Anti-smoking campaigns that have proved effective (Pechman and Reibling, 2000; Sly *et al.*, 2001, 2002; Wakefield *et al.*, 2003) have often involved frontal attacks financed by government agencies on the *bona fides* of the tobacco industry. This is an unusual enough occurrence in a capitalist society to have impressed teenagers, at least in the short run – although the campaigns have often proved politically unsustainable in the longer term (Givel and Glantz, 2000). Also more available in the nicotine field, though underutilised, has been the option of harm reduction through changing the mode of use of the psychoactive substance (Shiffman *et al.*, 1997).

As for alcohol, the WHO-CHOICE programme has estimated cost-effectiveness ratios for specific interventions, and for combinations of interventions (Shibuya *et al.*, 2003). Results for 'Europe-A' are shown in Table 11.5. Again, the cost-effectiveness calculations exclude the government revenue gained from the tax from the calculations.

4.3 Medication and Drug Policy Impact Studies

Compared to the considerable literatures in the alcohol and tobacco fields, the policy impact study literature is relatively undeveloped with respect both to illicit drug use and to medical use of prescription or over-the-counter psychoactive substances. The sustained effort by MacCoun and Reuter (2001) to assemble the evidence on the likely results of illicit drug legalisation in the US showed how weak the evidence base is in this area. A recent review (MacDonald, 2004) found agreement that there was some responsiveness to the price of illicit drugs, but that 'there is not yet a consensus on the possible range of price elasticities for certain drugs'. An authoritative US review of research on 'supply-reduction policy' noted that 'the required evidence is largely nonexistent. The problem is not just that the relevant studies have not been done. Systems for acquiring the needed data are inadequate or nonexistent'. The report's conclusion was stated in ringing terms: 'It is unconscionable for this country to continue to carry out a public policy of this magnitude and cost without any way of knowing whether and to what extent it is having the desired effect' (Manski *et al.*, 2001:143, 279).

The literature on the impact of changes in regulatory regimes for prescription psychoactive substances has primarily focused

TABLE 11.5 Comparative cost-effectiveness of tobacco interventions in 'Europe-A' (Shibuya *et al.*, 2003).

	Total DALYs saved (millions/year)	Average cost-effectiveness ratio ($/DALY)
Global average tax rate (44%)	2.0	44
Highest regional tax rate (75%)	4.8	18
Doubling the highest tax	6.9	13
Enforced bans on smoking in indoor public space	0.8	358
Comprehensive advertising ban	0.6	189
Counteradvertising campaigns	0.7	337
Nicotine replacement	0.7	2164

on the effects of shifts in prescription control systems on physicians' prescribing practices in the US (often referred to as 'triplicate prescription' requirements). A general finding was that the systems did reduce prescribing of the medications covered, but resulted in some substitution of more problematic medications which were not covered, and also some non-prescribing when it would have been appropriate (Weintraub *et al.*, 1991; Hoffman *et al.*, 1991; VanHaaren *et al.*, 2001; Wagner *et al.*, 2003; Ross-Degnan *et al.*, 2004; Simoni-Wastila *et al.*, 2004).

5 SCENARIOS FOR THE FUTURE

5.1 Recalibration of Availability in Terms of Potential for Harm

The Transform Drug Policy Foundation (2004) has recently put forward a discussion of 'options for control', to be used 'after the war on drugs'. The Foundation's 'time line for reform' anticipates that 'cannabis production and supply [will be] legalised and regulated' in the UK in the period 2007–2012, and that a group of 'coalition states' including Europe, Australia, Canada and South American states will opt out of the international treaties in the period 2013–2018.

Political systems have responded slowly to the over-regulation of cannabis and the under-regulation of alcohol and tobacco. For alcohol and tobacco, there are large economic interests at stake, which have fought against any increase in control, in the case of alcohol, quite successfully. For cannabis, as a drug included in the international drug-control system, any substantial change in status is politically very difficult, at least until there is a change of position by the US, as the prime mover of the international control system (Bullington, 2004; Bewley-Taylor, 1997). For both alcohol and cannabis, a shift in control status requires pushing against the general weight of public opinion.

A process of change, extending over 40 years and not yet ended, has altered the cultural–political position of cigarettes and other smoked forms of tobacco. Cigarette smoking is now associated with poverty and marginality. In most developed countries and some developing ones, cigarette smoking is in the process of being banned from public places. This has happened in Ireland, and Scotland will follow shortly. The arrangements proposed for England are not far short of a ban.

The *Framework Convention on Tobacco Control* (Taylor and Bettcher, 2000) commits its national parties to both internal and international policies. It can be expected to push forward the marginalisation of cigarette smoking in future years. Calls for outright prohibition (Ferrence, 2003) have so far been rare, but can be expected to increase. There is a need for thinking and research on alternatives for more restricted availability. Should cigarettes become a behind-the-counter item at the chemist's shop or in specific-purpose alcohol and tobacco shops? There is also an urgent need for thinking and research on policies concerning alternative nicotine products. The effects of allowing or encouraging other nicotine products, and other harm reduction strategies, need to be modelled and studied (Ferrence *et al.*, 2000; Warner, 2002).

For alcohol, substantial progress has been made in the specific area of drink-driving, which is less publicly acceptable in many countries and is subject to effective countermeasures. In recent years, the UK has lagged behind in this area. The UK blood alcohol limit of 0.08 per cent is one of the highest in Europe, and the UK has not moved to match Australia, for instance, in terms of the highly effective strategy of random breath-testing. In the coming 20 years, it is probable that the UK will catch up with progress internationally in this area.

The UK's public policy signals for alcohol more generally are mixed. Legislation reforming the alcohol licensing laws is pushing towards increasing availability, for instance in opening hours for pubs. On the other hand, it is increasingly apparent that problems from alcohol have been rising, and, across the political and prestige spectra, the media have been raising the alarm (eg Bowditch, 2004; Levy and Scott-Clark, 2004; Anonymous, 2006; Alleyne, 2004). The media unanimity probably portends a change in political direction in coming years.

At the international level, increasing calls can be expected for a framework convention on alcohol control, on the model of the tobacco convention, as many of the same issues arise. In the European Union, it can be expected that the strong tendency to view alcohol as an ordinary trade commodity will be tempered by the adoption and eventually the strengthening of an alcohol strategy.

5.1.1 Cannabis

The international drug conventions are a considerable impediment to reforming the status of cannabis. The UK has already been scolded by the International Narcotics Control Board for the relatively minor step, in full accord with the treaties, of moving cannabis to classification 'C', although the British Government did not accept these criticisms unchallenged (Travis, 2003). There are some signs of a more conservative European trend over cannabis. Switzerland has put on ice indefinitely the plans for a legal internal market there (Anonymous, 2004a), and the Swedish minister for justice returned from an EU meeting which adopted a common drug policy proclaiming that he 'would not be astonished' if all coffee shops in the Netherlands were closed by 2010 (Bøe, 2004; Anonymous, 2004b). But there is a clear longer-term trend in most parts of Europe towards greater acceptance of recreational cannabis use. In this context, there is a need for research to develop more specific tests, analogous to the blood-alcohol level for alcohol, of levels of current intoxication which affect driving behaviour. Consideration should also be given to means of discouraging types of cannabis use with greater health harm, in particular the combined smoking of tobacco and cannabis.

5.2 Substances of the Future?

Despite the pharmacological innovation of recent decades, traditional plant-derived substances dominate the legal and illegal psychoactive substance markets. Ecstasy (MDMA) is the single example of a substance which has come into wide use only since the 1960s. Periodic fads and fashions from new or revived substances can be expected, but the experience of recent decades suggests that markets for psychoactive substances are surprisingly conservative.

A common pattern in the history of psychoactive substances is the introduction of one substance as a 'cure' for another, followed by the discovery that the new substance also has substantial 'abuse potential'. Drug regulatory systems are aware of this history, so there is probably less likelihood of the pattern repeating itself today, at least with respect to substances which can be used for recreational highs.

There is more likelihood of new substances establishing themselves in performance enhancement. In sport, the increase in testing for sports doping and the establishment of the World Anti-doping Agency has resulted in a kind of 'arms race' in which those seeking to evade the system try out novel substances and approaches beyond the reach of the existing testing protocols (Carstairs, 2003). The success of Viagra and its competitors demonstrates that the demand for performance-enhancing substances reaches well beyond the remedying of disabilities. For other aspects of performance, too, notably wakefulness and intellectual performance, there is a substantial latent demand.

5.3 New Medications and other Treatments

Enormous resources have been devoted, particularly in the US, to developing new pharmacotherapies and other biomedical treatments for psychoactive substance-use problems (Midanik, 2004). But the experience of the past is that most of these medications will not be widely used (Room, 2004a). Stumbling blocks include 'patient compliance' – whether the medications will actually be welcomed and used by those being treated – and the ideological boundaries of what is considered acceptable as aims and means of care. The most successful pharmacotherapies have been maintenance medications such as methadone, buprenorphine and nicorette. For these, too, political acceptance has not been easy, since it involves accepting continued addiction.

The emphasis in new medications is shifting towards approaches that do not require continuing compliance by the 'patient', such as the development of drug vaccines and of depot forms of opioid antagonists using slow-release deposits in the patient's body. These medications lend themselves to compulsory regimes, whether imposed by the state or by worried parents seeking to protect their child from dangerous attractions. These raise substantial ethical, legal and social questions (Center for Cognitive Liberty and Ethics, 2004; Harwood and Myers, 2004; WHO, 2004: Chapter 7).

5.4 Erasing Borders

Improvements in communication and transport have made contacts between different cultures and jurisdictions routine. Governments find it increasingly difficult to control what crosses their national or regional borders. Internet shopping is increasingly transforming the availability of psychoactive medications, removing physician oversight as well as nullifying national controls (Spain *et al.*, 2001; Lineberry and Bostwick, 2004; St George *et al.*, 2004). Trade and common-market agreements have placed limits on the extent to which governments can control a national or local market, and the trend is for controls to weaken further. Thus, in the context of the European Union, in 2004 the European Commission filed a court case attacking Sweden's right to forbid cross-border Internet purchasing of alcoholic beverages (Eubusiness, 2004), and

another attacking UK Customs enforcement actions against those importing alcohol and tobacco products in excess of the guidelines on amounts for personal use (Gow, 2004). In the wider arena of the World Trade Organisation, the proposed agreements under the General Agreement on Trade in Services (GATS) threaten further restrictions on the ability of nations to control their domestic market in legal psychoactive substances (Grieshaber-Otto and Schacter, 2002). While the Framework Convention on Tobacco Control seeks to counter these trends specifically for tobacco products, the question of whether its provisions will supersede or be subordinated to the requirements of trade agreements remains unsettled (Parmentier, 2003).

5.5 Social and Personal Control

Broadening the net of individualised social control has been facilitated by technological innovations in wholesale drug-screening methods. Costs have come down but are still not trivial. The argument for drug testing in sports – that fairness requires that everyone compete with their 'natural body' – also potentially applies to competitive situations such as scholarship and professional examinations, bridge or chess tournaments, or even scientific discovery or warfare. Future years may see developments in this direction. In the US, particularly, random drug testing has been widely extended, with the intention of deterring drug use by denying those with positive tests access to such valued activities as employment or university student loans. But this strategy has encountered substantial resistance as an intrusion on civil liberties and privacy (Comer, 1994; Marx, 1998; Brunet, 2002; White, 2003; Center for Cognitive Liberty and Ethics, 2004).

The tendency in the present era seems to be for states to broaden the net of social control with individually applied measures. ASBOs in the UK are a manifestation of this trend. Finding the 'bad apples' and banning them from the premises has proved a politically more attractive alternative to maintaining controls on alcohol sales and marketing (Room, 2004b; Home Office, 2004).

6 AN OPPORTUNITY FOR RESEARCH – AND FOR EVIDENCE-BASED POLICIES

We may expect to see substantial changes in psychoactive substance policies in the coming years, and we may expect to be surprised at times by their direction and speed. An important step for the UK would be to make the commitment that these changes will be evidence-based. Experience suggests that forging a link between the policy process and the research community, so that a tradition of good policy impact studies and policy-oriented research is built up, requires careful attention and specific funding. Such an investment would allow the UK to move into a new era of evidence-based policy making, and would also make a contribution to the international knowledge base for action.

Acknowledgements

This report draws in part on Room (2000). My thanks to Neil Hunt and Robert MacCoun for useful comments.

References

Alleyne, R. (2004) Violence will rise if pubs are open all day, says Met chief. *Telegraph* 29 December. www.telegraph.co.uk/news/main.jhtml?xml=/news/2004/12/29/ndrink29.xml

Anonymous (1998) High anxieties: what the WHO doesn't want you to know about cannabis. *New Scientist* 21 February.

Anonymous (2004a) Parliament rejects decriminalisation of cannabis. Swissinfo, Swiss Radio International 15 June. www.mapinc.org/drugnews/v04/n866/a01.html

Anonymous (2004b) Clampdown could spell trouble for 'coffee shops'. Associated Press 20 November. www.cannabisnews.com/news/thread19851.shtml

Anonymous (2006) The sorry legacy of Labour's binge. Daily Mail 26 November. http://www.dailymail.co.uk/pages/live/articles/news/newscomment.html?in_article_id=369785&in_page_id=1787

Babor, T., Caetano, R., Casswell, S., Edwards, G., Giesbrecht, N., Graham, K., Grube, J., Gruenewald, P., Hill, L., Holder, H., Homel, R., Österberg, E., Rehm, J., Room, R., and Rossow, I. (2003) *Alcohol: no ordinary commodity – research and public policy*. Oxford: Oxford University Press.

Barrows, S. (1991) 'Parliaments of the people': the political culture of cafés in the early third republic. In: S. Barrows, and R. Room (eds), *Drinking: behavior and belief in modern history*. Berkeley: University of California Press: 87–97.

Bennett, J.M. (1996) *Ale, beer and brewsters in England: women's work in a changing world, 1300–1600*. Oxford: Oxford University Press.

Bewley-Taylor, D.R. (1997) *The US and international drug control 1909–1997*. London and New York: Pinter.

Bøe, S. (2004) Ett steg mot knarkstopp (A step towards stopping drugs). *Dagens nyheter* 20 November (1st section): 12.

Bowditch, G. (2004) How alcohol has slipped past the health regulators. *The Scotsman* 20 November.

Brunet, J.R. (2002) Employee drug testing as social control: a typology of normative justifications. *Rev Publ Personnel Admin* 22: 193–215.

Bruun, K. (1971) Implications of legislation relating to alcoholism and drug dependence. In: L.G. Kiloh, and D.S. Bell, (eds), *Proceedings, 19th International Congress on Alcoholism and Drug Dependence*. Australia [sic]: Butterworths: 173–181.

Bruun, K. (ed) (1982) *Alcohol policies in United Kingdom*. Stockholm: Stockholm University, Sociology Department, Studier i svensk alkoholpolitik (Studies in Swedish alcohol policy).

Bullington, B. (2004) Drug policy reform and its detractors: the United States as the elephant in the closet. *J Drug Issues* 34: 687–721.

Carstairs, C. (2003) The wide world of doping: drug scandals, natural bodies, and the business of sports entertainment. *Addict Res Theory* 11: 263–281.

Center for Cognitive Liberty and Ethics (2004) *Threats to cognitive liberty: pharmacotherapy and the future of the drug war*. Davis, CA: Center for Cognitive Liberty and Ethics. 11 May version. www.cognitiveliberty.org/issues/Pharmacotherapy.html

Chaloupka, F.J., Wakefield, M., and Czart, C. (2001) Taxing tobacco: the impact of tobacco taxes on cigarette smoking and other tobacco use. In: R.L. Rabin, and S.D. Sugarman, (eds), *Regulating tobacco*. Oxford: Oxford University Press: 39–71.

Chatterton, P. and Hollands, R. (2003) *Urban nightscapes: youth cultures, pleasure spaces and corporate power*. London: Routledge.

Chisholm, D., Rehm, J., van Ommeren, M., Monteiro, M., and Frick, U. (2004) The comparative cost-effectiveness of interventions for reducing the burden of heavy alcohol use. *J Stud Alcohol* 65: 782–793.

Comer, D. (1994) The case against workplace drug testing. *Organization Science* 5: 259–267.

EUbusiness (2004) EU to take Sweden to court over booze import laws: report. *EUbusiness* 13 July. http://www.eubusiness.com/Sweden/040713102232.7nuldmyo/

Ezzati, M., Lopez, A.D., Rodgers, A., Vander Horn, S., Murray, C.J.L., and the Comparative Risk Assessment Collaborating Group (2002) Selected major risk factors and global and regional burden of disease. *Lancet* 360: 1347–1360.

Ferrence, R. (2003) Learning from tobacco: bans on commercial availability are not unthinkable. *Addiction* 98: 720–721.

Ferrence, R., Slade, J., Room, R., and Pope, M. (eds) (2000) *Nicotine and public health*. Washington: American Public Health Association.

Fischer, B., Kendall, P., Rehm, J., and Room, R. (1997) Charting WHO goals for licit and illicit drugs for the year 2000: are we on track? *Public Health* 111: 271–276.

Foxcroft, D.R., Ireland, D., Lister-Sharp, D.J., Lowe, G., and Breen, R. (2003) Longer-term primary prevention for alcohol misuse in young people: a systematic review. *Addiction* 98: 397–411.

Frånberg, P. (1987) The Swedish snaps: a history of booze, bratt, and bureaucracy – a summary. *Contemp Drug Probl* 14: 557–611.

Gable, R.S. (2004) Comparison of acute lethal toxicity of commonly abused psychoactive substances. *Addiction* 99: 686–696.

Geelhoed, M.L.A. (2004) *Conclusions de l'avocat générale M.L.A. Geelhoed* [on cases C-434/02 and C-210/03]. Luxembourg: Court of Justice

of the European Communities. 7 September. http://curia.eu.int/jurisp/cgi-bin/form.pl?lang=en&Submit=Submit&alldocs=alldoc&docj=docj&docop=docor&docor=docor&docjo=docjo&numaff=C-434-02&datefs=&datefe=&nomusuel=&domaine=&mots=&resmax=10 – and click on "Opinion"

Gilljam, H. and Rosaria Galanti, M. (2003) Role of *snus* (oral moist snuff) in smoking cessation and smoking reduction in Sweden. With other papers and commentaries. *Addiction* 98: 1183–1207.

Givel, M.S. and Glantz, S.A. (2000) Failure to defend a successful state tobacco control program: policy lessons from Florida. *Am J Publ Health* 90: 762–767.

Gow, D. (2004) UK taken to court over booze cruises. *Guardian* 20 October. www.guardian.co.uk/guardianpolitics/story/0,,1331289,00.html

Grieshaber-Otto, J. and Schacter, N. (2002) GATS: impacts of the International 'Services' Treaty on health-based alcohol regulation. *Nordisk Alkohol- and Narkotikatidskrift* (Nordic Studies on Alcohol and Drugs), 19 (English supplement): 50–68. www.stakes.fi/nat/pdf/02/natsup-02.pdf

Hall, W., Room, R., and Bondy, S. (1999) Comparing the health and psychological effects of alcohol, cannabis, nicotine and opiate use. In: H. Kalant, W. Corrigall, W. Hall, and R. Smart (eds), *The health effects of cannabis*. Toronto: Centre for Addiction and Mental Health: 475–506.

Hammurabi (2000) *Code of Hammurabi*, translated by L.W. King. www.fordham.edu/halsall/ancient/hamcode.html

Harwood, R. and Myers, T.G. (eds) (2004) *New treatments for addiction: behavioral, ethical, legal and social questions*. Washington, DC: National Academy Press. www.nap.edu/books/0309091284/html/

Hibell, B. (1984) Ölkets betydelse för alkoholkonsumtionen bland unga och gamla (The importance of medium-strength beer for alcohol consumption among young and old). In: T. Nilsson (ed), *När mellanölet försvann* (When medium-strength beer disappeared). Linköping: Linköpings Universitet: 94–107.

Hilts, P.J. (1994) Is nicotine addictive? it depends on whose criteria you use. *New York Times*. 2 August. www.ukcia.org/research/addictive.htm

Hobbs, D., Hadfield, P., Lister, S., and Winlow, S. (2003) *Bouncers: violence and governance in the night-time economy.* Oxford: Oxford University Press.

Hoffman, R.S., Wipfler, M.G., Maddaloni, M.A., and Weisman, R.S. (1991) Has the New York state triplicate benzodiazepine prescription regulation influenced sedative-hypnotic overdoses? *N Y State J Med* 91: 436–439.

Home Office (2004) Anti-social behaviour orders; penalty notices for disorder. www.homeoffice.gov.uk/anti-social-behaviour/penalties/anti-social-behaviour-orders/ www.homeoffice.gov.uk/anti-social-behaviour/penalties/penalty-notices/

Hunter, J. (2002) English inns, taverns, alehouses and brandy shops: the legislative framework, 1495–1797. In: B. Kümin and B.A. Tlusty (eds), *The world of the tavern: public houses in early modern Europe.* Aldershot: Ashgate: 65–82.

Järvinen, M. (1991) The controlled controllers: women, men and alcohol. *Contemp Drug Probl* 18: 389–406.

Jha, P. and Chaloupka, F.J. (1999) *Curbing the epidemic: governments and the economics of tobacco control.* Washington, DC: World Bank. www.worldbank.org/tobacco/reports.asp

Jha, P., Paccaud, F., and Nguyen, S. (2000) Strategic priorities in tobacco control for governments and international agencies. In: P. Jha, and F. Chaloupka (eds), *Tobacco control in developing countries.* Oxford: Oxford University Press: 449–464.

Kaplan, J. (1970) *Marijuana: the new prohibition.* New York and Cleveland: World Publishing Co.

Kleiman, M.A.R. (1992) *Against excess: drug policy for results.* New York: Basic Books.

Lemert, E.M. (1962) Alcohol, values and social control. In: D.J. Pittman, and C.R. Snyder (eds), *Society, culture, and drinking patterns.* New York and London: Wiley: 553–571.

Levy, A. and Scott-Clark, C. (2004) Under the influence. *Guardian* 20 November. www.guardian.co.uk/weekend/story/0,,1354076,00.html

Lineberry, T.W. and Bostwick, J.M. (2004) Taking the physician out of 'physician shopping': a case series of clinical problems associated with internet purchases of medication. *Mayo Clinic Proceedings* 79: 979–982.

MacAndrew, C. and Edgerton, R. (1969) *Drunken comportment.* Chicago: Aldine.

MacCoun, R. (2004) Is the addiction concept useful for drug policy? In: R. Vuchinich, and N. Heather (eds), *Choice, behavioral economics, and addiction.* Oxford: Elsevier Science: 355–373. http://ist-socrates.berkeley.edu/~maccoun/MacCoun The Addiction Concept.pdf

MacCoun, R. and Reuter, P. (2001) *Drug war heresies: learning from other vices, times and places.* Cambridge: Cambridge University Press.

MacCoun, R., Reuter, R., and Schelling, T. (1996) Assessing alternative drug control regimes. *J Policy Analysis Management* 15: 330–352.

MacDonald, Z. (2004) What price drug use? The contribution of economics to an evidence-based drugs policy. *J Econ Surv* 18: 113–152.

Manski, C., Pepper, J., and Petrie, C. (eds) (2001) *Informing America's policy on illegal drugs: what we don't know keeps hurting us.* Washington, DC: National Academy of Sciences.

Marx, G. (1998) An ethics for the new surveillance. *The Information Society* 14: 171–185.

McDonald, D., Moore, R., Norberry, J., Wardlaw, G., and Ballenden, N. (1994) *Legislative options for cannabis in Australia.* National Drug Strategy Monograph 26. Canberra: Australian Government Publishing Service.

Midanik, L. (2004) Biomedicalization and alcohol studies: implications for policy. *J Publ Health Policy* 25: 211–228.

Moore, M.H. and Gerstein, D.R. (eds) (1981) *Alcohol and public policy: beyond the shadow of prohibition.* Washington: National Academy Press.

Office of National Drug Control Policy (1994) *National drug control strategy: reclaiming our communities from drugs and violence.* Washington, DC: Executive Office of the President.

Parmentier, R. (2003) *Tobacco control: don't trade away public health.* London: Action on Smoking and Health, 8 March. www.ictsd.org/pubs/external/tobacco.pdf

Partanen, J. (1975) On the role of situational factors in alcohol research: drinking in restaurants vs. drinking at home. *Drink Drug Pract Surveyor* 10: 14–16.

Pechman, C. and Reibling, E.T. (2000) Anti-smoking advertising campaigns targeting youth: case studies from USA and Canada. *Tobacco Control* 9 (Supplement II): 18–31.

Pierce, J.P., Gilpin, E.A., Emery, S.L., White, M.M., Rosbrook, B. and Berry, C.C. (1998). Has the

California tobacco control program reduced smoking? *J Am Med Assoc* 280: 893–899.

Rabin, R.L. and Sugarman, S.D. (eds) (2001) *Regulating tobacco*. Oxford: Oxford University Press.

Ramstedt, M. (2002) The repeal of medium-strength beer in grocery stores in Sweden: the impact on alcohol-related hospitalizations in different age groups. In: R. Room (ed), *The effects of Nordic alcohol policies: what happens to drinking and harm when alcohol controls change?* NAD Publication 42. Helsinki: Nordic Council for Alcohol and Drug Research: 117–131.

Room, R. (1973) The social psychology of drug dependence. In: D. Hawks (ed), *The epidemiology of drug dependence: report on a conference*. Copenhagen: WHO Regional Office for Europe: 69–75.

Room, R. (1989) Drugs, consciousness and self-control: popular and medical conceptions. *Int Rev J Psychiatry* 1: 63–70.

Room, R. (1990) Alcohol problems and the city. *Br J Addict* 85: 1395–1402.

Room, R. (1996) Drinking, violence, gender and causal attribution: a Canadian case study in science, law and policy. *Contemp Drug Probl* 23: 649–686.

Room, R. (2000) Control systems for psychoactive substances. In: R. Ferrence, J. Slade, R. Room, and M. Pope (eds), *Nicotine and public health*. Washington: American Public Health Association: 37–61.

Room, R. (2004a) 'What if we found the magic bullet?' Ideological and ethical constraints on biological alcohol research and its application. In: R. Müller, and H. Klingemann (eds) *From science to action? 100 years later: alcohol policies revisited*. Dordrecht: Kluwer: 153–162.

Room, R. (2004b) The impotence of reason in the face of greed, selfish ambition and moral cowardice. *Addiction* 99: 1092–1093.

Room, R. (2006) Drug policy and the city. *Int J Drug Policy* 17:136.

Room, R. and Rossow, I. (2001) The share of violence attributable to drinking. *J Subst Use* 6: 218–228.

Room, R., Jernigan, D., Carlini-Marlatt, B., Gureje, O., Mäkelä, K., Marshall, M., Medina-Mora, M.E., Monteiro, M., Parry, C., Partanen, J., Riley, L., and Saxena, S. (2002) *Alcohol and developing societies: a public health approach*. Helsinki: Finnish Foundation for Alcohol Studies and Geneva: World Health Organisation.

Roques, B.P. (chair) (1999) *La dangerosité de drogues: rapport au secrétariat d'État a la santé* (The dangerousness of drugs: report to the state secretariat for health). Paris: La documentation française – Odile Jacob.

Rorabaugh, W.J. (1981) *The alcoholic republic: an American tradition*. New York: Oxford University Press.

Ross-Degnan, D., Simoni-Wastila, L., Brown, J.S., Gao, X., Mah, C., Cosler, L.E., Fanning, T., Gallagher, P., Salzman, C., Shader, R.I., Inui, T.S., and Soumerai, S.B. (2004) A controlled study of the effects of state surveillance on indicators of problemtic and non-problematic benzodiazepine use in a medicaid population. *Int J Psychiatry Med* 34: 103–123.

Schechter, E.J. (1986) Alcohol rationing and control systems in Greenland. *Contemp Drug Probl* 15: 587–620.

Shibuya, K., Ciercierski, C., Guindon, E., Bettcher, D.W., Evans, D.B., and Murray, C.J.L. (2003) WHO framework convention on tobacco control: development of an evidence-based global public health treaty. *BMJ* 327: 154–157.

Shiffman, S., Gitchell, J., Pinney, J.M., Burton, S.L., Kemper, K.E., and Lara, E.A. (1997) Public health benefit of over-the-counter nicotine medications. *Tobacco Control* 6: 306–310.

Siegel, M. and Biener, L. (1997) Evaluating the impact of statewide anti-tobacco campaigns: the Massachusetts and California tobacco control programs. *J Soc Issues* 53: 147–168.

Simoni-Wastila, L., Ross-Degnan, D., Mah, C., Gao, X., Brown, J., Cosler, L.E., Fanning, T., Gallagher, P., Salzman, C., and Soumerai, S.B. (2004) A retrospective data analysis of the impact of the New York triplicate prescription program on benzodiazepine use in medicaid patients with chronic psychiaric and neurological disorders. *Clin Therapeut* 26: 322–336.

Single, E., Robson, L., Xie, X., and Rehm, J. (1998) Economic costs of alcohol, tobacco and illicit drugs in Canada, 1992. *Addiction* 93: 991–1066.

Sly, D.F., Hopkins, R.S., Trapido, E., and Ray, S. (2001) Influence of a counteradvertising media campaign on initiation of smoking: the Florida 'Truth' campaign. *Am J Public Health* 91: 233–238.

Sly, D.F., Trapido, E., and Ray, S. (2002) Evidence of the dose effects of an antitobacco counteradvertising campaign. *Prev Med* 35: 511–518.

South Australia (1978) Royal commission into the non-medical use of drugs. *Cannabis: A Discussion Paper*. Adelaide: Government Printer.

Spain, J.W., Siegel, C.F., and Ramsey, R.P. (2001) Selling drugs online: distribution-related legal/regulatory issues. *Int Marketing Review* 18: 432–449.

St George, B.N., Emmanuel, J.R., and Middleton, K.L. (2004) Overseas-based online pharmacies: a source of supply for illicit drug users? *Med J Australia* 180: 118–199.

Taylor, A.L. and Bettcher, D.W. (2000) WHO framework convention on tobacco control: a global 'good' for public health. *Bull WHO* 78: 920–929. whqlibdoc.who.int/bulletin/2000/Number%207/78(7)920-929.pdf

Transform Drug Policy Foundation (2004) *After the war on drugs: options for control*. Bristol: Transform Drug Policy Foundation. www.tdpf.org.uk/Policy General AftertheWaronDrugsReport.htm

Travis, A. (2003) High stakes. *Guardian* 16 April. society.guardian.co.uk/societyguardian/story/0,7843,937205,00.html

United Nations (1976) *Commentary on the convention on psychotropic substances, Vienna 21 February 1971*. New York: United Nations. The Convention's text is at http://www.incb.org/pdf/e/conv/convention_1971_en.pdf

United Nations Office of Drug Control (UNODC) (2004) *Single convention on narcotic drugs, 1961*. Vienna: United Nations Office of Drug Control. www.unodc.org/pdf/convention 1961 en.pdf

Van de Mheen, D. and Gruter, P. (2004) Interventions in the supply side of the local hard drug market: towards a regulated hard drug trade? The case of Rotterdam. *J Drug Issues* 34: 145–161.

VanHaaren, A.M., Lapane, K.L., and Hughes, C.M. (2001) Effect of triplicate prescription policy on benzodiazepine administration in nursing home residents. *Pharmacother* 21: 1159–1166.

Wagenaar, A.C. and Toomey, T.L. (2000) Alcohol policy: gap between legislative action and current research. *Contemp Drug Probl* 27: 681–733.

Wagner, A.K., Soumerai, S.B., Zhang, F., Mah, C., Simoni-Wastila, L., Cosler, L., Fanning, T., Gallagher, R., and Ross-Degnan, D. (2003) Effects of state surveillance on new post-hospitalization benzodiazepine use. *Int J Qual Health Care* 15: 423–431.

Wakefield, M., Flay, B., Nichter, M., and Giovino, G. (2003) Effects of anti-smoking advertising on youth smoking: a review. *J Health Comm* 8: 229–247.

Warner, K. (2002) Tobacco harm reduction: promise and peril. *Nicotine Tobacco Res* 4: 61–71.

Weintraub, M., Singh, S., Byrne, L., Maharaj, K., and Guttmacher, L. (1991) Consequences of the 1989 New York State triplicate benzodiazepine prescription regulations. *J Am Med Assoc* 266: 2392–2397.

White, T. (2003) Drug testing at work: issues and perspectives. *Subst Use Misuse* 38: 1891–1902.

World Anti-Doping Agency (WADA) (2003) *World anti-doping code*. Montreal: World Anti-Doping Agency. www.wadaama.org/rtecontent/document/code_v3.pdf

World Health Organisation (2004) *Neuroscience of psychoactive substance use and dependence*. Geneva: World Health Organisation.

CHAPTER

12

Sociology and Substance Use

Professor Neil McKeganey, Professor Joanne Neale, Charlie Lloyd and Dr Gordon Hay

1 EXECUTIVE SUMMARY

This report looks at the contribution of sociological research on substance use and misuse within the UK and considers possible future developments in this area over the next 20 years. Research in the area of substance misuse began in the UK with Stimson and colleagues' classic study of heroin users (Stimson and Ogborne, 1970; Stimson and Oppenheimer, 1982). In the mid- to late-1980s sociological research in this area was shaped primarily by the focus on studying drug users' HIV-related risk behaviour. More recently, research in this area has tended to focus on criminal justice concerns, including identifying the extent of drug-related offending, the prevalence of drug use and effective ways of tackling drug abuse.

1.1 Prevalence

There are indications that, while the overall proportion of the population consuming alcohol has not changed markedly in the recent past, alcohol consumption has increased in the case of both young people and women. In the case of illegal drug use, there are indications that the prevalence of abuse has increased dramatically in the last 50 years. In 1955, for example, there were 46 new cases on the Home Office Addicts Index. By 1995 this figure had increased to 14 735. The National Drug Treatment Monitoring System in the UK identified 128 969 drug users in contact with services in England and Wales in 2004. Overall, it has been estimated that there may be around 350 000 problematic drug users in the UK.

With regard to the future, we have identified a number of scenarios covering possible increases in the prevalence of problem drug use. These range from a high-prevalence scenario of around one million problem drug users by 2025, to a medium-prevalence scenario of around 750 000 problem drug users, a low-prevalence scenario of around 500 000 problem drug users, and a reducing-prevalence scenario of around 300 000 problem drug users. On the basis of the longer-term trend of problem drug use of the last 40 years, it is certainly not beyond the bounds of credibility that the number of problem drug users could increase three-fold to the one million level by 2025.

The impacts of a possible three-fold increase in prevalence, if it occurred, could be considerable. For example, the number of drug-related deaths per year could increase from around 2000 to around 6000 per year. There could be around 400 000 drug users who are Hepatitis-C positive and 10 000 who are HIV positive. There could be around 300 000 children with a drug-dependent mother in the UK. The economic and social cost of drug abuse could increase to around £35 billion a year. There could

be a substantial increase in drug-related crime to a level that would severely challenge the capacity of the police and other enforcement agencies to respond, and drug use and drug-related paraphernalia could become much more visible within public spaces.

Such an expansion in the level of problem drug use could result in a close interweaving between the legal and illegal economy to the point that it would be virtually impossible to distinguish between the two economies. In due course, interests associated with the illegal drugs trade could seek to secure growing local, and national, political influence. Public attitudes towards drugs and drug users could undergo substantial change, leading to the development of much harder or more tolerant attitudes towards those using illegal drugs. Similarly, drug policy could itself change dramatically, with much greater emphasis on prescribing heroin and cocaine, as well as other drugs of abuse, in order to reduce the extent of drug-related criminality.

1.2 Individual and Cultural Factors Influencing Drug Use

There are indications from sociological research that some forms of drug use have become increasingly normalised within the UK. This is evident from studies of young people, as well as from the growing to drugs within the advertising industry (e.g. Opium perfume). In terms of risk factors underpinning drug use and drug problems, those that have been identified include parental drug use, family disruption, social deprivation and child sexual and physical abuse. It is possible that changes in the prevalence of substance use and misuse could lead to significant changes in these risk factors and also to individuals who do not have the classic 'addict profile' of multiple social and family problems using and getting into difficulty with substances. Changes in youth transitions and, in particular, the lengthening of the period covered by youth and the delayed onset of adult responsibilities (associated in part with increases in the proportion of young people remaining in full-time education for longer) may have an important influence on changes in the pattern of legal and illegal drug use.

1.3 Treatment

Increasingly, service provision both for illegal drug users and those with alcohol problems is being delivered in the form of integrated packages of care that incorporate health, social and other forms of support, as well as drug misuse treatment. This is resulting in the expansion of 'wraparound' services encompassing housing, education, training, and employment. These developments seem set to continue as a result of a number of factors. For example, increased polydrug use may mean that it will not be possible for services to treat clients as simply 'heroin users', 'stimulant users' or 'problem drinkers'. Similarly, if the prevalence of drug use – and the numbers of individuals from more affluent, educated and middle-class backgrounds – increases, service users will tend to have greater purchasing power and more knowledge of the available treatment options. This will make them a more demanding client group that expects provision to be tailored more closely to their personal circumstances.

To date, the proportion of drug treatment clients over the age of 35 has been low in the UK and elsewhere. It is possible that, in future years, society will find itself dealing with large numbers of middle-aged and even elderly 'difficult-to-treat' addicts. This burgeoning new treatment group could jeopardise the willingness of the medical profession to prescribe opiates and injectable drugs for fear that some individuals will need this expensive treatment for many years. Equally, such initiatives could come to be seen as negative treatments of despair – simply warehousing large numbers of individuals who have been failed by the existing system in order to protect the community from their drug-related offending, while keeping them out of a criminal justice system that is already struggling to cope.

Inevitably, new forms of drug misuse will generate new pharmacological interventions that will require both clinical and non-clinical testing and assessment. Although the optimal nature and extent of non-medical treatments continue to be disputed, psycho-social and behavioural interventions play an important role in tackling addictions and an ever-increasing number of such treatments are emerging. A key aim for sociological research must be to learn more about how best to exploit their potential.

1.4 Conclusions

It is possible that over the next 20 years the illegal drug problem in the UK will expand beyond the capacity of society to cope. Drug use could become a commonplace and visible occurrence on the streets; drug-related offending could be at such a level that the individual freedoms of drug users could be severely curtailed; drug-producer countries could cease to be accepted in the international community; there could be an irremediable linking of the legal and illegal drug economy; and there could be an attempt to secure increasing political influence on the part of those operating at the uppermost levels of the illegal drug economy. These are in a sense the features of a worst-case scenario. Nobody knows whether illegal drug use will expand to the worst-case scenario of a threefold increase in problem drug user numbers in the UK or whether it will reduce. However, what is clear is that illegal drug use has expanded phenomenally in the past 50 years and it would seem very unlikely that the current best estimate of around 350 000 problem drug users in the UK represents the ceiling in terms of the prevalence of this problem.

If we are to avoid the point where drug abuse reaches a level that is beyond the capacity of society to cope with it (and we have no way of knowing what that point may be) there will be a need to substantially increase funding in the areas of drug prevention, drug treatment and drug enforcement and to ensure that interventions in each of these areas are maximally effective.

2 INTRODUCTION

This report looks at the contribution of sociological research on substance use and misuse within the UK. It is possible to view drug use as an individual behaviour in which a given person consumes a given drug and experiences the effects of that substance on his or her system. Sociology, however, reminds us that drug-using behaviours are not simply a matter of what the individual person does. Rather, drug use exists within a cultural context: some drugs are legal and some are not, some people have anti-drug attitudes and some have pro-drug attitudes, some people enjoy drugs that have a euphoric effect and others prefer drugs that have a depressive effect. As well as being substances in their own right, drugs can also be associated with a certain kind of image, for example, some substances may seem 'cool' and 'attractive', others may have the reputation of being 'dirty' and 'dangerous'. These social factors can influence what drugs are used, how they are used, who uses them, and the impact of drug use on society. Understanding these dimensions is the role of sociologists and it is their contribution that we look at in this report.

Section 3 provides a short overview of sociological research in the area. Section 4 examines what is known about the prevalence of drug use and considers possible changes in its prevalence over the next 20 years. In Section 5, we look at individual and sociocultural factors associated with the onset and progression of illegal drug use. We consider how these factors may change over the next 20 years and with what impact. Section 6 focuses on treatment, considering the effectiveness of existing treatments and the scope for new treatments as the drug problem itself evolves. Finally, in Section 7,

we draw our conclusions together and assess the nature and consequences of drug use in the future.

In any report on drug use and drug users, there are inevitably problems about the use of the terms 'drug user', 'drug abuser', and 'substance misuse', or 'substance use'. The sensitivities of language in this connection are difficult enough when one is referring only to illegal drugs. They are compounded when one is also talking about legal substances. Mostly, it will be obvious whether we are discussing legal or illegal drugs, but where this distinction is unclear we will refer to substance use and misuse. It is also important to acknowledge that, while sociology as a discipline can be clearly defined as 'the systematic study of human society, especially present day societies' (Hirsch et al., 2002), this does not mean that it is straightforward to identify the distinctive contribution of sociologists to studying substance use and misuse. Over the past 20 years, it has become increasingly commonplace for sociologists to work in multidisciplinary teams, and it is therefore often very difficult to identify the contribution of any single discipline.

3 SOCIOLOGICAL RESEARCH IN THE SUBSTANCE USE/MISUSE FIELD

Sociological research on substance use and misuse within the UK has gone through a number of overlapping phases during the last 30 years. The growth of illegal drug use in the 1960s had not led to the development of a major programme of substance use and misuse research, even by the 1970s. The picture was rather different in the United States, with a number of key researchers working on drug-use-related topics (Finestone, 1957; Sutter, 1966, 1969; Feldman, 1968; Preble and Casey, 1969). One of the most influential studies carried out in the US at this time was Howard Becker's classic *Outsiders* (1963). This ethnographic, and to an extent autobiographical, study outlined the ways in which neophyte cannabis users learn to interpret the experiences associated with their use of the drug and – in so doing – contribute a form of ethnocultural knowledge about the drug and its effects which in turn shapes future users' experiences.

Becker's account was resonant at that time with the upsurge of interest in the UK in qualitative sociological research. This interest influenced probably the first distinctively sociological study of drug use and drug users in the UK. Carried out by Stimson and colleagues (Stimson and Ogborne, 1970; Stimson and Oppenheimer, 1982), this pioneering work involved charting the experiences of individuals dependent on heroin. By following them over an extended period, Stimson was able to provide a detailed description of the impact of heroin use on individuals' lives. The study revealed that, while some users appeared able to incorporate heroin into their lives, others' involvement with the drug fundamentally damaged, and in some cases ended, their lives. This research raised important questions about heroin addiction, the services that users needed and the broader nature of drug policy in the UK.

At the time this research was undertaken, heroin use was largely confined to London. By the 1980s, research was charting a heroin epidemic that had spread to encompass a range of northern and Scottish cities. Parker et al. (1988) and Pearson (1987a) reported on heroin use in Liverpool, while Ditton and Speirits (1982) outlined its spread in Glasgow. These and other studies showed the spread of heroin use among socially excluded working-class males, and to a lesser extent females, across the UK.

In the 1980s, research on substance use and misuse in the UK underwent a transformation brought about by the fear that injecting drug users were at risk of spreading HIV infection (Bloor et al., 1992; Bloor, 1995). Evidence of rapid and widespread transmission of HIV among injecting drug users attending a general practice surgery in Edinburgh underlined those fears and led

to research on the prevalence of injecting drug use (Frischer et al., 1993), the extent and social determinants of drug injectors' HIV-related risk behaviour (Grund et al., 1991; McKeganey and Barnard, 1992) and the effectiveness of services designed to reduce drug injectors' HIV-related risk behaviour, including the impact of the newly developed needle and syringe exchange services (Stimson et al., 1988a, 1988b).

By the mid-1990s, fears that tens of thousands of injecting drug users within the UK would become HIV positive, and spread infection to the wider population, had receded. Attention switched back to the epidemic of drug use that had swept through the UK. More recent research has encompassed a much broader range of topics, including developing methods to better estimate the number of people using drugs (Frischer et al., 2001; Hay et al., 2001; Hickman et al., 2004b, 2004c); identifying the shifting patterns and forms of legal and illegal drug use among young people (Currie et al., 2003); understanding young people's routes into drug use (McIntosh et al., 2003a, 2003b, 2003c); understanding the place of legal and illegal drugs in youth culture (Parker et al., 1998); understanding recovery from dependent drug use and assessing the success of treatment services (Neale, 1998); looking at the impact of drug use on families (Barnard and Barlow, 2002; Barnard, 2003) and communities (McKeganey et al., 2004a); and looking at the policing of drugs and drug users (May et al., 2002). Much of the current and recent research effort in this area has been fuelled by concerns over drug- and alcohol-related offending and how this might be reduced.

3.1 Theorising Drug Use

As well as describing what drugs are used by what groups of people, sociologists have also sought, with varying success, to construct theories that account for why people use different substances. Whereas 'individualistic explanations' tend to assume that people who take drugs are suffering from some form of physiological or psychological illness or deficiency, sociologists have placed much greater influence on a range of social and cultural factors that explain patterns of drug-using behaviour in society. For example, emphasis has been given to the way individuals may be motivated to use illegal drugs as a result of their marginalisation from society, or because illegal drug use has become normalised within certain social groups, or as a result of the power of advertising.

One of the earliest theories of drug-using behaviours derived from the theoretical work of Robert Merton (1938). Merton argued that societies have valued goals (for example, wealth and status) and that individuals achieve these goals through socially structured channels (for example, good education and hard work). Where access to these objectives by legitimate means is denied, individuals may turn to illegitimate means to succeed. Alternatively, they may reject or 'retreat' from those things that are valued by society and the accepted ways of attaining them. For Merton (1938), drug use was a typical 'retreatist' behaviour. Building on Merton's work, Cloward and Ohlin (1960) later described drug users as 'double failures' – people who had failed in both conventional and illegitimate attempts to lead satisfactory lives and to get ahead in society.

The image of drug users as inadequate persisted until the mid-1960s. Thereafter, a number of largely American sociological studies (Finestone, 1957; Feldman, 1968; Fiddle, 1967; Preble and Casey, 1969; Sutter, 1972) challenged the belief that addiction was a 'pathology' and argued instead that drug users were normal self-determining individuals who had willingly chosen a lifestyle that just happened to be deviant. This lifestyle became known as the drug-using 'career'. The premise was that drug users actively adopted the 'street addict' identity and organised their behaviour, self-perception and sense of personal worth around that master status (Stephens, 1991).

The concept of drug use as a career relates closely to the labelling theory of sociologists

such as Howard Becker (1963). According to labelling theory, the more people are labelled as deviants, the more likely it is that they will behave like deviants and think of themselves as deviants. Many labelled deviants eventually become career deviants and join with other similar individuals to form deviant subcultures. The individuals within these subcultures may then become isolated from non-deviants and thus increasingly trapped within a separate antisocial identity. Authors such as Jock Young (1971) have argued that the state, the law and the media perpetuate this process by promoting negative stereotypical images of drug users. These negative images further reinforce deviant behaviour and labelling, resulting in deviancy amplification.

Such theorising emphasises the role played by broader social processes and structural factors in drug taking, a connection that was developed in the 1980s when various commentators (Peck and Plant, 1986; Dorn and South, 1987; Pearson, 1987a, 1987b; Parker et al., 1988) began to draw attention to the associations between opiate use and poor housing, unemployment, family breakdown and poverty. This more structural theoretical approach maintains that the individuals most at risk of becoming drug dependent are those who are politically and economically marginalised and most disaffected from family, school, work and the standard forms of leisure (Downes and Rock, 1998). This argument has been developed by Friedman in his work on the sociopharmacology of drug use (Friedman, 2002). He argues that drug use must be located in a broad socioeconomic context since social structures and processes affect the likelihood that individuals will use various substances.

Feminist commentators, meanwhile, have highlighted the marginalisation of women within theoretical explanations of substance use and misuse (Rosenbaum, 1981; Ettorre, 1992, 1994; Taylor, 1993; Pettiway, 1997). Authors such as Ettorre (1992), Sterck (1999) and Maher (1997) have rejected limited accounts of women as passive and sick individuals and instead identified them as social actors who consciously used dependent substances as a means of taking something for themselves, seeking pleasure, or coping with an oppressive situation. In this way, women's drug use was theorised as a move towards agency and self-definition that involved autonomy and assertiveness. Additionally, the diverse and complex responses of individual women to drug-related issues were emphasised (Taylor, 1993).

The importance of agency and self-definition – along with diversity and difference – are also central aspects of postmodernist theory. According to postmodernism, there was a revolutionary restructuring of society during the twentieth century. As a result, individuals have become less constrained by the structures of inequality and are now able to exercise choice far more than previously (Jones, 1997). Self-denial and prudence have been replaced by self-fulfilment and choice through a culture of consumption (Featherstone, 1991; Bauman, 1992). As Parker *et al.* (1995) have argued, postmodern society has become characterised by the fracturing of moral authority, increasing globalisation, an emphasis on consumption rather than production and a reshaping of class and gender relationships. This, it is claimed, has resulted in the normalisation of drug use where drug taking has become a regular and ordinary feature of everyday life (Shiner and Newburn, 1999; South, 1999).

But, despite these insights, sociological research has not yet provided a single definitive explanation of drug taking.

4 DEVELOPMENTS IN THE PREVALENCE OF SUBSTANCE USE AND MISUSE

In this section, we look at current and past information on the nature and extent of drug and alcohol use within the UK and anticipate possible developments over the next 20 years, particularly in relation to problem drug use. Perhaps the first thing to say is

that, overall, there is much less information available on the prevalence of either illegal drug use or alcohol use in the last 30 or so years than one might have expected. As a result, it is by no means easy or straightforward to portray either the past prevalence of these behaviours or their future development. Nevertheless, in this section we attempt to construct a number of possible scenarios covering future changes in prevalence and how these could impact on society in the next 20 years.

4.1 Alcohol

There is a range of surveys of varying size reporting information on levels of alcohol consumption in the UK. Key among these is the General Household Survey, which obtains information from over 20 000 individuals across the UK. The 2002 survey (Office for National Statistics, 2004) shows that 74 per cent of men and 59 per cent of women had consumed alcohol in the preceding week. These overall percentages are very similar to those for 1998. But there have been significant changes in alcohol consumption on the part of women and young people. In the case of women, the proportion reporting drinking 6–8 units of alcohol on at least one day within the last week increased from 24 per cent in 1998 to 28 per cent in 2002. Similarly, the proportion of women drinking more than 35 units of alcohol in the last week increased from 7 per cent in 1998 to 10 per cent in 2002.

4.2 Illegal Drugs

There has never been a consistent mechanism for measuring the prevalence of illegal drug use in the UK. The first system for monitoring such use was the Home Office Addicts Index, which started in the 1930s and terminated in 1997. The Addicts Index principally collated information on heroin addicts coming forward for treatment. In 1955, there were 46 new cases registered on the index. By 1995 this figure had increased to 14 735.

More recently the National Drug Treatment Monitoring System, which replaced the Addicts Index in 2001, has provided provisional figures for 2003/2004 showing a total of some 128 969 people in contact with drug treatment services in England and Wales (Department of Health, 2004). While this increase in registrations undoubtedly reflects the expansion in treatment services in the UK over that period, it also reflects the increase in illegal drug use from the 1960s through to the present day.

4.3 Current Prevalence Estimates

Prevalence estimates for the UK come from various studies carried out at the local (e.g. Brighton) or national (e.g. Scotland) level in different years. The most up-to-date estimates are for Scotland (Information and Statistics Division, 2004; Hay *et al.*, 2001), where the estimate refers to 2003, followed by England for 2001 (Frischer *et al.*, 2004) and Northern Ireland for 2000/2001 (McElrath, 2002). The most recent prevalence estimate for Wales was derived in 1994 (Wood *et al.*, 2000) and is now thought to be obsolete. The prevalence estimates for Scotland and Northern Ireland were derived using the capture–recapture method, whereas the England estimate combined capture–recapture estimates for Brighton, Greater Manchester, Liverpool and parts of London within a multivariate indicator method analysis.

The prevalence estimates are summarised, along with the rate per population aged 15–64, in Table 12.1.

These estimates primarily refer to problem heroin users. If it is assumed that the prevalence rate for England (8.91 per thousand) applies to Wales, Table 12.2 is the result.

On this basis, and using the most up-to-date prevalence information largely derived from 2001 data, there will already be over 350 000 problem drug users in the UK.

4.4 Past Trends in Problem Drug Use

Little is known about the past trends in problem drug use. The current best estimate of there being around 350 000 problem drug users in the UK is simply a point estimate referring to 2000. As we have indicated,

TABLE 12.1 Summary of most recent prevalence estimates.

Country	Number	Population (15–64 years)	Rate per 1000
England	287 670	32 292 156	8.91
Northern Ireland	828	1 095 309	0.76
Scotland	51 582	3 352 022	15.39

TABLE 12.2 Summary of most recent prevalence estimate, whole of UK.

Country	Number	Population (15–64 years)	Rate per 1000
England	287 670	32 292 156	8.91
Northern Ireland	828	1 095 309	0.76
Scotland	51 582	3 352 022	15.39
Wales	16 513	1 853 654	8.91
UK total	356 593	38 593 141	9.24

however, the number of problem drug users in treatment in the 1960s, as documented by the Addicts Index, numbered in the hundreds and not the hundreds of thousands. The number of actual problem drug users (as distinct from the number in treatment) is likely also to have been in the hundreds at that time.

How then did the prevalence of problem drug users rise from a low level in the 1960s to what was found at the beginning of the twenty-first century? The simplest assumption would be that prevalence of problem drug use increased steadily over the 40-year period. However, research that has attempted to estimate the incidence and prevalence of problem drug use on the basis of data on drug-related deaths has suggested that there may have been a rapid increase in the prevalence of problem drug use in the 1990s (De Angelis *et al.*, 2004).

Figure 12.1 represents four possible scenarios relating to the future prevalence of problem drug use in the UK. The top line represents a possible increase in prevalence from around 350 000 to 1 million. The second line represents a possible increase in prevalence from around 350 000 to 750 000; the third line represents a possible increase in prevalence from 350 000 to around 500 000 and the fourth line represents a possible decrease in prevalence from 350 000 to 300 000 by 2025.

We explore below a number of factors that might influence these future prevalence scenarios. Before doing so, it is worth considering the possible reasons why the prevalence of problem drug use might remain stable in the next 20 years.

4.4.1 Drug Production and Cultivation

One scenario where prevalence could remain constant over the next 20 years would be if the global production of heroin and cocaine was already at its maximum level

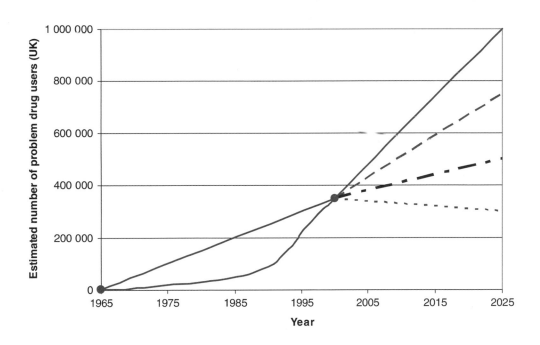

FIGURE 12.1 Possible trends in the prevalence of problem drug use in the UK. (—): from 350 000 to 1 million; (– – –): from 350 000 to 750 000; (— - —): from 350 000 to 500 000; (· · ·): from 350 000 to 300 000 by 2025.

and there was little in the way of stored drugs that could serve an increased level of usage. While the data on drug production and storage is by no means robust, the 2004 World Drug Report from the United Nations Office of Drugs and Crime identifies a willingness on the part of producer farmers to plant more – not fewer – illegal crops. The report also makes the case that reductions in the overall acreage allocated to illegal crops in countries such as Columbia and Afghanistan have been compensated for by improvements in production techniques which in turn have led to increases in overall yield (United Nations Office of Drugs and Crime, 2004).

4.4.2 Global Conflict

It is far from clear what impact global conflicts have on overall drug production and distribution. It is possible that global conflicts in the next 20 years might reduce levels of production within key areas with a corresponding depressive effect on drug user numbers. However, it is equally likely that such conflicts could see an increase in production and distribution. For example, the dismantling of the Taleban regime in Afghanistan resulted in an increase, at least in the short term, in heroin production. It is difficult to anticipate what further global conflicts might arise during the next 20 years or what impact they will have on drug production and consumption.

4.4.3 Change in Drug-using Behaviours

It is possible that the next 20 years could bring a major cultural shift in the social acceptability of illegal drug use, resulting in, for example, a move away from drug injecting on the part of individuals who might otherwise have started to inject drugs. At present we know relatively little about the choices individuals make about what drugs to use, in what contexts, and at what levels. In Scotland, two national drug-misuse

prevalence estimation studies carried out in 2000 and 2003 identified a reduction in the overall prevalence of problematic drug use from 55 800 to 51 582 (Hay *et al.*, 2005). These data remind us that the prevalence of problematic drug use can decrease even where it is not clear why such a reduction may have occurred.

4.4.4 Vulnerable Populations

Another possible scenario in which the number of problematic drug users could remain constant would be if the figure of around 350 000 represented the total vulnerable population. However, this seems unlikely. We know from recent prevalence estimation research that problematic drug use is more common in urban areas than in rural areas. This would suggest that, at minimum, there is room for expansion in the prevalence of problematic drug use in rural areas. We also know from recent prevalence estimation research that, while the overall prevalence of problematic drug use within the UK may be around 1 per cent, it is much higher in many urban centres such as London, Glasgow and Manchester. This suggests that we have not reached the absolute ceiling in terms of the prevalence of problem drug use in the UK.

4.4.5 Changes in Policy

It is possible that the changes in government policy with regard to illegal drug use could have a significant influence on the overall number of problem drug users within the UK. It is difficult to speculate at this stage the various ways in which prevalence may be influenced by specific changes in policy.

4.5 Possible Future Increase in the Prevalence of Problem Drug Use

We explore three factors below which individually and in concert could influence future increases in the prevalence of problem drug use in the UK. These are: changes in the gender balance in those using illegal drugs, changes in the age structure of those using illegal drugs, and changes in the level of drug use in rural areas in the UK.

4.5.1 Changes in the Gender Balance of Problem Drug Users

Most prevalence studies suggest that males make up approximately 70 per cent of problem drug users. On that basis, the current estimate of around 356 593 problem drug users will be made up of 249 615 men and 106 977 women. Studies looking at less problematic forms of drug use, particularly drug use within school samples, suggest that the gender gap is narrowing (European Monitoring Centre for Drugs and Drug Addiction, 2005).

If the gender gap closed completely, and women problem drug users caught up completely with men (at the prevalence levels found in 2001), there would be approximately 2 × 249 615 problem drug users, i.e. approximately 500 000 problem drug users in the UK (13 per 1000 of the population aged 15–64). If the current gender gap halved, there would be an additional 71 319 female problem drug users, taking the number of

female problem drug users to 178 296 (i.e. half way between the existing 106 977 estimate for the number of female problem drug users and the estimated 249 615 male problem drug users). This would result in an estimated 427 911 problem drug users in the UK. Finally, if the gender gap remained the same, the prevalence of problem drug use would remain at 350 000.

4.5.2 Changes in the Age Profile of Problem Drug Users

Most problem drug users are typically aged 20–30. There are two obvious ways in which changes in the age structure of the drug-using population could influence the overall number of problem drug users. First, the average age at which people begin to use drugs could decrease and, second, there could be an increase in the number of drug users aged over 30. To examine the possible effect of widening the age range, we can compare different scenarios using data from Greater Manchester in 2001 (Millar *et al.*, 2004).

Figure 12.2 demonstrates the prevalence rates found in three age ranges, 15–24, 25–34 and 35–64 (recalculated from the 35–54

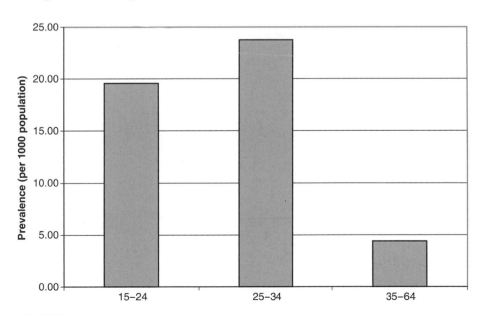

FIGURE 12.2   Prevalence of problem drug use in Greater Manchester, 2001, by age group.

prevalence rate used in the original publication). With an overall prevalence rate of
11.92 per 1000 population aged 15–64, the
prevalence in Greater Manchester is higher
than that estimated for the whole of England.
The area does, however, include some local
authority areas with lower prevalence, e.g.
7.19 per 1000 in Stockport, 7.68 per 1000 in
Bury and 7.91 per 1000 in Trafford.

As a worst-case scenario, if the extent of
problem drug use in the 15–24 age range rose
to the level found in the 25–34 age range (as
a result of a lowering of the average age at
which people use drugs) and the prevalence
in the 35–64 age range rose to half of that
currently seen in the middle age group, this
would increase the number of problem drug
users to just under 500 000. This scenario is
shown in Figure 12.3.

If the lower age range rose to match that
currently found in the 25–34 age range, and
the prevalence rate in the older age group
rose slightly to one-quarter of that currently
seen in the 25–34 age range, this would
increase the prevalence of problem drug use
in the UK to just under 400 000. Finally, if
the prevalence of problem drug use in the
15–24 age range rose to match that currently

found in the 25–34 age range (Scenario 2
in Figure 12.3), the number of problem
drug users in the UK would rise to 375 000
nationally.

4.5.3 Increase in the Prevalence of Problem Drug Use in Rural Areas

In this section, we look at the possible
impact on the overall prevalence of problem drug use in the UK of an increase in
the prevalence of problem drug use in the
rural areas. The possibility of a significant
increase in the prevalence of problem drug
use in rural areas was highlighted most
recently in research carried out by Hay and
colleagues in Scotland (Hay *et al.*, 2005). In
particular, Hay and colleagues showed that
while there had been a small decrease in the
overall prevalence of problem drug use in
Scotland in 2000–2003, prevalence in some of
the rural areas had increased markedly over
that period.

Previous research has estimated that the
prevalence of problem drug use in Greater
Manchester is around 11.92 per 1000 aged
15–64). The equivalent figure for parts of

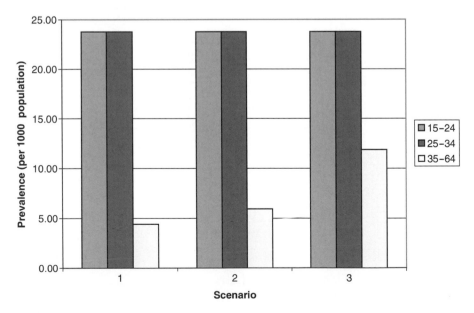

FIGURE 12.3   Possible prevalence of problem drug use, by age group, under three scenarios.

London has been identified as 24.8 per 1000 aged 15–64, while the figure for Liverpool is thought to be around 14.0 per 1000 aged 15–64 (Millar *et al.*, 2004; Hickman *et al.*, 2004c). The weighted average (weighted by population size) for these three areas is 18.45 per 1000 aged 15–64.

If the prevalence of problem drug use for England and Wales as a whole rose to the 18.45 per 1000 figure (based on the London, Liverpool and Manchester prevalence estimation work), the number of problem drug users in England and Wales would rise to around 630 000. Combining this estimate with the data from Scotland would give an overall figure of around 680 000 problem drug users in the UK by 2025. If the prevalence of problem drug use across England and Wales rose to the level already found in Scotland, this would result in there being approximately 580 000 problem drug users in the UK. But if the prevalence of problem drug use in rural England and Wales remained the same, the prevalence at the UK level would also remain at 350 000.

4.6 Overall Changes in Prevalence

It is possible that the prevalence of problem drug use in the UK by 2025 could fall below the current best estimate of 350 000 drug users. As we have already mentioned, the research by Hay and colleagues (2005) identified a small decrease in the prevalence of problem drug use in Scotland between 2000 and 2003. Similarly, the number of drug-related deaths in England and Wales also fell from 1571 in 1999 to 1388 in 2003 (National Statistics, 2005). These figures are potentially significant because data on drug-related deaths is often taken as a proxy measure of the overall prevalence of problem drug use. On the basis of the drug-related death figures, there is the possibility that we may have witnessed a small reduction in the overall prevalence of problem drug use in the UK in recent years and that this may continue. However, sitting alongside such a possibility is the fact that the prevalence of problem drug use in the UK has increased

markedly over the last 40 years. If these long-term trends continue it is entirely possible that we may witness the prevalence of problem drug use in the UK rising to between 500 000 and one million in the next 20 years.

While it is clearly not possible to predict the actual prevalence of problem drug use by 2025 it is important, from a sociological point of view, to explore the possible impact of a significant increase in problem drug use. In the remainder of this section, we consider the possible impact of the worst-case scenario of there being a three-fold increase in the number of problem drug users in the next 20 years. It is important to stress that the sorts of impacts we outline below could begin to be apparent in some parts of the UK in advance of a possible three-fold increase in problem drug user numbers.

4.7 What would be the Impact of the Worst-case-scenario Three-fold Increase in the Prevalence of Problem Drug Use in the UK?

4.7.1 Drug-related Deaths

Figures for 2000 for England and Wales suggest there were 1666 drug-related deaths (*Health Statistics Quarterly*, 2004). In the same year, there were 292 drug-related deaths in Scotland and 54 in Northern Ireland (drug-related deaths in Scotland in 2003, General Register Office for Scotland; personal communication for the Northern Ireland figure), giving a total of 2012. If the number of problematic drug users in the UK rose to one million, there could be approximately 6000 deaths a year.

4.7.2 Blood-borne Infection

HIV has remained low at around 1 per cent, among injecting drug users in most parts of the UK. But the situation in relation to hepatitis C is markedly different, with 35–40 per cent of injecting drug users thought to have contracted the infection in the UK (Health Protection Agency, 2003).

A three-fold increase in the prevalence of problematic drug use could mean somewhere in the region of 350 000–400 000 injecting drug users who are Hepatitis C positive and 10 000 who are HIV positive.

4.7.3 Childcare

The *Hidden Harm* report (Advisory Council on the Misuse of Drugs, 2003) suggests that there were 88 200 children in England and Wales and 17 900 children in Scotland who had a mother who was a problem drug user in 2000. No information is provided for Northern Ireland. On this basis, there are approximately 100 000 children with a drug-using mother in the UK. If the prevalence of problem drug use were to treble, it could be expected that the number of children with a drug-dependent mother would at least treble to 300 000. This estimate does not include children of drug-using fathers whose mother is not using drugs.

4.7.4 The Economic and Social Costs of Problem Drug Use

Christine Godfrey and colleagues (2002) from the University of York outlined an approach to calculating the economic and social costs of problem drug use in England and Wales in 2000. They estimated it at £10 402 per problem drug user, and the total social costs at £35 456 per user. (See also Chapter 13 of this volume.) If there are currently around 350 000 problem drug users in the UK, the total economic and social cost would be of the order of £12.8 billion per year. If there were one million problem drug users in the UK, the total economic and social cost would rise to £35.4 billion, an increase of over £22 billion.

The largest part of that cost is the estimated social costs associated with victims of crime, accounting for £24 billion. There are also additional healthcare costs (just over £1 billion), and benefit payments (just over £2 billion). The government's reactive spending on crime (as opposed to the social costs of victims of crime) would total £7 billion. These costs do not include the costs of treatment, currently estimated to be in the region of £500 million per year, which could also treble in the event of an increase in prevalence to the 1 million mark.

4.7.5 Drugs and Crime

Many key institutions are already struggling to cope with the impact of illegal drug use. Research in Scotland that involved interviewing and drug testing arrestees found that 80 per cent of those arrested reported having used an illegal drug within the last 12 months (McKeganey *et al.*, 2002a). Holloway *et al.* (2004), reporting similar research in England and Wales, found that between 1999 and 2002 around 65 per cent of tested arrestees were found to have used illegal drugs. The proportion of arrestees who tested positive for opiates and/or cocaine increased from 29 per cent in 1999 to 35 per cent in 2002. In this study, 85 per cent of arrestees using heroin, cocaine or crack reported having committed one or more property crimes in the last 12 months (Holloway *et al.*, 2004). Increasingly, then, policing in many areas is about policing the impact of the UK's drug problem. In the event of a three-fold increase in the size of the problematic drug-using population, it is difficult to see how the enforcement agencies could avoid being overwhelmed by drug-related offending without a very substantial increase in their own resources.

4.7.6 Public Visibility of Problematic Drug Use

At the present time, while problematic drug use may be fairly visible in some communities, public evidence of drug usage (discarded drug-injecting paraphernalia, individuals using drugs on the streets) is not that commonplace. If the UK did have a million problematic drug users, illegal drug use would become much more visible in public spaces, and many more families would have direct personal experience of a son, daughter, father or mother addicted to illegal drugs.

4.7.7 Interweaving of the Legal and Illegal Economies

In the event of a three-fold increase in the size of the problematic drug-using population, there would be increasing pressure to launder illegal drug money through the legal economy. Similarly, the success of efforts at seizing the assets of drug dealers is likely to mean that greater attention is devoted, on the part of those involved in the illegal drug economy, to concealing their assets in legitimate economic enterprises either in the UK or abroad. In time, it could become virtually impossible to distinguish between the legitimate and illegitimate economies and some local communities could become financially dependent on the illegal drug economy without knowing it.

4.7.8 Economic and Political Influence

With increasing economic influence being located within the hands of a small group of high-level drug suppliers and drug dealers, it is possible that a number of the key individuals involved could seek to exercise local political influence in order to protect their own enterprises (both legal and illegal) and, in time, seek to gain influence at the national political level.

4.7.9 Drug Policy

In response to these developments, it is possible that one might see radical changes in drug policy. In the event of a three-fold increase in the prevalence of problematic drug use, and a corresponding increase in the level of drug-related crime, there could be considerable pressure on doctors to prescribe heroin and/or cocaine as an effective crime-reduction measure (Dijkgraaf *et al.*, 2005). Alternatively, one might see pressures developing to use the technology of satellite tracking to limit the movement of known drug users. Equally, one might see the development of communities from which known drug users are excluded – with the information on who to exclude being determined through a policy of much wider drug testing.

4.7.10 Foreign Policy

At the present time, both the UK and the US governments provide substantial support to the governments of Afghanistan and Colombia to reduce the level of heroin and cocaine production (for example, encouraging heroin- and cocaine-producing farmers to produce different crops). However, the Global Drug Report from the United Nations Office of Drugs and Crime (2004) states, on the basis of a 2003 survey of Afghan farmers, that only 4 per cent of those surveyed reported an intention to decrease opium production, and 69 per cent indicated an intention to increase it.

If the production of heroin and cocaine was sustaining something of the order of a million drug users in the UK, and an equivalent number in the US, it is possible that the negative impact of drug abuse in these countries would be so great as to lead to increasing calls in both countries for much greater military intervention within drug-producing countries. Alternatively, in the face of continuing drug production in certain countries, there will be some who advise not an increase in military intervention but an increase in aid and other non-military government support in order to encourage local farmers to move away from illegal drug-crop production.

4.7.11 Changes in Public Attitudes

A trebling in the problematic drug-using population may lead either to greater tolerance of those who are using and dependent on illegal drugs, or to much greater tensions between those who are and those who are not dependent on them. Drug abuse could become a major fault line within our society.

4.8 Conclusion

In this section we fleshed out the possible impact of a three-fold increase in the prevalence of problematic drug use. As we indicated at the outset, there is no way of knowing whether we will witness an increase in prevalence of that order in the next 20 years, a plateauing in the number of drug user or a decrease in drug user numbers. On the basis of long-term trends, however, the scenario of a three-fold increase in problematic drug user numbers would not be beyond the bounds of credibility. This scenario gives rise to the question of whether society would always be able to cope with its illegal-drug-use problem irrespective of the size of that problem. At the present time, UK society does indeed cope, albeit at considerable cost, with what is thought to be an estimated 350 000 problematic drug users. It cannot be assumed that the same would be said if that figure doubled or trebled. Indeed, in the face of such an expansion, it is very likely that there would be communities within the UK whose very sustainability was called into question as a result of their local drug problem. The possibility of a further significant increase in the prevalence of problem drug use in the UK clearly underlines the importance of efforts aimed at reducing the number of problem drug users.

5 INDIVIDUAL SOCIAL AND CULTURAL FACTORS INFLUENCING DRUG USE

5.1 Public Attitudes

The last 20 years have seen a major change in public attitudes towards cannabis. In the 1983 British Social Attitudes Survey (Stratford et al., 2003), 12 per cent of respondents said that they thought cannabis should be legalised. By 2001, this figure had increased to 41 per cent. The growing liberalisation of public attitudes towards cannabis, however, is not matched by a similar shift in attitude towards heroin and ecstasy. In the 2001 survey, 87 per cent of respondents felt that heroin should remain illegal and 88 per cent felt that ecstasy should remain illegal – similar proportions to 1993 (Stratford et al., 2003).

Changes in public attitudes towards illegal drugs are likely to have been influenced by a wide range of social factors, including the representations of drugs and drug users in the media: and particularly through advertising.

Depictions of illicit drug use in film date back to the late nineteenth century (Blackman, 2004; Shapiro, 2003). There has also been a long history of widely publicised drug-dependent actors and actresses, drug overdoses and scandals. The same applies to the link between music and drugs (Blackman, 2004), from the early references to drug use in the blues of the 1930s through to the present day, again involving drug-dependent musicians, tragic drug-related deaths and public scandals. It is harder to gauge whether this represents an increasing trend. Given the proliferation and diversification in most modern media, research needs to do more than show greater references to drugs in current film, television, music and literature.

One important area where it seems almost undeniable that there has been an explosion in drug references is advertising. Blackman (2004) has claimed that drugs are now 'part of the mainstream economy: they provide a reservoir of images and ideas which can be exploited by advertisers to sell products'. Blackman points to the wide range of products that drug imagery has been used to sell: hemp products; mobile phones; perfumes (Opium and Addiction) and, perhaps most brazenly, computer games. Other clear examples are the fashion industry ('heroin chic') and the drinks industry, which has employed 'spaced-out' imagery to sell alcoholic drinks and 'natural highs' to sell soft drinks.

5.2 Changes in Youth Transitions to Adulthood

There have been major changes over the past 30 years in young people's transitions to adulthood (Coles, 2001; Jones, 2002). Until the 1970s, there were clear pathways and progressions for young people by which they achieved adult status. More recently, the loss of manual and semi-manual jobs in traditional industries and the huge rise in the proportion of women who work has led to much greater complexity and much greater uncertainty for young people's progression. These economic changes have been paralleled by many more young people staying on in education and a prolongation of the period when young people are economically dependent on their parents. In short, youth has been extended. This may explain some of the increases in drug-use prevalence referred to above (McCambridge and Strang, 2004).

5.3 Race

Household and school surveys of drug-use prevalence have repeatedly shown black and minority ethnic people to have lower rates of illegal drug and alcohol use than white people. However, an increasing proportion of second- and third-generation British Asians are using illegal drugs at least on a recreational basis.

5.4 Gender

Both men and women use drugs, but addiction research has focused largely on males. In the earliest ethnographic studies of heroin misuse conducted in the US (Finestone, 1957; Sutter, 1966, 1969, 1972; Feldman, 1968; and Preble and Casey, 1969), street addicts were portrayed as innovative, self-determining men who somehow managed to carve out an active role for themselves in an otherwise hostile world. This image was maintained in later research where male drug users were similarly described as busy, self-respecting individuals who actively confronted and purposely

responded to external constraints and life opportunities (Agar, 1973; Waldorf, 1973; Hanson et al., 1985; Johnson et al., 1985; Biernacki, 1979; Rosenbaum, 1981; Bourgois, 1996).

By contrast, female drug users have often been omitted from – or at best peripheral to – studies of drug misuse (Ettorre, 1992, 1994; Henderson, 1988; Pettiway, 1997; Rosenbaum, 1981; Taylor, 1993). When they have appeared, they have overwhelmingly been portrayed as victims or as weak, self-destructive and insecure individuals who were sicker, more deviant and more psychologically disturbed than their male peers (Colten, 1979; Ettorre, 1989, 1992; Pettiway, 1997). Until recently, female drug use has tended to be discussed in relation to a narrow range of 'women's issues' such as the effects of addiction on childbirth, child rearing and parenting (Glynn et al., 1983; Murphy and Rosenbaum, 1995), or the involvement of women drug users in prostitution (Freund et al., 1989; Perkins and Bennett, 1985).

As both the number of drug-using women and the number of female drug-misuse researchers have increased, information relating to gender differences in drug-taking behaviour has been emerging. Recent research has shown that women report shorter progressions from first drug use to dependence than men (Anglin et al., 1987; McCance-Katz et al., 1999), are more likely to share used injecting equipment and to have a sexual partner who is also a drug user (Barnard, 1993; Becker and Duffy, 2002; Donoghoe et al., 1992; Dwyer et al., 1994; Gossop et al., 1994; Powis et al., 1996). In addition, disproportionate numbers of drug-dependent women have suffered traumatic experiences such as sexual abuse, incest, domestic violence, or the death of a child or a stillbirth (Becker and Duffy, 2002; El-Bassel et al., 2000; Gilbert et al., 2001; Horgan et al., 1998). Likewise, female drug users experience particularly high levels of mental health problems, including low self-esteem, depression, anxiety and suicidal feelings (Becker and Duffy, 2002; Gilbert et al., 2001).

5.5 Changes in Risk Factors in the Development of Illegal Drug Use

5.5.1 *Parental Drug Use*

A large body of research has shown that substance-dependent people tend to have had substance-dependent parents (e.g. Lloyd, 1998; Rhodes *et al.*, 2003; Johnson and Leff, 1999). However, the relative importance of genetic predisposition and the family environment is not so clear. Interestingly, recent research on twins suggests that the genetic and environmental factors that influence risk for use and problematic use are 'largely or entirely nonspecific in their effect' and that the 'environmental experiences unique to the person largely determine whether predisposed individuals will use or misuse one class of psychoactive substances rather than another' (Kendler *et al.*, 2003).

5.5.2 *Family Disruption and Family Relationships*

While some studies have found an association between divorce or separation and drug use, including more problematic use (Rhodes *et al.*, 2003), a growing body of research seems to indicate that once family relationships are taken into account, family structure ceases to be influential (Friedman *et al.*, 2000; Spooner, 1999). It may be family relationship difficulties, rather than separation, that cause poor outcomes for children (Rogers and Prior, 1998). Similarly a number of studies have attempted to identify the type of parent–child relationships that are associated with problem use. Generalising from this growing literature, it would appear that lack of attachment and warmth, overprotection, rejection and possibly poor parental monitoring are associated with problem use (Spooner, 1999; Oxford *et al.*, 2000; Lee and Bell, 2003; Glavak *et al.*, 2003; Anderson and Eisemann, 2003).

These findings suggest that poorer parent–child relationships would be accompanied by greater vulnerability to substance dependence, along with a whole host of other

problems. There have been major changes in parenting in recent times in the UK, including recent growth in non-parental care due to changing trends in the employment of women. Men are more involved in parenting (especially in cases where the mother is working) and children appear to be increasingly protected (e.g. Ransom and Rutledge, 2005). Whether these changes have led – and will lead in the future – to changes in parental attachment or the other factors referred to above is an open question. However, policies that encourage parental attachment and warmth and discourage overprotection may prove important to prevent future problematic use.

5.5.3 *Child Sexual and Physical Abuse*

Since Lloyd's review in 1998, which concluded that there was 'a strong relationship between child sexual abuse and drug abuse', there has been a burgeoning in the literature in this subject area. Virtually all of these studies have focused on drug users in treatment (Westermeyer *et al.*, 2001; Berry and Sellman, 2001; Ballon *et al.*, 2001; Liebschutz *et al.*, 2002; Medrano *et al.*, 1999). Excluding one study with exceptionally high rates, self-reported sexual abuse rates vary between 50 per cent and 64 per cent for females and between 10 per cent and 24 per cent among males. Rates for physical abuse varied between 40 per cent and 55 per cent among females and between 23 per cent and 26 per cent among males. Given the much greater level of social awareness of these issues in recent times, it may be that rates will stabilise or decline.

5.5.4 *School*

Previous research has shown that poor performance at school, truanting, exclusion and attendance at pupil referral units (or 'continuation schools' in the US) are associated with problematic drug use. This conclusion has been verified by more recent work (Rhodes *et al.*, 2003; Goulden and

Sondhi, 2001). Many of these school-based factors cannot be seen in isolation from earlier family factors and the considerable body of evidence showing an association between conduct disorder and drug use.

The permanent exclusion rate in England has been decreasing in recent years. After 1997/8 it declined by 24 per cent to 9290 in 2002/3 (Department for Education and Skills, 2004a). Any substantial decrease in the truancy rate is likely to help prevent the escalation of drug use among those attending school who might otherwise be on the street during the day with time to kill.

5.5.5 Social Deprivation

Sociological research on the UK heroin epidemic of the 1980s recognised that these new drug problems were developing in the poorest areas of cities (Pearson, 1987a; Parker et al., 1988). Since then, a number of studies have shown deprivation to be linked to problem drug use (see Rhodes et al., 2003).

The connection between deprivation and problematic drug use is likely to be complex, but will probably involve parenting. Bringing up a child in deprived circumstances is more stressful and difficult than in well-off circumstances (Utting, 1995). There is also the issue of access to drugs. Longitudinal research on young people in the US has shown that exposure to cocaine is more widespread in more deprived neighbourhoods (Crum et al., 1996). Class A drug markets are likely to develop in areas where crime and disaffection with police are high (Lupton et al., 2002). Thus exposure to drugs like heroin is likely to be more common in socially excluded communities (Webster et al., forthcoming).

The proportion of children brought up in 'poverty' is declining (Sutherland et al., 2003). While this may have an eventual impact on problematic drug use, it is difficult to avoid the conclusion that without a dramatic rise in the fortunes of some of the more deprived areas of the country, there is likely to be a continuing escalation in the use of such drugs as heroin and cocaine.

6 TREATMENT

There is now a wide range of readily accessible drug services within the UK, including in-patient drug detoxification and residential rehabilitation, methadone and other substitution programmes and non-clinical interventions such as counselling and group work. In addition, new types of treatment such as vaccines, ultra-rapid detoxifications, memory extinction and transcranial magnetic stimulation are emerging. In this chapter, we examine research on the impact of drug treatment services and consider how treatment may need to evolve if it is to address changes in the pattern and profile of drug use.

In medical research, it is commonly assumed that the gold standard in measuring what works is the randomised control trial (RCT). The drug-misuse treatment field has had its fair share of clinical experiments. However, there are difficulties in conducting highly controlled evaluations with groups of addicts. It is almost impossible to ensure that any given individual only receives one specific treatment, and there are ethical issues in withholding support from someone simply to maintain a rigorous evaluation methodology. Additionally, drug treatment programmes can be very diverse and comprise non-medical as well as medical components, making systematic comparisons difficult.

Alongside RCTs, the effectiveness of drug treatment services has been assessed using longitudinal outcome studies. They have consistently provided research evidence that the major treatment modalities (methadone prescribing, residential services, and drug-free out-patient support) are effective in reducing illicit drug use, reducing the incidence of crime-related behaviour, and supporting improvement in physical health, mental health, and social functioning (Fletcher and Battjes, 1999).

In the criminal justice field, longitudinal studies of prison drug treatment programmes have also shown positive outcomes in terms of relapse and recidivism rates (Field, 1992; Inciardi et al., 1997;

Knight *et al.*, 1997; Martin and Player, 2000; Martin *et al.*, 2003; Pelissier *et al.*, 1998; Shewan *et al.*, 1994; Wexler *et al.*, 1990). Despite this, there is worrying evidence that the availability of drug treatment provision in prisons is insufficient to meet need, and drug users' perceptions of the help they receive while in jail is poor (Neale and Saville, 2004). Furthermore, the long-term success of relatively new criminal justice interventions – such as drug courts, arrest referral schemes and the drug treatment and testing order (DTTO) – has yet to be proven. An evaluation of DTTOs concluded that there was a low completion rate which probably reflected the challenges faced by local services in keeping chaotic drug users on an intensive and highly structured programme (Audit Commission, 2002).

Current sociological drug-misuse research highlights the importance of 'process' factors (as opposed to simple 'outputs' and 'outcomes') in drug service evaluation (Neale and Saville, 2004). Key process factors relate to how services are delivered and the attitudes of service providers. According to one qualitative study, positive service attributes include offering a broad range of services, having staff with specialist drugs knowledge, being accessible, having a good attitude towards drug users, encouraging open and honest working relationships, being willing to listen and being supportive and understanding (Neale, 1998).

Qualitative studies have also examined the barriers drug users can face when attempting to access help. An Australian study of women who self-managed change in their alcohol and other drug dependence found that the principal barriers to accessing treatment included social stigma and labelling, lack of awareness of the range of treatment options, concerns about childcare, the perceived economic and time costs of residential treatment, the confrontational models used by some treatment services, and stereotypical views of clients (Copeland, 1997).

A recent Home Office report on women drug users and drug service provision argued that female drug users have specific experiences and needs that are not always recognised or met by service providers (Becker and Duffy, 2002). These relate to pregnancy and childcare, sex-working, sexual and physical abuse and mental health needs. A Home Office study by Sangster *et al.* (2002) found that drug services in the UK have also failed to develop in ways that would make them more accessible to black and ethnic-minority people. This research argued that there is a place for specialist drug services, but mainstream providers must also develop accessible and appropriate support that recognises the diversity of needs across ethnic groups.

In terms of alcohol treatment, the new alcohol harm-reduction strategy for England (Prime Minister's Strategy Unit, 2004) identifies a range of appropriate interventions. It concludes that no particular treatment is more effective than any other in responding to alcohol problems, but different types of treatment are appropriate for different types of individual. Accordingly, more co-ordinated arrangements for commissioning and monitoring standards and for tailoring treatment to differing individual needs and motivations are required.

Increasingly, service provision for both illegal drug use and alcohol problems is being delivered in the form of integrated packages of care that incorporate general health, social and other forms of support, as well as drug misuse treatment (National Treatment Agency, 2002). This is resulting in an expansion of 'wraparound' housing, education, training and employment services. Although such developments have yet to be thoroughly evaluated, the complexity and extent of problems accompanying addiction are likely to mean that enabling service users to achieve relatively simple goals, such as moving into paid employment or retaining secure accommodation, will prove very difficult (Kemp and Neale, 2005). The success or failure of integrated models of care and add-on services may therefore need to be judged by small incremental steps rather than by large-scale change.

As support services become more individ-ualised and involve a wider range of care providers, qualitative research – particularly that incorporating service users' views – will have an increasing role to play in ser-vice evaluation. Moreover, the importance of user-centeredness can be expected to intensify for two further reasons. More poly-drug use means that it will not be possi-ble to treat drug service clients as simply 'heroin users', 'stimulant users' or 'prob-lem drinkers'. And if the prevalence of drug use – and the numbers of individuals from more affluent, better-educated and middle-class backgrounds – increases, service users will tend to have greater purchasing power and knowledge of the available treatment options. This will make them a more demanding client group that expects provi-sion to be tailored closely to their personal circumstances.

6.1 Looking to the Future in Drug Treatment Research

In the future, sociologists must build on existing research evidence to increase under-standing of how services might better help vulnerable and marginalised subgroups of drug users, the families and carers of drug users, and the communities in which drug users live. Equally, it will be necessary to investigate and evaluate a broader range of drug treatments than has been the case hitherto.

International research suggests that the provision of safe injecting rooms (SIRs) reduces drug users' mortality and other health risks. However, theoretical and sim-ulation evidence has indicated that SIRs can also diminish incentives to refrain from drug use by reducing the risk of drug-related death (Clarke, 2001). Though SIRs are not currently available in the UK, this may change during the next 20 years as the UK government comes to face the prospect of problematic drug use becoming much more visible in public spaces.

Recently, the UK government has given guarded endorsement to the use of pre-scribed injectable opioid drugs to a minority of (mainly older) heroin misusers who have failed to respond to other treatment (Drug Strategy Directorate, 2002; National Treat-ment Agency, 2003). Where such treatments are occurring, there is a clear need for them to be carefully monitored and evaluated.

To date, the proportions of drug treatment clients over 35 years have been low in the UK and elsewhere. It is possible that in future, society will find itself dealing with large numbers of middle-aged and even elderly 'difficult-to-treat' addicts. This burgeoning new treatment group could jeopardise any nascent willingness in the medical profes-sion to prescribe opiates and injectable drugs for fear that some individuals will need this expensive treatment for many years. Equally, such initiatives could come to be seen as neg-ative treatments of despair – simply ware-housing large numbers of individuals, who have been failed by the existing system, in order to protect the community from their ill-doings while keeping them out of a criminal justice system that is bursting at its seams.

Both of these possibilities highlight the importance of future research into the preva-lence and treatment needs of older drug users. However, at the opposite end of the age spectrum, society must deal with ever-younger drug users. It is here that the boundary between treatment and preven-tion is most blurred. Although the effective-ness of drug prevention programmes has been widely contested, research indicates that drug education – if delivered in the proper context and in the appropriate way – can reduce drug misuse or at least delay the onset of experimentation (DrugScope, 2004). Building on this evidence, the Depart-ment for Education and Skills (2004b) now provides detailed guidance on what schools should be doing in this area and efforts are being made to equip young people with core life skills that will protect them against drug taking.

Inevitably, new forms of drug misuse will generate new pharmacological interventions that will require both clinical and non-clinical testing and assessment. Currently, good substitution therapies for many drugs (such as synthetic drugs, crack cocaine and cannabis) are not available. In years to come, this treatment gap will probably disappear as pharmaceutical technologies advance. Even if suitable treatment drugs are not developed, vaccinations against specific forms of drug taking will almost certainly appear. Vaccines to help nicotine users (NicVax) and cocaine users (TA-CD) break their addictions are already being developed.

Although the optimal nature and extent of non-medical treatments continue to be disputed (Wodak, 2001), psychosocial and behavioural interventions play an important role in tackling addictions and an ever-increasing number of such treatments are emerging. A key aim for sociological research must be to learn more about how best to exploit their potential.

The importance of mutual aid in recovery processes is clearly reflected in the popularity of Alcoholics Anonymous (AA) and Narcotics Anonymous (NA). But mutual-aid practices are increasingly varied. For example, there are trends towards the political organisation of addicts, the professionalisation of mutual-aid movements and the globalisation of recovery mutual aid via the Internet. Nowadays, mutual-aid groups differ markedly (White, 2004) and more information about their functions and capabilities is needed.

Finally, it is important to highlight the role that local communities might play in tackling drug problems in the future. Involving communities in developing locally based initiatives through the imaginative use of existing and planned network partnerships is a cornerstone of the UK drug strategy (Home Office, 1998). Despite this, sociological research has sounded a note of caution by criticising romantic and idealised notions of 'community'. Communities exist within communities and attempts to present a unified front can obscure the many differences between people (Cockburn, 1977; Cowley et al., 1977; McClenaghan, 2000;

Peterson, 1994). While community-based responses to drug problems are to be welcomed, the success of such initiatives may depend upon first re-establishing a sense of safety within local neighbourhoods and, second, increasing understanding and trust between local people who use drugs and those who do not (McKeganey et al., 2004a).

7 CONCLUSIONS

In this review we have covered a wide range of areas to do with the sociology and the social impact of drug use and abuse. We have looked at issues to do with how sociologists have understood drug use; past and possible future changes in the prevalence of legal and illegal drug use; factors associated with individuals' drug use; and the impact of treatment services in meeting the needs of people who get into difficulty as a result of their drug use.

In terms of looking to the next 20 years, one of the key issues we have considered is the possible increase in overall prevalence of problem drug use. While it is not possible to say with any certainty what the level of illegal drug use will be in 2025, we can speculate, on the basis of past increases in prevalence, that the next 20 years may witness a three-fold increase in prevalence. Such an increase would not be beyond the realm of possibility and could come about as a result of such factors as the level of drug use among females equalling that among males, a reduction in the age of onset of illegal drug use, a lengthening of drug-using careers, and an increase in the level of drug use in rural areas. These are all developments of which we are starting to see the early signs at the present time (Hay et al., 2005; McKeganey et al., 2004b; European Monitoring Centre for Drugs and Drug Addiction, 2005).

The result of such a development could be that within the next 20 years the prevalence of problematic drug use in the UK could increase from around the 350 000 to one million. Again, while it is not possible to be precise as to the impact of such an increase, there clearly would be significant effects on health services, on the police, on domestic drug policy and on foreign policy.

It is possible that any significant expansion in the use of heroin, cocaine and any new drugs yet to be developed might occur among new social groups whose 'risk profile' is very different from those who are currently using these drugs. These individuals may be less likely to resort to crime to fund their drug use and, when they do develop problems associated with their drug use, they may be more responsive to treatment than current problematic drug users. It is possible that the prevalence of problem drug use in the UK could remain at its current level, although we think this is an unlikely outcome.

The impact of any significant increase in the prevalence of problem drug use is itself likely to be influenced by the nature of any policy developments in this area. If heroin and cocaine became legal, for example, one would not necessarily expect to see anything like the connection between problematic drug use and crime which is commonplace today. However, the legalisation of these drugs could see a much greater expansion in their use to the point where the level of their consumption would be on a par with current levels of alcohol and tobacco use.

In the next 20 years there may also be marked changes in the nature of drug treatment services, with less focus on addiction and more focus on intoxication (Caulkins et al., 2003). There may be a need for drug treatment services to be much more responsive to the greater consumer power and knowledge of a large group of users who do not have the traditional risk profile which includes abuse and social exclusion. Equally, there will be a need to identify exactly what 'treatment' means for individuals who are not yet addicted but who may be on the road to addiction. Other demographic changes are also likely to influence the nature of drug treatment, including the decreasing age of onset of illegal drug use as well as

individuals who have remained drug dependent into their 60s and 70s.

The field of prevention might also undergo dramatic change. Drug prevention technology today is somewhat underdeveloped. It is possible that the introduction of cheap, non-invasive, drug-testing kits might fundamentally change the terrain of drug prevention, allowing services to focus directly on those who are using specific substances at a point well before they get into difficulty with those substances. Similarly, it may be that widespread drug testing itself reduces the overall prevalence of drug use. We might see widespread erosion of the rights of individuals as a result of their drug use (McKeganey, 2004).

If there was anything like a three-fold increase in the level of drug-related offending, there would be a very strong push to limit the freedom of known drug users, both those who have become addicted to certain drugs and mere users of specific substances. We already accept the principle of requiring drug users to undergo treatment as part of their processing by the criminal justice system. It may be that any significant expansion in drug-related offending would call forth initiatives to limit drug users' movements, possibly using the technology of satellite tracking.

In the face of these sorts of developments, there is likely to be a need to increase the support for those working in the drug treatment, drug prevention and drug enforcement fields. There will be a growing need to support professional practice in each of these areas to ensure that professional practice is based on clear evidence of 'what works'. This will necessitate much greater investment in research to establish the effectiveness of different approaches to tackling society's drug problem.

7.1 Acknowledgements

The work of preparing this review was undertaken on the basis of a grant from the Department of Trade and Industry as part of the Foresight Project Brain Science,

Addiction and Drugs Project. The views contained in this report are those of the authors and should not be attributed to the funding body. The authors would, however, like to acknowledge the support and advice of the Foresight team in undertaking this review.

References

Advisory Council on the Misuse of Drugs (2003) *Hidden harm: responding to the needs of the children of problem drug users.* London: HMSO.

Agar, M. (1973) *Ripping and running. A formal ethnography of urban heroin addicts.* New York and London: Seminar Press.

Anderson, P. and Eisemann, M. (2003) Parental rearing and individual vulnerability to drug addiction: a controlled study in a Swedish sample. *Nord J Psychiatry* 57(2): 147–156.

Anglin, M.D., Hser, Y.I., and McGlothlin, W.H. (1987) Sex differences in addict careers: becoming addicted. *Am J Drug Alcohol Abuse* 13: 59–71.

Audit Commission (2002) *Changing habits: the commissioning and management of drug treatment services for adults.* London: Audit Commission.

Ballon, B.C., Courbasson, C. and Smith, P.D. (2001). Physical and sexual abuse issues among youths with substance use problems. *Can J Psychiatry* 46: 617–621.

Barnard, M. (1993) Needle sharing in context: patterns of sharing among men and women injectors and HIV risks. *Addiction* 88: 805–812.

Barnard, M. (2003) Between a rock and a hard place: the role of relatives in protecting children from the effects of parental drug problems. *Child Family Social Work* 8: 291–299.

Barnard, M. and Barlow, J. (2002) Discovering parental drug dependence: silence and disclosure. *Children and Society* 17: 45–56.

Bauman, Z. (1992) *Intimations of modernity.* London: Routledge.

Becker, H. (1963) *Outsiders: studies in the sociology of deviance.* New York: Free Press.

Becker, J. and Duffy, C. (2002) *Women drug users and drugs service provision: service level responses to engagement and retention.* London: Home Office.

Berry, R. and Sellman, J.D. (2001). Childhood adversity in alcohol- and drug-dependent women presenting to out-patient treatment. *Drug Alcohol Rev* 20: 361–367.

Biernacki, P. (1979) Junkie work, 'hustlers' and social status among heroin addicts. *J Drug Issues* 9: 535–551.

Blackman, S. (2004). *Chilling out: the cultural politics of substances consumption, youth and drug policy.* Maidenhead, Berkshire: Open University Press.

Bloor, M. (1995) *The sociology of HIV transmission.* London: Sage Publications.

Bloor, M., McKeganey, N., Findlay, A., and Barnard, M. (1992) The inappropriateness of psychosocial models of risk behaviour to understanding HIV-related risk behaviour among Glasgow male prostitutes. *AIDS Care* 4: 131–137.

Bourgois, P. (1996) *In search of respect: selling crack in El Barrio.* Cambridge: Cambridge University Press.

Caulkins, J., Reuter, P., Iguchi, M., and Chiesa, J. (2003) *Drug use and drug policy futures. Insights from a colloquium.* Philadelphia: Rand Corporation.

Clarke, H. (2001) Some economics of safe injecting rooms. *Aust Econ Rev* 34: 53–63.

Cloward, R. and Ohlin, L. (1960) *Delinquency and opportunity.* Chicago: Free Press.

Cockburn, C. (1977) *Local state: management of cities and people.* London: Pluto Press.

Coles, B. (2001). *Joined-up youth research, policy and practice: a new agenda for change.* Leicester: Youth Work Press.

Colten, M.E. (1979) A description and comparative analysis of self-perceptions and attitudes of heroin-addicted women. In: US Department of Health, Education and Welfare, *Addicted women: family dynamics, self-perceptions, and support systems.* Rockville, MD: National Institute on Drug Abuse: 7–36.

Copeland, J. (1997) A qualitative study of barriers to formal treatment among women who self-managed change in addictive behaviours. *J Subst Abuse Treat* 14: 183–190.

Cowley, J., Kay, A., Mayo, M., and Thompson, M. (1977) *Community or class struggle.* London: Stage 1.

Crum, R.M., Lillie-Banton, M., and Anthony, J.C. (1996). Neighbourhood environment and opportunity to use cocaine and other drugs in late childhood and early adolescence. *Drug Alcohol Depend* 43: 155–161.

Currie, C., Fairgrieve, J., Akhtar, P., and Currie, D. (2003) Scottish Schools Adolescent Lifestyle and Substance Use Survey (SALSUS) national report: smoking, drinking and drug use among

13- and 15-year-olds in Scotland in 2002. Edinburgh: TSO.

De Angelis, D., Hickman, M., and Yang, S. (2004) Estimating long-term trends in the incidence and prevalence of opiate use/injecting drug use and the number of former users: back-calculation methods and opiate overdose deaths. *Am J Epidemiol* 160: 994–1004.

Department for Education and Skills (2004a). *Permanent exclusions from schools and exclusion appeals in England.* London: Department for Education and Skills.

Department for Education and Skills (2004b) *Drugs: guidance for schools.* London: Department for Education and Skills.

Department of Health (2004) Provisional statistics from the national drug treatment monitoring system in England and Wales 2001/2002 and 2002/2003.

Dijkgraaf M.G.W., van der Zanden, B.P., de Borgie, C.A.J.M., Blanken, P., van Ree, J.M. and van den Brink, W. (2005) Cost utility analysis of co-prescribed heroin compared with methadone maintenance treatment in heroin addicts in two randomised trials. *BMJ* 330: 1297.

Ditton, J. and Speirits, K. (1982) *The rapid increase of heroin addiction in Glasgow during 1981.* Glasgow: Department of Sociology, University of Glasgow.

Donoghoe, M., Dorn, N., James, C., Jones, S., Ribbens, J., and South, N. (1987) How families and communities respond to heroin. In: N. Dorn and N. South (eds), *A land fit for heroin? Drug policies, prevention and practice.* Basingstoke and London: Macmillan Education Ltd.

Dorn, N. and South, N. (eds) (1987) *A land fit for heroin? Drug policies, prevention and practice.* Basingstoke and London: Macmillan Education Ltd.

Downes, D. and Rock, P. (1998) *Understanding deviance: a guide to the sociology of crime and rule breaking*, 3rd edition. Oxford: Oxford University Press.

DrugScope (2004) Does drug education stop drug use? http://www.drugscope.org.uk/druginfo/drugsearch/faq_template.asp?file=%5Cwip%5C11%5C1%5C2%5Ceducation.html (accessed 18 August 2004).

Drug Strategy Directorate (2002) *Updated drug strategy 2002.* London: Home Office.

Dwyer, R., Richardson, D., Ross, M.W., Wodak, A., Miller, M.E., and Gold, J. (1994) A comparison of HIV risk between women and men who inject drugs. *AIDS Ed Prev* 6: 379–389.

El-Bassel, N., Gilbert, L., Schilling, R., and Wada, T. (2000) Drug abuse and partner violence among women in methadone treatment. *J Fam Viol* 15(3): 209–228.

Ettorre, E. (1989) Women, substance abuse and self-help. In: S. MacGregor (ed.), *Drugs and British society: responses to a social problem in the eighties.* London and New York: Routledge.

Ettorre, E. (1992) *Women and substance use.* New Brunswick, New Jersey: Rutgers University Press.

Ettorre, E. (1994) What can she depend on? Substance use and women's health. In: S. Wilkinson and C. Kitzinger (eds), *Women and health: feminist perspectives.* London: Taylor and Francis.

European Monitoring Centre for Drugs and Drug Addiction (2005) *Differences in patterns of drug use between men and women.* Lisbon: European Monitoring Centre for Drugs and Drug Addiction.

Featherstone, M. (1991) *Consumer culture and postmodernism.* London: Sage.

Feldman, H. (1968) Ideological supports to becoming and remaining a heroin addict. *J Health Social Behav* 9: 131–139.

Fiddle, S. (1967) *Portrait from a shooting gallery.* New York: Harper and Row.

Field, G. (1992) Oregon prison drug treatment programmes. In: C. Leukfield, and F. Tims (eds), *Drug abuse treatment in prison and jails.* Washington, DC: National Institute of Drug Abuse.

Finestone, H. (1957) Cats, kicks and color. In: H. Becker (ed.), *The other side.* New York: The Free Press.

Fletcher, B.W. and Battjes, R.J. (1999) Introduction to the special issue: treatment process in DATOS. *Drug Alcohol Depend* 57: 81–87.

Freund, M., Leonard, T.L., and Lee, N. (1989) Sexual behavior of resident street prostitutes with their clients in Camden, New Jersey. *J Sex Res* 26: 460–478.

Friedman, S.R. (2002) Sociopharmacology of drug use: initial thoughts. *Int J Drug Policy* 13: 341–347.

Friedman, A.S., Terra, A., and Glassman, K. (2000). Family structure versus family relationships for predicting substance use/abuse and illegal behaviour. *J Child Adol Subst Abuse* 10(1): 1–16.

Frischer, M., Leyland, A., Cormack, R. *et al.* (1993) Estimating population prevalence of injection drug use and HIV infection among injection drug users in Glasgow. *Am J Epidemiol* 138(3): 170–181.

Frischer, M., Hickman, M., Kraus, L., Mariani, F., and Wiessing, L. (2001) A comparison of the different methods for estimating the prevalence of problematic drug misuse in Great Britain. *Addiction* 96: 1465–1476.

Frischer, M., Heatlie, H., and Hickman, M. (2004). *Estimating the prevalence of problematic and injecting drug use for drug action team areas in England: a feasibility study using the multiple indicator method.* Home Office Online Report 34/04. www.homeoffice.gov.uk/rds/pdfs04/rdsolr3404.pdf

Gilbert, L., El-Bassel, N., Rajah, V., Foleno, A., and Frye, V. (2001) Linking drug-related activities with experiences of partner violence: a focus group study of women in methadone treatment. *Violence Victims* 16(5): 517–536.

Glavak, R., Kuterovac-Jogodic, G., and Sakoman, S. (2003). Perceived parental acceptance-rejection, family-related factors and socio-economic status of families of adolescent heroin addicts. *Croatian Med J* 44(2): 199–206.

Glynn, T.J., Wallenstein Pearson, H., and Sayers, M. (1983) *Women and drugs.* Rockville, MD: National Institute on Drug Abuse.

Godfrey, C., Eaton, G., McDougall, C., and Culyer, A. (2002) *The economic and social costs of class A drug use in England and Wales, 2000.* London: Home Office Research Study 249.

Gossop, M., Griffiths, P., and Strang, J. (1994) Sex-differences in patterns of drug taking behavior: a study at a London community drug team. *Br J Psychiatry* 164: 101–104.

Goulden, C. and Sondhi, A. (2001). *At the margins: drug use by vulnerable young people in the 1998/99 Youth Lifestyles Survey.* London: Home Office Research Study 228.

Grund, J.P.C., Kaplan, C.D., and Adriaans, N.F.P. (1991) Needle sharing in the Netherlands: an ethnographic analysis. *Am J Public Health* 81: 1602–1607.

Hanson, B., Beschner, G., Walters, J.M. and Bovelle, E. (eds) (1985) *Life with heroin: voices from the inner city.* Lexington, MA: Lexington Books.

Hay, G., McKeganey, N., and Hutchinson, S. (2001) *Estimating the national and local prevalence of problematic drug use in Scotland.* Edinburgh: Scottish Executive.

Hay, G., Gannon, M., McKeganey, M., Hutchinson, S., and Goldberg, D. (2005) *Estimating the national and local prevalence of problem drug misuse in Scotland.* Edinburgh: ISD Scotland.

Health Protection Agency (2003) *Shooting up infections among injecting drug users in the United Kingdom 2002. An update 2003.* London: Health Protection Agency.

Health Statistics Quarterly (2004) Spring 21: 59.

Henderson, S. (1988) Living with the virus: perspectives from HIV-positive women in London. In: N. Dorn, S. Henderson, and N. South (eds), *AIDS: women, drugs and social care.* London: Falmer.

Hickman, M., Griffin, M., Mott, J., Corkery, J., Madden, P., Sondhi, A., and Stimson, G. (2004a) Continuing the epidemiological function of the addicts index: evidence from matching the Home Office addicts index with the national drug treatment monitoring system. *Drug-Educ Prev Polic* 11(2): 91–100.

Hickman, M., Higgins, V., Bellis, M., Tilling, K., Walker, A., and Henry, J. (2004b) Injecting drug use in Brighton, Liverpool and London: best estimates of prevalence and coverage of public health indicators. *J Epidemiol Comm Health* 58: 766–777.

Hickman, M., Higgins, V., Hope, V., and Bellis, M. (2004c) *Estimating prevalence of problem drug use: multiple methods in Brighton, Liverpool and London.* Home Office Online Report 36/04. www.homeoffice.gov.uk/rds/pdfs04/rdsolr3604.pdf

Hirsch, E.D., Kett, J.F., and Trefil, J.S. (2002) *New dictionary of cultural literacy.* 3rd edition. Haughton Mutilin.

Holloway, K., Bennett, T., and Lower, C. (2004) *Trends in drug use and offending: the results of the New-ADAM Programme 1999–2004.* London: Home Office Findings: 219.

Home Office (1998) *Tackling drugs to build a better Britain: the government's ten-year strategy for tackling drugs misuse Cm 3945.* London: The Stationery Office.

Horgan, A., Cassidy, C.E., and Corrigan, A. (1998) Childhood sexual abuse histories in women with drug and alcohol misuse disorders. *Ir J Psycholog Med* 15(3): 91–95.

Inciardi, J.A., Martin, S.S., Butzin C.A., Hooper, R.M., and Harrison, L. (1997) An effective model of prison-based treatment for drug-involved offenders. *J Drug Issues* 27: 261–278.

Information and Statistics Division (2004) *Drug misuse statistics Scotland, 2004.* Edinburgh: ISD. www.drugmisuse.isdscotland.org/publications/04dmss/04dm ss.htm

Johnson, J.L. and Leff, M. (1999). Children of substance abusers: overview of research findings. *Pediatrics* 1030: 1085–1099.

Johnson, B.D., Goldstein, P.J., Preble, E., Schmeidler, J., Lipton, D.S., Spunt, B., and Miller, T. (1985) *Taking care of business: the economics of crime by heroin abusers.* Lexington, MA: Lexington.

Jones, G. (1997) Youth homelessness and the 'underclass'. In: R. Macdonald (ed.), *Youth, the 'underclass' and social exclusion.* London and New York: Routledge.

Jones, G. (2002). *The youth divide. Diverging paths to adulthood.* York: Joseph Rowntree Foundation.

Kemp, P. and Neale, J. (2005) Employability and problem drug users. *Critical Social Policy* 25: 28–46.

Kendler, K.S., Jacobson, K.C., Prescott, C.A. and Neale, M.C. (2003). Specificity of genetic and environmental risk factors for use and abuse/dependence of cannabis, cocaine, hallucinogens, sedatives, stimulants and opiates in male twins. *Am J Psychiatry* 160(4): 687–695.

Knight, K., Simpson, D.D., Chatham, L.R., and Camacho, L.M. (1997) An assessment of prison-based drug treatment: Texas in-prison therapeutic community program. *J Offend Rehab* 24: 75–100.

Lee, J. and Bell, N.J. (2003). Individual differences in attachment-autonomy configurations: linkages with substance use and youth competencies. *J Adol* 26: 347–361.

Liebschutz, J., Savetshy, J.B., Saitz, R., Horton, N.J., Lloyd-Travaglini, C., and Samet, J.H. (2002). The relationship between sexual and physical abuse and substance abuse consequences. *J Subst Abuse Treat* 22: 121–128.

Lloyd, C. (1998). Risk factors for problem drug use: identifying vulnerable groups. *Drugs: Ed Prev Polic* 5(3): 217–232.

Lupton, R., Wilson, A., May, T., Warburton, H., and Turnbull, P.J. (2002) *A rock and a hard place: drug markets in deprived neighbourhoods.* Home Office Research Study 240. London: Home Office.

Maher, L. (1997) *Sexed work gender race and resistance in a Brooklyn drug market.* Oxford: Oxford University Press.

Martin, C. and Player, E. (2000) *Drug treatment in prison: an evaluation of the RAPt treatment programme.* Winchester: Waterside Press.

Martin, C., Player, E., and Liriano, S. (2003) Results of evaluations of the RAPt drug treatment programme. In: M. Ramsay (ed.), *Prisoners' drug use and treatment: seven research studies.* Home Office Research Series. London: Home Office.

May, T., Warburton, H., Turnbull, P.J., and Hough, M. (2002). *Times they are a-changing: policing of cannabis.* York: Joseph Rowntree Foundation.

McCambridge, J. and Strang, J. (2004). Patterns of drug use in a sample of 200 young drug users in London. *Drugs: Ed Prev and Polic* 11(2): 101–112.

McCance-Katz, E.F., Carroll, K.M., and Rounsaville, B. (1999) Gender differences in treatment-seeking cocaine abusers: implications for treatment and prognosis. *Am J Addict* 8: 300–311.

McClenaghan, P. (2000) Social capital: exploring the theoretical foundations of community development education. *Br Ed Res J* 26(5): 565–582.

McElrath, K. (2002) *Prevalence of problem heroin use in Northern Ireland.* Belfast: Queens University.

McIntosh, J., Gannon, M., McKeganey, N., and MacDonald, F. (2003a) Exposure to drugs among pre-teenage schoolchildren. *Addiction* 98. 1615–1623.

McIntosh, J., MacDonald, F., and McKeganey, N. (2003b) Dealing with the offer of drugs: the experiences of a sample of pre-teenage schoolchildren. *Addiction* 98(7): 977–986.

McIntosh, J., MacDonald, F., and McKeganey, N. (2003c) The initial use of drugs in a sample of pre-teenage schoolchildren: the role of choice, pressure and influence. *Drugs: Ed Prev Polic* 10(2): 147–158.

McKeganey, N. (2004) *Random drug testing of schoolchildren: a shot in the arm or a shot in the foot for drug prevention?* York: Joseph Rowntree Foundation.

McKeganey, N. and Barnard, M. (1992) *AIDS, drugs and sexual risk: lives in the balance.* Buckingham: Open University Press.

McKeganey, N., Connelly, C., Knepil, J., Norrie, J., and Reid, L. (2002a) *Interviewing and drug testing of arrestees: a pilot of the arrestee drug abuse monitoring methodology*. Edinburgh: Scottish Executive Central Research Unit.

McKeganey, N., Neale, J., Parkin, S., and Mills, C. (2004a) Communities and drugs: beyond the rhetoric of community action. *Probation J* 51(4): 343–361.

McKeganey, N., McIntosh, J., MacDonald, F., Gannon, M., Gilvarry, E., McArdle, P., and McCarthy, S. (2004b) Preteen children and illegal drugs. *Drugs: Ed Prev Polic* 11(4): 315–327.

Medrano, M.A., Zule, W.A., Hatch, J., and Desmond, D.P. (1999). Prevalence of childhood trauma in a community sample of substance-abusing women. *Am J Alcohol Abuse* 25 (3): 449–462.

Merton, R.K. (1938) Social structure and anomie. *Am Soc Rev* 3: 672–682.

Millar, M., Gemmel, I., Hay, G., and Donmall, M. (2004) *The dynamics of drug misuse: assessing changes in prevalence*. Home Office Online Report 35/04. www.homeoffice.gov.uk/rds/pdfs04/rdsolr3504.pdf

Murphy, S. and Rosenbaum, M. (1995) The rhetoric of reproduction: pregnancy and drug use. *Contemp Drug Prob* 23: 581–585.

National Statistics (2005) *Health statistics quarterly*. Palgrave.

National Treatment Agency (2002) *Models of care for treatment of adult drug misusers*. London: National Treatment Agency.

National Treatment Agency (2003) *Injectable heroin (and injectable methadone): potential roles in drug treatment*. London: National Treatment Agency.

Neale, J. (1998) Drug users' views of drug service providers. *Health Soc Care Commun* 6: 308–317.

Neale, J. and Saville, E. (2004) Comparing the effectiveness of community and prison-based drug treatments. *Drugs: Ed Prev Polic* 11: 213–228.

Office for National Statistics (2004) *Living in Britain. Results from the 2002 General Household Survey*. London: Office for National Statistics.

Oxford, M.L., Harachi, T.W., Catalano, R.F., and Abbott, R.D. (2000). Preadolescent predictors of substance initiation: a test of both the direct and mediated effect of family social control factors on deviant peer associations and substance initiation. *Am J Drug Alcohol Abuse* 27(4): 599–616.

Parker, H., Bakx, K., and Newcombe, R. (1988) *Living with heroin. The impact of a drugs 'epidemic' on an English community*. Milton Keynes and Philadelphia: Open University Press.

Parker, H., Measham, F., and Aldridge, J. (1995) *Drug futures: changing patterns of drug use among English youth*. Research Monograph 7. London: Institute for the Study of Drug Dependence.

Parker, H., Aldridge, J., and Measham, F. (1998). *Illegal leisure: the normalisation of adolescent drug use*. London: Routledge.

Pearson, G. (1987a) *The new heroin users*. Oxford: Basil Blackwell.

Pearson, G. (1987b) Social deprivation, unemployment and patterns of heroin use. In: N. Dorn and N. South (eds), *A land fit for heroin? Drug policies, prevention and practice*. Basingstoke and London: Macmillan Education Ltd.

Peck, D.F. and Plant, M.A. (1986) Unemployment and illegal drug use: concordant evidence from a perspective study and national trends. *BMJ* 293: 929–932.

Pelissier, B.M.M., Gaes, G., Rhodes, W., Camp, S., O'Neil, J., Wallace, S., and Saylor, W. (1998) *TRIAD drug treatment evaluation project six-month interim report*. Washington, DC: Federal Bureau of Prisons Office of Research and Evaluation.

Perkins, R. and Bennett, G. (1985) *Being a prostitute*. Boston: Allen and Unwin.

Peterson, A.R. (1994) Community-development in health promotion: empowerment or regulation? *Aust J Pub Health* 18(2): 213–217.

Pettiway, L.E. (1997) *Workin' it: women living through drugs and crime*. Philadelphia: Temple University Press.

Powis, B., Griffiths, P., Gossop, M., and Strang, J. (1996) The differences between male and female drug users: community samples of heroin and cocaine users compared. *Subst Use Misuse* 31: 529–543.

Preble, E. and Casey, J. (1969) Taking care of business: the heroin user's life on the streets. *Int J Addiction* 1: 1–24.

Prime Minister's Strategy Unity (2004) *Alcohol harm reduction strategy for England*. London: Cabinet Office.

Ransom, S. and Rutledge, H. (2005). *Including families in the learning community: family centres and the expansion of learning*. York: Joseph Rowntree Foundation.

Rhodes, T., Lilly, R., Fernandez, C., Giorgino, E., Kemmesis, U.E., Ossebaard, H.C., Lalam, N.,

Faasen, I., and Spannow, K.E. (2003) Risk factors associated with drug use: the importance of 'Risk environment'. *Drugs: Ed Prev Polic* 10(4): 303–329.

Rogers, B. and Prior, J. (1998) *Divorce and separation. The outcomes for children*. York: Joseph Rowntre Foundation.

Rosenbaum, M. (1981) *Women on heroin*. New Brunswick, New Jersey: Rutgers University Press.

Sangster, D., Shiner, M., Patel, K., and Sheikh, N. (2002) *Delivering drug services to black and ethnic-minority communities*. London: Home Office.

Shapiro, H. (2003). *Shooting stars: drugs, Hollywood and the movies*. London: Serpent's Tail.

Shewan, D., Macpherson, S., Reid, M.M., and Davies, J.B. (1994) *Evaluation of the Saughton drug treatment reduction programme: main report*. Occasional Paper No. 12. Edinburgh: Scottish Prison Service.

Shiner, M. and Newburn, T. (1999) Taking tea with Noel: the place and the meaning of drug use in everyday life. In: N. South (ed.), *Drugs: cultures, controls and everyday life*. London: Sage Publications.

South, N. (1999) Debating drugs and everyday life: normalisation, prohibition and 'otherness'. In: N. South (ed.), *Drugs: cultures, controls and everyday life*. London: Sage Publications.

Spooner, C. (1999). Causes and correlates of adolescent drug abuse and implications for treatment. *Drug Alcohol Rev* 18: 453–457.

Stephens, R.C. (1991) *The street addict role: a theory of heroin addiction*. Albany: State University of New York Press.

Sterck, C. (1999) *Fast lives: women who use crack cocaine*. Florida: Temple University Press.

Stimson, G.V. and Ogborne, A.C. (1970) Survey of addicts prescribed heroin at London clinics. *Lancet* 30: 116–136.

Stimson, G. and Oppenheimer, E. (1982) *Heroin addiction, treating and control*. London: Tavistock.

Stimson, G., Alldrit, L., Donoghoe, M., and Lart, R. (1988a) *Injecting equipment exchange schemes final report*. London: Goldsmiths College.

Stimson, G., Alldrit, L., Dolan, K., and Donoghoe, M. (1988b) Syringe exchange schemes for drug users in England and Scotland. *BMJ* 296: 1717–1719.

Stratford, N., Gould, A., Hinds, K., and McKeganey, N. (2003) *The measurement of changing public attitudes towards illegal drugs in Britain*. London: Economic and Social Research Council.

Sutherland, H., Sefton, T., and Piachaud, D. (2003). *Poverty in Britain: the impact of government policy since 1997*. York: Joseph Rowntree Foundation.

Sutter, A. (1966) The world of the righteous dope fiend. *Issues Criminol* 2(2): 177–222.

Sutter, A.G. (1969) Worlds of drug use on the street scene. In: D.R. Cressey and D.A. Ward (eds), *Delinquency, crime and social process*. New York: Harper and Row.

Sutter, A.G. (1972) Playing a cold game: phases of a ghetto career. *Urban Life Cult* 1: 77–91.

Taylor, A. (1993) *Women drug-users: an ethnography of a female injecting community*. Oxford: Clarendon Press.

United Nations Office on Drugs and Crime (2004) *World Drugs Report Volume 1 Analysis*, Vienna.

Utting, D. (1995). *Family and parenthood: supporting families, preventing breakdown*. York: Joseph Rowntree Foundation.

Waldorf, D. (1973) *Careers in dope*. New Jersey: Prentice Hall.

Webster, C., Simpson, D., MacDonald, R., Abbas, A., Cieslik, M., Shildrick, T., and Simpson, M. (2006) *A critical case study of young adulthood and social exclusion*. London: Policy Press.

Westermeyer, J., Wahmanholm, K., and Thuras, P. (2001) Effects of childhood physical abuse on course and severity of substance abuse. *Am J Addict* 10: 101–110.

Wexler, H.F., Falkin, G.P., and Lipton, D.S. (1990) Outcome evaluation of a prison therapeutic community for substance abuse treatment. *Crim Just Behav* 17: 71–92.

White, W.L. (2004) Addiction recovery mutual aid groups: an enduring international phenomenon. *Addiction* 99: 532–538.

Wodak, A. (2001) Drug treatment for opioid dependence. *Aust Presc* 24: 4–6.

Wood, F., Bloor, M., and Palmer, S. (2000) Indirect prevalence estimates of a national drug-using population: the use of contact-recontact methods in Wales. *Health Risk Soc* 2: 47–58.

Young, J. (1971) *The drugtakers: the social meaning of drug use*. London: MacGibbon and Kee.

Economics of Addiction and Drugs

Jonathan Cave and Christine Godfrey

1 EXECUTIVE SUMMARY

There are many misconceptions about the consumption and control of illicit drugs, including that drug users are unresponsive to price; that controlling licit substance use may encourage young people to switch to illegal drugs; and that availability controls are likely to be more effective than measures to reduce demand. Economics provides both theories and empirical evidence to explore factors influencing current drug use, the costs to society of the harm they create and the cost-effectiveness of different policy options.

This summary sets out the results of this review in addressing the Foresight project's questions.

1.1 What will be the Psychoactive Substances of the Future?

Economists do not have the answer to this question but can provide insight into how the markets for different drugs may ebb and flow. In particular, the importance of social factors is considered alongside economic incentives, such as price and income, to yield more comprehensive and complex models of the current and future behaviours of consumers and suppliers of drugs. An important aspect of this work is how different groups in society may make different demands for policies, the richer groups potentially demanding more restrictions, while the poor bear more of the costs of drug use. The analysis of drug adoption also provides a way to see the characteristics of future substances in terms of their impact, whether on the individual, social groupings or markets. The models can also predict whether new drugs will drive out existing ones or find a niche in separated or polydrug-using clusters.

1.2 What are the Effects of Using Psychoactive Substances?

The economic impact of problem drug use is sizeable, with Class A drug users estimated to generate social costs of £12 billion in 2000. These effects are spread across individuals, families, communities and society more generally. The problematic rather than the occasional user seems to be responsible for the majority of these costs, but this may partly reflect data deficiencies. Also, for novel drugs, longer-term health and dependency impacts associated with problematic use may take time to emerge. Governments may need to adopt a precautionary approach to any drug with a dependence potential. The theoretical demand models also shed light on how social groupings, information, economic constraints and policy affect drug-use choices by affecting perceived costs and benefits, and by triggering simplified or myopic decision making.

1.3 What Mechanisms do We have to Manage the Use of Psychoactive Substances?

In a departure from conventional wisdom, both economic theory and empirical evidence suggest that drug prices influence demand. Also, there are a number of complementary relationships between licit and illicit substances. This suggests that policies can be devised to affect individual behaviour. Controlling supply has proved harder, and theoretical models highlight a number of reasons for the sometimes seemingly contradictory outcomes of the application of narrow policy options without an analysis of complete market interactions. Policy effects may well be localised and insignificant in the short run, but much more substantial after network effects and social change have taken hold. The analysis suggests that gateway and cross-drug effects are significant, but are also potentially reversible, so that policy should be both targeted on the most cost-effective drugs and patterns of use and be adaptive to emerging evidence on changing prices and habits. Economics also suggests that drug use follows punctuated and/or cyclical paths, so that policies should 'lead' or 'follow' the cycle. Finally, the analysis suggests that policy should take account of and try to influence structures on both the supply and demand sides of the market, if only to avoid such 'rebound' effects as the social isolation of drug-using clusters or inadvertent support for suppliers' attempts to limit entry and enforce market discipline. Where effective treatments exist, their use saves costs to society. But the incentives for industry to develop effective treatments for novel drugs may be lacking until serious and sizeable problems have begun to emerge.

2 INTRODUCTION

The current consumption of both licit and illicit drugs is seen to have a range of economic impacts, and there is general concern about costs arising both as a direct result of their use and from measures such as enforcement, education and treatment put in place in an attempt to reduce these problems. Economics has a set of tools whose application goes beyond simply quantifying the problem. This review aims to explore the role of economics in explaining changes in drug use, predicting expected and unexpected impacts of policy changes and evaluating the overall worth of different policy options.

A wide range of psychoactive substances are used in society and most are subject to some legal controls. The focus of this review are the currently controlled psychoactive substances in the UK. Good data on illegal markets where such controlled substances are traded are hard to obtain. But useful insights can be drawn from theory, and from the empirical analysis of legal addictive goods such as alcohol and tobacco. Also, some studies have explored interactions between licit and illicit markets, in particular whether changes in restrictions on the use of legal drugs such as alcohol and tobacco affect the demand for or supply of illicit ones.

Section 3 gives a brief overview of models of addictive goods and their potential for explaining both drug-use patterns and the impact of different policy options. Existing empirical studies of the size of the UK market, the costs associated with drug problems and factors that influence consumers and suppliers of illicit drugs are reviewed in section 4 and conclusions drawn regarding implications for future trends. Section 5 reviews the empirical literature

on the cost-effectiveness of different policy instruments. Sections 3–5 bring together existing knowledge; section 6 speculates about how embedding the most novel theories in social models could be more useful in exploring scenarios about the future diffusion of new and existing drugs and resulting consequences and policy options.

3 THE ROLE OF ECONOMIC THEORY

3.1 The Basic Economic Model and its Application to Addictive Goods

Economics is built on demand and supply, determined by rational, informed (but constrained) choice and reconciled by markets. In making choices, rational consumers are expected to take all current and future costs and benefits of their actions into account, but generally are not expected to take account of the impact of their actions on others, nor of the external costs (or benefits) of their choices. External costs make market-clearing consumption higher than is socially optimal. There is potential for government intervention to improve overall welfare, providing its costs do not exceed its benefits, by reducing external social impacts or by helping economic agents to internalise them.

Addictive goods challenge this simple model in two ways. In an extreme model of addiction, users would be incapable of effective choices, making them insensitive to price or their own income. The rational addiction model (Becker and Murphy, 1988), explored below, is an attempt to find a middle ground, suggesting how consumers can rationally pursue their welfare, even if they are aware of the nature of dependence and how this may influence their future choices. Another issue is the role of information about the effects of existing and novel addictive substances. The risks of some licit drugs such as cigarettes may be relatively well known, but just how well informed are consumers

TABLE 13.1   Which costs count under different assumptions?

	Addicted	Not addicted
Unaware of adverse consequences	Private + external costs + production resources	Private and external costs
Aware of adverse consequences	External costs + ? (dependent on views of rationality of addiction)	External costs

Source: Buck *et al.*, 1996.

about risks of other licit drugs such as alcohol, or of illicit drugs that have been available for a number of years, or of novel drugs with an unknown risk potential? Lack of information about adverse consequences creates a need to include some private costs in decisions about government intervention (see Table 13.1). It could be argued that 'non-rational' addicted consumers are not getting optimal utility from their consumption and are therefore diverting productive resources that could increase overall welfare.

Clearly one issue raised by novel substances, or indeed novel consumption patterns, is the difficulty of estimating potential longer-term effects, particularly on individual health but also on dependence potential. The continuing debate about the potential effects of marijuana illustrates these difficulties. In a recent overview, Pacula (2005) argues that accumulating evidence of the impact of marijuana on educational achievement translates into reduced future earnings in addition to the costs of treating health-related consequences for those, albeit a small proportion, developing a dependency problem.

Table 13.2 illustrates the economic impacts of drug use, and the groups in society that may bear some of its costs. Within the economic model, costs falling on families and carers are often treated as 'private' but the nature of dependence – particularly severe dependence – would suggest that normal models of agreed intra-household choice do not apply. A number of other issues influence the distinction between private and external costs. The basic economic model takes an individualistic approach to

consumption decisions. However, economic models of collective behaviour take account of the interactions between individuals. This has some parallel in the debate about whose costs count. If individuals 'care' about the impacts of drug use on others, this may affect social welfare and how societies value the consequences of addictive behaviour. In particular, what value is given by society to the risks of death from drug taking? Should this and other individual values form part of the 'costs' of drugs to society that prompt government action? These considerations determine the choice and level of government policies in drug markets. They can help make explicit some assumptions being made in often simplistic debates about the legal status of different drugs. They also provide a framework for scenario analyses to explore the potential impact on overall social welfare. The evidence that has attempted to put values to some of the internal and external costs of illicit drugs in the UK is reviewed in Section 4.

3.2 Addiction, Choice and Demand for Illicit Drugs

Rational choice means that each actor has a feasible set of options – determined by constraints – that can be ranked according to preferences. Personal choices involve such matters as consumption (of licit and illicit goods and services), investment (in the form of savings, education, etc.) and supply (particularly labour supply and criminal activity). The points of analysis – where economics touches issues relating to

TABLE 13.2 Economic impacts of drug use.

Bearer of cost	Examples of impact
Users	Premature death Loss of quality of life – mental and physical health, relationships, etc. Impact on educational achievement, training opportunities, etc. Excess unemployment and loss of lifetime earnings
Families/carers	Impact on children of users Transmission of infections Intergeneration impact on substance use Financial problems Concern/worry for users Caring for substance users or substance users' dependants
Other individuals directly affected	Victims of drink/drug driving and other accidents, substance-related violence, substance-related crime Transmission of infections from substance users
Wider community effects	Fear of crime Environmental aspects of drug markets – needles, effects of drug dealing in community, etc.
Industry	Sickness absence Theft in the workplace Security expenditure to prevent substance-related crime Productivity losses Impact of illicit markets on legitimate markets
Public sector	Healthcare expenditure Criminal justice expenditure Social care services Social security benefits

Source: Godfrey *et al.*, 2002.

psychoactive substances – involve:

- the preferences themselves – how past consumption affects preferences, the accuracy with which choices are assessed, the rate at which the future is discounted, preferences for investment and supply as well as consumption, externalities, etc.;
- the feasible set – prices and income (returns on investment and supply activities);
- income-generating activities;
- the choice process – this includes time-consistency, the influence of context and cues, alternative models of 'addictive choice' and the handling of risk, uncertainty and incomplete information.

A variety of models explore individual choices to consume drugs and undertake other actions associated with drug taking, such as crime. All these models establish connections between behaviour and economic influences (price, purity, etc.). But they differ in the nature of these connections, and thus in their predictions regarding new drugs, and importantly, policy impacts. They also differ in their consistency with neuroscience, psychology and the empirical evidence. Among the characteristics that such models should explain are:

- users do not follow monotone behaviour patterns – they frequently abstain for short periods but relapse in the long run

(Goldstein, 2001; O'Brien, 1997; Trosclair et al., 2002);

- users often develop compulsive use patterns, even when prolonged use reduces or reverses the hedonic benefits of drug taking;
- consumption, quitting and relapse are often triggered by contextual cues;
- users often recognise their behaviour as a mistake, but see themselves as lacking self-control. In other words, they believe they would have been better off had they not taken drugs;
- users often resort to precommitment strategies to control their behaviour, for example, by consuming other drugs that block or interfere with the pleasurable aspects of their drug of choice, or entering treatment or rehabilitation centres;
- drug use responds to economic factors, though the extent and timing of this response may be problematic. There is evidence of forecasting, with users reducing their current consumption to limit vulnerability to anticipated future price increases;
- drug use is affected by the attention paid to consumption choices. For instance, recovering addicts can overcome temporary cravings if they are reminded of adverse effects – even when they are well aware of these effects. Conversely, distractions that mask such knowledge (eg rave environments) can increase the likelihood of use. (This suggests that attention-management strategies may be a useful adjunct to addiction therapies, and also that there is value in information-exchange activities even when the message is not 'new'. Of course, an overly familiar message may not attract attention.);
- there are strong and systematic differences in patterns of use and response to environmental changes between different drugs and methods of administration and between individuals.

The rational addict model (Becker and Murphy, 1988) asserts that drug use, like other behaviour, forms part of a solution to a global expected lifetime-utility maximisation. Preferences (even time preference) may change in complex ways as a result of past behaviour, but the rational agent takes this into account by working backwards from all possible ends of life. In this view, drug taking is an individual problem in the absence of prohibition and the only societal problems arise from externalities. Drug taking thus enhances welfare (at least *ex ante*) and externality problems can be dealt with by suitable government action.

This model does not imply that 'rational' addicts are happy with the choices they've made and the life they lead. Welfare improvements are only expectations, and many may well 'lose the gamble' they've undertaken. Nevertheless, on aggregate, the 'winners' could compensate the losers and still have enough left over for a risk premium.

The empirical predictions are quite strong. Users should seek out the lowest-cost way of meeting their demand discount the future geometrically at the same rate for drugs and for all other goods be risk-averse (because expected utility is concave) have no problems of self-command (doing things that they expect to regret) and thus have no need to 'play games against their future selves' as Schelling (1980) puts it.

The model has been extended to account for observed behaviour (MacDonald, 2004). This adds learning and regret, and endogenous determination of time preference. Experiments show that heroin produces higher rates of time preference (discounting) than other reinforcers. Ex-addicts report a fear of relapse so that treatment by managing contingencies is effective even when the monetary rewards are far smaller than the costs of the drug habit (Bretteville-Jensen, 1999).

Other models invoke time-inconsistent preferences – typically by biasing utility towards the present, for instance, via hyperbolic discounting (O'Donaghue and Rabin, 1999, 2000; Gruber and Koszegi, 2001). In such models, small immediate rewards may be preferred to later, more substantial rewards for only a short period before they are available. Choices made in advance will tend to favour deferred rewards. Under these conditions, precommitment strategies that remove the power to revisit choices or which mask cues that might raise the possibility of choice are in the individual's long-term interest. Individual strategies may be consciously economic (eg by limiting the discretionary spending power of vulnerable persons), social (by choosing a different group of friends or living situation) or cognitive (eg by making consumption choices more deliberate, and thus sensitive to scientific information, and limiting impulse purchases). Consumers may rationally demand government action to reduce their choices. Becker *et al.* (2004) recently extended this welfare analysis to suggest that restrictive policies, such as prohibition, could be preferred by the rich and that such policies' costs fall disproportionately on the poor.

These models are all based on changing individual preferences. A different approach considers changes in the way individuals perceive choices and translate preferences into actions. A simple and tractable approach, largely consistent with neurological science and the stylised facts above, incorporates different cognitive states, triggered by cues in the environment in ways that reflect past experience. In 'cold' states, individuals take a wide range of information into account and behave in 'rational' ways, using attention, foresight and memory. In 'hot' cognitive states, individuals' decisions are simplified by ignoring alternatives and consequences. Such 'shortcuts' are not inherently irrational or suboptimal. The brain is a finite mechanism, and cognitive decisions can have substantial opportunity costs. So many repeated behaviours are reduced to routines chosen by rough-and-ready rules of thumb, backed by 'wake-up rules' that identify situations where explicit decisions are needed.

Melioration models (Herrnstein and Prelec, 1992; Heyman, 2003) attempt to reconcile compulsive aspects of drug taking (consistent with a disease model of addiction) and its responsiveness to prices and adverse effects (consistent with learning and rational addiction). The analysis is based on four observations. First, repeated consumption decreases future values of both the drug and competing activities. Second, the frequency of an activity depends on its relative attractiveness, so drug taking that makes alternative behaviours less attractive can increase, even if its own utility declines. Third, psychological experiments (Heyman and Tanz, 1995) suggest that reinforcement is relative to a frame of reference, which can change to favour suboptimal choices. Fourth, while local frames of reference favour excessive drug use, the reverse is true of global frames of reference.

Of further interest is the relationship between different drugs. Some substitutability within classes of drugs (eg stimulants or depressants) may be expected. If prices of one depressive drug rose, consumers would switch to a substitute. However, the empirical literature suggests more complementarity, and a rise in polydrug use has been observed. Complementarity among drugs creates analytical problems for microeconomic analysis and can lead to equilibria that are inefficient – dominated by one or a few drugs – or that fail to exist at all.

A second phenomenon is the so-called 'gateway effect' (DiNardo and Lemieux, 1992; Chaloupka *et al.*, 1999a; Pacula, 1997) whereby initiation into one substance leads to the use of another. This suggests targeting patterns for enforcement activity. It may be more efficient to target the gateway drug (or activity) than the eventual drug. However, 'rational addiction' models of polydrug abuse suggest that this effect could be reversed, depending on the relative attractiveness of either drug to novice users as well as any asymmetric spillover from using one drug to using another. Gateway effects are not simple and gateways do not always work in a single direction. Therefore, changes in relative alcohol and cannabis prices, for example, could lead to their changing places as gateway drugs to one another or to 'hard drugs'. Similarly, where peer group effects are important, gateway trajectories may differ from group to group.

3.3 Supply and Markets

Supply-side points of analysis involve:

- underlying motivation – usually assumed to be profit maximisation, but others – eg political or ideological – may require different treatment;
- available 'technology' for turning inputs into output. Inputs include raw materials, labour, capital, etc., but also complementary activities such as (for illicit substances) money-laundering, intimidation of rivals, corrupt services and other means of managing law enforcement and other risk;
- investment;
- financial constraints.

The 'supply chain' stretches from international or source-country supply, processing, transhipment and money-laundering markets to domestic wholesale and retail (even street-level) markets. At street level, the separation of supply and demand breaks down; user and seller activity may best be modelled as a way to reduce the cost of obtaining drugs.

The supply chain can be analysed in terms of:

- structure – in particular, the degree and distribution of market power, both upstream and down. This measures the extent to which market players are able to control their environment, and thus the degree to which deep pockets or other forms of influence may immunise them from policy impacts or even allow them to exploit policy to limit competition;
- conduct – suppliers of illicit substances have a range of strategies at their disposal. Many of these (eg predatory behaviour, use of violence, bribery, etc.) are of direct policy concern.

Drug markets have different supply-side and market dynamics from conventional markets and other illicit markets in terms of turnover, price and quality variability, violence, corruption and the extent of rents and social costs. The unavailability of legal channels for dispute resolution may predispose illicit drug markets to violence and corruption. This is reinforced on both sides: law enforcement pressure may reduce the expected costs of violence while the cost of violent market regulation may make corruption more attractive.

The general tendency to concentration has some important drivers. Law enforcement pressure may control market entry and the accumulation of 'learning economies'. In addition, law enforcement limits consumer search and can make punishments more credible and thus reduces the temptation to renege on cartel agreements. On the other hand, the threat of disruption at any level of the market makes one-to-one connections risky, so monopoly is, on the whole, less likely and less resilient than oligopoly.

The legal risks that inhibit price search also reduce the effectiveness of consumer recourse and reputations in promoting quality, so competitive forces may well produce low prices and variable quality. The conventions of supply (eg fixed prices for unobservable 'doses') mean that supply shocks are transmitted to those least able to bear them. This may magnify adverse health consequences.

3.4 Conclusions

3.4.1 What are the Psychoactive Substances of the Future?

There is a growing literature on the dynamics of drug-taking behaviour and associated harms and optimal policies. It involves both representations of individual drug-taking decisions and models of collective behaviour. Individual economic models provide predictions about the impact of changes in prices and provide some guidance as to the economic legitimacy of restrictive government policies. They also help explain some of the observed unanticipated consequences of policy actions. The potential to analyse the ranges and interactions of policy changes suggests an important role for economic modelling in future scenario analyses.

Existing collective models recognise the crucial importance of social interactions for intentions with regard to drugs and the eventual results of acting on those intentions. The prevalent form of collective modelling likens drug use to epidemic disease. Choices about drugs are strongly influenced by information and incentives from interactions with peer groups, educators, medical personnel, mass media, authority figures, etc. These influence all-important inputs to the demand models: price expectations, beliefs about the likelihood and severity of risks, tastes for particular experiences, coping strategies for managing adverse effects or future behaviour and even the 'framing' of drug-use decisions: what consequences are considered, how they are evaluated and weighted, and how uncertainty (as well as risk) is incorporated. But beyond this focus on social determinants of drug use lies a deeper issue; that drug use itself as a social ritual determines the social environment as much as it is determined by it. The importance of such an approach in exploring the patterns of drug adoption is explored in section 6.

3.4.2 What will the Future Impact of Psychoactive Substance be?

Current economic models highlight uncertainty about the future impact of different illicit markets. The inherent instability of these markets can lead to health and other consequences for users, beyond the direct harms to individuals, families, communities and society in general from dependent drug use. However, chronic problems may only become apparent after consumption has been prevalent in a large enough group of the population for a long enough period of time. The emerging evidence on marijuana may or may not parallel the case of tobacco, where the full health impact has only been fully measured some 50 years after

the mass adoption of cigarette smoking (Doll et al., 2004). Economic theory gives some guidance on a precautionary principle for governments to follow, in that individuals may 'rationally' demand some constraints on their behaviour.

3.4.3 What Interventions will be Available in the Future?

The predictions from economic models are that consumers are likely to respond to changes in market incentives and be responsive to policy options, but social factors are also important.

4 THE EMPIRICAL PICTURE

4.1 Data Issues

Finding data on illegal activities will always be challenging. In addition, it has not been a tradition of economic research to test and retest models. New theoretical models and empirical estimates are sometimes presented without rigorous statistical testing, and without refuting previous theoretical models. This makes empirical economic evidence difficult to review systematically. Specific definition and measurement issues arise around prices and levels of use.

Measuring prices higher up the value chain is complicated by complex contingent payment arrangements, money-laundering costs, etc. A survey can be found at Caulkins and Reuter (1999). Table 13.3 shows a breakdown of US cocaine prices. A recent analysis taking account of some of these complexities suggests that black-market prices of cocaine are 2–4 times the likely legal market prices in the US and that the corresponding multiple is 6–19 for heroin (Miron, 2003). However, care should be used in extrapolating these figures because, for both drugs, prices and purity differ between Europe and the US and among European countries.

Certainly, the prices of illicit substances are high. This means (Kleiman, 1997) that elasticities cannot safely ignore income

TABLE 13.3   Components of drug prices.

Component	Per cent of retail price
Wholesale (farmgate) price	1
Importation[1]	12
Retail labour[2]	13
Higher-level labour	3
Seizure of drugs and assets[3]	8–11
Money-laundering costs	2–4
Packaging, processing, inventory	4
Compensation for prison risk[4]	24
Compensation for violence risk	33
Taxes	0

1. Differential between the source-country and landed price;
2. Illegality forces substitution of costly labour for efficient capital equipment and requires extensive vigilance;
3. Based on seizures at all levels, evaluated at wholesale cost;
4. Incarceration valued at average income, measured by survey.

Source: Caulkins and Reuter (1998).

effects. Also, an addict who responds to price increases by committing more crime is not showing inelastic demand but increasing discretionary income to pay the difference. Price changes should also significantly affect heavy users' behaviour, as has been found for alcohol users. While light users may respond to price increases by reducing consumption, heavy users may reduce other consumption (eg housing, food) or commit more crime. Price rises may move some across the boundary from light to heavy use and criminal activity.

Many components – especially farmgate prices – are so small that policies targeting them are unlikely to achieve much impact. Most costs are unmonetised risk compensation – so accounting profits are likely greatly to exceed economic profits. Accounting losses will almost never induce exit. Also, differences in tolerance for non-monetary costs favour market domination by the less risk-averse (or even risk-seeking). Thanks to this adverse selection,

supply-side policies that impose risk may have attenuated or perverse effects. Young, poorly educated and violence-prone males are most likely to tolerate such costs. So the association of violence and drugs may not wholly be due to the struggle for profit.

The second problem is determining consumption patterns. Except for tobacco, almost all drugs have highly asymmetric consumption following 'Pareto's 80:20 law' – 80 per cent of consumption accounted for by 20 per cent of the user population. Heavy users who account for most demand and its attendant problems are likely to be under-sampled in population surveys, and data and analysis are almost certain to be dominated by light or occasional users. However, convenient samples of problem drug users, such as those arrested or seeking treatment, are not representative either. Such samples may 'over-represent' problems and consumption (see discussion by Pudney in Bramley-Harker, 2001).

4.2 Size of the UK Illicit Drug Market

An obvious first empirical estimate is the size of the UK illicit market. However, few research studies are available. Bramley-Harker (2001) took data from arrestees. The NEW-ADAM (New English and Welsh Arrestee Drug Abuse Monitoring) data measured problem drug use prevalence and estimated expenditure from a sample of arrestees with data collected by means of structured interviews and urine samples. Population surveys were used to estimate numbers of occasional users. The results suggest that in 1998 a regular heroin user spent about £16 500 per year on all drugs and a regular crack user £21 000. Occasional users' estimated expenditure (£1.9 billion) was much lower than regular users' (£4.7 billion). The total estimate for the UK market (£6.6 billion), while sizeable, is still smaller than alcohol expenditure for the same year (£32 billion). The NEW-ADAM data point to a surprisingly high number of crack cocaine users but the overall expenditure figure was similar to a previous Office for National

Statistics estimate based on seizure data [between £4.3 billion and £9.9 billion (Groom *et al.*, 1998)].

4.3 Measuring the Impact of Illicit Drug Use

Economic models distinguish between private costs of drug use and externalities borne by others in society. There are major gaps in the UK information (Culyer *et al.*, 2001). Some large international studies have attempted to estimate the external costs of illicit drug use in comparison to those from licit drugs. In general, the costs of illicit substances, while substantial, are smaller than for alcohol and tobacco. They are generally dominated by crime, health and productivity costs.

4.3.1 Individual Impacts

There is a general lack of UK data on personal impacts (good or bad) and their valuation. Some data are available on mortality, morbidity and loss of earnings, including epidemiological data on premature mortality from different licit and illicit drugs. Tobacco accounts for the largest number of premature deaths at 106 000 per year in the UK (Twigg *et al.*, 2004), alcohol accounts for 22 000 in England (Rannia, 2003) and illicit drugs between 1000 and 3000 (Advisory Council on the Misuse of Drugs, 2000). However, tobacco deaths tend to occur at a later age than those from alcohol or illicit drugs. In terms of life years, the percentages lost to alcohol and tobacco are approximately equal and far greater than from illicit substances.

More robust evidence is emerging on the impact of substance use, especially problem use, on employment (for example, MacDonald and Shields, 2004). US research also highlights the impact of early substance misuse on educational attainment. These two factors could suggest substantial impacts on the lifetime legitimate earnings of substance misusers. Pacula (2005), for example, suggests that early marijuana use may reduce future earnings by 2 per cent.

4.3.2 Externalities

Few studies attempt empirical estimates of families' costs such as the lost earnings of carers. Rather, empirical studies include some public sector resource costs. For example, care of problem Class A drug users' children was estimated to cost £63 million and healthcare for neonates £4.3 million per year in England and Wales for 2000 (Godfrey *et al.*, 2002).

Workplace costs of all drugs are of considerable interest but hard to quantify (Godfrey and Parrott, 2005). Some drugs consumed in or close to working time have a direct impact on productivity. Some workers may feel stimulants help productivity, although the long-term productivity impact of most drugs remains unproven. Previous excess use can also lead to workplace problems. These potential effects can alter drug users' behaviour as they attempt to get desired effects in leisure time while ensuring they are fit for work. The long-term impact of such polydrug use is largely unknown.

Most empirical attention has been given to the public sector impacts of different substances. The most recently published costs of Class A drug use in England and Wales are reproduced in Table.13.4. The total shown of £12 billion per year is based on the medium estimate of users and costs and taken from Godfrey *et al.* (2002). Estimates for premature

TABLE 13.4 Costs of Class A drug use in England and Wales, 2000.

Item	Cost (£ billion)
Healthcare	0.35
Premature death	1.02
Workplace/drug driving	No data available
Other social	0.06
Crime	10.56
Total	11.99

Source: Godfrey *et al.*, 2002.

death were calculated using willingness to pay. However, premature death is not a large component of Class A drug-use costs, which are dominated by crime costs (88 per cent of the total). Also, in contrast to alcohol, problem drug users account for almost all estimated cost (99 per cent) of Class A drug use. However, this study could not find data to estimate the potential impacts of drug driving or workplace drug use. Costs for different types of drug user varied substantially, with young recreational users estimated to cost £36 per user and older regular users only £3 per user, in contrast to the much larger estimate of £35 500 for each problem drug user.

4.4 What Factors Influence Illicit Drug Demand?

4.4.1 Own Price

While limited in number and mainly US-based, most published studies find significant relationships between the price and consumption of marijuana, heroin and cocaine (see reviews in Pacula and Chaloupka, 2001; Godfrey, 2001; Saffer and Chaloupka, 1999a). Available studies suggest that raising the prices of any of these drugs will reduce drug use, but there are differences in the size of the effects between studies. For example, heroin price elasticity ranged from −0.27 to −1.5 and cocaine from −0.44 to −2.5, although estimates for most drugs centre around −1.0. Most studies use population survey data. The research gives support to the rational addiction model.

Two more recent studies (Dave, 2000a, 2000b) used drug arrestee and hospital admission data. Again, price was found to significantly affect heroin and cocaine use, although estimated price elasticities were lower (between −0.1 and −0.3) than the population studies. Similarly Bretteville-Jensen and Sutton (1996) and Bretteville-Jensen (2003) used data from more problematic users and found significant price impacts for Norwegian data. Interesting in these

studies was a division between users and user/dealers, with user/dealers having lower price elasticity. Animal and human experimental studies confirm these findings on the impact of price for both occasional and regular users (Petry and Bickel, 1999; Sumnall et al., 2004).

It is difficult to draw conclusions from the available literature about the relative price effects across different groups of the drug-using population. Recent work suggests that pregnant users are price-sensitive (Corman et al., 2004), with a $10 increase in pure cocaine price estimated to reduce use by 12–15 per cent.

There are some parallels to the study of licit drug demand, where more data has led to a focus on the impact of price on different aspects of behaviour, particularly the starting and stopping of different drugs. With licit drugs, prices across different brands or types of the same drug can be explored. Patterns tend to be complex, with brand-conscious consumers tending to adopt patterns of behaviour within age cohorts but also proving price-sensitive within these patterns.

4.4.2 Cross-price Elasticities

Of particular policy interest is the impact of changes in the price of one drug on the consumption of others, particularly across the licit–illicit divide. Several studies attempt to explore such cross-price effects. In particular, studies have considered the relationship between prices and restrictive policies affecting alcohol and marijuana consumption. Studies have generally been based on US youth population surveys (see review in Williams et al., 2004). The majority of these studies found complementarity between these two drugs, suggesting that restrictions or higher prices for alcohol will reduce both drinking and marijuana consumption. There have been similar findings for Australia (Cameron and Williams, 2001). However, these studies have some inconsistencies, the complementarity being stronger in younger age groups than in ethnic minorities or women, although the latest study found a similar relationship for college students (Williams *et al.*, 2004).

Other studies examine the relationships between cigarettes and marijuana; cocaine and marijuana; alcohol and heroin; and alcohol and cocaine (Chaloupka *et al.*, 1999b; Farrelly *et al.*, 1999; Saffer and Chaloupka, 1999a). All found complementarities.

A related issue is the gateway hypothesis of a set pathway from one drug to another. The evidence is currently inconclusive.

4.4.3 Income

As discussed above, the relationship between drug use and income is complex, especially for problem users who may finance use through criminal and drug-dealing activities. Bretteville-Jensen and Sutton (1996) estimated an income elasticity of 0.47 from their survey of non-dealing heroin users in Norway, suggesting income increases will raise drug use. They also found that drug users reduced their illegal income when legitimate income (from work or social benefits) rose.

4.4.4 Enforcement

Many demand studies also explore the impact of street-level enforcement on drug demand, to test whether changing use or low-level-dealing penalties or decriminalisation of possession also affects use by changing the effective price. The results have been mixed, partly due to data difficulties. Policies themselves may be influenced by use levels. There also seems to be some difference between older populations where decriminalisation has an effect and younger populations where no such effects have been found (Pacula and Chaloupka, 2001).

More recent studies, which have attempted to control for such effects, tend to find more positive policy impacts. Desimone and Farrelly (2003), for example, found that increases in either cocaine or marijuana

arrest probabilities decreased demand for both drugs for both adult and juveniles in the US. But Williams (2004) found that Australian marijuana decriminalisation only increased use among males over 25, and did not affect young males or females.

4.4.5 Information

Pacula *et al.* (2000) investigated the impact of perceptions of drug-related harm on marijuana consumption in the US. They found that the perception of harm had increased and these changed perceptions reduced demand. In Sweden it was found that young people may overestimate longer-term health risks of licit drugs such as alcohol and tobacco (Lundberg and Lindgren, 2002) but can be unaware of some shorter-term impacts, consistent with some theoretical models.

4.4.6 Social Factors

Most empirical models are based on individual data and models. There have been attempts to explore some peer effects and an interesting study of college drinking in the US suggests that changing the demographic mix of a college has a direct impact on the rate of problem drinking (Wechsler and Kuo, 2003).

4.5 Empirical Evidence on Supply Behaviour

There is a much smaller economic literature on suppliers' behaviour. The literature has focused on the impact of enforcement expenditure on market outcomes and this literature is briefly reviewed in section 5. As suggested above, it may be difficult to influence retail prices by untargeted interdiction policies. Theory would suggest considerable scope for profit and market concentration. Caulkins *et al.* (1999) found profit margins in US markets varying from 50 per cent to less than 10 per cent. In exploring potential supply–demand interactions,

Saffer and Chaloupka (1999b) did find that police drug-control spending affects supply as well as demand.

4.6 Conclusions

4.6.1 What will the Future Impact of Psychoactive Substance be?

What can be learnt from the estimates of illicit drug market size and the value of associated problems? Regular (and often problematic) users dominate spending and problems created. However, this may simply reflect current drugs of misuse or a lack of knowledge of longer-term impacts. Even with marijuana, the emerging evidence is that costs are associated with problem use, either impeding schooling or later, when dependence emerges. However, not enough is known about regular users and the impact of their use in the workplace or in situations such as driving that are risky both to users and the rest of society.

Tobacco costs are more evenly spread and patterns of alcohol drinking are related to a complex set of problems connected with both acute and chronic use.

4.6.2 What Interventions will be Available in the Future?

Economic evidence on demand suggests that consumers of illicit drugs respond to incentives in a similar way to users of other goods and services. Prices and regulations affect demand for both licit and illicit drugs. In general, drugs are complementary, so relaxing policies on any one drug may increase the consumption of all substances. In particular, concerted policy to change sentiment among emerging cohorts does seem to have the potential to shift demand.

While these economic and policy factors shouldn't be ignored, social factors influencing preferences are likely to play a large part in determining overall consumption patterns. Demographic shifts may influence consumption in the short term, although globalisation and the diffusion of

habits mean that trends in use spread across populations. We have less evidence about suppliers' behaviour but markets seem to adapt to changing preferences.

Demand for interventions across income groups and generational cohorts raises interesting future scenarios. Current evidence points to similar demand and supply factors across different drugs. Indeed, there has been a growth of polydrug use among consumers and some evidence of suppliers becoming more concentrated on this demand.

5 COST-EFFECTIVE MANAGEMENT OF SUBSTANCE MISUSE

Economists use economic evaluation techniques to compare the costs and consequences that occur in different policy scenarios. Current evidence is briefly reviewed for enforcement; treatment approaches; workplace policies and school-based information relevant to the UK. The brief nature of the review partly reflects the lack of good quality research worldwide on the cost-effectiveness of these interventions. It is too early to draw definitive conclusions about the detailed aspects of current drug policy but important to note that evidence will not be accumulated without well designed evaluative studies designed to include economic elements.

5.1 Enforcement

In the UK, as in most other countries, interventions designed to reduce the availability of drugs take a substantial share of drug policy expenditure. Recent years have seen a sizeable increase in expenditure on treatment and currently the share for enforcement has fallen from over 50 per cent in 2001 to below 40 per cent (Godfrey et al., 2005).

Demand studies suggest that increasing the probability of arrest may impact on demand. The supply literature suggests that availability measures only have a limited impact on the overall size of the market (see review in MacDonald, 2004). For example, no evidence was found to suggest a major police initiative had an impact on drug use or prices in London (Best *et al.*, 2001). Models of the cost-effectiveness of availability compared to treatment approaches have consistently suggested that treatment would provide better value for money than enforcement. However, combining more sophisticated modelling techniques using social models of demand and taking account of the temporal patterns of adoption of new drug consumption patterns suggest that the relative cost-effectiveness of policies may vary over this diffusion process (Behrens *et al.*, 1999).

5.2 Treatment

Reviews of drug treatment and rehabilitation, mainly for heroin users, suggests that treatment saves society far more than it costs (Cartwright, 2000; McCollister and French, 2003). Most of the empirical studies have been undertaken in the US but a number of UK studies, such as the National Treatment Outcome Research Study (NTORS), have suggested similar benefits (Coid *et al.*, 2000; Gossop *et al.*, 1998) with a reduction in social costs of about 9–15 times the spending on drug treatment in the two years following treatment (Godfrey *et al.*, 2004). A simulation model estimating the impact of increases in the numbers of problem drug misusers in community-based methadone treatment of 10 000 a year over the next five years predicted a reduction in the social costs of drug misuse of £3–4 billion (Godfrey *et al.*, 2005). Current policy does involve increasing the numbers in treatments of all types, not just community-based methadone treatment, through a number of different schemes, such as arrest referral and other components of the Drug Interventions Programme. Given the potential savings from reduced crime and other benefits from treatment such programmes could be cost-effective and indeed

cost-saving. In the absence of primary evaluations of such policies, simulation models do provide one means of evaluating these different components of current programmes. Unfortunately the research on the costs and therefore the cost-effectiveness of different means of attracting problem drug users into the treatment system is very limited.

While studies of the economic costs and benefits of treatment have provided evidence on the overall worth of increasing levels of treatment, far less is known about the comparative worth of different treatment approaches. While a number of studies have recently been completed or are under way (e.g. UKCBTMM Project Group, 2004), this is an important area for future research.

For the future, there is considerable scope for the development of pharmacotherapies and psychosocial approaches. Effective treatments are likely to be cost-effective, given the high social costs associated with problem drug users. Novel approaches that reduced the potential development of dependence could also be worthwhile. However, the history of securing resources for heroin addiction suggests that it may be difficult to secure investment in such treatments. Similarly it is important to conduct research into the different means of attracting and retaining problem drug misusers into the treatment system.

5.3 School-based and Other Prevention Policies

Systematic reviews of the effectiveness of school-based programmes directed at reduced alcohol consumption suggest that most have limited effectiveness and are costly (eg Foxcroft *et al.*, 2003). Caulkins *et al.* (1999) indicate, however, that if effective school-based interventions can be devised, they may also prove to be cost effective despite their high cost. Other types of study on the demand for illicit drugs reviewed above do suggest that young people are influenced by perceptions of harm. While school-based interventions may remain an important source of information, but are not necessarily expected to change drug-related behaviour, other approaches may prove more promising. However, measuring the impact of any prevention programme on behaviour rather than just awareness is challenging and needs to take account of the other factors influencing demand. There is fertile grounds for new research building upon theoretical insights reviewed in the previous section and taking into account potential models of drug adoption.

5.4 Interventions in the Workplace

Drug misuse could have various impacts in the workplace, as suggested in sections 3 and 4. This is also an area where there are commercial interests in devising tests and policies for employers. However, the evidence of the cost-effectiveness of such policies in reducing drug use is very limited. In particular, drug testing of employees may be a useful selection device for employers, selecting employees with a range of characteristics such as risk aversion, rather than controlling the use itself (Godfrey and Parrott, 2005). As a setting, it does provide an opportunity for treatment interventions, which could provide some payback for employers.

5.5 Conclusions

There are no simple policy solutions to reduce demand and, given that this demand will respond to changing market conditions, policy initiatives may have to be commensurate with these changes and external factors such as globalisation. Prevention programmes will need to be evaluated taking such factors into account and realistic goals for the impact of such programmes on population level data set.

Dependent individuals have generally been shown to have the highest social costs and treatment for such individuals has been shown to be cost-saving for society. There is considerable scope for devising novel treatments but the commercial incentives for

developing this business are currently small. The commercial response to drug taking has focused on devising interventions for employers.

6 PATTERNS OF DRUG ADOPTION

An important part of the growing literature on the dynamics of drug taking is a theoretical treatment of collective behaviour, calibrated to empirical data.

These models of collective behaviour display common phenomena, with greater or lesser fidelity, including:

- S-shaped adoption paths,
- cascade or 'herd' behaviour,
- 'punctuated' paths of long periods of slow and localised change separated by brief periods of profound or discontinuous adjustment,
- path-dependence or hysteresis (locally irreversible change),
- cycles.

Everingham and Rydell (1994) present a simple model of market dynamics based on a division between poor, heavy users of a drug, and light users who may be poor or rich. These groups have potentially different elasticities with respect to price, information and other factors. Poor, heavy users can finance their purchases through legitimate work, property crime or drug sales to rich users. Considering only the third of these, a fall in rich users' demand will constrain the income – and consumption – of poor heavy users. But if their drug use reduces their legitimate income, their need to increase their own drug sales may bid down drug prices. The same analysis suggests that legal sanctions may increase the attractiveness of short-term employment in drug markets relative to activities such as education.

More recent models (for example, Behrens et al., 1999, 2002) take account of the twin forces of contagion (promoting drug use) and prior observation (deterring it).

Endogenously influenced forces pulling in opposite directions can easily lead to cycles.

It is possible to extend this view in several directions. First, 'contagion' from non-users can discourage drug use, as policies aimed at decreasing the social acceptability of drug use recognise. Second, contagion (in either direction) is opposed by cohesion with social contacts.

A third factor, as Behrens *et al.* (2002) point out, is that drug reputations reflect both current use and memories or prior observation of heavy users. This is analogous to the 'stock of addiction' variable in rational addiction models – with the significant difference that its present value may respond negatively to past increases. In addition, recent experiences that depress the 'reputation' of a drug may switch to a positive impact as the experience recedes, consistent with psychological evidence that compulsive addicts try to recreate 'that first fine careless rapture'. (A similar effect could be obtained simply by attaching a positive weight to the first experience and using negative discounting.)

Individual preferences for drug use may also display unobserved – or partially observed – heterogeneity. Individuals observe each other's actions, not their underlying tastes. This by itself can generate multiple equilibria and cycles. A series of control-theoretic models that take account of age distributions (eg Almeder *et al.*, 2004) and intertemporal drug-supply decision (eg Feichtinger and Tragler, 2002) also produce cycles and multiplicity. Moreover, people differ in proximity and the salience or persuasiveness of their experience. Changes in collective behaviour reflect the structure, strength and direction of societal ties. Indeed, networks depend on behaviour. One justification for standard epidemiological models of drug adoption is that addicts gradually form networks consisting almost entirely of other drug users. In the beginning, this involves some recruitment of existing social contacts, marking the contagious phase. Eventually there are few left to infect. This slows propagation by limiting 'outside' contacts, but – by embedding users in like-minded groups – reduces 'benign contagion' from non-users and may increase the 'infectiousness' of contact with non-users. This is consistent with evidence that successful quitting typically involves a change of acquaintances.

6.1 Theoretical Modelling of Drug-adoption Patterns

Treating drug adoption as a social phenomenon sheds light on the progress and likely outcomes of both new-drug introduction and policy efforts to control use or adverse effects. The models in this section extend the epidemiological literature, in ways consistent with individual addiction models and evidence on the growth, spread and decline of drug 'epidemics'.

The underlying ideas are that drug decisions are influenced by:

- individual tastes,
- drug-taking prevalence and the strength of 'peer pressure',
- perceptions of risks and costs.

The models take account of the impact of direct and indirect observation on peer pressure and risk assessment as well as 'objective' information. The structure and strength of those connections – and even the underlying taste for the drug – are influenced by drug use. A simple chain of models captures these phenomena – at least qualitatively – and many features noted in section 3, while remaining tractable enough for scenario studies and policy simulations.

6.2 A Simple Model with One Drug and a Large, Fully Connected Population

The first model incorporates unobserved and heterogeneous tastes; price, risk information, legal and societal disincentives; 'peer pressure'; and drug use among the peer groups. There is uncertainty about others' tastes but people make the choices they intend. This essentially static model shows multiple equilibria and can be used as the basis for dynamic analysis (illustrated in the discussion).

We begin with the decision to consume a single drug; the individual's relative utility for drug use is:

$$U_i(\theta_i, \overset{\omega}{\pi}, v, \rho, \Gamma) = \theta_i[1 + v\pi_i(\Gamma)] - \rho \quad (13.1)$$

where:

θ_i	the individual's intrinsic taste for the drug
v	peer-pressure effect: social pressure or social drug consumption
ρ	anticipated price/risk: health, legal, workplace, social, purchase price, etc.
$\overset{\omega}{\pi} = (\pi_1, \ldots, \pi_n)$	the vector of drug use prevalence across the population
Γ	the social network: a set of connected pairs (i, j)
$\pi_i(\Gamma)$	drug use prevalence among one's network neighbours (i.e $\{j : (i,j) \in \Gamma\}$)

This model makes very strong symmetry assumptions, uses a particularly simple reduced form and is limited to 'rational addiction' in the sense that only preferences change – though it departs from the standard model in taking account of others' consumption. The purpose is to demonstrate that some unexpected qualitative features can arise in a simple setting.

In the simplest model, everyone is connected to everyone else and the population is large enough so that each experiences the general level of prevalence π. Because tastes differ, all do not make the same choice; the drug will be consumed by those with sufficient taste for the experience: $\theta_i \geq \theta^*$, where the critical value of taste satisfies:

$$\theta^*[1 + v\pi] = \rho \quad (13.2)$$

If taste is distributed between q_- and q_+ according to cumulative distribution $F(F(\theta)$ is the proportion whose taste does not exceed θ), $\pi = 1 - F(\theta^*)$, so:

$$1 - F^{-1}(\pi) = \frac{\rho}{[1 + v\pi]} \quad (13.3)$$

In a second version of this model, expected price/risk is influenced by learning from others. This utility function is:

$$U_i(\theta_i, \overset{\omega}{\pi}, v, \rho, \Gamma) = \theta_i[1 + v\pi_i(\Gamma)] - \rho(1 - \beta\pi_i(\Gamma)) \quad (13.4)$$

where β measures peer learning. The equilibrium condition is:

$$1 - F^{-1}(\pi) = \frac{\rho(1 + \beta\pi)}{[1 + v\pi]} \quad (13.5)$$

Figure 13.1 shows the (common) left-hand side of equations 13.3 and 13.5, plotted with their right-hand sides (for the case $F =$ cumulative normal with mean $= -5$ and variance $= 5$; $\rho = 20$; $v = 6$).

This shows multiple equilibria and that *stable* equilibrium prevalence falls as peer learning about price/risk becomes more important.

For some values, there is a unique equilibrium. The actual structure of the results also depends on the range of tastes:

$$\rho > (1 + \pi)\theta \quad (13.6)$$

$$\theta_+ > \rho \quad (13.7)$$

Condition 6 says that the lowest-preference person would not take the drug even if all their peers did; 7 says that the highest-preference person would consume even if none of their peers did. For the (unbounded) normal distribution, both hold trivially.

If both conditions hold, the multiple equilibrium situation shown in Figure 13.1 is possible. If neither holds, there is likely to be a unique equilibrium.

Figure 13.2 shows the structure of the equilibrium set as a function of price/risk and peer effects.

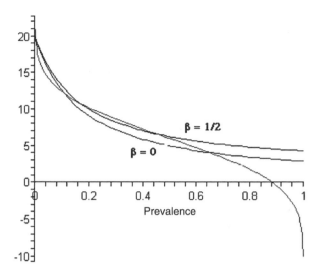

FIGURE 13.1 Sample plot of equilibrium prevalence in simple model.

Stronger peer effects produce multiple equilibria; catastrophic jumps and S-shaped paths. The model becomes more interesting with endogenous changes in the peer and price/risk effects. Drug use may reinforce an individual's tendency to pay attention to their peer group. Although network structure is fixed, an individual's ties to users may strengthen as a result of their own use or if increasing social isolation introduces social considerations into primarily hedonic or utilitarian drug-use decisions. This can move the individual into the multiple-equilibrium part of the diagram and reinforce choices. The behaviour of individuals with similar tastes and price/risk perceptions might diverge as peer effects strengthen.

More striking effects come from endogenous changes in perceived price/risk. If users' experience and close acquaintance with heavy users increase these perceptions (eg through increased expenditure needs and negative observations) and vice versa for non-users, the model implies

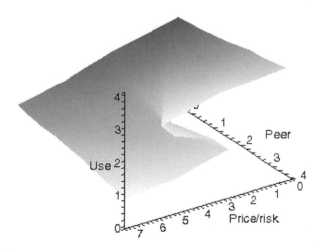

FIGURE 13.2 Multiple equilibria in the drug-adoption model.

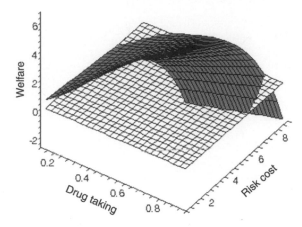

FIGURE 13.3   Prevalence, price/risk and welfare.

anticlockwise cycles in drug prevalence. As with memory-contagion models, these cycles may be localised and optimally addressed by policy that 'follows the cycle'.

Welfare

Total welfare can be expressed as:

$$W = (1 + \nu\pi) \int_{\theta^*}^{\theta} \theta f(\theta)d\theta - \rho(1 - F(\theta^*)) \quad (13.8)$$

Using $\pi = 1 - F(\theta^*)$ to eliminate the critical taste parameter θ^*, we get:

$$W = (1 + \nu\pi) \int_{1-F^{-1}(\pi)}^{\theta_+} \theta f(\theta)d\theta - \rho\pi \quad (13.9)$$

This implicitly normalises the welfare of non-users to 0, takes no account of welfare decreases (mistakes) associated with drug-taking beyond those modelled with price/risk, and does not model different levels of individual consumption – only population prevalence. The model only implies multiple equilibria for given values of price/risk and peer effects, so we can plot welfare as a function of these parameters and drug taking (Figures 13.3 and 13.4).

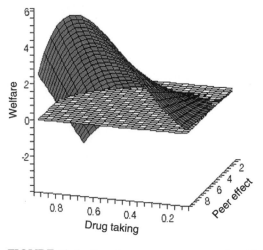

FIGURE 13.4   Prevalence, peer pressure and welfare.

A few other phenomena can tractably be handled by simple variants of this model. One concerns information about prevalence and price/risk. If individuals rely on general rather than direct experience, users will be a representative sample of the taste distribution. In one sense, the results are broadly similar – roughly S-shaped time-paths of adoption or remission, with 'catastrophic' jumps when peer effects are large. However, the behavioural response to policy changes may be different – in the absence of peer effects, an increase in perceived price/risk will have much less effect than in the 'strategic' model, but if peer effects are large, increases in price/risk will always reduce prevalence, while in the strategic model modest price/risk increases may increase prevalence.

6.3 A Dynamic Model with Fixed Tastes

Treating drug use as conventional behaviour sheds light on the interaction of drug-use choices and social contacts. This dynamic model is based on the twin phenomena of cohesion with one's reference group and contagious 'heterodox' behaviour. The underlying possibilities are based on the previous model. Choice dynamics reflect, in addition, the stylised facts of addictive behaviour in section 3 including the possibility of mistakes. A first model examines formation and welfare properties of 'conventional' behaviour for a given social pattern; the next subsection combines this with evolving social linkages.

From equation 13.4, the payoffs to drug-taking choices between any two socially-linked individuals are demonstrated in Table 13.5.

Consider a network of individuals making repeated choices over time. We assume that:

- at any moment, each person has a certain probability of re-examining their choice;
- that person will try to adopt the best reply to neighbours' choices and will succeed with probability $1 - \mu$;
- with probability μ, they will make the 'wrong' choice.

This defines a Markov process on the population's drug-taking behaviour $\overset{\omega}{\pi}$.

An individual will wish to adopt the drug if 'most' of their neighbours do:

$$\pi_i(\Gamma) \geq (\rho - \theta_i)/(\theta_i \nu - \rho\beta) \qquad (13.10)$$

To begin, we assume that all people have the same tastes (θ) and that every person is connected to everyone else. The limit of this distribution will be a single behaviour, which will involve only experimental drug taking if, and only if, abstinence is risk-dominant:

$$\theta < \rho(2 + \beta)/2 + \nu \qquad (13.11)$$

Abstinence is socially efficient if:

$$\theta < \rho(1 + \beta)/1 + \nu \qquad (13.12)$$

In this model:

- if peer pressure is stronger than peer learning ($\nu > \beta$), abstinence is stable when it is optimal, but may be stable even when suboptimal;
- if peer pressure is weaker than peer learning ($\nu < \beta$), abstinence is optimal when it is stable, but may be optimal even when unstable;

This provides some simple policy prescriptions. Because optimality here ignores externalities, stabilising abstinence may be desirable in broader circumstances. Policy can affect perceived price/risk by: conventional law-enforcement cost- or risk-imposing strategies that target users, action against dealers that makes price, quality or availability more uncertain, and education, especially peer reinforcement of risk information. Policy, for example youth policy, can also affect peer pressure. It is even

TABLE 13.5 The simple 2-player drug-use game.

Player 2 takes drug

		Yes	No
Player 1 takes drug	Yes	$(\theta_1(1 + \nu) - \rho(1 + \beta), \theta_2(1 - \nu) - \rho(1 + \beta))$	$(\theta_1 - \rho, 0)$
	No	$(0, \theta_2 - \rho)$	$(0,0)$

possible – through provision of localised healthcare, law enforcement or price/purity information – to alter the strength of the peer-learning effect (β).

Ignoring the dynamics of social interaction, a 'rational addiction' policy would have to alter these parameters to the point where

$$\theta < \rho \min \left\{ 1, \frac{1+\beta}{1+\nu} \right\} \qquad (13.13)$$

This involves strictly more policy intervention unless the peer-pressure effect (ν) exactly equals the peer-learning effect (β) – but these are at least partly susceptible to policy intervention!

If peer pressure dominates peer learning, it is easier to make abstinence stable, achieving the desired result through non-cooperative evolution. Otherwise, it is easier to make abstinence optimal (among users), achieving the desired result through co-operative (or bargaining) means.

Speed of convergence to the stable outcome depends – in this model at least – on the frequency with which choices are revisited and the fidelity with which they are realised. This directly reflects the cue-conditioned cognition model (see section 3). The dynamics can also be adapted for asymmetry between quitting and relapse – changing rates of onset or recovery but not the ultimate stable state.

Risk-dominant behaviour will eventually prevail in any symmetric network. Other 'geometries' can have clusters or pockets of drug use in an abstinent population – or vice versa. Clustering (small worlds of individuals all of whose friends are likely to be friends of each other) is more likely in certain groups, and has two effects on adoption. It slows propagation, but, within groups, peer effects are likely to be very strong. These impacts are borne out by empirical experience and suggest further forms of educational and youth policy intervention.

When tastes differ, the analysis becomes more complicated, but some general observations can be made. Even with relatively few 'high-taste' individuals, a cluster can 'tip' into drug taking if the proportion is large enough (it may well take more than one 'rotten apple'). Vulnerability is reduced if those with middling tastes for the drug have many outside connections to others with low to middle tastes or in clusters with relatively few high-taste individuals. The same holds for abstinence in populations where high taste is prevalent.

Adoption or remission are, in general, neither uniform nor monotone. Beyond the stochastic aspects, a given cluster may 'get stuck' for a long period until external changes trigger rapid change. Policy interventions, whether global or localised, do not produce a constant stream of effects but instead have tipping points and delayed impacts that must work through the network as a whole before producing observable changes. On the other hand, the impacts, when they come, may well be profound.

6.4 Endogenous Tastes and Structures

The previous sections treated tastes (θ_i) and structure (Γ) as fixed. Neither assumption is likely to survive contact with the real world. Network analysis has already developed a treatment of endogenous structures based on chance encounters: unlinked parties may form a link if each benefit by doing so. Links dissolve if either party wishes to end the association. This defines a Markov process – this time on societal structures – whose limiting outcomes may be considered stable. One simple application would hold drug-taking behaviour constant; stable and efficient networks are likely to differ sharply. This may be desirable if individuals take insufficient account of externalities (involving other people, times or random consequences). It also suggests that even well-informed and foresightedly rational individuals might fail to form 'optimal' social contacts.

To gain deeper insight, it is desirable to combine these models – to let drug-taking behaviour and social interactions change on the same timescale. Such models can, under the right conditions, reconcile efficiency and stability and produce lower drug use. But this is not inevitable.

One would expect drug adoption to increase the proportion of high-taste individuals among a given person's contacts, and ultimately to increase clustering as individuals sharing a common link are brought into contact. At the same time, links with low-taste individuals – at least non-users – may fall away. This fits heroin users' lifecycle contagion patterns, with simple implications for crime rates, treatment effectiveness and external costs. Policies that enhance clustering – for example, by driving users underground – can have two opposed effects. The first is to reduce the chances and depth of contact between experienced drug users and non-users. The second is to make such contacts more 'dangerous' because the individual making contact with such a cluster is more likely to be influenced by the drug user than vice versa. In addition, under policy and societal conditions that knit drug-using clusters tightly together, drug use provides a ready-made entrée to a tightly-knit cluster, which may be attractive to members of more scattered groupings.

A second useful extension is endogeneity of tastes. It is perfectly feasible to make tastes a function of past consumption behaviour. This is consistent with the individual models of addiction in which preferences change (eg the rational addiction models), but has not been explored here.

6.5 Polydrug Models

The model given above concentrates on a single drug. There is no difficulty in principle in extending this to the case of multiple or combined drug use. While space does not permit a comprehensive treatment, two interesting phenomena can be treated.

Consider different 'drugs' ($k = 1, \ldots, K$), where some may involve combinations (to handle complementarities easily). The utility function generalises to:

$$U_i(\theta_i, \overset{\varpi}{\pi}, v, \rho, \Gamma) = \sum_k \left[\theta_i^k \left[1 + \sum_{k'} v_k^{k'} \pi_i^{k'}(\Gamma) \right] - \rho^k \left(1 - \sum_{k'} \beta_k^{k'} \pi_i^{k'}(\Gamma) \right) \right]$$

(13.14)

where:

θ_i^k	individual i's intrinsic taste for drug k
$v_k^{k'}$	peer-pressure effect of prevalence of drug k' use on taste for drug k
ρ^k	anticipated price/risk for drug k
$\overset{\varpi}{\pi} = (\pi_1, \ldots, \pi_n)$	the vector of drug use prevalence across drugs and population
$\beta_k^{k'}$	peer learning effect of observing drug k' use on price/risk of drug k
$\pi_i^k(\Gamma)$	prevalence of drug k use among i's network neighbours

Under suitable assumptions, 'diagonal' outcomes will survive – if peer effects are strong enough then cohesion will stabilise homogeneous behaviour. The Markov analysis used in section 6.3 can be adapted as follows. As before, individuals have random chances to re-evaluate their behaviour and succeed with some probability, resulting in a Markov process whose limiting distribution defines the stable outcomes. In the single-drug model, the population would drift away from one pattern if enough people made 'mistakes' – by choosing the other. Here, there are more possibilities, and thus various ways in which a group could change from one state (say abstinence) to another (say heroin use):

- a sufficient proportion could experiment with heroin use to cause the others to change by peer pressure;

- a sufficient proportion could experiment with another drug to make heroin a 'best reply' to the mixed behaviour of the group;
- a sufficient proportion could experiment with another drug (say crack) to tip the group into its use, from which heroin use could be reached by a smaller step.

In the formal analysis, the stability of a transition from one outcome to another is measured by the smallest number of 'mistakes' required to follow one of the above paths. The stable outcomes are those which are easiest to fall into and hardest to fall out of.

There are situations where the transition from abstinence to stable drug use runs through another drug – this is an example of a gateway effect, and depends as much on the network structure of users as on physiological complementarities between the intermediate and eventual drugs. There are situations of stable polydrug abuse – again, these can arise purely through societal interactions. The trajectories and stable states depend on cross-drug peer and learning effects, so that they can be reversed by policies (or information) that change relative prices, risks or social acceptability, such as 'fashion' cascades, as with heroin chic. In addition, policy effects can be attenuated: a policy that inhibits one route into adoption of a particular drug may simply displace the dynamics to the next 'shortest' route.

The same model can be used to simulate the impacts of introducing (or withdrawing) drugs.

6.6 Conclusions

The models discussed in this section show that a wide range of policies and types of drugs and drug use can be analysed in a unified way. They capture societal interactions in a flexible but transparent way and thus help bridge the gap between individual models of conventional microeconomics (and some psychological and physiological models) and collective models coming from sociology and criminology.

The models do not, by themselves, shed light on the psychoactive substances of the future, but they do shed light on how the characteristics of such substances and incumbent patterns of use will influence which potential substances are taken up and what the impacts are likely to be. However, the abstract nature of the models means that they are more suited to scenario exploration than prediction. They are best used in conjunction with scenarios to put flesh on the narrative bones, add colour and detail and provide a link between 'rounds' of scenario interaction.

In addition to the impacts associated with the prevalence of drug use, these models can shed light on induced changes in social structures. Such changes – in particular the formation of 'small worlds' around drug use – can be profoundly important in determining a range of other societal outcomes, including implications for non-drug crime, health, education and workplace productivity.

The models also suggest a wide range of interventions such as:

- those aimed directly at the evolution and spread of drug behaviours;
- the interactive effects of law enforcement, informative and treatment interventions.

They can also lead to a dynamic view of policy intervention that shows how to make policies 'follow the cycle' and how to achieve better results by exploiting network dynamics (for example, by making optimal outcomes stable) and the potential for cooperative progress within the affected community (by making stable outcomes optimal).

6.7 For the Future

The economic evidence and modelling surveyed in this section is more useful for exploring the future than for predicting it. In particular, it offers a range of inputs for scenario-based exploration. A scenario, in this context, is a partially-specified description of a possible future which can be used to draw out hidden implications of current knowledge and data, explore the logical consistency of findings based on different data, perspectives and methods, integrate a range of different policy options and objectives, explore how key stakeholders are likely to respond to unfolding challenges, and increase the validity and clarity with which future options and developments are understood.

A scenario is based around four main elements:

- key uncertainties – important aspects of the future that are either unknown at present or unknowable in the sense that they have not yet happened;
- relationships between key variables and parts of the system;
- levers – the policy and strategic options that will act through these relationships;
- measures – the terms in which system behaviour is described and evaluated.

Further aspects include descriptive details and a narrative thread. There are so many possible futures that descriptions tend to be either confusing or banal. A scenario should encapsulate a single idea or possibility and convey it clearly and convincingly. This idea may involve a specific mechanism (such as the importance of learning or social interaction to drug adoption, the implications of cue-conditioning or self-strategising or gateway and polydrug interactions), a novel policy lever such as the conscious use of uncertainty-generating strategies to 'steer' individual decisions, or new measures (for example, of the structural characteristics of drug supplies, estimates of rents and value added, estimates of the distribution of use across groups).

Scenario exploration can follow one or both of two routes: 'forecast' analysis, which starts from the present and tries to identify possible 'landing places' and their likelihood and desirability; and 'backcasting' analysis, which starts from a desired (or feared) future and works out what must have happened in order to realise it. The useful results are the identification and prioritisation of key areas of uncertainty, highlighting key relationships whose operation might lead to efficiencies or unintended consequences, policy sets – policy combinations, priorities and contingent strategies, and relevant measures – indicators or measurements derived from existing or fresh data, together with an understanding of what they do and do not tell us.

In this setting, the empirical results surveyed above can be used to produce coherent starting points for constructing the basic elements and to add convincing colour to the narrative thread that explains the main idea.

The theoretical models, by contrast, can be used to illustrate qualitative features or to make quantitative predictions. In scenario exploration, they can be used in the initial description to produce graphic or other illustrations of spillovers and other effects to help link the various parts of the narrative and draw attention to holistic consistency. They can also be used in an iterative exploration of the scenario involving alternative policies or resolutions of key uncertainties. Finally, they can be used to produce quantitative measures to aid in policy evaluation – though not (given data and econometric limitations and the profound gaps between the measured past and the explored future) in specific detail.

More concrete observations can be made of the demand-and-supply aspects of drug use. On the demand side, economic evidence supports the importance of choice and thus the relevance of 'economic' variables relating to individual beliefs about risks attached to drug use, price and income effects, the impact of supply, price and quality uncertainty, the interaction of drug use with education and health, and the importance of peer effects and learning in conveying and appropriately reinforcing good decisions.

On the supply side, the evidence suggests that targeting of specific drugs, market locations and levels, key players and supplier strategies (eg money-laundering or the use of violence) can play a key role in changing the performance of drugs markets. It also suggests reasons why the possibility of users becoming dealers at the local level may be important for the ability of policy to discourage drugs trafficking by imposing costs, how supply uncertainty may affect prices, qualities and market efficiency and whether the prevalence of minimally refined agricultural products (eg the 'big three' of heroin, cocaine and cannabis) is likely to be threatened by 'high-tech' alternatives.

References

Advisory Council on the Misuse of Drugs (2000) *Reducing drug-related deaths*. London: The Stationery Office.

Almeder, C., Caulkins, J., Feichtinger, G., and Tragler, G. (2004) An age-structured single-state drug initiation model: cycles of drug epidemics and optimal prevention programs. *Socio-Economic Planning Sciences* 38(1): 91–109.

Becker, G. and Murphy, K. (1988) A theory of rational addiction. *J Political Econ* 96(4): 675–700.

Becker, G., Murphy, K., and Grossman, M. (2004). *The economic theory of illegal goods: the case of drugs*. NBER Working Paper 10976. Cambridge, Mass: National Bureau of Economic Research.

Behrens, D., Caulkins, J., Tragler, G., Haunschmied, J., and Feichtinger, G. (1999) A dynamic model of drug initiation: implications for treatment and drug control. *Math Biosci* 159: 1–20.

Behrens, D., Caulkins, J., Tragler, G., and Feichtinger, G. (2002) Why present-oriented societies undergo cycles of drug epidemics. *J Econ Dynam Control* 26: 919–936.

Best, D., Strang, J., Beswick, T., and Gossop, M. (2001) Assessment of a concentrated, high-profile police operation: no discernible impact on drug availability, price or purity. *Br J Criminol* 41: 738–745.

Bramley-Harker, E. (2001) *Sizing the UK market for illicit drugs*. Research, Development and Statistics Directorate Occasional Paper 74. London: Home Office.

Bretteville-Jensen, A. (1999) Addiction and discounting. *J Health Econ* 18: 393–407.

Bretteville-Jensen, A. (2003) Heroin consumption, prices and addiction: evidence from self-reported panel data. *Scand J Econ* 105: 661–679.

Bretteville-Jensen, A. and Sutton, M. (1996) *Under the influence of the market: an applied study of illicitly selling and consuming heroin*. Discussion Paper 147. York: Centre for Health Economics, University of York.

Buck, D., Godfrey, C., and Sutton, M. (1996) Economic and other views of addiction: implications for the choice of alcohol, tobacco and drug policies. *Drug Alcohol Rev* 15: 357–368.

Cameron, L. and Williams, J. (2001) Substitutes or complements? Alcohol, cannabis and tobacco. *Econ Rec* 77: 19–34.

Cartwright, W. (2000) Cost–benefit analysis of drug treatment services: review of the literature. *J Mental Health Pol Econ* 3: 11–26.

Caulkins, J., Rydell, P., Everingham, S., Chiesa, J., and Bushway, S. (1999) *An ounce of prevention: a pound of uncertainty*. Santa Monica, CA: Drug Policy Research Center, RAND.

Caulkins, J. and Reuter, P. (1998) What can we learn from drug prices? *J Drug Issues* 28(3): 593–612.

Caulkins, J. and Reuter, P. (1999) The meaning and utility of drug prices. *Addiction* 91: 1261–1264.

Chaloupka, F., Grossman, M., and Tauras, J.A. (1999a) The demand for cocaine and marijuana by youth. In: F. Chaloupka, M. Grossman, W.K. Bickel, and H. Saffer (eds), *The economic analysis of substance use and abuse: an integration of econometric and behavioural economic research*. Chicago: University of Chicago Press: 133–155.

Chaloupka, F., Pacula, R., Farrelly, M., Johnston, L., O'Malley, P., and Bray, J. (1999b) *Do higher cigarette prices encourage youth to use marijuana?* NBER Working Paper 6938. Cambridge, Mass: National Bureau of Economic Research.

Coid, J., Carvell, A., Kittler, Z., Healey, A., and Henderson, J. (2000) *The impact of methadone treatment on drug misuse and crime*. Home Office Research Study 120. London: Home Office.

Corman, H., Noonan, K., Reichman, N., and Dave, D. (2004) *Demand for illicit drugs by pregnant women*. NBER Working Paper 10688. Cambridge, Mass: National Bureau of Economic Research.

Culyer, A., Eaton, G., Godfrey, C., Koutsolioutsos, H., and McDougall, C. (2001) *Economic and social cost of substance misuse in the United Kingdom: review of the methodological and empirical studies of the economic and social costs of illicit drugs*. York: Centre for Criminal Justice Economics and Psychology, University of York.

Dave, D. (2004a) *The effects of cocaine and heroin price on drug-related emergency department visits.* NBER Working Paper 10619. Cambridge, Mass: National Bureau of Economic Research.

Dave, D. (2004b) *Illicit drug use among arrestees and drug prices.* NBER Working Paper 10648. Cambridge, Mass: National Bureau of Economic Research.

Desimone, J. and Farrelly, M. (2003) Price and enforcement effects on cocaine and marijuana demand. *Econ Inq* 41: 98–115.

DiNardo, J. and Lemieux, T. (1992) *Alcohol, marijuana and American youth: the unintended effects of government regulation.* NBER Working Paper 4212. Cambridge, Mass: National Bureau of Economic Research.

Doll, R., Peto, R., Boreham, J., and Sutherland, I. (2004) Mortality in relation to smoking: 50 years' observations on male British doctors. *BMJ* doi:10.1136/bmj.38142.554479.AE (published 22 June).

Everingham, S. and Rydell, C.P. (1994) *Modeling the demand for cocaine.* Santa Monica, CA: RAND.

Farrelly, M., Bray, J., Zarkin, G., Wendling, B., and Pacula, R. (1999) *The effects of prices and policies on the demand for marijuana: evidence from the National Household Surveys on drug abuse.* NBER Working Paper 6940. Cambridge, Mass: National Bureau of Economic Research.

Feichtinger, G. and Tragler, G. (2002) Multiple equilibria in an optimal control model for law enforcement. Proceedings of the Steklov Institute of Mathematics, Moscow. *Am Math Soc* 236: 449–460.

Foxcroft, D.R., Ireland, D., Lister-Sharp, D.J., Lowe, G., and Breen, R. (2003) Longer-term primary prevention for alcohol misuse in young people: a systematic review. *Addiction* 98: 397–411.

Godfrey, C. (2001) Modelling drug markets: empirical evidence available from economic studies. In: EMCDDA *Scientific Report: Expert Meeting on Drug Markets and Modelling.* 23–24 October 2000. www. emcdda.europa.eu/?fuseaction=public. Attachment Download &nNodeID=1947

Godfrey, C. and Parrott, S. (2005) The extent of the problem and the cost to the employer. In: H. Ghodse (ed.), *Addiction at work: tackling drug misuse in the workplace.* Aldershot: Gower.

Godfrey, C., Eaton, G., McDougall, C., and Culyer, A. (2002) *The Economic and social costs of class A drug use in England and Wales, 2000.* Home Office Research Study 249. London: Home Office.

Godfrey, C., Stewart, D., and Gossop, M. (2004) Economic analysis of the costs and consequences of drug misuse and its treatment: two-year outcome data from the National Treatment Outcome Research Study (NTORS). *Addiction* 99: 687–707.

Godfrey, C., Parrott, S., Eaton, G., Culyer, A., and McDougall, C. (2005) Can we model the impact of increased drug treatment expenditure on the UK drug market? In: B. Lindgren and M. Grossman (eds), *The economics of substance use.* New York: Elsevier.

Goldstein, A. (2001) *Addiction: from biology to drug policy.* 2nd edition. New York: Oxford University Press.

Gossop, M., Marsden, J., and Stewart, D. (1998) *NTORS at one year: the National Treatment Outcome Research Study – changes in substance use, health and criminal behaviours at one year after intake.* London: Department of Health.

Groom, C., Davies, T., and Balchin, S. (1998) Developing a methodology for measuring illegal activity for the UK national accounts. *Economic Trends* 536(July).

Gruber, J. and Koszegi, B. (2001) Is addiction 'rational'? Theory and evidence. *Q J Econ* 116(4): 1261–1303.

Herrnstein, R. and Prelec, D. (1992) A theory of addiction. In: G. Loewenstein and J. Elster (eds), *Choice over time.* New York: Russell Sage Foundation.

Heyman, G.M. (2003) Consumption-dependent changes in reward value: a framework for understanding addiction. In: R.E. Vuchinich, and N. Heather (eds), *Choice, behavioural economics and addiction.* Oxford: Pergamon Press.

Heyman, G.M. and Tanz, L.E. (1995) How to teach a pigeon to maximize overall reinforcement rate. *J Exp Anal Behav,* 64: 277–297.

Kleiman, M. (1997) The problem of replacement and the logic of drug law enforcement. *Drug Policy Anal Bull* 3: 8–10.

Lundberg, P. and Lindgren, B. (2002) Risk perceptions and alcohol consumption among young people. *J Risk Uncertainty* 25: 165–183.

McCollister, K.E. and French, M.T. (2003) The relative contribution of outcome domains in the total economic benefit of addiction interventions: a review of first findings. *Addiction* 98: 1647–1659.

MacDonald, Z. (2004) What price drug use? The contribution of economics to an evidence-based drugs policy. *J Econ Surveys* 18: 113–140.

MacDonald, Z. and Shields, M. (2004) Does problem drinking affect employment? Evidence from England. *Health Econ* 13: 139–155.

Miron, J. (2003) The effect of drug prohibition on drug prices: evidence from the markets for cocaine and heroin. *Rev Econ Stat* 85: 522–530.

O'Brien, C. (1997) A range of research-based pharmacotherapies for addiction. *Science* 278: 66–70.

O'Donoghue, T. and Rabin, M. (1999) Doing it now or later. *Am Econ Rev* 89: 103–124.

O'Donoghue, T. and Rabin, M. (2000) *Addiction and present-biased preferences*, Manuscript, Berkeley.

Pacula, R. (1997). *Adolescent alcohol and marijuana consumption: is there really a gateway effect?* NBER Working Paper 6384. Cambridge, Mass: National Bureau of Economic Research.

Pacula, R. (2005). Marijuana use and policy: what we know and have yet to learn. *NBER Reporter*. Research Summary (Winter).

Pacula, R. and Chaloupka. F. (2001) The effects of macro-level interventions on addictive behaviour. *Subst Use Misuse* 36(13): 1901–1922.

Pacula, R., Grossman, M., Chaloupka, F., O'Malley, P., Johnston, L., and Farrelly, M. (2000) *Marijuana and youth*. NBER Working Paper 7703. Cambridge, Mass: National Bureau of Economic Research.

Petry, N. and Bickel, W. (1999) A behavioural economic analysis of polydrug abuse in heroin addicts. In: F. Chaloupka, M. Grossman, W. Bickel, and H. Saffer (eds), *The economic analysis of substance use and abuse*. Chicago: National Bureau of Economic Research, University of Chicago Press.

Rannia, L. (2003) Alcohol misuse: how much does it cost? London: Strategy Unit, Cabinet Office.

Saffer, H. and Chaloupka, F. (1999a) The demand for illicit drugs. *Econ Inq* 37: 401–411.

Saffer, H. and Chaloupka, F. (1999b) *State drug control spending and illicit drug participation*. NBER Working Paper 7114. Cambridge, Mass: National Bureau of Economic Research.

Schelling, T. (1980). The intimate contest for self-command. *The Public Interest* (Summer): 94–118.

Sumnall, H., Tyler, E., Wagstaff, G.F., and Cole, J.C. (2004) A behavioural economic analysis of alcohol, amphetamine, cocaine and ecstasy purchasers by polysubstance misusers. *Drug Alcohol Depend* 76: 93–99.

Trosclair, A., Huston, C. Pederson, L., and Dillon, I. (2002) Cigarette smoking among adults – United States, 2000. *Morbid Mortal Weekly Report*, 51(29): 642–645.

Twigg, L., Moon, G., and Walker, S. (2004) *The smoking epidemic in England*. London: Health Development Agency.

UKCBTMM Project Group (2004) *The effectiveness and cost-effectiveness of cognitive behaviour therapy for opiate misusers in methadone maintenance treatment: a multicentre, randomised, controlled trial*. Final Report to the Research and Development Directorate, Department of Health, as part of the Drug Misuse Research Initiative. November.

Wechsler, H. and Kuo, M. (2003) Watering down the drinks: the moderating effect of college demographics on alcohol use of high-risk groups. *Am J Public Health* 93: 1929–1933.

Williams, J. (2004) The effects of price and policy on marijuana use: what can be learned from the Australian experience? *Health Econ* 13: 123–137.

Williams, J., Pacula, R., Chaloupka, F., and Wechsler, H. (2004) Alcohol and marijuana use among college students: economic complements or substitutes? *Health Econ* 13: 825–843.

14

Problem Gambling and Other Behavioural Addictions

Jim Orford

1 EXECUTIVE SUMMARY

A broad view of addictions gives an important place to behavioural addictions such as excessive eating, excessive exercising, hypersexuality, Internet and other technological addictions, shopping addiction and various forms of gambling. The most researched is gambling, which now has a substantial and rapidly growing literature.

1.1 Explanations for Gambling Addiction

In that literature there is support for explanations for gambling addiction at the biological, personal, learning and cognitive process, and social levels. These are summarised in Table 14.1. Although research has mostly been confined to the study of factors at only one of those levels, a number of cross-cutting themes are emerging:

1. One of the strongest of these themes links learning processes and the importance of availability and accessibility, the particular vulnerability of adolescents and an early start to gambling, and the role of family members.
2. A closely related theme links emotional reward from gambling, emotions associated with processes such as 'chasing losses' and the experience of 'near misses', the association with substance use and misuse, and the possible role of brain

TABLE 14.1 Explanations for gambling addiction, showing some cross-cutting themes.

Social	Learning and cognitive	Biological	Personal
Availability/accessibility[1]	Monetary reward[1]	Genetics	Psychoanalytical
Adolescent vulnerability[1]	Emotional reward[1,2]	Neurotransmitter brain systems[2]	Personal functions[1]
Parental influence[1]	Chasing losses[2]		Locus of control[1]
Substance use[2]	Near misses[2]	Prefrontal cortical brain systems[3]	Impulsivity[3]
Income	Discounting of delayed reward[3]		
Ethnicity	Cognitive biases and illusions		

[1,2,3] Indicate cross-cutting themes 1, 2 and 3.

neurotransmitter systems such as the mesolimbic dopamine system.

3. And another theme links impulsivity as a personal characteristic and the possible involvement of the ventromedial prefrontal cortex of the brain.

An additional area that stands out in the gambling field is concerned with cognitive biases and illusions, including the failure to understand randomness, the 'gambler's fallacy' and the illusion of control.

The available evidence allows us to speculate about which behavioural addictions may be most troublesome in the next 10–20 years. Technological innovation is now so rapid that legislation has difficulty keeping up. Two new forms of gambling that may have considerable addiction liability – fixed-odds betting terminals and betting exchanges – came on the scene while the new Gambling Act was being considered. They add to developments such as Internet gambling and spread betting, as well as numerous new variations of traditional forms of gambling such as bingo and casino table games, which are likely to increase their addiction liability. The Gambling Bill encourages industry innovation and would legalise new forms of gambling or new ways of accessing gambling that are likely to increase addiction potential. These include casino resorts, gambling machines with unlimited stakes and prizes, and British Internet gambling sites.

The most troublesome addictions in the near future could be forms of gambling and other types of consumption that combine certain features:

- easy availability, particularly when opportunities are so many that they become part of national life, such as gambling machines in pubs and shopping malls and gambling via personal computers,
- rapidly achieved, intense emotional reward,
- the opportunity for continuous play or a rapid return to play.

The liability of addiction will be enhanced by features that add to the entrapment potential of the activity, such as betting on the same numbers, having an illusion of control, believing that one is nearly winning or is improving performance, or getting to know other participants, perhaps in an Internet chat room. Activities that could carry greatest future risks of behavioural addiction include those shown in Box 14.1.

Box 14.1 Activities that may carry greatest future risk for behavioural addiction.

Gambling machines types A and B
Gambling on Internet sites
Pornography on the Internet
Internet games, chat rooms etc.
Shopping
Eating

1.2 Preventing and Treating Behavioural Addictions

Ways of preventing and treating behavioural addictions that are likely to be most common in coming decades are summarised in Box 14.2. It should be recognised that certain activities with addiction potential are particular risks for women (excessive eating, shopping addiction, excessive gambling-machine playing).

Box 14.2: Ways of managing behavioural addiction in the future.

Assess and advertise addiction liability
Limit availability of dangerous activities,
    especially for children and adolescents
Identify addiction as it develops
Make treatment available

With the exception of some specialist services for people with eating disorders (which are often oriented towards anorexia and severe cases of bulimia), the provision of treatment for behavioural addiction has scarcely been considered, and research lags far behind that on treatment for substance addictions. Potentially effective forms of treatment will in many cases be similar to those for substance addiction, including psychological treatments such as cognitive behaviour therapy and certain pharmacological treatments. The involvement of family members is recommended and mutual-help organisations such as Gamblers Anonymous have a role to play. The spectrum of forms of help available should include telephone support, self-help manuals, and treatments that range in intensity from very brief to residential.

2 INTRODUCTION TO THE CONCEPT OF BEHAVIOURAL ADDICTION

'Addiction' is an apt, commonly understood word to use with respect to appetites – desires and inclinations – that have got out of hand and become excessive. But the word has become overly identified with drugs that have an effect on the central nervous system. A broader view places at least some behavioural addictions on an equal footing with drug addictions. The present author has developed this line of thinking, arguing that the field is better defined by the term 'excessive appetites' than 'drug dependencies' (Orford, 2001a,b).

Excessive eating is a good example of a phenomenon that is included in this more broadly-defined field. Various patterns of excessive eating have been described, referred to as binge eating, binge eating disorder, bulimia nervosa or bulimarexia (Leon and Roth, 1977; Wardle and Beinart, 1981; Fairburn and Wilson, 1993; Hay et al., 1996). They are associated with extreme preoccupation with food and weight, the episodic consumption of enormous amounts of food in short periods of time, a sense of lack of control over eating during the episode, guilt, shame, depression and self-condemnation following such 'binges', compensatory behaviours such as self-induced vomiting or the use of medications to prevent weight gain, self-initiated attempts at behavioural control, recommendations for restraint from others, hiding and hoarding food, lying to others about eating activities, and stealing food or money to buy it (Hamburger, 1951; Morganstern, 1977; American Psychiatric Association, 1994). Excessive eating appears to be much more common among women than men, although male cases have been described (eg Wilps, 1990; Tanofsky *et al.*, 1997). It has also been suggested that exercise can become excessive to the point of addiction (Farrar, 1992; Veale, 1987; Yates, 1991; Cox and Orford, 2004) and that excessive eating and exercising often co-occur (Yates, 1991).

Another behavioural addiction that challenges the narrow view of the field is hypersexuality or 'sex addiction'. The evidence is overwhelming that ordinary sex can for many people become difficult to control. The evidence comes from the nineteenth- and early twentieth-century literature on 'nymphomania' (Groneman, 1994); autobiographies and biographies; more recent, detailed accounts of the phenomenon (eg Carnes, 1983; Goodman, 1998); and the existence of 12-step groups such as Sex Addicts Anonymous and Sexual Compulsives Anonymous (Goodman, 1998). What is referred to here is heterosexual activity of a perfectly legal kind, ie ordinary sex that can become compulsive (usually involving multiple partners and running health, social and other risks in the process), in other words what is sometimes referred to as 'hypersexuality', and not, for example, sex with minors or non-consensual sex. The parallel with alcohol addiction is therefore a very close one, ie something which in moderation is enjoyable and relatively harmless, and engaged in by most people, but which for some people becomes excessive.

Another form of behaviour that was recognised by psychiatrists nearly a hundred years ago as one of the 'manias' ('oniomania' in this case), and which has received more attention in the last 10 years, is excessive shopping (Lee and Mysyk, 2004; Dittmar, 2004). It is characterised by chronic, repetitive purchasing, often of goods that are hoarded and underused; preoccupation with shopping; irresistible, intrusive and senseless impulses to buy; unsuccessful attempts to control the activity; feelings of guilt and depression following an episode; and harmful consequences, especially debt (Black, 1996;

Lejoyeux *et al.*, 1999; Lee and Mysyk, 2004; Dittmar, 2004). Excessive eating and buying have been reported predominantly among women, and have been reported to co-occur significantly (eg Faber *et al.*, 1995).

Whether such behaviours are true addictions has been questioned, but most of the questions raised could equally be asked of drug addictions. There has been much debate over whether excessive eating, buying or gambling are best categorised as 'addictions', 'compulsions' or 'impulsive control disorders' (Orford, 2001a; Lee and Mysyk, 2004). Another question that has been raised in the context of excessive buying (Lee and Mysyk, 2004), but which is equally pertinent in the case of addictive substances, is whether labelling such behaviour on the part of an individual as an addiction diverts attention from relevant societal issues. In the case of excessive buying, those issues would include the construction of shopping malls, rising consumerism generally with increased pressures to buy, and the increasing normalisation of indebtedness. Such considerations are highly relevant to any attempt to predict what addictions might increase in future.

Another set of behavioural addictions are what Griffiths (1999) has called 'technological addictions', including addiction to television, video and computer games, computer use generally, and the Internet specifically. The way in which use of the Internet can get out of control for some people, bringing their behaviour into conflict with other needs and activities, has been described by Shaffer (1996) and Young (1998), among others.

Box 14.3 lists a number of criteria for the recognition of a behavioural addiction, adapted from Griffiths (2002). These criteria are very similar to those used in definitions of drug dependence, which, according to these criteria, would form a subset of addictions. Then all forms of addiction, whether involving the ingestion of a substance or not, would be seen as behavioural addictions.

3 GAMBLING ADDICTION

Gambling addiction fits the criteria shown in Box 14.3 particularly well and much of the remainder of this review will focus on it.

There are a number of reasons for this choice. The evidence of the potential addictiveness of gambling is widespread and of long standing (France, 1902; Squires, 1937; Barker and Miller, 1968; Lesieur, 1984; Custer and Milt, 1985; Griffiths, 1990; Orford *et al.*, 2003). Indications that a person is experiencing addiction to gambling include the sheer amount of the gambling activity, the person's concern about its excessiveness, the strength of desire for and preoccupation with gambling, a feeling of loss of control, and economic, social and psychological harms. Those harms include debt, poor work performance and loss of employment, criminality (especially theft, fraud and embezzlement), marital and family disharmony and separation, stress-related physical symptoms, and depression and attempted and completed suicide (Lesieur, 1984; Lorenz and Yaffee, 1984; Custer and Milt, 1985; Ladouceur *et al.*, 1994; Blaszczynski and Farrell, 1998; Meyer and Stadler, 1999). Box 14.4 provides very brief extracts from case vignettes, one of a man addicted to horse-race gambling (Barker and Miller, 1968), while the others are quotations from two adolescent gambling-machine addicts (Griffiths, 1993a).

Box 14.3 A possible set of criteria for defining behavioural addiction.

1. The behaviour is engaged in at an abnormally high frequency and/or volume.
2. The behaviour is highly salient, as indicated by a preoccupation with the object of the activity or the means of acquiring it, feelings of craving for the object that are experienced as irresistible, or experience of distress when the activity is stopped or prevented.
3. The experience of the behaviour being out of one's control, unsuccessful attempts to control the activity, or behaviour aimed at reducing the harmful effects of the behaviour.
4. The subjective experience of mood modification in association with the behaviour or use of the behaviour to avoid or reduce an unpleasant mood state.
5. The behaviour brings conflict with family members or other people, as indicated by lying to others about the activity, stealing from others to support the activity, or criticism from others about the behaviour.
6. The behaviour is causing harms in other life areas such as finance, education or work, and physical or mental health.

Box 14.4 Cases of gambling addiction.

He had gambled in 'betting shops' for more than 2 years and had lost over £1200. Initially he ascribed his gambling mainly to boredom, but he had recently gambled to repay his debts, which exceeded £100. His usual practice was to spend all his salary (£15 to £30 per week) in a betting shop on Saturdays. He invariably reinvested his winnings on horses and returned home with nothing so that his wife and children went without food, clothes and fuel ... Matters came to a head when he put his own money and the complete pay packet of a sick friend (who had asked him to collect his pay) on one horse and lost £40. This resulted in 18 months' probation. His gambling had been causing serious marital difficulties and was affecting the health of his wife and his eldest son. He was referred for treatment by his doctor (Barker and Miller, 1968: 288–289).

While I was playing fruit machines there were no good experiences, only bad, such as stealing money from my family and robbing chip shops, phone boxes and tills in shops (male, aged 17; Griffiths, 1993a).

... any dinner, bus fare money went into fruit machines during school hours. When I started my full time job ... as a cashier, my weekly wages of £75 went ... in a few hours. I needed more money therefore I stole from the cash till ... I am now going to court (female, aged 16; Griffiths, 1993a).

The first British adult prevalence survey of gambling and problem gambling, covering over 7000 individuals, was conducted in 1999/2000 (Sproston *et al.*, 2000; Orford *et al.*, 2003) and the first national prevalence study of problem gambling among adolescents was reported by Fisher (1999). The mutual-help organisation Gamblers Anonymous is nearly 50 years old and has existed in the UK for over 40 years. The diagnosis 'pathological gambling' first appeared in the *Diagnostic and Statistical Manual* (DSM) of the American Psychiatric Association (APA, 1994) in its third edition in 1980. Since the revised third edition in 1987, the diagnostic criteria have been specifically modelled on alcohol and drug dependence (Castellani, 2000). A number of standard screening questionnaires exist, including the two that were used in the British adult Gambling Prevalence Survey: the South Oaks Gambling Screen (SOGS, Lesieur and Blume, 1987) the most commonly used internationally; and a scale based on the DSM-IV criteria. A screen for adolescents, also based on DSM-IV criteria, was used by Fisher (1999), the DSM-IV-J.

Two international academic journals exist that are specifically devoted to gambling and problem gambling (the *Journal of Gambling Studies* and *International Gambling Studies*) and the leading British journals on addiction (*Addiction* and *Addiction Research and Theory*) regularly carry articles on excessive gambling. Although the literature on gambling addiction is small beside that on alcohol, tobacco and other forms of drug addiction, it is substantial and rapidly growing. One of the attractions of studying behavioural addictions is that it '... can serve as an informative model for substance dependence since it represents a similar addictive disorder, but it does not carry the confounding issue of exogenous drug effects on brain substrates' (Bechara, 2003: 44). In that sense excessive gambling can be seen as a prototypical addiction.

There are a number of distinct forms of gambling, and 13 were included in the British Gambling Prevalence Survey. Some, such as the National Lottery draw, appear to be associated with a lower risk of excess, while other forms appear to be more risky. According to the British Gambling Prevalence Survey, these include gambling-machine playing, betting on horse races, private betting, and particularly betting on dog races, placing bets on other events with a bookmaker, and playing table games in a casino. Different forms of gambling vary in numerous ways, including size of maximum possible win, the possibility of continuous play, the element of skill or judgement involved and the frequency and immediacy of payout (Raylu and Oei, 2002). Different theories of the most addictive elements involved exist, but the most addictive forms of gambling seem to be those that are most accessible, allow continuous play, and pay out quickly and frequently.

As a result of technological and commercial innovations, and proposed legislative changes of a generally liberalising kind, the British gambling scene is currently changing rapidly. It embraces many types of gambling that vary in their structures and the settings in which they are carried out. For example, the National Lottery is a game of pure chance with purchases made once or twice a week or less often at readily available high street outlets. Football pools, which lost to the Lottery their previous position as the main long-odds, jackpot form of British gambling, have similar characteristics, but involve an element of knowledgeable choice, although many players treat it as a purely chance game (Forrest, 1999). Horse-race gambling away from the race course (off-course betting) only became legal in 1960, since when the high street betting office has become a prominent feature of British life. Gambling machines have also been permitted in a wide variety of locations, including pubs, since 1960. They can be played continuously, they pay out quickly, and are believed by some players to involve a considerable skill element.

Since the 1968 Gaming Act, casinos have been tightly controlled in Britain in terms of permission to set them up, membership, and permitted activities other than gambling. Bingo and betting on dog races at urban racing stadiums are yet other forms of gambling that have been part of the British gambling scene for many years, in those cases appealing particularly to people in lower occupational-status categories, and, in the case of bingo, particularly to women (Dixey, 1996).

In many other countries the amount of money estimated to have been staked on all gambling activities escalated dramatically during the last decades of the twentieth century (Wynne and Shaffer, 2003). In Britain the total amount stated was £42 billion, of which £7.3 billion was gross gambling yield to the industry after subtracting winnings (KPMG, 2000). During that period the gambling industry proposed further innovations, many of which were approved by the Gaming Board. New features of gaming machines that made them more attractive and encouraged the view that skill was involved, opportunities to bet in betting offices on a wider range of sporting events, increases in maximum prizes through connected games (eg in bingo), rollovers, and new types of casino game, were all introduced. Following the report of the Gambling Review Body (2001), the recent Gambling Act encourages such innovation and continued expansion of the gambling industry (Department for Culture, Media and Sport, 2002, 2003). It proposes to lift some of the restrictions on setting up new casinos, and the law regulating how casinos operate, in the expectation that the number of casinos will increase and 'casino resorts' will become established.

With the future of addiction in mind, the most important developments may lie in new ways of gambling that may have increased addiction potential. Prominent among those is Internet gambling, both placing bets via the Internet and playing 'virtual' games operated solely on the Internet. The British Gambling Prevalence Survey found that only a very small proportion of British gambling was conducted via the Internet at the turn of the century (Sproston et al., 2000), but it was widely estimated that it would grow rapidly. Under the new Gambling Act, British-operated Internet gambling sites would become legal, being licensed and regulated by the planned Gambling Commission. Technological developments in telecommunications such as more sophisticated mobile telephones, and digital interactive TV, may also impact on gambling in unforeseen ways (KPMG, 2000).

Spread betting is another comparative newcomer, starting as a form of betting on financial markets and later becoming a way of betting on the outcome of sporting events. It is still offered by specialist companies and regulated separately from other forms of gambling, by the Financial Services Authority (Gambling Review Body, 2001). The unique quality – and risk – of spread betting lies in the fact that the potential loss can be far greater than the amount of money staked. The British Gambling Prevalence Survey found that, although fewer people who had bet in that way, their losses were greater than for most other forms of gambling (Sproston et al., 2000).

An example of industry innovation, using modern technology, is fixed-odds betting terminals (FOBTs), which have been developed since the report of the Gambling Review Body on which the new Gambling Act is based, instantly becoming common in betting offices. Offering casino-style games such as roulette and blackjack via machines, their status has been subject to legal action between the Gaming Board and the Association of British Bookmakers. The former argued that they were gaming machines, the latter that they were a form of betting activity. An agreement was reached in November 2003. Betting offices will be able to offer no more than four machines of any kind, the maximum prize on FOBTs will be £500 and maximum stake £100, only roulette will be allowed and the speed of play will be restricted. One view is that this agreement will prevent unrestricted proliferation. Others argue that it has set a precedent which will be impossible to reverse (Joint Committee on the draft Gambling Bill, 2004).

One of the proposals in the Gambling Act, which almost certainly has implications for gambling addiction is the provision for a new, fourth, category of gambling machines. These 'category A' machines, to be permitted only in casinos, will have unlimited stakes and prizes. Much committee time has been devoted to considering the permissible number of such machines per casino (Joint Committee on the draft Gambling Bill, 2004). By most theories of the addictive elements in gambling, such machines would be regarded as particularly risky.

Another controversial development, too recent to be discussed by the Gambling Review Body, is the setting up of 'betting exchanges'. They enable punters to bet directly with each other, rather than with bookmakers, via an operator who matches opposite bets and takes a commission. Modern technology has made this possible on a scale not previously anticipated and the exchanges have recently become an important and lucrative element in the gambling industry. Indeed, one of the largest exchanges, Betfair, was given the Queen's Award for Enterprise in 2003. The exchanges challenge the business model of the existing bookmaking industry and might pose risks for the integrity of racing and other sports. The British Gambling Prevalence Survey found that private betting was one of the forms of gambling most associated with problems (Sproston *et al.*, 2000).

If the availability hypothesis is valid, as is generally believed, the combination of rapid technological development and liberalising legislation will lead to an increase in gambling addiction.

4 ACCOUNTING FOR THE DEVELOPMENT OF A BEHAVIOURAL ADDICTION SUCH AS GAMBLING

4.1 Explanations at the Biological Level

A number of studies, including the British Gambling Prevalence Survey, have found a significantly raised prevalence of problem gambling among the children of problem gamblers (Walters, 2002). The stronger, adoption method of estimating possible genetic influence has not been used, but the two twin studies that have been carried out do suggest some role for genetics. The larger study, of over 3000 male–male twin pairs, of which both twins served in the US military during the Vietnam era (Eisen *et al.*, 1998) suggested that inherited factors plus shared environmental experiences might explain 46–55 per cent of the variance in reports of pathological gambling symptoms depending on the criteria used. The much smaller study involved 155 young adult twin pairs identified from state birth records in Minnesota, USA (Winters and Rich, 1998). That study is interesting because of its suggestion that the role of genetics might be very different for men and women, for different types of gambling activity, and for different gambling criteria. Differences between monozygotic ('identical') and dizygotic ('non-identical') twins were evident only for the more popular, readily available, high-potential-payout forms of gambling, and the differences emerged mostly for men and not for women except with gambling machines.

A number of studies have searched for abnormalities of one or other of the main neurotransmitter brain chemicals that might be involved in gambling, particularly serotonin, noradrenalin and dopamine, and for variants of genes associated with the functioning of those neurochemical systems (Ibánez *et al.*, 2003). A small number of studies have reported findings suggesting abnormality of serotonin response among 'pathological gamblers', but these have been inconsistent and even opposite, one finding evidence for raised, and one for lowered, sensitivity (National Research Council, USA, 1999). Roy *et al.* (1988) failed to support a role for serotonin but did find evidence for a greater-than-normal concentration of noradrenalin or a metabolite of it in the cerebrospinal fluid, blood and urine of 'pathological gamblers', and a more recent study has produced similar findings (Bergh *et al.*, 1997, cited by the National Research Council, 1999). A group of Spanish researchers has reported an abnormality in male pathological gamblers of the serotonin transporter gene 5HTT and, also in males, a variant of the monoamine oxidase A gene, which may have implications for serotonergic or dopaminergic transmission (Ibánez *et al.*, 2003).

A group in the US has focused on genes associated with the brain dopamine system, a focus of addiction research generally (eg Wise, 1994), finding variations in D1 and D2 receptor genes (Comings *et al.*, 1996, 1997), although Ibánez *et al.* (2003) stress the preliminary nature of this work. The mechanisms that are being proposed are probably not specific to gambling, but rather are common to a variety of addictions (eg Comings *et al.*, 1997). The involvement of the brain dopamine system in gambling addiction is further supported by reports that some Parkinson's disease sufferers, treated with dopamine replacement therapy such as levodopa, develop 'pathologic gambling' (Molina *et al.*, 2000) and others show signs of addiction to the dopamine replacement medication (Lawrence *et al.*, 2003). Reports of possible effectiveness in the treatment of gambling addiction with naltrexone, an opioid receptor antagonist with a likely effect on the mesolimbic dopamine pathway (National Research Council, 1999; Grant *et al.*, 2003) may provide some further evidence of overlapping neurobiological mechanisms in gambling and substance addiction.

Others have proposed neurocognitive abnormalities. Bechara (2003) has suggested impairment of a certain kind of decision making, associated with lesions of the ventromedial prefrontal cortex, as a model for addictions including gambling addiction. Indeed, the task that was developed for testing that type of decision making, which involved the ability to switch from choosing cards from a pack associated with early experiences of reward to those from packs that became more productive as time went on, was known as the 'gambling task' before it was ever used with participants with addiction problems. Subsequently, those

with substance and gambling addictions have been found to display abnormalities on that task (Petry, 2001; Cavedini *et al.*, 2002; Bechara, 2003). That line of work is helping to make a connection between neurocognitive findings in gambling and modern neurocognitive theories of addiction more generally. These are beginning to see a role for both mesolimbic reward motivational systems and frontal cortical inhibitory or self-control systems (Lubman *et al.*, 2004).

Chambers and Potenza (2003) have attempted to explain why the prevalence of problem gambling is so high among adolescents (Shaffer and Hall, 1996; Fisher, 1999). They suggest that gambling addiction is one of a number of conditions to which adolescents are vulnerable because they share the characteristic of impulsivity (see below). The link with adolescence, they suggest, is due to a particular robustness of the mesolimbic dopamine system at that stage of development combined with the immaturity of the inhibitory brain systems.

The possibility that gamblers might experience withdrawal symptoms when they stop gambling has been investigated (Wray and Dickerson, 1981; Rosenthal and Lesieur, 1992; Orford *et al.*, 1996). The most commonly experienced symptoms on cessation of gambling are psychological, such as restlessness, irritability, depressed mood, insomnia and headaches. The timing of these 'symptoms' suggests that they are more likely to be related to the recent experience of loss, feelings of indecision about continued gambling, or worry and preoccupation about debts and other gambling-related harms, rather than to cessation of gambling *per se*.

4.2 Explanations at the Personal Level

The possibility that there may be personal vulnerabilities to gambling addiction has been studied from a number of angles. Psychoanalysts have proposed that gambling served the functions of rebellion against parental authority and distraction from guilt (Rosenthal, 1987). Bergler (1958) who, unlike other psychoanalysts, had studied a considerable number of cases, came to the view that gambling addicts were gambling, not to win, but rather with the unconscious wish to lose. His 'wish to lose' theory became popular, particularly with Gamblers Anonymous.

From studies using observational methods, including participant observation, ideas have emerged about the personal functions that gambling might serve. They include that gambling, involving taking a chance, represents a pleasurable alternative to the routine and boredom of life; that gambling represents a milieu in which gamblers can appear to exercise control, show composure and exercise intelligent choice, uncover information (eg about horses), appear knowledgeable and 'beat the system'; that gambling is equivalent to play; that for regular casino players the casino becomes 'encompassing', providing a place for players to watch television, eat, meet friends, gamble and have a drink; and in the British amusement arcade setting, that players could, depending on age and personality, display leadership or following behaviour (Goffman, 1967; Newman, 1972; Rosecrance, 1988; Ocean and Smith, 1993; Fisher, 1993a).

The personality trait approach has been used most often, although with mixed success. One of the most studied traits has been 'sensation seeking', but results have been inconsistent and sometimes opposite (Raylu and Oei, 2002). 'Locus of control' has fared somewhat better. Studies have either found gambling groups to be higher than normal on external locus of control (holding the belief that rewards result from luck, chance, fate, the influence of powerful others, or are unpredictable) or found no differences (Walker, 1992), although Carroll and Huxley, 1994, later found young dependent machine players to be more internally controlled. The most popular trait in recent years has been 'impulsivity'. A number of studies have reported positive findings for impulsivity but they represent a very mixed bag of research designs and samples.

The personality trait approach is beset with difficulties. The leading ideas, such as sensation seeking and impulsivity, overlap, and a number of different measures exist for the same trait. Furthermore, the literature is a small one and largely consists of a number of unrelated studies that vary in the ages of the participants, whether the index gambling group consists of problem gamblers, regular gamblers or simply gamblers, whether the sample is all male or includes women, the type of gambling, and the location of the research. A particular personality trait might be more important at an early or late stage in the development of a gambling problem but not at other stages, might be more important for men than for women or vice versa, or might be significant in the case of some forms of gambling and not others. Furthermore, traits such as sensation seeking, impulsivity and locus of control have often been found on close study to consist of a set of inter-related components. Petry (2001) found three independent factors in an analysis of results from several impulsivity scales: impulse control, novelty seeking, and time orientation.

Studies often contain the assumption that personality traits are long standing, possibly originating in childhood or even having genetic origins, and that they are antecedents of problem gambling. That is only an assumption and an equally convincing argument could be made that signs of impulsivity, for example, are a consequence of the development of a gambling problem. However, the only predictive study, by Vitaro et al. (1999), found that impulsivity in 12–14-year-olds predicted problem gambling at age 17 after controlling for early gambling behaviour and other relevant variables.

4.3 Learning Processes

Complementary to the search for personality traits associated with gambling are approaches that consider the development of addictive gambling as a process. Foremost among such theories is the idea that people become conditioned or 'learn' the habit of gambling as a consequence of the 'rewards' obtained, the basic notion of conditioning through reinforcement. Gambling resembles the behaviour observed in animal models so closely that a behavioural learning analysis seems an obvious contender for explaining, at least in part, how gambling might become a problem (Cornish, 1978; Griffiths, 1995; Knapp, 1997; Elster, 1999; Orford, 2001a,b). A careful analysis suggests that gambling mostly operates on a random ratio schedule of reinforcement; a special case of the variable ratio schedule, which is known to lead to particularly persistent behaviour (Knapp, 1997). This schedule makes financial reward from a given play especially unpredictable. The more you play, the greater the chance of having a win, but you don't know when, and the chances of a win on the next play do not increase the greater the run of losses.

An account of the potential addictiveness of gambling from a learning perspective would be incomplete without including the secondary reinforcing of the conditioning by association with a whole host of apparently neutral cues surrounding gambling occasions. These include race commentaries in betting offices, the colours, shapes and noises that make up the atmosphere of a casino, and the lights, sounds and other stimuli built into gambling machines and the arcades that house them (Griffiths, 1993b, 1995). Sharpe *et al.* (1995) provided experimental evidence of such conditioning, in the form of psychophysiological responses, in the case of problem gamblers watching videos depicting gambling or imagining themselves winning.

Emotional rewards from gambling are widely thought to be as important as financial ones. Arousal, in the form of increases in heart rate, has been found in a number of studies to be associated with real (as opposed to simulated) machine or horserace gambling (eg Leary and Dickerson, 1985; Coventry and Norman, 1997; Coventry and Hudson, 2001). What problem gamblers often say about the emotional changes during gambling resembles reports of the taking of amphetamines (Hickey *et al.*, 1986). But for some people, or under some circumstances, gambling has been described, not as a stimulant, but as a kind of 'self-medication', as an 'anaesthetic' or a form of 'escape seeking' (Lesieur and Rosenthal, 1991; Jacobs, 1993; Elster, 1999). The association between problem gambling and depression is relevant here. Lesieur and Rosenthal (1991) found some evidence that escape-seeking gambling was more common among women than among men.

4.4 Cognitive Processes

Cognitive approaches to gambling have taken a number of different directions. One is concerned with the degree to which people are 'risk-averse' or the opposite, and the conditions of risk and mood under which people take more or fewer risks (Nygren, 1998). Another approach concerns the 'expectancies' that people hold regarding the effects that an activity is likely to have for them, for example, general positive expectancies or more specific arousal expectancies (Walters and Contri, 1998). A paradigm that has become popular recently is 'delay discounting'. The methodology involves finding out how much a delayed reward is 'worth' to the participant compared to an immediate reward. It is known that the worth of monetary reward drops with increasing delay, according to a hyperbolic function. A study by Petry and Caserella (1999) supported the hypothesis that the fall-off in the value of rewards with increasing delay would be greatest for problem gamblers with substance problems, intermediate for substance misusers without gambling problems, and least for controls. Petry and Caserella suggested that this rapid discounting of delayed rewards may be one index of impulsivity.

The cognitive approach that has featured most strongly in relation to gambling is to do with mental biases and illusions. The varieties of irrationality evident in gambling have been well described by a number of writers on the subject (eg Ladouceur and Walker, 1996; Rogers, 1998) and are shown in Box 14.5. For example, most people have a poor understanding of probability, tending to underestimate high frequency events and

---

Box 14.5 Common cognitive biases and distortions that occur during gambling (based on Ladouceur and Walker, 1996; Rogers, 1998).

Overestimation of probability of large
    prizes
Belief that short runs of events should
    appear 'random'
The gambler's fallacy
Entrapment
Belief in hot and cold numbers
Unrealistic optimism
Perceived luckiness
Superstitious thinking
Illusion of control
Erroneous beliefs
Biased evaluation of outcomes

---

overestimate low-frequency ones, and generally show overconfidence in their judgements of probability (Rogers, 1998). The 'representativeness heuristic' refers to the assumption that small samples of events (such as a short run of plays or bets) are representative of all events or of a much longer run. Some combinations of UK National Lottery numbers are, erroneously, considered to be less likely than others (eg 1, 2, 3, 4, 5, 6; Ladouceur and Walker, 1996). Failure to grasp the point that each event in a series of random events is independent of all others underlies a form of irrationality that has earned the title of the 'gambler's fallacy'. Roulette players often believe that certain numbers are due because they have not recently come up (Ladouceur and Walker, 1996) and National Lottery players often believe that recently drawn numbers are less likely to come again soon (Coups *et al.*, 1998; Rogers and Webley, 1998). There is evidence that a high proportion of National Lottery players choose the same numbers every week, and that many feel the need to bet repeatedly on the same numbers through fear of missing a potential win on numbers in which much has already been 'invested'. This has been referred to as one of the ways in which gambling brings about 'entrapment' (Rogers, 1998).

The idea of the 'illusion of control' was first introduced by Langer (1975). She and others have shown that gamblers bet more when they believe they have greater control, for example, when playing against an apparently less-confident competitor, when given an early experience of winning, or when allowed to throw the roulette ball themselves (Langer and Roth, 1975; Ladouceur and Mayrand, 1987). Both Carroll and Huxley (1994) and Griffiths (1995) found that young problem machine gamblers differed from non-problem gamblers in having a greater belief in the role of skill in machine gambling, and in giving overestimates of the amounts of money they were likely to win.

A form of entrapment often thought to be of central importance in problem gambling is 'chasing one's losses' (Lesieur, 1994; Dickerson, 1990; Orford *et al.*, 1996). It includes within-session chasing but also between-session chasing which may be more discriminating of problem gamblers (O'Connor, 2000). In O'Connor's (2000) particularly thorough study of chasing, the most important behavioural signs appeared to be increasing the size of bets or stakes after a loss, or after a win, plus continuing to bet instead of stopping after a loss.

So called 'near misses' (more correctly referred to as 'near wins') were thought by his participants to be particularly important in encouraging chasing. Near misses, which are built into almost all forms of gambling in one way or another, were first highlighted by Reid (1986). He noted that some commercial gambling activities, notably fruit machines and scratch card lotteries, were designed to ensure a higher-than-chance frequency of near misses. A fruit machine might show two winning symbols in the payout line with a third visible just above or below. Reid theorised that a near miss could produce some of the excitement of a win, and in that way a player was not so much constantly losing but constantly nearly winning. Another suggestion is that the near miss might be motivating because it produces frustration or 'cognitive regret' (Griffiths, 1995). Lotteries provide ample opportunities for experiencing near misses and small wins (Miers, 1996). Technological developments are likely to increase the frequency of near win experiences.

4.5 Explanations at the Social Level

The evidence from several countries, including the UK, is that adolescence is a time of particular vulnerability to problem gambling. Prevalence figures are often several times higher for adolescents than for adults (Shaffer and Hall, 1996; Fisher, 1999). There is also evidence that the earlier the age a child or adolescent starts to gamble, the greater is the risk of problems related to gambling in later adolescence and adulthood (Griffiths, 1990; Fisher, 1996; National Research Council, 1999). Interviews with some of the participants in the British Gambling Prevalence Survey who scored above the threshold on one or other of the two problem gambling screening instruments that were used (White *et al.*, 2001; Orford *et al.*, 2003) gave a clear indication of what the interviewees believed to be the mechanisms involved. They emphasised the role played by other people, particularly parents, who set a norm for gambling, conveying a positive image of gambling, taking a keen interest in it and making it appear an attractive and acceptable activity, often coaching youngsters in how to gamble. The influence of the peer group has been less studied, but there is some evidence to support the idea that, as adolescence progresses, more gambling is conducted with friends rather than family and that the influence of the peer group becomes important (Fisher, 1993b; Coups *et al.*, 1998; Gupta and Derevensky, 1998; National Research Council, 1999).

In terms of ethnic group, a number of studies find the rate of problem gambling among indigenous peoples in Canada, New Zealand and the US to be several times higher than that found in the rest of the population (Raylu and Oei, 2004), as have studies of minority or immigrant groups in Australia, Sweden and the US (National Research Council, 1999; Rönnberg *et al.*, 1999; Welte *et al.*, 2001; Raylu and Oei, 2004).

Other variables that might influence the development of gambling addiction include household income. British studies show that people with lower incomes spend a higher proportion of them on gambling (Miers, 1996; Shepherd *et al.*, 1998; Grun and McKeigue, 2000; Orford *et al.*, 2003). In Britain and the US there is evidence of a tendency for people with lower incomes to be over-represented among problem gamblers (National Research Council, 1999; Orford *et al.*, 2003).

Gambling is positively correlated with other potentially addictive activities such as tobacco, alcohol and drug consumption. One set of studies attests to this relationship among adolescents (Fisher, 1993b, 1999; Griffiths and Sutherland, 1998; Gupta and Derevensky, 1998). A further type of study that supports this link has examined the co-occurrence of gambling problems and substance problems among adults receiving treatment (Martínez-Pina *et al.*, 1991; Abbott and Volberg, 1992; Giacopassi *et al.*, 1998; National Research Council, 1999). Gambling and alcohol consumption might be linked because intoxication might facilitate heavier gambling. The best experimental study of this possibility, by Kyngdon and Dickerson (1999), supported that hypothesis. Increased use of alcohol might be a response to problems created by excessive gambling. Both might be related to stress or part of a larger constellation of behaviours indicative of non-conformity to norms of moderation.

Part of the stereotype of problem gambling is that it is overwhelmingly male. Figures for those seeking treatment in the US tend to confirm that picture, as do population surveys, such as the British Gambling Prevalence Survey, which found a rate of problem gambling two to three times as high among men as women. But in US surveys, the median percentage of women among problem and pathological gamblers was found to be nearly 40 per cent (National Research Council, 1999). More than one population survey has found that the scope of men's gambling is greater than women's (Hraba and Lee, 1996; Sproston *et al.*, 2000). The type and location of women's gambling is different from that of men, and bingo stands out as an activity favoured more by women than men (Hraba and Lee, 1996; Rönnberg *et al.*, 1999; Sproston *et al.*, 2000). In Australia, it has been suggested that along with a normalisation of gambling has come a 'feminisation', that the proportion of women among help-seekers has risen, and that machine gambling has increasingly become a problem for women (Trevorrow and Moore, 1998; Crisp *et al.*, 2000).

In complete contrast to person-centred explanations for gambling problems are 'supply side' explanations. They see the availability, accessibility and ecology of gambling as the main causes of varying rates of problem gambling across geographical areas, such as the different states of Australia or the US, or across time periods (eg before and after the inauguration of a state or national lottery, the opening of a particular casino, or the introduction of a new gambling venue such as riverboat casinos in the US). The evidence for the availability hypothesis has been considered by official review bodies in Australia (Australian Productivity Commission, 1999), the US (National Research Council, 1999) and the UK (Gambling Review Body, 2001). Each concluded that increased availability of opportunities to gamble was associated with more gambling and more problem gambling. Among the evidence is a particularly thorough study carried out before and after the opening of a new casino in Niagara Falls, Canada (Room *et al.*, 1999; Turner *et al.*, 1999) and a study of household expenditure on gambling (problem gambling was not assessed) before and after the inauguration of Britain's National Lottery (Grun and McKeigue, 2000).

5 AVAILABILITY OF TREATMENTS FOR BEHAVIOURAL ADDICTIONS

Other than treatment for gambling and for 'eating disorders', treatment for behavioural addictions is minimal in the UK and elsewhere. In the case of gambling problems, the need for treatment and the form it might take have been considered by experts in the UK (Bellringer, 1999; Griffiths and MacDonald, 1999) and to a greater extent in the US (eg McCown and Chamberlain, 2000). Both the issues and the treatments have their parallels in the field of treatment for substance misuse. The main difference is that problem gambling treatment is lagging behind by 20–30 years at least, despite the inclusion of 'pathological gambling' in psychiatric classifications such as that of the American Psychiatric Association for a quarter of a century (see earlier).

Meta-analyses of outcome evaluation studies of psychological treatments have been carried out by Blaszczyski and Silov (1995), López-Viets and Miller (1997) and by the US National Research Council (1999). All found that this field was at a very early stage of development. But reviewers have drawn encouraging conclusions about likely outcomes from treatment. López-Viets and Miller (1997) concluded that it was not uncommon for two-thirds of problem gamblers to be abstinent or to be controlling their gambling at 6- or 12-month follow-ups. The best of those studies was a follow-up of 274 people treated in Minnesota, USA (Stinchfield and Winters, 1996, cited by the National Research Council, 1999). The treatment in that study used a multi-modal approach, self-help groups, and family counselling. Abstinence rates of 43 per cent at the 6-month follow-up and 42 per cent at 12 months were reported, with an additional 20 per cent (at 6 months) and 24 per cent (at 12 months) gambling in a controlled way.

A variety of types of psychosocial treatments have been tried. Currently it is behavioural, and particularly cognitive-behavioural, forms of treatment that have started to receive closer attention and about which reviewers have tended to be most positive. An example is the treatment tested by Sylvain *et al.* (1997) in a small trial. The central element of this treatment was the correction of erroneous perceptions about gambling, theoretically based on the idea of cognitive distortions maintaining gambling, especially the 'illusion of control'. Other elements of treatment were problem-solving training, social-skills training, and relapse prevention.

As in the treatment of substance addictions, it has been widely recommended that family members, who are often affected by a gambling problem, should be involved in treatment to improve outcomes both for the gambler and for family members (eg Bellringer, 1999; Griffiths and MacDonald, 1999; National Research Council, 1999; Petry and Armentano, 1999; McCown and Chamberlain, 2000).

A recent review of pharmacological treatments for pathological gambling (Grant *et al.*, 2003) also found that field to be at an early stage of development, with few double-blind controlled trials, often poor description of patients, inconsistent use of outcome measures, and small numbers of participants. Evidence for effectiveness is therefore only preliminary. Most supported, as noted earlier, are selective serotonin reuptake inhibitors (SSRIs) such as fluvoxamine, with some support for naltrexone (National Research Council, 1999; Grant *et al.*, 2003), although Grant *et al.* (2003) warn that naltrexone can be dangerous for the liver outside a rather narrow therapeutic dose range. Also used have been mood stabilisers such as lithium and carbamazepine, although Grant *et al.* (2003) stated that no clear conclusions about their efficacy could be drawn from existing evidence. They suggested there might be a role for atypical antipsychotic medications, which have received some clinical support, and for the drug acamprosate which has not been formally studied in relation to gambling but has been the subject of recent research with alcohol dependence. Their general recommendation is to combine pharmacological treatments with psychological therapies, which they consider have demonstrated promising results.

Rather than focus on treatment type, others have focused on the intensity, setting or modality of treatment. Possibilities vary from telephone helplines and brief treatments to hospital in-patient treatment. In the UK, the national organisation GamCare has a telephone helpline staffed for 12 hours a day by trained volunteers. It received 1700 calls in its first 12 months (Bellringer, 1999; Griffiths *et al.*, 1999). The National Research Council (1999) reported that similar helplines were operating in 35 US states. Brief treatments have taken the form of mailed self-help manuals with or without a face-to-face or telephone interview (Dickerson *et al.*, 1990; Hodgins *et al.*, 2001). As with substance addictions, there is evidence that some people with gambling problems can make positive changes without any treatment at all (Marotta, 1999; Hodgins and el-Guebaly, 2000).

At the other end of the spectrum is residential treatment. In the USA, the first specialised treatments for people with gambling problems were in-patient hospital treatment programmes. Although their number is tiny compared to such programmes for people with alcohol or drug problems, there are now a number of such facilities across the USA, and, for some authors (eg McCown and Chamberlain, 2000), hospitalisation is the treatment of choice. In Britain, there is only one specialised residential facility for problem gamblers, the Gordon House Association (named after its founder Gordon Moody). Rather than a hospital, Gordon House (now two houses, in fact) is a house in an ordinary street, run in conjunction with a voluntary sector housing association, where treatment includes a therapeutic programme described in detail by Bellringer (1999).

Outside the professional treatment field, Gamblers Anonymous (GA), of which Bellringer (1999) estimated that there were around 200 meetings each week in Britain and Ireland, is one of the largest concentrations of experience and knowledge of problem gambling in Britain. Meetings of GamAnon, for partners, parents, and family and friends of problem gamblers, often take place at the same time and at the same venue, but in a separate room. Most of those who have written from their experience of treating problem gambling have been very positive about GA, writing of it as an important component of the help that is available (eg Bellringer, 1999; McCown and Chamberlain, 2000). The treatment evaluation literature has been more cautious, pointing to a very small number of studies (eg Brown, 1985; Stewart and Brown, 1988, based on a study in Scotland) suggesting that drop-out rates are high and follow-up abstinence rates low. It would be inappropriate to conclude much from such a small number of studies, and in any case it is not agreed that a self-help organisation like GA can or should be evaluated in the same way as a professional treatment.

Most writers on treatment for gambling problems have noted the underrepresentation in treated samples of women and of members of ethnic-minority groups (eg National Research Council, 1999). Particularly surprising is the almost complete absence of reference in the literature to the treatment of adolescent problem gambling. In Britain this lack has been discussed and more appropriate ways of meeting the treatment needs of adolescents suggested (Griffths and MacDonald, 1999; Griffths, 2002).

6 CONCLUSION: CURRENT SCIENCE CAPABILITY AND DEVELOPMENTS IN THE NEXT 10 YEARS

Two developments are taking place at the present time which together make a strong case for placing behavioural addictions near the centre of our thinking over the next 10 years or so. The first is the growing awareness of the dangers to society and its citizens posed by addiction to activities that do not involve the ingestion of a substance. As well as gambling, sex addiction, with its implications for the nation's sexual health, is one example. Eating addiction in the form of binge eating disorder is another, with obvious implications for the nation's health.

The other quite recent development is the appearance of biological and psychological models of addiction which, unlike earlier models, can embrace non-substance addictions with ease. For these models the distinction between substance and non-substance addictions is less important than for earlier generations of addiction models such as that based on neuroadaptation and withdrawal relief. What is currently lacking is for addiction researchers who have specialised in either substance or non-substance addictions to extend their work to include both.

There is a small but growing science capability in gambling and gambling addiction. Small but active groups with special expertise in psychosocial and biological aspects exist in Australia, where the prevalence of gambling addiction is the highest recorded, and the US and Canada. In the UK there is a small number of active individuals. Other European countries with some capacity are Spain, where concern has been high and there is an active biological group in Madrid; Italy, with a biological group in Milan; the Netherlands; and Sweden, which, besides the UK, is the only European country to have mounted a national prevalence study.

A further shortcoming is the overspecialisation of addiction research. The present author agrees with Goudriaan et al. (2004: 137) who wrote:

> It would be interesting to combine neuropsychological, physiological, neuroimaging and neurochemical studies, in order to discover if abnormalities in the different kinds of studies are related to each other.

They were writing about gambling research, but the same applies to addiction research more generally. It is arguably not only different kinds of biobehavioural laboratory research that need to be combined, but also research on biological, psychological and social factors, to reflect a full bio-psycho-social model of addiction. We need to develop the capability, not only to combine work on substance and non-substance addictions, but also to carry out work that combines disciplines and research methods – linking the laboratory, the clinic and the community, combining experimental with non-experimental methods of both quantitative and qualitative kinds, and crossing the boundaries between social science, psychology and neuroscience – in ways that are not happening at present.

Acknowledgements

I should like to gratefully acknowledge help received from Dana Samson, Research Fellow in the School of Psychology at the University of Birmingham, who introduced me to the work of Bechara on impaired decision making and gambling; Dr Phil Terry, Senior Lecturer in the Birmingham School of Psychology, who gave time at an early stage to discussion of the possible neuropharmacology of gambling; and to Mrs Pat Evans who prepared draft and final versions of the review.

References

Abbott, M.W. and Volberg, R.A. (1992) *Frequent gamblers and problem gamblers in New Zealand: Report on Phase 2 of the National Survey.* Auckland: National Research Bureau Ltd.

American Psychiatric Association (1994) *Diagnostic and statistical manual of mental disorders,* 4th edition. Washington DC: APA.

Australian Productivity Commission (APC) (1999) *Australia's gambling industries.* Report No. 10, Canberra: Ausinfo.

Barker, J. and Miller, M. (1968) Aversion therapy for compulsive gambling. *J Nerv Ment Dis* 146: 285–302.

Bechara, A. (2003) Risky business: emotion, decision-making, and addiction. *J Gambl Stud* 19: 23–51.

Bellringer, P. (1999) *Understanding problem gamblers: a practitioner's guide to effective intervention.* London: Free Association Books.

Bergh, C., Eklund, T., Soedersten, P., and Nordin, C. (1997) Altered dopamine function in pathological gambling. *Psychol Med* 27: 473–475.

Bergler, E. (1958). *The psychology of gambling.* London: Harrison.

Black, D.W. (1996) Compulsive buying: a review. *J Clin Psych* 57: 50–54.

Blaszczynski, A. and Farrell, E. (1998) A case series of 44 completed gambling-related suicides. *J Gambl Stud* 14: 93–109.

Blaszczynski, A. and Silov, D. (1995) Cognitive and behavioral therapies for pathological gambling. *J Gambl Stud* 11: 195–220.

Boyer, M. and Dickerson, M. (2003) Attentional bias and addictive behaviour: automaticity in a gambling-specific modified Stroop task. *Addiction* 98: 61–70.

Brown, R.I.F. (1985) The effectiveness of Gamblers Anonymous. In: W.R. Eadington (ed.), *The gambling studies: Proceedings of the Sixth National Conference on Gambling and Risk Taking* 5: 258–284.

Carnes, P. (1983) *Out of the shadows: understanding sexual addiction.* Minnesota: CompCare Publishers.

Carroll, D. and Huxley, J.A.A. (1994) Cognitive, dispositional, and psychophysiological correlates of dependent slot machine gambling in young people. *J Appl Soc Psychol* 24: 1070–1083.

Castellani, B. (2000) *Pathological gambling: the making of a medical problem.* New York: State University of New York Press.

Cavedini, P., Riboldi, G., Keller, R., D'Annucci, A., and Bellodi, L. (2002) Frontal lobe dysfunction in pathological gambling patients. *Biol Psychiatry* 51: 334–341.

Chambers, R.A. and Potenza, M.N. (2003) Neurodevelopment, impulsivity, and adolescent gambling. *J Gambl Stud* 19: 53–84.

Cocco, N., Sharpe, L., and Blaszczynski, A.P. (1995) Differences in preferred level of arousal in two sub-groups of problem gamblers: a preliminary report. *J Gambl Stud* 11: 221–229.

Comings, D.E., Rosenthal, R.J., Lesieur, H.R., Rugle, L.J., Muhleman, D., Chiu, C., Dietz, G., and Gade, R. (1996) A study of the dopamine D2 receptor gene in pathological gambling. *Pharmacogenetics* 6: 223–234.

Comings, D.F., Gade, R., Wu, S., Chiu, C., Dietz, G., Muhleman, D., Saucier, G., Ferry, L.,

Rosenthal, R.J., Lesieur, H.R., Rugle, L.J., and MacMurrary, P. (1997) Studies of the potential role of the dopamine D1 receptor gene in addictive behaviors. *Mol Psychiatry* 2: 44–56.

Copello, A., Orford, J., Hodgson, R., Tober, G., and Barrett, C. On behalf of the UKATT Research Team (2002) Social Behaviour and Network Therapy: basic principles and early experience. *Addict Behav* 27: 345–366.

Cornish, D. (1978) *Gambling: a review of the literature and its implications for policy and research.* Home Office Research Study 42, London: HMSO.

Coups, E., Haddock, G., and Webley, P. (1998) Correlates and predictors of lottery play in the United Kingdom. *J Gambl Stud* 14: 285–303.

Coventry, K.R. and Hudson, J. (2001) Gender differences, physiological arousal and the role of winning in fruit machine gamblers. *Addiction* 96: 871–879.

Coventry, K.R. and Norman, A.C. (1997) Arousal, sensation seeking and frequency of gambling in off-course horse racing bettors. *Br J Psychology* 88: 671–681.

Cox, R. and Orford, J. (2004) A qualitative study of the meaning of exercise for people who could be labelled as 'addicted' to exercise – can 'addiction' be applied to high frequency exercising? *Addic Res Theory* 12: 167–188.

Crisp, B.R., Thomas, S.A., Jackson, A.C., Thomason, N., Smith, S., Borrell, J., Ho, W., and Holt, T.A. (2000) Sex differences in the treatment needs and outcomes of problem gamblers. *Res Social Work Practice* 10: 229–242.

Custer, R. and Milt, H. (1985) *When luck runs out: help for compulsive gamblers and their families.* New York: Facts on File Publications.

Department for Culture, Media and Sport (2002) *A safe bet for success: modernising Britain's gambling laws.* London: The Stationery Office.

Department for Culture, Media and Sport (2003) Draft Gambling Bill: Policy document, Cm. 6014-IV.

Dickerson, M. (1990) Gambling: the psychology of a non-drug compulsion. *Drug Alcohol Rev* 9: 187–199.

Dickerson, M., Hinchy, J., and Legg England, S. (1990) An evaluation of a minimal intervention for media-recruited problem gamblers. *J Gambl Stud* 6: 87–102.

Dittmar, H. (2004). Understanding and diagnosing compulsive buying. In: R. Coombs (ed.), *Addictive disorders: a practical handbook.* New York: Wiley.

Dixey, R. (1996) Bingo in Britain: an analysis of gender and class. In: J. McMillen (ed.), *Gambling cultures.* London: Routledge: 136–151.

Eisen, S.A., Lin, N., Lyons, M.J., Scherrer, J.F., Griffith, K., True, W.R., Goldberg, J., and Tsuang, M.T. (1998) Familial influences on gambling behavior: an analysis of 3,359 twin pairs. *Addiction* 93: 1375–1384.

Elster, J. (1999) Gambling and addiction. In: J. Elster and O. Skog (eds), *Getting hooked: rationality and addiction.* Cambridge: Cambridge University Press.

Faber, R.N., Christenson, D.A., de Zwaan, M., and Mitchell, J. (1995) Two forms of compulsive consumption: comorbidity of compulsive buying and binge eating. *J Cons Res* 22: 296–304.

Fairburn, C.G. and Wilson, G.T. (1993) Binge eating: definition and classification. In: C.G. Fairburn and G.T. Wilson (eds), *Binge eating: nature, assessment and treatment.* New York: Guilford 3–14.

Farrar, J.E. (1992) Excessive exercise. In: J.E. L'Abate, J.E. Farrar and D.A. Serritella (eds), *Handbook of differential treatments for addictions.* Boston: Allyn and Bacon: 242–251.

Fisher, S. (1993a) The pull of the fruit machine: a sociological typology of young players. *Sociol Rev* 41: 447–474.

Fisher, S. (1993b) Gambling and pathological gambling in adolescents. *J Gambl Stud* 9: 277–288.

Fisher, S. (1996) *Gambling and problem gambling among casino patrons: a report to a consortium of the British casino industry.* University of Plymouth.

Fisher, S. (1999) A prevalence study of gambling and problem gambling in British adolescents. *Addict Res* 7: 509–538.

Forrest, D. (1999) The past and future of the British football pools. *J Gambl Stud* 15: 161–176.

France, C. (1902) The gambling impulsive. *Am J Psychology* 13: 364–407.

Gambling Review Body, Department for Culture, Media and Sport (2001) *Gambling Review Report.* Norwich: HMSO.

Giacopassi, D., Vandiver, M., and Stitt, B.G. (1998) College student perceptions of crime and casino gambling: a preliminary investigation. *J Gambl Stud* 13: 353–361.

Goffman, E. (1967) *Interaction ritual.* New Jersey: Doubleday.

Goodman, A. (1998) *Sexual addiction: an integrated approach*. Connecticut: International Universities Press.

Goudriaan, A.E., Oosterlaan, J., de Beurs, E., and Van den Brink, W. (2004) Pathological gambling: a comprehensive review of biobehavioral findings. *Neurosci Biobehav Rev* 28: 123–141.

Grant, J.E., Kim, S.W., and Potenza, M.N. (2003) Advances in the pharmacological treatment of pathological gambling. *J Gambl Stud* 19: 85–109.

Griffiths, M. (1990) Addiction to fruit machines: a preliminary study among young males. *J Gamb Stud* 6: 113–126.

Griffiths, M. (1993a) Factors in problem adolescent fruit machine gambling: results of a small postal survey. *J Gambl Stud* 9: 31–45.

Griffiths, M. (1993b) Fruit machine addiction in adolescents: a case study. *J Gambl Stud* 9: 387–399.

Griffiths, M. (1995) *Adolescent gambling*. London: Routledge.

Griffiths, M. (1999) Internet addiction: fact or fiction? *The Psychologist: Bull Br Psychol Soc* 12: 246–250.

Griffiths, M. (2002) *Gambling and gaming addictions in adolescence*, London: Blackwell.

Griffiths, M. and MacDonald, H.F. (1999) Counselling in the treatment of pathological gambling: an overview. *Br J Guid Couns* 27: 179–189.

Griffiths, M. and Sutherland, I. (1998) Adolescent gambling and drug use. *J Comm Appl Social Psychol* 8: 423–427.

Griffiths, M., Scarfe, A., and Bellringer, P. (1999) The UK national telephone gambling helpline – results on the first year of operation. *J Gambl Stud* 15: 83–90.

Groneman, C. (1994) Nymphomania: the historical construction of female sexuality. *Signs: J Women Cul Soc* 19: 337–367.

Grun, L. and McKeigue, P. (2000) Prevalence of excessive gambling before and after introduction of a national lottery in the United Kingdom: another example of the single distribution theory. *Addiction* 95: 959–966.

Gupta, R. and Derevensky, J.L. (1998) Adolescent gambling behavior: a prevalence study and examination of the correlates associated with problem gambling. *J Gambl Stud* 14: 319–345.

Hamburger, W. (1951) Emotional aspects of obesity. *Med Clin North America* 35: 483–499.

Hay, P., Fairburn, C.G., and Doll, H.A. (1996) The classification of bulimic eating disorders: a community-based cluster analysis study. *Psychol Med* 26: 801–812.

Hickey, J.E., Haertzen, C.A., and Henningfield, J.E. (1986) Simulation of gambling responses on the addiction research center inventory. *Addict Behav* 11: 345–349.

Hodgins, D.C., Currie, S.R., and el-Guebaly, N. (2001) Motivational enhancement and self-help treatments for problem gambling. *J Consult Clin Psychol* 69: 50–57.

Hodgins, D.C. and el-Guebaly, N. (2000) Natural and treatment–assisted recovery from gambling problems: a comparison of resolved and active gamblers. *Addiction* 95: 777–789.

Hraba, J. and Lee, G. (1996) Gender, gambling and problem gambling. *J Gambl Stud* 12: 83–101.

Ibánez, A., Blanco, C., de Castro, I.P., Fernandex-Piqueras, J., and Saiz-Ruiz, J. (2003) Genetics of pathological gambling. *J Gambl Stud* 19: 11–22.

Jacobs, D.F. (1993) Evidence supporting a general theory of addiction. In: W.R. Eadington and J.A. Cornelius (eds), *Gambling behavior and problem gambling*. Reno: University of Nevada.

Joint Committee (House of Lords/House of Commons) on the Draft Gambling Bill (2004) London: The Stationery Office.

Knapp, T.J. (1997) Behaviorism and public policy: B.F. Skinner's views on gambling. *Behav Social Issues* 7: 129–139.

KPMG (2000) *The economic value and public perceptions of gambling in the UK*. Report for Business In Sport and Leisure.

Kyngdon, A. and Dickerson, M. (1999) An experimental study of the effect of prior alcohol consumption on a simulated gambling activity. *Addiction* 94: 697–707.

Ladouceur, R. and Mayrand, M. (1987) The level of involvement and the timing of betting in gambling. *J Psychol* 121: 169–175.

Ladouceur, R. and Walker, M. (1996) A cognitive perspective of gambling. In: P.M. Salkovskis (ed.), *Trends in cognitive and behavioural therapies* New York: Wiley: 89–120.

Ladouceur, R., Boisvert, J.M., Pepin, M., Lorangere, M., and Sylvain, C. (1994) Social cost of pathological gambling. *J Gambl Stud* 10: 399–409.

Langer, E.J. (1975) The illusion of control. *J Personality Social Psychol* 32: 311–328 (cited by Carroll and Huxley, 1994).

Langer, E.J. and Roth, J. (1975) Heads I win, tails it's chance: the illusion of control as a function of the sequence of outcomes in a purely chance task. *J Personality Social Psychol* 32: 951–955.

Lawrence, A.D., Evans, A.H., and Lees, A.J. (2003) Compulsive use of dopamine replacement therapy in Parkinson's disease: reward systems gone awry? *Lancet* 2: 595–604.

Leary, K. and Dickerson, M.G. (1985) Levels of arousal in high and low frequency gamblers. *Behav Res Ther* 23: 635–640.

Lee, S. and Mysyk, A. (2004) The medicalization of compulsive buying. *Social Sci Med* 58: 1709–1718.

Lejoyeux, M., Haberman, N., Solomon, J., and Adès, J. (1999) Comparison of buying behaviour in depressed patients presenting with and without compulsive buying. *Comp Psychiatry* 40: 51–56.

Leon, G. and Roth, L. (1977) Obesity: psychological causes, correlations, and speculations. *Psychol Bull* 84: 117–139.

Lesieur, H.R. (1984) *The chase: the career of the compulsive gambler.* Rochester, Vermont: Schenkman.

Lesieur, H.R. (1994) Epidemiological surveys of pathological gambling: critique and suggestions for modification. *J Gambl Stud* 10: 385–397.

Lesieur, H.R. and Blume, S.B. (1987) The South Oaks Gambling Screen (SOGS): a new instrument for the identification of pathological gamblers. *Am J Psychiatry* 144: 1184–1188.

Lesieur, H.R. and Rosenthal, R.J. (1991) Pathological gambling: a review of the literature (prepared for the American Psychiatric Association Task Force on DSM-IV committee on disorders of impulse control). *J Gambl Stud* 7: 5–39.

López-Viets, V.C. and Miller, W.R. (1997) Treatment approaches for pathological gamblers. *Clin Psychol Rev* 17: 689–702.

Lorenz, V.C. and Yaffee, R.A. (1984) Pathological gambling: medical, emotional and interpersonal aspects, paper presented at Sixth National Conference on Gambling and Risk Taking, Atlantic City, New Jersey, December.

Lubman, D.I., Yücel, M., and Pantelis, C. (2004) Addiction, a condition of compulsive behaviour? Neuroimaging and neuropsychological evidence of inhibitory dysregulation. *Addiction* 99: 1491–1502.

McCown, W.G. and Chamberlain, L.L. (2000) *Best possible odds: contemporary treatment strategies for gambling disorders.* New York: Wiley.

McCusker, C.G. and Gettings, B. (1997) Automaticity of cognitive biases in addictive behaviours: further evidence with gamblers. *Br J Clin Psychol* 36: 543–554.

Marotta, J.J. (1999) *Recovery from gambling with and without treatment.* Unpublished thesis, University of Nevada.

Martínez-Pina, A., De Parga, J.L.G., Vallverdu, R.F., Planas, X.S., Mateo, M.M., and Aguado, V.M. (1991) The Catalonia survey: personality and intelligence structure in a sample of compulsive gamblers. *J Gambl Stud* 7: 275–299.

Meyer, G. and Stadler, M.A. (1999) Criminal behavior associated with pathological gambling. *J Gambl Stud* 15: 29–43.

Miers, D. (1996) The implementation and effects of Great Britain's National Lottery. *J Gambl Stud* 12: 343–373.

Molina, J.A., Sainz-Artiga, M.J., Fraile, A., Jimenez-Jimenez, F.J., Villanue Orti-Pareja, M., and Bermejo, F. (2000) Pathologic gambling in Parkinson's disease: a behavioral manifestation of pharmacologic treatment. *Move Dis* 15: 869–872.

Morganstern, K. (1977) Cigarette smoke as a noxious stimulus in self-managed aversion therapy for compulsive eating: technique and case illustration. In: J. Foreyt (ed.), *Behavioral treatments of obesity.* Oxford: Pergamon.

National Research Council, National Academy of Sciences, Committee on the Social and Economic Impact of Pathological Gambling (1999). *Pathological gambling: a critical review.* Washington DC: National Academy Press.

Newman, O. (1972). *Gambling: hazard and reward.* London: Athlone Press.

Niaura, R., Goldstein, M., and Abrams, D. (1991) A bioinformational systems perspective on tobacco dependence. *Br J Addict* 86: 593–597.

Nygren, T.E. (1998) Reacting to perceived high- and low-risk win–lose opportunities in a risky decision-making task: is it framing or affect or both? *Motivation Emotion* 22: 73–98.

Ocean, G. and Smith, G.J. (1993) Social reward, conflict, and commitment: a theoretical model of gambling behavior. *J Gambl Stud* 9: 321–339.

O'Connor, J. (2000) *An investigation of chasing behaviour.* Unpublished PhD thesis, University of Western Sydney, Macarthur.

Orford, J. (2001a) *Excessive appetites: a psychological view of addictions.* 2nd edition. Chichester: Wiley.

Orford, J. (2001b) Addiction as excessive appetite. *Addiction* 96: 15–31.

Orford, J., Morison, V., and Somers, M. (1996) Drinking and gambling: a comparison with implications for theories of addiction. *Drug Alcohol Rev* 15: 47–56.

Orford, J., Sproston, K., Erens, B., and White, C., and Mitchell, L. (2003) *Gambling and problem gambling in Britain.* London: Brunner-Routledge.

Petry, N.M. (2001) Substance abuse, pathological gambling, and impulsiveness. *Drug Alcohol Depend* 63: 29–38.

Petry, N.M. (2003) Discounting of money, health, and freedom in substance abusers and controls. *Drug Alcohol Depend* 71: 133–141.

Petry, N.M. and Armentano, C. (1999) Prevalence, assessment, and treatment of pathological gambling: a review. *Psychiatric Serv* 50: 1021–1027.

Petry, N.M. and Casarella, T. (1999) Excessive discounting of delayed rewards in substance abusers with gambling problems. *Drug Alcohol Depend* 56: 25–32.

Potenza, M.N., Leung, H.C., Blumberg, H.P., Peterson, B.S., Fulbright, R.K., Lacadie, C.M., Skudlarski, P., and Gore, J.C. (2003) An fMRI stroop task study of ventromedial prefrontal cortical function in pathological gamblers. *Am J Psychiatry* 160: 1990–1994.

Raylu, N. and Oei, T.P. (2002) Pathological gambling: a comprehensive review. *Clin Psychol Rev* 22: 1009–1061.

Raylu, N. and Oei, T.P. (2004) Role of culture in gambling and problem gambling. *Clin Psychol Rev* 23: 1087–1114.

Reid, R.L. (1986) The psychology of the near miss. *J Gambl Behav* 2: 32–39.

Rogers, P. (1998) The cognitive psychology of lottery gambling: a theoretical review. *J Gambl Stud* 14: 111–134.

Rogers, P. and Webley, P. (1998) *It could be us! A cognitive and social psychological analysis of individual and syndicate-based national lottery play in the UK.* Unpublished manuscript, University of Exeter.

Rönnberg, S., Volberg, R.A., Abbott, M.W., Moore, W.L., Andrén, A., Munck, I., Jonsson, J., Nilsson, T., and Svensson, O. (1999) *Gambling and problem gambling in Sweden.* Report no. 2 of the National Institute of Public Health Series on Gambling.

Room, R., Turner N.E., and Ialomiteanu, A. (1999) Community effects of the opening of the Niagara Casino. *Addiction* 94: 1449–1466.

Rosecrance, J. (1988) *Gambling without guilt: the legitimation of an American pastime.* Pacific Grove, California: Brooks/Cole.

Rosenthal, R.J. (1987) The psychodynamics of pathological gambling: a review of the literature. In: T. Galsk (ed.), *The handbook of pathological gambling.* Springfield, Illinois: Charles C. Thomas.

Rosenthal, R.J. and Lesieur, H.R. (1992) Self-reported withdrawal symptoms and pathological gambling. *Am J Addict* 1: 151–154.

Roy, A., Adinoff, B., Roehrich, L., Lamparski, D., Custer, R., Lorenz, V., Barbaccia, M., Guidotti, A., Coster, E., and Linnoila, M. (1988) Pathological gambling: a psychobiological study. *Arch Gen Psychiatry* 45: 369–373.

Shaffer, H.J. (1996) Understanding the means and objects of addiction: technology, the internet, and gambling. *J Gambl Stud* 12: 461–469.

Shaffer, H.J. and Hall, M.N. (1996) Estimating the prevalence of adolescent gambling disorders: a quantitative synthesis and guide toward standard gambling nomenclature. *J Gambl Stud* 12: 193–214.

Sharpe, L., Tarrier, N., Schotte, D., and Spence, S.H. (1995) The role of autonomic arousal in problem gambling. *Addiction* 90: 1529–1540.

Shepherd, R., Ghodse, H., and London, M. (1998) A pilot study examining gambling behaviour before and after the launch of the National Lottery and scratch cards in the UK. *Addict Res* 6: 5–12.

Sproston, K., Erens, B., and Orford, J. (2000) *Gambling behaviour in Britain: results from the British Gambling Prevalence Survey.* London: The National Centre for Social Research.

Squires, P. (1937) Fyodor Dostoevsky: a psychopathographical sketch. *Psychoanal Rev* 24: 365–388.

Stewart, R.M. and Brown, R.I.F. (1988) An outcome study of Gamblers Anonymous. *Br J Psychiatry* 152: 284–288.

Sylvain, C., Ladouceur, R., and Boisvert, J.M. (1997) Cognitive and behavioral treatment of pathological gambling: a controlled study. *J Consult Clin Psychol* 65: 727–732.

Tanofsky, M.B., Wilfley, D.E., Spurrell, E.B., Welch, R., and Brownell, K.D. (1997) Comparison of men and women in binge eating disorder. *Int J Eating Dis* 21: 49–54.

Tiffany, S.T. (1990) A cognitive model of drug urges and drug-use behavior: role of automatic and nonautomatic processes. *Psychol Rev* 97: 147–168.

Trevorrow, K. and Moore, S. (1998) The association between loneliness, social isolation and women's electronic gaming machine gambling. *J Gambl Stud* 14: 263–284.

Turner, N.E., Ialomiteanu, A., and Room, R. (1999) Checkered expectations: predictors of approval of opening a casino in the Niagara community. *J Gambl Stud* 15: 45–70.

Veale, D.M.W. (1987) Exercise dependence. *Br J Addict* 82: 735–740.

Vitaro, F., Arseneault, L., and Tremblay, R.E. (1999) Impulsivity predicts problem gambling in low SES adolescent males. *Addiction* 94: 565–575.

Walker, M.B. (1992) *The psychology of gambling.* Oxford: Butterworth-Heinemann.

Walters, G.D. (2002) Behavior genetic research on gambling and problem gambling: a preliminary meta-analysis of available data. *J Gambl Stud* 17: 255–271.

Walters, G.D. and Contri, D. (1998) Outcome expectancies for gambling: empirical modeling of a memory network in federal prison inmates. *J Gambl Stud* 14: 173–191.

Wardle, J. and Beinart, H. (1981) Binge eating: a theoretical review. *Br J Clin Psychol* 20: 97–109.

Welte, J., Barnes, G., Wieczorek, W., Tidwell, M., and Parker, J. (2001) Alcohol and gambling pathology among US adults: prevalence, demographic patterns and comorbidity. *J Stud Alcohol* 62: 706–712.

White, C., Mitchell, L., and Orford, J. (2001) *Exploring gambling behaviour in-depth: a qualitative study.* London: National Centre for Social Research.

White, N.M. (1996) Addictive drugs as reinforcers: multiple partial actions on memory systems. *Addiction* 91: 921–949.

Wilps, R.F. (1990) Male bulimia nervosa: an autobiographical case study. In: A.E. Andersen (ed.), *Males with eating disorders.* New York: Brunner/Mazel.

Winters, K.C. and Rich, T. (1998) A twin study of adult gambling behavior. *J Gambl Stud* 14: 213–225.

Wise, R.A. (1994) A brief history of the anhedonia hypothesis. In: C.R. Legg and D. Booth (eds), *Appetite, neural and behavioural bases.* Oxford: Oxford University Press: 243–263.

Wray, I. and Dickerson, M. (1981) Cessation of high frequency gambling and withdrawal symptoms. *Br J Addict* 76: 401–405.

Wynne, H.J. and Shaffer, H.J. (2003) The socioeconomic impact of gambling: the Whistler symposium. *J Gambl Stud* 19: 111–121.

Yates, A. (1991) *Compulsive exercise and eating disorders: toward an integrated theory of activity.* New York: Brunner/Mazel.

Young, K.S. (1998) *Caught in the net: how to recognise the sgns of Internet addiction and a winning strategy for recovery.* New York: Wiley.

15

Ethical Aspects of Developments in Neuroscience and Drug Addiction

Richard Ashcroft, Alastair V. Campbell and Ben Capps

1 EXECUTIVE SUMMARY

Foreseeable progress in neuroscience[1] – specifically the study of how chemicals alter an individual's genotype and phenotype – may have a significant impact on the treatment of addiction. This review focuses on the ethical strands of the debate, looking tentatively at how we can manage the use of psychoactive substances in the future to best advantage for the individual, the community and society. There is significant potential for great social and individual benefit from developments in this area – but these need to be evaluated alongside some potentially significant risks of harm or limitations on individual freedom that might undermine the value or acceptability of these developments. However, drug misuse puts anyone who does it at risk.

In this report, we look at the use of both licit and illicit substances that have a potentially addictive element, and some of the interventions that may become important in the treatment of such substance addiction. We identify why these interventions may be used for both sanctioned and illegal purposes and define what questions should be asked of ethics in light of what benefits or harms may be evident at this stage. We have had to be selective in our discussion, confining it to a representative selection of specific developments that may potentially be employed for both medical and non-medical purposes. We look in detail at developments in the prevention and treatment of drug addiction, such as vaccinations (Section 3); the use of genetic data to predict the effects of drugs on individuals, and how genetics may predispose one to addiction (Section 4); the use of neural imaging to identify past, present and potential addicts (Section 5); and the consequences of the use of medicinal drugs for non-medical reasons, such as cognitive enhancement (Section 6).

2 ETHICAL ISSUES OF POTENTIAL CLINICAL APPLICATIONS: THE NEXT 20 YEARS?

The misuse of drugs, both legal and illegal, presents society with a number of significant problems. Health impact on addicts include chronic conditions such as cirrhosis, lung cancer and HIV (Hall and Carter, 2004; World Health Organisation (WHO), 2004), and acute or short-term effects such as overdose. Drug misuse is also linked to risk taking and, in many cases, to criminal and antisocial behaviour. The misuse of potentially addictive drugs and the resulting harms have a complex impact on the relationship between the individual and society (Aust and Condon, 2003; Aust and Smith, 2003; Crombag and Robinson, 2004), raising issues of the addict's behaviour and their capacities to act responsibly (Kleiman, 2003; Morse, 2004; for legal issues see Ashworth, 2003; Mason et al., 2003). However, contemporary debates have focused on the biological and neurological alteration of the brain associated with addiction, as this is the area where we are gaining most new knowledge, rather than on the social sciences (Cami,

2003; Hall et al., 2003a, 2004a; Leshner and Koob, 1999; Murry, 2004; Nutt, 1997; Uhl, 2003).

While there are undoubtedly good prospects for significant benefits to individuals and to society from advances in understanding and technologies in this area, there is also some uncertainty about the moral implications of these developments. Many of the ethical questions concerning neuroscience and addiction research have been given renewed emphasis by the negative connotations, including stigmatisation and discrimination, associated with drug misuse (Copeland, 1997). Here we do not comment on research ethics per se, since the literature is well established in this area. In neuroscience and addiction research, special concern should be devoted to confidentiality and privacy, because of the nature of illicit drug misuse and the circumstances and behaviour sometimes associated with addiction, the capacity for informed consent in addicts and their voluntary participation in therapeutic and non-therapeutic research (for example, while intoxicated or in emergency situations and raising issues of 'best interests'[2]; Bosk, 2002; Charland, 2002; Cohen, 2002; Hall et al., 2003b), the constitution of the research team, especially with regard to members' competency to deal with comorbid conditions and criminal activity, and incentives to participate in research (eg socio-economic constraints; McCrady and Bux, 1999); and possible coercion to participate (eg from attending medical professionals).

In this report, we concentrate on some major avenues of research that are of interest because of their potentially imminent and significant application to human subjects. We are concerned with unpacking such developments within an ethical framework broadly conceived around 'human rights',[3] and which essentially protects one's autonomy – the capacity to lead one's life according to one's own values – including emergent principles such as competency, consent, privacy and confidentiality.[4] Autonomy is not to be understood as mere 'independence' from others, nor as the 'freedom to do whatever one wants'. Rather, it is the capacity to make decisions for oneself, without undue influence, interference or coercion from others, and without harming or imposing excessively on others (O'Neill, 2002). Respect for the autonomy of a given person entails the requirement to respect the autonomy of others; all human rights jurisprudence is consistent on this issue. In the body of this chapter, we discuss various situations where the respect for autonomy of a given person and the respect for the autonomy of others requires balancing.

While our emphasis is on the autonomy-undermining effects of addiction, and therefore may suggest an overly paternalistic attitude to protecting people from drug misuse, ie doing something in someone's best interests without concerning oneself too much with whether the person wants this or not, certain psychoactive substances may have therapeutic uses and other benefits. For example, drugs that improve alertness or maximise concentration may allow people to make more choices concerning their potential aspirations. Therefore, while we focus on the addictive component of drug misuse, there may develop socially approved reasons why drugs may legitimately be used if the risk of addiction is reduced (so the benefits of the drug outweigh the risk of addiction) or removed entirely.

We do not look at individual aspects of why one tries or starts misusing potentially addictive drugs, the reasons why an addict embarks on a particular type of behaviour, nor how society should deal with addicts (implicating the so-called 'moral' and 'medical' models of addiction; see Ashcroft and Franey, 2004; Hall et al., 2004a; Husak, 2004; Leshner, 1997; Morse, 2000; Watson, 1999). We are presuming that the goals of the new developments are to either treat addiction (ie addiction is a disease); to limit the effects of a drug on the individual (and therefore potentially 'cure' addiction)[5]; or to prevent or reduce the risks of developing an addiction.

3 VACCINATIONS AND DRUG MISUSE

At present, treatments aimed at stopping the craving felt by addicts or to prevent relapse can be modestly effective (Hall, 2002).[6] Their success can improve significantly when used alongside behavioural and counselling services (Kavanagh et al., 2004; WHO, 2004). These treatments are designed to reduce the intake of the drug, prevent craving in periods of abstinence, and to reduce relapse. Research has concentrated on developing drugs with fewer adverse side-effects, and genotyping may better match patients to existing pharmacological treatments for addiction (Hall et al., 2004a; McGregor and Gallate, 2004).

Recent attention has been directed to developing a means of inactivating the drug before it can gain access to the central nervous system. These vaccines are designed to block or significantly reduce the effects of certain drugs on the brain[7] by inducing antibody formation, producing an effect similar to vaccination against infectious disease. Removing the 'high' may reduce the craving for the drug. Furthermore, vaccination may stop a person from becoming addicted in the first place by removing the incentive to take the drug.

Vaccination poses a range of ethical issues in its own right, and is also a good model for thinking about the ethics of treating and preventing addiction by other means.

There have been recent advances in the potential vaccination of individuals from common drugs of misuse such as cocaine (Centre for Cognitive Liberty and Ethics (CCLE), 2004; Carrera et al., 2004; Hall and Carter, 2004; Kantak, 2003); alcohol (CCLE, 2004); tobacco and nicotine (CCLE, 2004; Hall, 2002; Kantak, 2003); marijuana (CCLE, 2004); and methamphetamine (Kantak, 2003). (See generally National Research Council (NRC), 2004; WHO, 2004.)

Although it is presently not known whether these treatments will have any side-effects, they may have better rates of compliance than existing oral drugs. They would be administered less often than conventional drugs, perhaps every six months, and could not be 'switched off' during their relatively prolonged effectiveness (Hall and Carter, 2002). This creates the problem that should anything go wrong with the treatment, it may be difficult to reverse the vaccine and also that such treatments would only affect the neurobiological effects of the drug. They would leave untouched any underlying behavioural pathology or dependency (Cohen, 1997).[8] So vaccination would have to be accompanied by counselling and support.[9]

A vaccine would have to be efficient and safe. It should also be selectively discriminatory, so that it would not unintentionally immunise against beneficial drug uses such as pain relief. If these criteria were met, the ethically significant questions would concern the balance between individual freedom and public welfare. First, however, issues of privacy and confidentiality must be raised.

3.1 Privacy and Confidentiality

There are few concerns about vaccinating a genuinely consenting addict to alter the progress of their addiction or prevent relapse after discontinued drug use. But questions arise about confidentiality and privacy. For example, if the cocaine vaccine or its antibodies were identifiable in tests, a positive result would betray a status open to stigmatisation.[10] The risk is that non-addicts, vaccinated because of a predisposition to addiction (see Section 4), as well as ex-addicts and actual addicts, might all be grouped together because of the presence of the vaccine antibodies. The fear of stigmatisation should be weighed against the potential benefits from treatment (Sommerville, 2002). As we shall see, this may be a question of a choice to have treatment or forced treatment to protect others. Confidentiality regarding the presence of antibodies that may rightly or wrongly associate the status of a recovered addict with that of an actual addict is

essential, as is self-determination in allowing the individual to decide who can have access to this information.

3.2 Who Should be Vaccinated?

A key distinction would be between those who are voluntarily vaccinated and those who are required to be vaccinated.

Vaccinations have traditionally been directed at a whole population, but there may often be reasons to target individual communities that have a high propensity to some disease.

In the case of psychoactive substance use, vaccination could be used to prevent and treat the health effects of drug misuse, and also to control the use of illegal drugs, since the costs of drug misuse for society are high. Vaccination could be used:

- as an aid to coping with drug withdrawal and possible relapse,
- to vaccinate persistent drug users,
- to vaccinate potential users.

3.2.1 A National Drug Vaccination Programme?

Population-wide vaccination programmes have been largely successful in decreasing the incidence of certain diseases, and have removed some almost entirely. Could a nationwide drug vaccination programme be implemented to reduce the incidence of drug addiction?

There are a number of arguments against such a measure. First, the vast majority of people do not misuse drugs, nor will they ever be exposed to them. Even among those who take a potentially addictive drug, addiction is not certain. It is therefore questionable whether mass vaccination would be justified in light of the relative risks, and compared with the cost and potential harms of repeated vaccination. It is also possible that certain beneficial aspects of medicinal drug use, such as pain control, which uses the active components of some drugs of misuse, would become ineffective in those vaccinated.

Some potentially harmful drugs, such as alcohol, also serve a socially beneficial role, and although regulated (to promote responsible use), their (mis)use is not prohibited in adults, though some resulting behaviour may be criminalised. It would be considered paternalistic and intrusive to vaccinate against their use. Would other drugs be viewed differently? In determining an appropriate balance between individual rights and social stability, a difficult choice may need to be made between restricting or removing the right to self-determination from the vast number of individuals not at risk in order to prevent the misuse of drugs by a minority.

We all have the right to live our lives relatively free from the interference, however well-meaning, of others and of the state. But equally, we do not have the right to inflict harm on others. The difficult balance in legislation and public policy between allowing and encouraging individual freedom and restricting that freedom to protect others will continue to be controversial – it is the very stuff of modern politics. In this area, the issues are complex because our interests in public safety and the prevention and detection and punishment of crimes against the person and against property seem to conflict with our interests in privacy and self-determination. This is a particularly acute problem since the interventions under discussion here are medical, and social trends since the 1950s have encouraged a very rights-based approach to medical treatment. Many doctors, for instance, will be loath to use their skills in the service of what they might see as a non-medical issue. Equally, many doctors will see the preventive approach as appropriate, particularly given their experience of treating the consequences of drug overdose or alcohol-related violence and injury. And this debate is likely to be repeated throughout society, not just within the medical profession. One outcome of this sort of debate may be a swing back away from the privileging of individual autonomy or personal rights in medical ethics as much as in criminal justice. However, it is impossible to discern how likely this is – or how far it could go. Insofar as vaccination forms part of medical practice, vaccination will be constrained, in competent persons at least, by the requirement that the vaccinee consent to vaccination. If vaccination is court-mandated, with the doctor carrying out the vaccination at the request of the court, such interventions will still normally require informed consent (and would normally be optional, with other more traditional punishments or rehabilitative measures as the alternatives). A challenging policy issue would concern the vaccination of mentally non-competent individuals; in such cases much more would lie on the judgement of the individual doctor that this vaccination was in the medical best interests of the vaccinee as well as being court-approved.

If it is not justifiable to vaccinate the entire nation, it could be feasible, and more affordable, to target certain groups within it. While there may be legitimate reasons to screen a certain population for a realistic link to addiction (based on ethnic, social or comorbid grounds), groups could be selected on more dubious arguments. What groups are candidates for vaccination? It is evident that areas of social deprivation or of high 'visible minorities' have a higher prevalence of drug use (Aust and Condon, 2003). Likewise, their inhabitants are disproportionately represented within the criminal justice system in connection with drug-related crime (see Khan, 1999). There may be certain groups that would benefit from directed vaccinations based on consensual and willing participation. But we must be very wary of the use of (mis)information to further alienate, stigmatise or discriminate against vulnerable groups, and of the risk of causing further social problems by such actions (see Aust and Condon, 2003).

3.2.2 The Vaccination of Consenting Adults

Even with a competent adult volunteering to participate in a vaccination programme, we must consider issues of confidentiality and privacy. Entering a drugs programme in a voluntary capacity could leave the participant open to stigmatisation and discrimination. Nor are the benefits and disbenefits of volunteering for treatment as clear cut as one may expect. The individual has to consider taking up a 'patient's role' and being seen to be part of the world of drug use. The vaccination will probably need periodic renewal and it may perpetuate withdrawal, adding to the relative unattractiveness of vaccination compared with taking the drug itself (Ashcroft and Franey, 2004; Nutt and Lingford-Hughes, 2004).

Moreover, addicts are often addicted to, or at least using, more than one drug, and there is often comorbidity between drug misuse and other mental conditions, such as depression (McGregor and Gallate, 2004). Vaccination would not be a treatment for addiction itself, and would need to be used alongside other interventions, for example, counselling, for prolonged abstinence from drug misuse. This is demonstrated by the relatively low success rate of existing drugs used in addiction therapy, which at most have only modest outcomes in long-term abstinence (Nutt and Lingford-Hughes, 2004).[11]

It is also possible that restrictions on the health service provision of such treatments would apply for cost reasons. They could include measuring compliance and willingness, and possibly requiring further rehabilitative measures.[12]

Finally, making vaccination available to episodic drug users raises the concern that they could use the drug and experience the 'high' in the knowledge that there may be a fast track out of addiction (Ashcroft and Franey, 2004), at least for those able to afford it.

Using a vaccine that palliates the addictive effects of drugs may allow people to use such substances for pleasure and not risk the harms of addiction,[13] or may create socially acceptable uses for previously addictive drugs. In the case of pleasure drugs, the possible social changes that this development may promote are unknown. Speculatively, it may lead to increased use of drugs for pleasure on the perceived availability of a 'quick fix'.[14] This raises the question of whether policies should continue to counter such use when the benefits outweigh the harms. The outcome may either be that more people come to perceive present paternalistic measures as unwarranted, or that spiralling drug use per se would lead to stricter legislative measures.

On a positive note, the use of drugs that are no longer addictive may lead to the expansion of or changes in the range of socially approved purposes. The potential use of such drugs in employment, for example, in maintaining alertness in driving, or commercial flight, may be significant for their social acceptance.

3.2.3 Coerced Vaccination of Addicts Who Use Illegal Drugs

Perhaps the most controversial questions raised by the vaccination of individual populations relate to the use of force (Ridgely *et al.*, 2004). Since this is a medical intervention, the spectre of people being treated against their wishes is raised.[15] Does addiction to an illegal drug give the state the right to impose vaccination? It could be justified as providing an alternative to sanctions such as prison. The underlying assumptions are that treating an offender's drug dependence will reduce the likelihood of their reoffending, and so reduce the associated criminal activity; and that coerced treatments, based on the disease model of addiction, are in the best interests of the addict. The former assumption relates to the public interest in controlling and reducing crime; the latter relates to paternalistically overriding the choices of the addict in their best interests (whatever the addict him or herself may think about them!).

There are two types of addict to mention here: those who, in addition to breaking the law by taking an illegal drug, are involved in activities that are antisocial or illegal[16]; and those who take the illegal drug but are not breaking any further laws – the crime committed is the taking of the drug.[17] Should these two groups be treated differently should vaccination ever become possible?

It is not unknown for methadone or other remedial measures, such as attendance at a support group, to be attached to a court judgement or housing-support programme. Might similar constraints be put on offenders who are also suffering from mental health problems, or who are claiming social security payments for unemployment or are homeless and seeking housing? Such choices may help or push offenders towards a more acceptable way of life, perhaps involving stable employment or housing for 'clean' individuals. However, there is evidence that coerced or compulsory drug treatment doesn't always work (Newman, 1974).

If a safe vaccine were available, it could either be offered in addition to a prison sentence or fines, or as an alternative[18] to more severe punishment, for example, as a requirement of probation as opposed to imprisonment. But both approaches have the problem that they fail to meet the requirements of informed consent. A choice between imprisonment or a medical intervention is clearly coercive (see CCLE, 2004). Would the addict make the same choice if he or she were not in this situation? And what are the ethical concerns of the medical profession's involvement in such measures (British Medical Association (BMA), 2001)?[19] On the other hand, from the point of view of criminal justice, coercion is an essential element of punishment, and the coercive element of this offer, while questionable from the point of view of medical ethics is perhaps unproblematic from the point of view of penal ethics. And indeed many convicted offenders and many victims of crime may prefer the vaccination approach to imprisonment as a way of dealing with the causes of crime and the personal problems frequently involved at the root of criminal behaviour.

If a criminal justice system is seeking to deter or prevent serious crime, it is unlikely that any addict would be 'offered' the vaccine as an alternative to the sentencing option, because knowing that there is an alternative to prison would not deter drug misuse or drug-related crime.[20] But a retributive theory of punishment, claiming that any punishment is justified because the offender has committed a wrong act and that the degree of punishment should be in proportion to the crime, may point to a different answer (Ten, 2004). In this case, we may offer the addict who commits no further crimes the option of vaccination, along with other sanctions such as community service, since the wrong act is taking the drug, and this may therefore be the most appropriate level of punishment.[21] This would also be consistent with a 'reformist' theory of criminal justice, which sees its role as the rehabilitation of offenders. Additionally, imprisonment may reinforce addictive behaviour, cause the addict to switch to more dangerous drug habits, and expose them to further harms such as HIV and hepatitis. Control of drugs within prisons is a recognised problem worldwide.[22]

3.2.4 Addictions to Legal Drugs

In the case of the misuse of drugs that are regulated but not prohibited, such as alcohol and tobacco, one must be careful that the status of addict does not become a crime. Of course, the uncontrollable use of legal drugs leads to criminal activities – such as antisocial behaviour, theft, violence and domestic violence – but this doesn't necessary follow.

In the case of legal drugs and where no additional crimes have been committed, the option of vaccination must be voluntary, since the addict is not breaking any law. Such a vaccination would normally be provided as part of a wider treatment plan. This may not be the case where criminal convictions follow from problem drug use short of addiction (for example, driving while under the influence of a psychoactive drug). In such situations, we can foresee vaccination being offered as part of the rehabilitation or punishment of the offender.

3.2.5 Pregnant Mothers

The main issue here is whether a case could ever be made to compel a pregnant mother to be vaccinated in her own interests and those of the child. The concern is that drug misuse may harm the foetus or continuation of the pregnancy, or that the child will be born with an addiction or addiction-related condition (Godding *et al.*, 2004). Vaccination if offered as a treatment, and taken by choice, by an addicted pregnant mother could protect her child; but what would be the possible outcome if treatment was forced, and on what grounds may this be ethical, if at all?

One side of the argument holds that, because the woman has decided that she wants to carry the pregnancy to term, she has responsibilities for the health of the foetus. This may be matched by the state's perceived duty to protect all human life – including the foetus – from intentional harms. The other side of the argument holds, in line with the present understanding in UK law,[23] that the foetus has no legal status. This suggests that neither the state nor the pregnant woman has any moral responsibilities towards the foetus except, in the case of the woman, those that she wishes to take on.

Somewhere between these competing claims is the argument that compelling the mother could only lead to further difficulties in her pregnancy, such as adverse effects on the foetus, the course of the pregnancy, and for the mother's health (Ridgely *et al.*, 2004). Coercive programmes may persuade pregnant addicts to avoid or not present themselves for prenatal care due to unwanted testing and treatment (NRC, 2004: 185).

The key issue is whether society or the state have any accountability to promote responsible pregnancies that protect the mother, the foetus, or both, and, if it does,

how far these measures can go. Some would argue that as society has to deal with the consequences of births of babies affected by maternal drug and alcohol use, it has some right to intervene to limit harm to the unborn caused in this way. Society already does intervene in a variety of ways to promote child health in the womb – through encouraging the taking of folic acid supplements and the offer of antenatal classes and antenatal screening, for instance. On the other hand, society has tended to reject approaches that would penalise mothers for actions during pregnancy which might harm their unborn child – from the decriminalisation of abortion to the rejection of so-called 'wrongful life' suits by the courts. The spectre of eugenics and the prospect of children suing their parents for negligence are considered by many to be stern warnings against taking such a coercive or punitive approach to maternal behaviour during pregnancy.

3.2.6 The Vaccination of Children

A further significant question is whether a strategy for immunising individuals before they try a drug should include children. As Nutt and Lingford-Hughes (2004) point out (drawing on the paradigm of child vaccination), 'cocaine dependence is more damaging to many individuals than measles'. The term 'vaccine' may also be unfortunate because it could raise unrealistic expectations among parents of complete drug protection ('immunity') for their children.

The question is not simple. It needs to consider both enrolment into a vaccination programme as a targeted population and as an individual. In the case of the former, one might look at targeting all minors as an 'at-risk' group, or use socioeconomic indicators that suggest that certain groups of minors are susceptible to drug addiction. In the case of individual vaccinations, the significant question could be whether it would be permissible for parents to have their children vaccinated in their children's best interests.[24] In all these cases, the vaccination would be pre-emptive and parental concerns that their children could be exposed to drugs in the future could fuel the programme. Can a case be made to immunise children against a potential future of drug use?

If the vaccine requires repeat injections (as seems likely), one risks the possibility of conditioning children to injecting substances. Furthermore, one has to ask when such a programme would begin, what it would cost, and the competence of the person being treated. There may be a point when the child wishes to discontinue the treatment. Would it still be worthwhile to force the adolescent to accept the injections, with consequences to medical and parental relationships?

Perhaps the greatest concern would be the intrusion into the life of a child – not just at the time of the vaccination but also into his or her future behaviour. Hasman and Holm (2004) argue that drug misuse is not an infection and therefore the discomfort and risk of harm to the child is not justified. The vaccination is a violation of the child's ability to assess the benefits and harms for himself or herself. This denial of important decision-making capacities for the child, they argue, limits the child's right to an open future. They conclude that whether such a decision does limit the future options of the child will be contestable.

However, as Hall (2002) has pointed out, objections to the 'open future' argument depends on a gross overestimation of the efficiency of childhood vaccination against addiction. For example, an adult who has been vaccinated as a child but who was determined to become addicted still could. It would simply be more expensive to do so.

3.3 The Potential Effects of Vaccination

Vaccinations could potentially affect the individual in two ways. First, they may alter the individual's 'mind' itself. Drug vaccinations, by their very nature, are 'mind-altering' in that they change the functioning of the brain. This is not the same as a vaccine that produces antibodies to ward off infection. Instead, it has been described as the use of pharmacotherapy to expand the '... drug war battlefield ... to a new terrain directly *inside* the bodies and brains of drug users' (CCLE, 2004: 6). This, according to the CCLE (2004: 4), is a 'threat to cognitive liberty', since one may be able to eliminate the desire to use illegal drugs, and thus the conscious actions of addicts or potential addicts.

One may, however, question these claims of 'mind-altering' effects. The vaccines are meant to change biological function transiently and affect the brain indirectly by attenuating the effects of psychoactive drugs. Indeed, it is intended that such vaccines will operate outside the brain, targeting and mopping up the drug before it enters the central nervous system, therefore not affecting the brain directly in the way that neuropharmaceutical drugs do (Hall, 2002).

The concern for the CCLE is that vaccines may be used to control the conscious actions of individuals even before they themselves act on them. Furthermore, vaccinations for drug use could be applied further, by vaccinations against other lifestyle choices (enforcing social conformity) and addictive behaviour such as gambling.

One must look at the potential responses of the actual, reformed or potential addict to the presence of the vaccine. Will those on vaccine programmes try to overcome the vaccination, thus risking overdose or harm from increased doses of the drug and its contaminants (Nutt and Lingford-Hughes, 2004)?[25] Or will they switch to other drugs? There are also risks, demonstrated in the completion of methadone maintenance treatment programmes, that tolerance can be reduced. So if the patient relapses, they overdose because they have no tolerance to the heroin at the levels they used to take, and can't judge the amount they need (Darke and Hall, 2003; Strang et al., 2003).

However, it is also important to consider that, when taken by choice, vaccines could provide a valuable addition to the available treatments for those dependent or addicted to any given drug which is causing medical and social harm.

4 GENETICS AND INDIVIDUALISED INFORMATION

Pharmacogenetics, the study of the biological response and effects of different drugs on the individual, and pharmacogenomics, the examination of the genome and gene–gene interactions with regard to drugs, offer the possibility of 'genomic medicine', tailoring drugs to the individual and foreseeing the likely effects that they may have – including a potential susceptibility to addiction (Burke *et al.*, 2002; Roses, 2004). Pharmacogenetics and pharmacogenomics have the potential to allow us to foresee and avoid side-effects and tailor treatment regimes more accurately to patients' needs. 'Predictive genomic medicine' may give us insights into an individual's likelihood of addiction or of developing a drug-related disease, allowing individual choices and societal policies based on genetic predispositions (Crabbe and Phillips, 1998). It is also possible that advances in genomics will drive down the current spending of the health service on treatment, cutting down on expensive treatment in favour of detection and avoidance programmes (Richards, 2003a). Specific to drug addiction, pharmacogenomics may identify genetic profiles with greater or lesser susceptibility to the action of the drug, while behavioural genomics could identify genetic profiles with greater or lesser susceptibility to addictive behaviour. Therefore, someone could be highly susceptible to becoming drunk on alcohol, but not likely to become addicted to alcohol; or less than usually susceptible to the effects of alcohol, but likely to develop an addiction to it. All of these possibilities have advantages and disadvantages from an ethical point of view.

It is important that the ethical issues of genetic research on addictive disorders are considered, because:

- the predictive nature of genetic information has the potential to affect people's lives adversely;
- genetic information carries implications not just for individuals, but also for families, communities and populations;
- genetic information has the potential to be used to stigmatise and victimise, but also to be used for treatment and improving individuals' safety and welfare.

Questions that have arisen in the context of addiction and genetic information are:

- should an individual be responsible for their actions if they know of a genetic predisposition to addiction or drug-related disease?
- how would a family (or community) respond to a member with a genetic disposition to addiction (raising issues of the misattribution of blame and guilt, and the subsequent effects, to relationships)?
- should parents be responsible in using measures to detect 'predispositions' to addiction and to prevent it by whatever means in their children?

At present we know very little about the answers to these questions, and part of the reason for this is that society at large is only now beginning to handle genetic information about risk, disease and behaviour on a regular basis. What we can infer on the basis of existing knowledge about the social response to genetic information may be relatively unreliable as society changes in response to the wealth of new genetic knowledge we are garnering. However, it is plausible that the available repertoire of responses to addiction and lay theories of what it is and how it is acquired or treated, being based on long-standing lay theories of free-will and responsibility, will shape how genetic explanations are understood, rather than being radically overhauled by such new kinds of explanation.

4.1 Understanding Genetic Information

Advances in understanding the genetic basis of disease through the establishment of genetic databases and the mapping of the human genome make genomic medicine (ie medicine organised around the systematic use of genetic information in diagnosis, prognosis and treatment) a realistic but probably distant proposition. In the case of single-gene conditions, where most progress in gene detection has occurred, few effective interventions are available and, as a whole, they are relatively rare in the population. The more common multifactoral diseases are dependent on complex gene-environment relationships and are not open to the same simple analysis (Hall *et al.*, 2004b).

Regardless of these biological hurdles, genomic medicine could potentially be used to inform or regulate an individual's use of certain drugs. This possibility presents us with questions of privacy, confidentiality, discrimination, and the misuse and usefulness of probabilities. For instance, how will knowing genetic susceptibility to addiction or drug-related disease change the behaviour of individuals? How will drug and drug-related disease screening programmes affect individuals and groups? And how should genetic information be given to 'at risk' individuals?

There is strong evidence to suggest that genetic factors play a role in the effects of drugs on the person, such as their absorption, metabolism and excretion, and these will sometimes correspond to a susceptibility to a drug-related disease (for example, see Lerman and Niaura, 2002; Mohn *et al.*, 2004; Nestler and Landsman, 2001; O'Loughlin *et al.*, 2004; Thun *et al.*, 2002; Tyndale, 2003). Advances in pharmacogenetics may allow researchers to identify genes and gene products that are implicated in addiction, tolerance, sensitisation, dependence, craving and relapse.[26] From this information, pharmacogenomic research may identify genes that represent a higher probability of addiction and indicate how large a dose, or doses, of a drug may cause addiction in the first place.

The genetic basis of addiction reflects genetic traits that influence one's behaviour with regard to drug taking and any resultant addiction. The effect will depend on the genotype and environmental cues and stresses, as well as the specific effects of any drug on an individual. These two factors are linked in addiction. So, for example, an addiction may need to be 'triggered' in any individual, but the sensitivity of the trigger may depend on the type of drug taken, how much and how often, as well as the user's genetic basis. A certain gene or group of genes may reveal a disposition to addiction to a given substance or behaviour, but perhaps not to others, and its effect may be different for different individuals.

It has been postulated that the mapping of the human genome and the use of genetic technology, such as gene chips – or DNA array technology – to allow the rapid identification of thousands of gene products will facilitate the identification of potential addicts (Nestler and Landsman, 2001). This emphasis on 'gene chasing', while potentially offering more effective and lower risk therapies, also raises concerns, such as a potential underemphasis on the social mechanisms of exposure to drugs.

One of the dangers is in the 'folk' understanding of genetic traits, which emphasises a deterministic understanding of genotype and phenotype. We have to acknowledge the complex interaction of genetics, behaviour (and therefore life choices) and environment on an individual's phenotype and genotype (Neil Holtzman interviewed in Richards, 2003b).

The already complex interaction between drug addiction, genes and the environment may be further complicated by the genetic factors involved in diseases themselves. Certain diseases may be caused, catalysed or compounded by the interaction of certain drugs with 'disease' genes. Furthermore, the likelihood of taking a drug, the amount taken and the duration of use may depend on other genetic factors, including those related to addiction.[27] It may become possible to screen the population to identify individuals who may be predisposed to developing specific diseases, some of which may be related to drug taking (Marteau and Lerman, 2001). Such information may be used to benefit the individual by developing safer, better-targeted and more efficient treatments for illness and other medical conditions. It may also be used to inform people of their genetic susceptibility to disease, which may motivate them to change their behaviour (Nuffield Council on Bioethics (NCB), 2003). But this evidence must be considered alongside the use of a specific drug, how and where it is taken, how it affects that individual, and a myriad of other environmental cues.

Finally, the identification of 'genes for . . . ' has been partly responsible for the creation of medical conditions out of what had previously been considered to be the normal difficulties an individual might face. So-called 'medicalisation' has been argued to have taken place in the characterisation of, for example, general anxiety disorder (GAD), social anxiety disorder and the gendered condition of 'female sexual dysfunction' (in response to female sexual anxieties and the move to promote impotence drugs) (Brownsword, 2003). Behaviour currently viewed as normal such as shyness (or GAD) may, in the future, be reclassified as pathological and be investigated for medical intervention. The concern here is that while people who are concerned about these traits or behaviours will be encouraged to see them as medical problems rather than as something to do with their own personal attitudes and behaviours, or to see something which may from some points of view be valuable or desirable as problematic and requiring change. That these shifts in perception may be driven principally by market-seeking commercial behaviour,

rather than principally by patients' or consumers' needs, has been a consistent worry in modern societies. It is surprisingly difficult to separate out what is 'genuine' and what is 'invented' in discussing these kinds of need or desire, however. The outcome may be that the perspective that 'genes' cause disease will lead to pressure to purchase remedies for these conditions and that it becomes the individual's responsibility to take measures to avoid them, rendering it unnecessary for the community to address them.[28] Yet, on the other hand, the relationship between biological theories, commercial interests and social wants is complex and difficult to predict or disentangle. There is a legitimate public and commercial interest in trying to understand and provide remedies for conditions that are debilitating or undermining for those who undergo them. We might question whether shyness is really a medical condition; but that is not to dispute that shyness is not something which shy people find deeply upsetting or disempowering. One consequence of the 'medicalisation' of shyness may be the growth of a market parallel to that of medicine which frankly and openly accepts 'lifestyle' conditions as its central concern. What would be controversial would be the boundary between lifestyle and healthcare interventions, especially given public funding of the latter but not the former.

Genetic factors in addiction and disease prevalence raise the opportunity for research to be misused or misunderstood (Hall *et al.*, 2002). People may pay attention to genetic risk factors when environmental factors are far more significant, or far easier to manipulate, or both. For instance, if there was a genetic risk factor for smoking-related lung cancer (or addiction to nicotine), some might argue that this means that people without these risk factors can smoke safely (or nonaddictively). Yet the baseline risk to people of regular tobacco smoking is very high, and these genetic risk factors merely make it worse.

A further risk inherent in genetics and addiction studies is that the interpretation of research may compound influences one way or another. The identification of susceptibility genes for addiction or addiction-related diseases would tempt individuals who lacked these genes to misuse drugs 'safely', while those with the genes might be dissuaded from trying drugs.

But there are a number of problems with such a simple interpretation. It fails to recognise that the effects of drugs vary from person to person. Individuals may vary in their sensitivity to the active ingredients' effects, in their tolerance of them and in the severity of their withdrawal.

There are benefits from genetic studies, however, not least that individuals at risk of becoming dependent or who have a higher susceptibility to a certain disease can be identified and warned and appropriate health-care measures taken, including screening for the disease. Side-effects can be avoided, preventive steps by individuals and society can be better undertaken and understood, and potentially a more sophisticated and perhaps more tolerant approach taken to the care and support of people at risk or in the grip of destructive behaviours.

4.2 Genes and Behaviour

How will genetic information alter an individual's behaviour? With Huntington's disease, the late onset of the condition can be preceded by prolonged periods of waiting, putting potential carriers of the gene in a situation of uncertainty about their own future. Among those who chose to be tested and were positive for the Huntington's gene, there was a reported higher rate of suicide as a result of a fatalistic response to the onset of the disease (Terrenoire, 1992). Screening alongside genetic counselling has been shown to reduce this. The ethical concern is whether those affected individuals had a right to know, or not know, future probabilities, so that they could make, or not make, important decisions on the basis of the best available knowledge (which is relevant in this case with regard to passing the gene on to their children); or whether

they have a responsibility to know the results of such tests so that they can make conscientious decisions. Yet these risks may not materialise; and we should also consider that in many cases people will choose to avoid passing on genetic 'conditions' such as shyness, addictions, or other behavioural traits to potential children. This may be achieved by choosing not to have genetically related children or screening gametes to be used in IVF, or through screening or terminating existing embryos or foetuses. This may not be because the conditions necessarily create problems for society, but because they create problems for individuals, either because of uncertainty in their own actions or of how they feel society sees these actions.

This leads us onto the potential risk of measures being imposed on individuals. A positive result to a test for a potential predisposition could validate forced measures by the state. We may also see the 'treatment' of previously normal behaviour through medical interventions, increasing the anxieties of individuals who fail to measure up to this new 'normalisation', and diverting funds and support from improvements in environmental and socioeconomic circumstances. State intervention is not necessarily bad – it is bad only where the intervention is ineffective, or bad value for money, or unjust, or unaccountable. The role of the state in using coercive treatment or prevention measures needs to be controlled by a robust and functioning democracy, and by adherence to human rights norms. Sometimes this might involve the imposition of coercive measures in the public interest. More often than not, coercion will not be necessary, or will be outweighed by other factors.

With regard to drug use and addiction, learning of a genetic risk factor for addiction may create a fatalistic attitude to drug use, but, unlike in the previous example, these predispositions are multifactoral and, at most, provide only an assessment of how likely a person is to develop an addiction or how difficult it will be to overcome it. Nonetheless, for some people, the idea that someone has a genetic risk factor for addiction may be interpreted as meaning that this person is completely unable to control their behaviour and so should have his or her rights strictly limited on the grounds of danger to self or others. This would be a dramatic overreaction to information which is at most likely to give information about relative risks. Yet this does underscore how difficult it is to think about the relationship between physical determinism (everything I do is caused by my physical make-up) and free will. Genetics and neuroscience may add little to this debate other than a new idiom for talking about it. In the context of drug addiction, this debate may have two outcomes: individuals will not try to stop taking the drug, or they may turn to other forms of help.[29]

What needs to be demonstrated and understood is that genetic information may allow an individual to decide that certain activities may put them at risk, and that changing their behaviour may reduce this risk – and not that there is no point in changing behaviour. Such use of genetic information is not new. Family histories have been used for some time to highlight risks, although there is evidence that genetic knowledge of a predisposition does not necessarily change behaviour (Terrenoire, 1992). While it is commonly asserted that a 'gene for ...' actually means a tip in the balance of probabilities, which may be very small if one considers environmental causes and life choices, a swing in the other direction – that one does not have the 'gene' – may lead to increased reassurance that drug misuse will not harm one. The key message should be that drug misuse puts anyone who does it at risk. Genetic factors may merely alter the likelihood of side-effects, overdose, addictiveness or the direct psychoactive effects of the drug. For most drugs, however, the basic pattern of response will not vary much between specific individuals with specific variations in genetic make-up.

Key to this debate will be how genetic information is presented and explained to individuals (including the task of effectively portraying data on 'risk') and how this motivates individuals to change their lifestyles (including the effects of anxiety, demoralisation and fatalistic attitudes).

4.3 Population Genetics

We discussed the implications of directing vaccination programmes towards certain populations in Section 3.2.1. One use of genomic information is to confirm genetic differences, in the context of this report those relating to susceptibility to addiction, the processes of addiction, and diseases associated with addiction in different populations. The benefit of such an approach is to identify individuals or populations who may be more susceptible, and then to take measures to treat, monitor, or pre-emptively avoid the onset of such disorders (Risch et al., 2002). However, whether such information is useful is debatable.

The ethical question is how do policy makers evaluate and decide on the weight placed on such data? As we have already emphasised, predispositions have both a genetic and an environmental aspect, and this corresponds to a risk. How society deals with this risk is dependent on incomplete data, or data which are highly complicated to interpret, and on cultural values. This is important because of the sensitivity of discussions about inequalities on the basis of perceived genetic 'evidence' of ethnic differences. One must avoid naïve inferences about genetic causation without evidence (Risch et al., 2002). Furthermore, the importance to be placed on such information must be carefully considered, as should the means of dissemination of such findings. Here, it is important to emphasise the qualitative variables that present risk factors[30] for diseases, treatment responses and adverse effects of pharmacological agents, allowing tailored treatments. The highlighting of such beneficial applications of genomics will be important in the study of addiction.

4.4 Modifying the Human Genome

It may become possible to alter the genes of an individual in order to alter their addictive behaviour. Neuropharmacological interventions already exist for this purpose and are more easily accomplished than genetic interventions (Farah and Wolpe, 2004). Gene therapy interventions that alter genes in situ to change the mechanisms of addiction may be difficult to achieve, like other gene therapies, whereas it is comparatively easy to inject a pharmacotherapeutic drug to counter the effects of addiction, once the basis of addiction is known.

One controversial means of achieving changes in genetic susceptibility to addiction that may be possible in the future would be at the preimplantation stage of embryogenesis. It would involve 'knocking out' or selecting some genes before the embryo developed. Apart from the complex arguments concerning embryo selection and termination, this raises ethical concerns similar to those mentioned in vaccinating children – that of a 'right to have an open future' (Section 3.2.6). Given that the use of this technology to avoid even serious genetic disease is socially controversial at present, it may well not be brought far into development. Yet it is perfectly possible that society would take a more actively welcoming approach to the use of preimplantation genetic diagnosis (PGD) to prevent the birth of babies with 'socially harmful' genes. The history of eugenics suggests that social support for this kind of application of genetics can be widespread. Equally, it is arguable that this gives us powerful reason to avoid the development or use of PGD technology for such purposes.

5 NEURAL IMAGING

Brain imaging technologies may be used to study the effects of drugs and the neurobiological consequences of chronic drug use (Hall *et al.*, 2004a; for review see Farah and Wolpe, 2004). It may become possible to use imaging to identify former, current and potential addicts. Such screening has the potential added benefit of being more immediately accessible and less expensive than screening for drug antibodies. It doesn't necessarily raise any further ethical issues than those already raised in this report, although there may be concerns in other areas of neuroscience concerning medical intrusions into individual preferences, and the shaping of social and moral attitudes (Farah and Wolpe, 2004).

The questions to focus on in the context of this report are whether an addict can competently enrol to take part in novel imaging research, since this is the most likely group to be targeted for research; and what the data will be used for, and by whom (bringing to the fore issues of privacy and confidentiality). For example, can characteristic patterns of brain activity in childhood and adolescence predict increased risk of addiction in later life (Hall *et al.*, 2004a)?

We still have to ask whether such medical interventions will be used in the best interests of the patient. Will imaging be used to identify addicts against their will (similar to a lie detector test) and then used in coercive measures in the legal or employment fields (with questionable success[31]) or for insurance purposes? And will it be used to identify those at risk of addiction and to justify non-consensual or intrusive measures, or to selectively abort foetuses that have certain brain signatures in utero (Lavine, 2002; Stevenson and Goldworth, 2002)?

Notwithstanding all these ethical questions, it is still likely that neural imaging will provide further information about the mechanisms of drug action, the mechanisms of addiction, and the impact of long-term drug use, which will be useful both in the diagnosis of disease and in the development and targeting of treatment. Questions will continue to be asked about whether in the future it might be possible to use imaging to excuse or explain drug-related behaviours in the court system, but much of the information provided by brain scanning will be insufficiently sensitive to provide detailed explanations of particular behaviours by most people. The impact of these technologies is likely to be felt most strongly in basic science and research into treatment.

6 PERFORMANCE, COGNITIVE ENHANCEMENTS AND DRUG ADDICTION

Future developments in psychopharmacology may allow specific psychological changes to be induced by targeted neurochemical interventions in the chemical events that underlie cognition and emotion (Farah *et al.*, 2004). The effects would not normally be hereditary – unless they altered the germ cells in some way – and would more often be temporary, or at least reversible (although this is an aspect that must be resolved). However, these drugs may alter what the human species can achieve, by making them 'better than well', and it is this aspect that we are interested in here.

There are great pressures to succeed in everyday life. Passing an exam or completing a job have financial and career consequences that can encourage the individual to enhance their chances of success. Furthermore, once success is achieved, there is the added concern for the user of returning to normalcy, which could be an incentive to continued drug use. This dependency on a drug for improved performance may at least prolong drug use and increase the chance of an addiction developing. Success may involve encouraging states of mind, including concentration, anxiety and mood, and metabolic alteration such as stimulation to reduce tiredness and bradycardia[32] to induce calmness. Further potential targets for pharmacological enhancement would include memory, executive function, appetite and libido. If these treatments work, there are many potential users, and a concern that this new breed of drugs may have abuse potential. Research into the mechanisms of addiction will give a better idea of how realistic this fear of

creating new addictions is, and how far this fear should outweigh the likely benefits of new drugs.

It is already apparent that drugs that are developed to treat a specific medical condition are being used for purposes for which they were not intended. Most, if not all, medicinal drugs have unwanted side-effects, and this sometimes includes addiction, but these are outweighed by the benefits of treatment. When the same drugs are used by those who are not ill for the purpose of enhancement above 'normal', this balance is not evident. The use of such drugs for this purpose is not necessarily novel (see Farah and Wolpe, 2004). But future developments may mitigate or remove some of the adverse effects of drugs, such as addiction and tolerance, which could mean increased interest in taking such drugs, both for medical[33] and non-medical reasons.

One example is the use of drugs that are normally prescribed to treat attention-deficit hyperactivity disorder (ADHD), such as methylphenidate (Ritalin). It is evident that this drug is being used by young people to help them with exams. This has led to a continuing debate over the increase in the use of Ritalin in schools and misuse in university settings and in other adult groups (Farah, 2002; Farah and Wolpe, 2004; Farah *et al.*, 2004; Rowland *et al.*, 2002). There is circumstantial evidence of addiction in some users.[34]

Other drugs developed for the treatment of memory and cognition defects (such as Alzheimer's disease) may be used to improve cognitive abilities in individuals who are not significantly cognitively impaired (Elliott, 2003; Hall, 2003). Critics of the wider use of such drugs argue that fuzzy diagnostic criteria are being used as an additional reason for 'treatment'. But, again, one must question whether there is a significant gap between, for example, using memory-enhancing drugs to slow down normal deterioration to a 'disease' state, and using it to enhance 'normal' capacities. Selective serotonin reuptake inhibitors, which are used to treat depression, are being used by people who are not depressed to alter their mood and personality (Fukuyama, 2002). To continue the list, beta-blockers are used to remove nervousness in stressful situations (Gems, 1999); modafinil (Provigil), which is normally used for narcolepsy, can make users more alert; and Prozac and similar drugs can be used to make people less shy, less compulsive and more confident (Gems 1999; see also Farah and Wolpe, 2004, who note that clinical trials investigating the effects of such drugs on healthy individuals, as opposed to affected individuals, are relatively rare).

6.1 Possible Personal Harms of Enhancement

The possible concerns from such use are two-fold. First, are there health harms that may be experienced by those who misuse such drugs? Second, are there adverse social impacts of the wider use of such drugs (Farah; 2002)? Addiction may play a role in both of these concerns, since uncontrolled use may lead to problems with drugs similar to those that we already have experience with

Many drugs developed for medical use have side-effects, and these may be outweighed by the medical benefits of the drug (Hall *et al.*, 2004b). Are the benefits of enhanced cognitive ability to be measured in the same way? Furthermore, such neural enhancements modify a complex system, and may cause unforeseen long-term problems. Enhancement in early life, for example, of memory, could exaggerate declining capacities later in life (Farah and Wolpe, 2004). Psychopharmacological enhancements to remove unwanted memories that may present serious debilitating effects in the individual, may be possible; but what would the consequences be for wanted memories or brain functioning? Or should we individually value memories, regardless of their content, as part of what we are? Many people would want to eliminate traumatic or embarrassing memories. It is far from clear how such technologies would be

used, whether they would be beneficial or harmful, and what impact they would have on individuals and society. On the one hand, it may be useful to eliminate the memory of the horrors of war or sexual assault; on the other hand, it could be equally useful to eliminate the memory of some criminal activity so as to be able to lie more convincingly under oath (or brain scan!).

The NCB has argued that we should be concerned about 'medicalising' human behaviour (NCB, 2002: 135). As we saw earlier, the diagnosis of the risk of a type of disease related to drug misuse may lead to fatalistic behaviour; likewise, the novel reclassification of types of behaviour, such as 'shyness', may lead to a desire to correct one's predicament by using enhancing drugs.

A great deal has been written on questions of what it is to be human and whether enhancement alters this in some way (see Farah, 2002; Fukuyama, 2002). Concerns have been expressed that such an approach diverts attention away from the value of life and its natural imperfections (see Farah and Wolpe, 2004). It may alter our comprehension of our responsibilities and encourage us to think of our actions as chemical reactions in the brain, and regarding personal inadequacies or deviancy as imperfections to be fixed through chemical means. There are also questions of desert or merit. Is it justifiable to improve oneself through hard work, perhaps by exercise to improve blood flow to the brain, but not to achieve the same results by taking a drug?

Some argue that efforts to improve the capacities of the human species do not raise significant problems, since industrialisation and other periods of intense progress have also had this effect. Furthermore, it is argued, we have for some time used numerous substances, such as alcohol, tobacco and caffeine, to alter mood and capacities. Enhancers could also instigate change for the better if properly managed. People might achieve more by improving their concentration or cognition, and this may be compensated for in schools by changing the emphasis to understanding and problem solving over recall tests.

Perhaps it could be argued that we should intervene in some aspects of use such as sports, where the use of enhancement drugs is termed 'cheating'. But in this case, what is the real difference between sport and workplace or university competition? The drugs are designed in both cases to provide a competitive edge. Perhaps, then, we should control their use by some individuals, as we regulate the use of sports enhancement drugs. The most immediate candidates would be children, on the grounds that they may not fully understand the impact of drug misuse (not that we do, at least presently!), and that they have longer for the adverse effects to develop over time.[35]

Conversely, should we regulate the use of such drugs for some groups, for example, with those who work in situations where enhanced concentration may save lives, make action safer, or increase output? If neurological enhancement can improve performance in certain activities, and this makes them safer (in pilots or long-distance drivers, for example), is there an ethical imperative for regulators to insist on their use?

Perhaps tellingly, the new drugs of enhancement are already being seen in a negative way and there is resistance to their use in those who do not need them for some medical condition (Wolpe, 2002).[36] The main concern seems to be that such drug use may expose individuals to unexpected consequences, and that such problems will alter the very nature of being – the mind (Wolpe, 2002).

6.2 Possible Social Harms of Enhancement

A different kind of argument against enhancement is based on issues of justice and equality. This approach shifts our attention to the continuing inequalities in our society, and the potential for new forms of discrimination through unequal access to enhancements.

One question for policy is whether we should prohibit the use of such drugs on the basis of the harms–benefit calculus, or concede that, while there may be adverse effects in such drug use, it is the individual's responsibility to take these drugs appropriately (Caplan, 2002). There are others who could be forced into taking such drugs. Children may be a particular concern and we might need to question the wisdom of parents who think that giving such drugs to them is in their best interests. But it is possible that the haunting visions of the eugenics movements in the twentieth century drive such concern. Why separate self-development through education (which itself may be biased towards different sections of the community) from the use of biotechnology?

Another issue is a possible increase in social inequalities through enhancement technologies. It may be argued that such enhancement may be used to enable individuals to better deal with injustices and discomfort in the world, instead of doing something about them. Furthermore, public acceptance of enhancement may make it impossible to reject it, especially for, say, underperforming children or employees with dangerous jobs, or as a remedy for poor cognitive performance.

These inequalities already exist but that is not a compelling reason to defend coercion (Caplan, 2002, 2003). There are already medical interventions that are only universally available to those who can pay – for example, IVF treatment – and the only means to remove this inequality would be to make it universally available or prohibit it (Hall *et al.*, 2004b).

6.3 Herbal Remedies

A number of herbal drugs have been associated with neurological effects such as cognitive enhancement (Sehgal and Hall, 2002). Ginseng has been associated with memory improvement, while ginkgo biloba appears to improve the concentration of those who take it, although there are some questions concerning the experimental evidence (see Ernst, 2000, 2003; Farah *et al.*, 2004; Farah and Wolpe, 2004; Solomon *et al.*, 2002). Research into the effects of these drugs is leading to developments in their medical use for treatment in dementia and other brain-compromising illnesses.

These drugs can chemically alter the brain, and therefore behaviour, but they are not regulated in the same way as conventional pharmaceuticals. Despite the mixed evidence of their effectiveness, such drugs sell well, possibly because of folk belief about the greater safety of 'natural' neuroenhancements. They are not formally regulated or monitored for detrimental effects (Sehgal and Hall, 2002), despite evidence that they have, among other undesirable effects, addictive elements such as craving, overdose and withdrawal, especially after long-term use (Dean *et al.*, 2003; Garges, *et al.*, 1998; Sehgal and Hall, 2002).

One means of controlling drug use is to allow potential users to make informed decisions once they are aware of the risks. But this option is not possible if such drugs are not included in standard pharmacological tests and regulation. This is evidently a problem both for potential users and the medical professional, where questions regarding adverse effects have yet to filter through (Ernst, 2003; Shaw *et al.*, 1995).

6.4 Other Possible Social Consequences of Enhancement

Drugs of various kinds have always been used in human societies for a wide variety of non-medical purposes – as stimulants, social disinhibitors, aids to relaxation, and so on. It would be inappropriate to think of the new drugs, or of new ways of using drugs, purely negatively. However, our focus here has been on problem drug use. While allowing for this, we note that one consequence of the introduction of a new drug or way of using drugs can be the evolution of new social forms of life around this new 'social technology'. These new

forms of life may be seen as positive by some and negative by others, who perhaps fear that these new forms of life are disruptive of existing ways of life or social values. The current debate about enhancement technologies illustrates this tension very clearly, as does the debate about the non-medical merits and demerits of cannabis use (especially in the 1970s) and ecstasy (3,4-methylenedioxymethamphetamine (MDMA)) use in the early 1990s. We have very little evidence or plausible predictive social science that would allow a prospective moral assessment of new drugs as social technologies, and we can't do much more than draw attention to this rather different perspective. We are cautiously confident, however, that core values such as autonomy, avoidance of drug- (or drug-use-) related harm to others, and avoidance of drug dependency will remain central to future assessments of drugs and their uses.

7 CONCLUSIONS

Advances in treatment for addiction or mental health disorders are to be welcomed, whether through vaccinations or a greater understanding of genetics. However, the use of such advances must be balanced against certain key ethical questions.

This report has highlighted the ethical questions that arise from prominent developments in neuroscience, drug use and addiction. Such developments include vaccination against addictive drugs, screening for genetic factors influencing response to drugs or disposition to addictive behaviour, brain imaging, and the use of drugs to enhance human performance. We have concentrated on areas of worry, risk and concern, since these (in reality or in perception) are likely to drive regulation and public debate, unless there is, for each technology, some overwhelming or exciting benefit which captures the public imagination. The discussions that follow this report should raise the question: Which (if any) of the technologies now being developed in neuroscience can legitimately be put into practice and with what ethical limitations? The rapid development of new medical applications often raises specific anxieties, which in this report have been repeatedly highlighted as concerns for autonomy in individuals' capacities for self-determination (consent, confidentiality, and the like). This sometimes has the effect of overemphasising the idea that progress inevitably (or uncontrollably) leads to negative consequences, often at the cost of individual rights and freedoms for the benefit of society. It is therefore important for analysis of the issues to demonstrate that science is not necessarily going to be used for malign or discriminatory purposes. Indeed, there are benefits for individual rights, such as improved autonomy through better treatments and management of conditions, as well as knowledge of one's genetic susceptibilities. We have concentrated on drug-related (and more generally technology-related) harms, and specifically those related to the harms and risks of drug addiction, because our analysis is based on a liberal, human-rights-oriented framework of analysis, in which personal autonomy and avoidance of harm to (innocent) others are central.

We have throughout had to generalise, either because experimental detail is lacking, or more often, because of a lack of space. This leaves a number of questions to be asked about specific drugs of misuse.

First, we must assess the cost-effectiveness, and medical effectiveness of and, where necessary, compliance with, the interventions mentioned, in comparison with existing interventions and management strategies. Key to this ethical discussion are the different aspects of safety with regard to different neurochemical interventions.

Second, the issue of coercive treatment (for example, of vaccination against addiction as an alternative to harsher penalties) could raise serious issues about the balance of individual autonomy and social harm or benefit. Even if such imposed treatment were effective, it might be considered a serious violation of more basic human rights.

The choice of such interventions by an individual fully informed of the risks and benefits is quite a different matter ethically, and offering a treatment should not be ruled out. It may be highly effective as a means of clinically managing addiction, since consent in light of situational constraints may still be valid.

In most cases (except for clearly 'out of it' states or during periods of severe craving) an addict can still give real consent, ie weigh up the consequences of action or inaction. The difficulty would arise if an individual were forced to accept treatment, once addicted or to prevent addiction. It is unclear whether this would lead to demonstrable benefits for that person in the short term. There may be some longer-term benefits. For example, medical professionals may consider that a certain treatment would palliate an addiction, and this, in the long term, would be in the addict's interests. But would these long-term benefits justify measures to override autonomy from the perspective of best interests or public good? Under the present principles of medical ethics, the answer would probably be 'no', since the harms to self-determination would be considerable. Similarly, violating individual liberty rights for long-term social goals would rarely be supported by current norms of medical ethics. But medical ethics is only one perspective here, as we have noted above: public interests in public safety and criminal justice have also to be considered, although these are, if anything, even more controversial and open to political and ethical disagreement.

Third, as long as information on the health harms of certain drugs for enhancement is properly disseminated and understood[37] (which at present is perhaps not the case), some would dispute whether we should try to legislate against their personal use, though it may need regulation as we have for medicines and alcohol. They might argue that it is difficult to see how society can justifiably concentrate on limiting the actions of an individual to temporarily improve their cognitive capacity through artificial means, when existing, and more pressing, social inequalities exist.[38] And indeed, using neurological enhancement drugs may not differ substantially from other forms of 'mental' enhancement technology, such as education. Furthermore, safe means of temporarily enhancing one's cognitive abilities, including a remote risk of causing an addiction, may allow a person to expand what they can achieve in everyday life. This may not necessarily be a bad thing, since society can adapt to provide appropriate measures of management (for example, by modification of existing tests and exams). It may also make some human activities safer, although questions regarding the justification for choosing chemical rather than social mechanisms (eg reduced working hours to minimise fatigue) to achieve this effect should be addressed.

Finally, how is knowledge of a genetic susceptibility to addiction going to affect any one individual? These are issues for experimental and clinical physiology to address in detail.

Significantly, it will be difficult to inform each person with certainty what 'genetic susceptibility' actually amounts to; how their (change in) behaviour will alter the effects of a drug; and, indeed, how any drug will affect any one individual, given the different biological, chemical and neurological effects of the drug itself and its context. Such information, carefully managed and given to the patient, and responsibly used by that individual, could present significant advantages for our life choices. Equally, it could be burdensome to live with and hard to interpret for individuals and indeed for society. Careful evaluation is needed to study the social and personal impacts of new technologies, just as much as their technical and economic impacts.

NOTES

1. The functional study of neurology, including all component parts from the neurones, to the brain and central nervous system.

2. The autonomy of the addict enrolled in research may become of increased importance in discussions concerning their ability to consent to certain procedures, insofar as the thesis that 'addiction is a brain disease' comes to dominate research and public discourse on addiction. Such an understanding of addiction may constrain researchers' ability to undertake certain types of research, and the means to justify it, on, for example, persons who are still actively addicted or who have 'recovered' from addiction, and the ability for addicts to give free and informed consent (Charland, 2002).

3. Since the Human Rights Act 1998, it has become increasingly important to present issues of ethics in terms of legal rights. These rights are often vague expressions of intent, and it is the responsibility of the law courts to unpack their exact meaning for Government policy (McHarg, 1999).

4. Watershed declarations, such as those at Nuremberg and Helsinki, stress that the rights of individuals must not be detrimentally subordinated to the advancement of science, medicine or society (Capron, 1999).

5. The use of such medical interventions will rest significantly on the demonstration of their safety and efficiency. This presupposes that research studies evaluating such treatments can be done, since if it is accepted that drug addicts lack the capacity to give consent to participate in research, then forward progress on these lines may be in doubt.

6. Relapse rates in the first year of treatment of almost all drugs of addiction is of the order of 70 per cent (Hall and Carter 2002a, 2004; Nutt and Lingford-Hughes, 2004).

7. Either by 'mopping up' the drug from the blood by binding a blocking antibody to it (the antibody-drug complex cannot enter the brain, although the vaccine is only effective as long as there is enough of the antibody to bind); or by a catalytic antibody which moves to the brain and binds to the cocaine, stopping its effect on

the reward system. For a description of both approaches, see Nutt and Lingford-Hughes (2004). The use of such strategies on actively addicted people may be better termed as simple treatment, since the preventative aspect is lost.

8. The realistic use of vaccines may also depend on the quantity of the drug typically taken by an addict. For example, an alcohol vaccine may not work because of the sheer quantities typically taken (measured in grams of alcohol), because a vaccine will typically only mop up drug molecules on the basis of milligram doses. So they may be effective on drugs taken in smaller amounts, such as heroin, cocaine and nicotine.

9. The most effective way of helping tobacco users quit involves a combination of pharmacotherapy with advice and behavioural support (Coleman, 2004).

10. In the case of HIV, the possible stigmatising effects of the virus have led to mechanisms to preserve individuals' status. Express consent is required for testing for its presence in blood; and clinics that can preserve anonymity can be used by those at risk of exposure (Danziger, 1994; Worthington and Myers, 2003).

11. Nutt and Lingford-Hughes put relapse at about 70 per cent or more in the first years for the treatment of almost all drugs of addiction.

12. The National Institute for Health and Clinical Excellence (NICE) guidance for the prescription of anti-smoking drugs (nicotine replacement therapy) and bupropion (Zyban) recommends that repeat prescriptions for these drugs should only be given to addicts that show a commitment to quitting, with those who fail to demonstrate such a commitment having to wait for six months before trying again (NICE, 2002).

13. By tackling the problem of addiction, drug misuse will still be harmful to the individual. Other health harms, including death from experimenting with combinations of psychoactive substances, which is a significant and increasing cause of premature death, will remain a substantial concern.

14. There is anecdotal evidence that heroin dependence could be 'cured' within 24 hours using general anaesthesia and naltrexone. Similarly optimistic views are expressed in *The Heroin Century* (Carnwarth and Smith, 2002).

15. The question is how subtle coercion, which may be justified in limited circumstances (eg 'All education contains some element of persuasion, even if it is no more than persuading people to pay attention to the issues being discussed', Campbell, 1991: 22), differs from that which is aggressive to the point of being 'no option'. It is also important to note where the coercion originates, since, for example, that from a concerned family member or friend may differ in nature to that from the paternalistic intentions of the state.

16. We are only talking about criminal activities in which the harm caused is foreseeable and is a controllable effect of the crime, ie the addict knows or has good reason to believe that, through their criminal actions, it is likely that it will lead to the harms in question, and therefore it is within their power to prevent, or lessen the probability of their occurrence. A further distinction to make is that the crime is, more often than not, directly associated with the outcome (unlike drug use and possible criminal activity), in that there is often not an intervening action.

17. So-called 'victimless crime'. Indeed, a libertarian may argue that the freedom of the individual to pursue pleasure is a right that should not be challenged unless it conflicts with the well-being of other persons. Of course, it could be argued, as has been, that there is no such thing as victimless crime.

18. The 'alternative' here may be framed as 'rehabilitative' or 'treatment-oriented', as opposed to being 'punishment'. It may also be that the vaccine is 'offered' to offenders who are convicted of drug- or alcohol-related crimes even where

there is no evidence for addiction – for example, those convicted of drunk or drugged driving. Here, the emphasis is more clearly on retributive justice (punishment) and prevention of reoffending than on treatment for an illness. This may increase the stigma attached to use of the vaccine if it is seen mainly as a tool of criminal justice.

19. The law does not recognise that a prison environment may itself undermine an individual's freedom to give or refuse consent (Mason *et al.*, 2003: S1 0.74). Furthermore, in the field of medical law, consent to treatment from a competent adult obtained by coercion is invalid.

20. It may also be used to protect inmates or prevent drug use by inmates in prisons, where drug use is a significant problem. It is possible that vaccines could be used in institutions such as the armed forces, where problem drug use is a significant concern relative to the effectiveness of personnel on duty.

21. Assuming 'criminals' are not in control of their 'drug' consumption, therefore it should be 'treated', and not punished. But then, could criminal activities associated with drug consumption be considered as out of their control? Perhaps the distinction can be made that the consumption of a drug and the drug-related crime cannot be allowed to continue because of the harm caused, whereas sole drug consumption does not cause harm (there is no victim) except to the individual.

22. See the WHO's Health in Prisons Project homepage for comprehensive information. www.hipp-europe.org/resources/INDEX.HTM (accessed 23 May 2005).

23. Unless it is born alive, thus there is no civil action available to the foetus in the UK for its negligent death (while *in utero*, it remains a 'person-in-waiting') (Mason *et al.*, 2003: S5.31).

24. Parents already make choices 'on behalf' of their children that will affect their lives as adults, such as diet and education.

25. Although the increased intake to induce the 'high' may also be a financial deterrent to users (Nutt and Lingford-Hughes, 2004).

26. For example, with regard to addiction to tobacco, genes have been associated with increased likelihood of smoking, smoking more cigarettes, and a lower likelihood of stopping smoking (Hampton, 2004).

27. Genes have been associated with possible candidate diseases caused by tobacco, such as heart disease and cancer, and these have been associated with a smoking addiction. Additionally, there are presently a number of genes associated with specific forms of cancer. In some cases, changes in behaviour and medical interventions have been shown to reduce the chances of disease-related mortality (Hampton, 2004).

28. It has been argued that genotyping for known conditions is only justified when there is an effective intervention to prevent the disorder in those who possess the susceptibility genes (Hall *et al.*, 2002). At present, no effective interventions exist in the form of pharmacotherapy. However, a potential addiction or the risk of a disease caused by addiction may be avoided if the individual alters their behaviour or avoids exposure to a potentially addictive drug. This presents problems when the individual is in a position that means they can't avoid the drug, such as living in a deprived area where drug misuse may be more evident.

29. A study has shown the prevalence of both of these attitudes in nicotine use. Although individuals were more amenable to effective cessation methods, they put less importance on the use of willpower (Wright *et al.*, 2003). This underlines concerns that genetic risks are perceived as immutable, weakening the belief that changing behaviour will reduce risks (Marteau and Lerman, 2001).

30. An epidemiological 'risk' may be associated either directly or indirectly with addiction or drug-related diseases, but 'fixed' at birth (for example, sex or

ethnicity), or acquired during life, for example, exposure to the drug itself. In the case of addiction research, it will be a mixture of both elements that will be important, because a person can't become addicted to something they have neither taken nor been exposed to. This information would be of great importance in medical interventions, drug prescription and addiction.

31. French *et al.* (2004) analyse in detail the pros and cons of workplace testing in pre-employment screening and post-employment surveillance.

32. Slowing of the heart rate.

33. Including less serious conditions, for example, mild depression and various eating disorders (Farah and Wolpe, 2004). This also may lead to increased medicalisation of conditions not previously seen as needing 'treatment'.

34. But one must be sceptical of such claims of 'phantom epidemics', more often than not confined to the popular media.

35. It should be borne in mind that using neurological enhancement drugs might cause collateral damage to the brain. While, for example, we enhance memory, a side-effect may be impairment to, or trade-off with, another capacity.

36. And, again, to highlight the potential contradictions – marijuana is presently seen as harmful (hence the legalisation of its use) while there are potential medical benefits.

37. It is unlikely that all psychoactive drugs will be entirely safe, and they will always present some risk to certain users (Hall, 2004). Potential addiction is one such risk.

38. Indeed, a ban on such use may itself be more coercive in legally stopping others from enhancement, than the effect of the (possible) gradual social acceptance of drug enhancements.

References

Ashcroft, R.E. and Franey, C. (2004) Further ethical and social issues in using a cocaine vaccine: response to Hall and Carter. *J Med Ethics* 30: 341–343.

Ashworth, A. (2003) *Principles of criminal law,* 4th edition. Oxford: Oxford University Press.

Aust, R. and Condon, J. (2003) *Geographical variations in drug use: key findings from the 2001/2002 British Crime Survey.* London: Home Office.

Aust, R. and Smith, N. (2003) *Ethnicity and drug use: key findings from the 2001/2002 British Crime Survey.* London: Home Office.

Bosk, C. (2002) Obtaining voluntary consent for research in desperately ill patients. *Med Care* 40: Supplement V-64-V-68.

British Medical Association (BMA) (2001) *The medical profession and human rights: handbook for a changing agenda.* London: Zed Books and BMA.

Brownsword, R. (2003) Causes for concern and causes of action: a comment on 'pushing drugs'. *Washburn Law J* 42: 601–614.

Burke, W., Atkins, D., Gwinn, D., Guttmacher, A., Haddow, J., Lau, J., Palomaki, G., Press, N., Richards, C.S., Wideroff, L., and Wiesner, G.L. (2002) Genetic test evaluation: information needs of clinicians, policy makers, and the public. *Am J Epidemiol* 156: 311–318.

Cami, J. (2003) Drug addiction. *N Engl J Med* 349: 975–986.

Campbell, A.V. (1991) Education or indoctrination? The issues of autonomy in health education. In: S. Doxiadis (ed.), *Ethics in health care education.* Wiley: London.

Caplan, A. (2002) No-brainer: can we cope with the ethical ramifications of new knowledge of the human brain? In: S. Marcus (ed.), *Neuroethics: mapping the field.* New York: Dana Press: 95–106.

Caplan, A. (2003) Is better best? *Sci Am* 389: 84–85.

Capron, A. (1999) Ethical and human rights issues in research on mental disorders that may affect decision-making capacity. *N Engl J Med* 340: 1430–1434.

Carnwarth, T. and Smith, I. (2002) *The heroin century.* London: Routledge.

Carrera, M., Kaufmann, G.F., Mee, J.M., Meijler, M.M., Koob, G.F., and Janda, K.D. (2004) Treating cocaine addiction with viruses. *Proc Natl Acad Sci* 101: 10416–10421.

Centre for Cognitive Liberty and Ethics (CCLE). (2004) *Threats to cogitative liberty: pharmacotherapy and the future of the drug war.* Davis, California: CCLE.

Charland, L. (2002) Cynthia's dilemma: consenting to heroin prescription. *Am J Bioethics* 2: 37–47.

Cohen, P.J. (1997) Immunisation for prevention and treatment of cocaine abuse: legal and ethical implications. *Drug Alcohol Depend* 48: 167–174.

Cohen, P.J. (2002) Untreated addiction imposes an ethical bar to recruiting addicts for non-therapeutic studies of addictive drugs. *J Law Med Ethics* 30: 73–81.

Coleman, T. (2004) ABC of smoking cessation: use of simple and behavioural support. *BMJ* 328: 397–399.

Copeland, J. (1997) Barriers to formal treatment among women who self-managed change in addictive behaviours. *J Subst Abuse Treat* 14: 183–190.

Crabbe, J.C. and Phillips, T.J. (1998) Genetics of alcohol and other abused drugs. *Drug Alcohol Depend* 51: 61–71.

Crombag, H. and Robinson, T.E. (2004) Drugs, environment, brain and behaviour. *Curr Dir Psychological Sci* 13: 107–111.

Danziger, R. (1994) Discrimination against people with HIV and AIDS in Poland. *BMJ* 308: 1145–1147.

Darke, S. and Hall, W. (2003) Heroin overdose: Research and evidence-based intervention. *J Urban Health* 80: 189–200.

Dean, A., Moses, G., and Vernon, J. (2003) Suspected withdrawal syndrome after cessation of St. John's wort. *Annals Pharmacother* 37: 150.

Elliott, C. (2003) *Better than well: American medicine meets the American dream.* New York: W.W. Norton.

Ernst, E. (2000) Herbal medicines: where is the evidence? *BMJ* 321: 395–396.

Ernst, E. (2003) Herbal medicines put into context. *BMJ* 327: 881–882.

Farah, M. (2002) Emerging ethical issues in neuroscience. *Nat Neurosci* 5: 1123–1129.

Farah, M. and Wolpe, P. (2004) Monitoring and manipulating brain function: new neuroscience technologies and their ethical implications. *Hasting Centre Report* 43: 35–45.

Farah, M., Illes, J., Cook-Deegan, R., Gardner, H., Kandel, E., King, P., Parens, E., Sahakian, B., and Wolpe, P. (2004) Neurocognitive enhancement: what can we do and what should we do? *Nat Rev Neurosci* 5: 421–425.

French, M.T., Roebuck, M.C., and Alexandre, P.K. (2004) To test or not to test: do workplace drug testing programmes discourage employee drug use? *Soc Sci Res* 33: 45–63.

Fukuyama, F. (2002) *Our posthuman future: consequences of the biotechnology revolution.* New York: Farrar Straus and Giroux.

Garges, H., Varia, I., and Doraiswamy, M. (1998) Cardiac complications and delirium associated with valerian root withdrawal. *J Am Med Assoc* 280: 1566–1567.

Gems, D. (1999) Book reviews: the face of the future: enhancing human traits: ethical and social implications, edited by Erik Parens. *Nature* 397: 222–223.

Godding, V., Bonnier, C., Fiasse, L., Michel, M., Longueville, E., Lebecque, P., Robert, A., and Galanti, L. (2004) Does *in utero* exposure to heavy maternal smoking induce nicotine withdrawal symptoms in neonates? *Ped Res* 55: 645–651.

Hall, W. (2002) The prospect for immunotherapy in smoking cessation. *Lancet* 360: 1089–1091.

Hall, S. (2003) The quest for a smart pill. *Sci Am* 289: 36–45.

Hall, W. (2004) Feeling 'better than well'. *EMBO Reports* 5: 1–5.

Hall, W. and Carter, L. (2002) *Ethical issues in trialing and using a cocaine vaccine to treat and prevent cocaine addiction.* Technical Report No. 140. Executive Summary. National Drug and Alcohol Research Centre. NSW, Australia. Available at: www.ndarc.med.unsw.edu.au/ndarc.nsf/.

Hall, W. and Carter, L. (2004) Ethical issues in using a cocaine vaccine to treat and prevent cocaine abuse and dependence. *J Med Ethics* 30: 337–340.

Hall, W., Madden, P., and Lynskey, M. (2002). The genetics of tobacco use: methods, findings and policy implications. *Tob Control* 11: 119–124.

Hall, W., Carter, L., and Morley, K. (2003a) Addiction, neuroscience and ethics. *Addiction* 98: 867–870.

Hall, W., Carter, L., and Morley, K. (2003b) Addiction, ethics and freedom. *Addiction* 98: 873–874.

Hall, W., Carter, L., and Morley, K. (2004a) Neuroscience research on the addictions: a prospectus for future ethical and policy analysis. *Addict Behav* 29: 1481–1495.

Hall, W., Morley, K., and Lucke, J. (2004b) The prediction of disease risk in genomic medicine. *EMBO Reports* 5: (special issue) S22–S26.

Hampton, T. (2004) Genes harbour clues to addiction, recovery. *JAMA* 292: 321–322.

Hasman, A. and Holm, S. (2004) Nicotine conjugate vaccine: is there a right to a smoking future? *J Med Ethics* 30: 344–345.

Husak, D. (2004) The moral relevance of addiction. *Subst Use Misuse* 39: 399–436.

Kantak, K.M. (2003) Vaccines against drugs of abuse: a viable treatment option? *Drugs* 63: 341–352.

Kavanagh, D., Andrade, J., and May, J. (2004) Beating the urge: implications of research into substance-related desires. *Addict Behav* 29: 1359–1372.

Khan, K. (1999) Commentary: race, drugs and prevalence. *Int J Drug Policy* 10: 83–88.

Kleiman, M. (2003) The 'brain disease' idea, drug policy and research ethics. *Addiction* 98: 871–872.

Lavine, D. (2002) MR imaging of fetal central nervous system abnormalities. *Brain Cognition* 50: 432–448.

Lerman, C. and Niaura, R. (2002) Applying genetic approaches to the treatment of nicotine dependence. *Oncogene* 21: 7412–7420.

Leshner, A.I. (1997) Addiction is a brain disease and it matters. *Science* 278: 45–47.

Leshner, A.I. and Koob, G. (1999) Drugs of abuse and the brain. *Proc Assoc Am Phys* 111: 99–108.

Marteau, T. and Lerman, C. (2001) Genetic risk and behavioural change. *BMJ* 322: 1056–1059.

Mason, J., McCall Smith, R., and Laurie, G. (2003) *Law and medical ethics*, 6th edition. London: LexisNexis Butterworths.

McCrady, B. and Bux, D. (1999) Ethical issues in informed consent with substance abusers. *J Consult Clin Psychol* 67: 186–193.

McGregor, I. and Gallate, J. (2004) Rats on the grog: novel pharmacotherapies for alcohol craving. *Addict Behav* 29: 1341–1357.

McHarg, A. (1999) Reconciling human rights and the public interests: conceptual problems and doctrinal uncertainty in the jurisprudence of the European Court of Human Rights. *Modern Law Rev* 62: 671–696.

Mohn, A.R., Yao, W.D., and Caron, M.G. (2004) Genetic and genomic approaches to reward and addiction. *Neuropharmacology* 47 (Supplement 1): 101–110.

Morse, S. (2000) Hooked on hype: addiction and responsibility. *Law Philos* 19: 3–9.

Morse, S. (2004) Medicine and morals, craving and compulsion. *Subst Use Misuse* 39: 437–460.

Murry, T. (2004) Ethical issues in immunotherapies and depot medications for substance abuse. In: National Research Council and the Institute of Medicine of the National Academies, *New treatment for addiction: behavioural, ethical, legal, and social questions.* Washington: National Academies Press: 188–212.

National Research Council (NRC) and the Institute of Medicine of the National Academies (2004). *New treatments for addiction: behavioural, ethical, legal and social questions.* Washington, DC: National Academies Press.

National Institute for Clinical Excellence (NICE). (2002) *2002/021 – NICE recommends use of smoking cessation therapies: press release.* Thursday 11 April.

Nestler, E. and Landsman, D. (2001) Learning about addiction from the genome. *Nature* 409: 834–835.

Newman, R. (1974) Involuntary treatment for drug addiction. In: P.G. Bourne (ed.), *Addiction.* New York: Academic Press: 113–126.

Nuffield Council on Bioethics (NCB). (2002) *Genetics and human behaviour: the ethical context.* London: Nuffield Council on Bioethics.

Nuffield Council on Bioethics (NCB). (2003) *Pharmacogenetics: ethical issues.* London: Nuffield Council on Bioethics.

Nutt, D. (1997) The neurochemistry of addiction. *Hum Psychopharmacol* 12: S53–S58.

Nutt, D. and Lingford-Hughes, A. (2004) Infecting the brain to stop addiction? *Proc Nat Acad Sci* 101: 11193–11194.

O'Loughlin, J., Paradis, G., Kim, W., DiFranza, J., Meshefedjian, G., McMillan-Davey, E., Wong, S., Hanley, J., and Tyndale, R. (2004) Genetically decreased *CYP2A6* and the risk of tobacco dependence: a prospective study of novice smokers. *Tobacco Control* 13: 422–428.

O'Neill, O. (2002) *Autonomy and trust in bioethics* Cambridge: Cambridge University Press.

Richards, T. (2003a) Putting genetics in perspective. *BMJ* 322: 1005–1006.

Richards, T. (2003b) Three views of genetics: the enthusiast, the visionary, and the sceptic. *BMJ* 322: 1016–1017.

Ridgely, M., Iguchi, M., and Chiesa, J. (2004) The use of immunotherapies and sustained-release formulations in the treatment of drug addiction: will current law support coercion? In: National Research Council and the Institute of Medicine of the National Academies. *New treatment for addiction: behavioural, ethical, legal, and social questions.* Washington: National Academies Press: 173–187.

Risch, N., Burchard, E., Ziv, E., and Tang, H. (2002) Categorisation of humans in biochemical research: genes, race and disease. *Genome Biol* 3(7):comment2007.1–007.12: 1–12.

Roses, A. (2004) Pharmacogenetics and drug development: the path to safer and more effective drugs. *Nat Rev Genetics* 5: 645–656.

Rowland, A., Umbach, D., Stallone, L., Naftel, A., Bohlig, E., and Sandler, D. (2002) Prevalence of medication treatment for attention deficit hyperactivity disorder among elementary school children in Johnston County, North Carolina. *Am J Public Health* 92: 231–234.

Sehgal, A. and Hall, J. (2002) Herbal medicines: harmless or harmful? *Anaesthesia* 57: 947–948.

Shaw, D., Kolev, S., House, I., and Murray, V. (1995) Should herbal medicines be licensed? *BMJ* 311: 451–452.

Solomon, P., Adams, F., Silver, A., Zimmer, J., and DeVeaux, R. (2002) Ginkgo for memory enhancement: a randomised controlled trial. *J Am Med Assoc* 288: 835–840.

Sommerville, A. (2002) Commentary: is testing for HIV without consent justifiable? *BMJ* 325: 1226–1227.

Stevenson, D. and Goldworth, A. (2002) Ethical considerations in neuroimaging and its impact on decision-making for neonates. *Brain Cognition* 50: 449–454.

Strang, J., McCambridge, J., Best, D., Beswick, T., Bearn, J., Rees, S., and Gossop, M. (2003). Loss of tolerance and overdose mortality after inpatient opiate detoxification: follow-up study. *BMJ* 326: 959–960.

Ten, C. (2004) Crime and punishment. In: P. Singer (ed.), *A companion to ethics.* Oxford: Blackwell Publishing: 366–372.

Terrenoire, G. (1992) Huntington's disease and the ethics of genetic prediction. *J Med Ethics* 18: 75–78.

Thun, M., Henley, S., and Calle, E. (2002) Tobacco use and cancer: an epidemiologic perspective for geneticists. *Oncogene* 21: 7307–7325.

Tyndale, R.F. (2003) Genetics of alcohol and tobacco use in humans. *Ann Med* 35: 94–121.

Uhl, G.R. (2003) Are over-simplified views of addiction neuroscience providing too simplified ethical considerations? *Addiction* 98: 871–874.

Watson, G. (1999) Excusing addiction. *Law Philosophy* 19: 589–619.

Wolpe, R. (2002) Treatment, enhancement, and the ethics of neurotherapeutics. *Brain Cognition* 50: 387–395.

World Health Organisation (WHO). (2004) *Neuroscience of psychoactive substance use and dependence.* Geneva: WHO.

Worthington, C. and Myers, T. (2003) Factors underlying anxiety in HIV testing: risk perceptions, stigma, and the patient-provider power dynamic. *Qual Health Res* 13: 636–655.

Wright, A., Weinman, J., and Marteau, T. (2003) The impact of learning of a genetic predisposition to nicotine dependence: an analogue study. *Tobacco Control* 12: 227–230.

16

History and the Future of Psychoactive Substances

Virginia Berridge and Tim Hickman

1 EXECUTIVE SUMMARY

The psychoactive substances of the future and responses to them will be the inheritors of the past. The past is not 'another country'. It is predictive of the issues and responses of the future and their implications.

The future may be marked by greater consumerism and individualism and a more hedonistic culture, with rising consumption of drugs and alcohol, or by greater puritanism in society. Both trends are visible and one may counterbalance the other.

There will always be new drugs that emerge and are considered to be problematic and addictive. These substances, like morphine and cocaine in the nineteenth century, are often uncritically welcomed and are used as 'cures' for addiction or other medical conditions. These new problem drugs are likely to emerge through pharmaceutical innovation. How their use is viewed will depend on a range of factors far removed from the pharmacological effects of the substance itself. Such factors, their value and their implications should be reviewed as part of any risk assessment. The simple use of the concept of addiction to categorise these complex interactions may not always be helpful.

Drug effects are highly dependent on individual circumstances and expectations. In the past, there has been an absence of concern about drug effects that would now be termed addiction.

Lay assessment of drug effects and the balancing of different drugs is possible without formal professional intervention. Society's assessment of drug effects is conditioned by who is using the drug and the social threat such use is seen to pose.

Policy alone is not the answer, but must be carefully timed to fit with social acceptability and culture. There will be conflicting trends in policy, with liberal and punitive approaches coexisting and balances between them realigning over time. Stages of policy making may occur where different policies are appropriate, given different points in a process of cultural change. Such processes will interact with culture, and culture and policy will reinforce one another. There is cultural change over the last half century towards the reduced use of some legal substances such as tobacco, counterbalanced by a rise in other substance use. A balance of interests, for example, involving pressure groups and industry, should be retained in policy making in order to avoid 'over-destabilising' culture.

Restrictive policies can work, but they must fit with popular support and have support from economic interests. Clear scientific and media messages are also important.

The availability of replacement substances, under medical or lay control, plays a role in containing harmful use.

It is important to retain substances seen as problematic or addictive in the future within a normal market rather than a black-market model, which is much more difficult to regulate.

It is important to define what the interaction between policy and culture is intended to achieve. Harm can be amplified by greater restriction of those who continue to use. Cultural change can begin locally and can transfer to a national scale. Transferring models from one national culture into a different one is often inappropriate.

2 INTRODUCTION

Different societies have responded differently to psychoactive substances and the nature of those responses has changed over time. History offers us plenty of examples of the arrival of new substances and how their arrival was dealt with. It also offers us examples of successful containment of 'epidemics' of drug use, of the rise and fall of particular substances, and of changes in how the use of those substances has been conceptualised.

All these changes can be analysed and explained. Those explanations, and the shifting historical patterns of substance use and regulation, offer food for thought for an exercise which is aiming to illuminate possible future patterns. They offer an insight into how problems have been conceptualised and responded to, and what different mixes of regulation and culture have produced.

For this review we concentrate on three main substances – those regulated in western societies as illicit drugs (including the opiates, cannabis and cocaine); alcohol; and tobacco. They offer a range of issues for consideration which can then be applied to possible future developments (Berridge, 2001). We range widely in terms of time up to the near present and bring together historical examples of substances that are often considered separately.

3 WHAT WILL BE THE PSYCHOACTIVE SUBSTANCES OF THE FUTURE?

Undoubtedly there will be new psychoactive substances in the future. There are plenty of examples of new drugs (morphine, codeine and cocaine in the late nineteenth century, LSD in the 1940s, Valium in the 1960s, ecstasy in the 1990s) emerging from old ones through technological innovation. Throughout history, drug use has ebbed and flowed and different substances have been perceived as problems at different stages in time. These processes will continue in the future.

It is important to remember at the outset that new drugs, or new methods of use, or the involvement of different types of people seen as social threats, have never failed to arouse disproportionate attention from social and medical commentators. Some forms of drug use may arouse particular fear, while other allied forms arouse little comment, in part because the consumers are seen as less threatening. The association of drugs and race, for example, has a long history, which we discuss below. Such issues raise questions about who is defining a particular drug-using phenomenon and why. Concepts associated with drug use have changed and will continue to change over time. They are not timeless and value-free. The concept of addiction also has a history, changing both its compass and its given significance, according to the concerns of the society of the time.

Our point is that attitudes and responses towards psychoactive substances have been socially constructed. They are not, and never have been, direct reactions to unambiguously medical or pharmacological problems. In this section, we analyse some of the issues which have led to changing attitudes towards particular substances and how they have come to be seen as threats. We make a dual argument. On the one hand, it is clear that there were problems associated with the use of some of these substances; but, on the other hand, responses to those problems have been dependent on a range of factors far removed from the effects of the drugs themselves. The effects are also subject to mediation by social factors, as we will see in section 4.

Our key themes are:

- changing cultures of use
- the role of technology
- professional interests
- scientific theories and the concept of addiction
- economic interests
- internationalism.

3.1 Changing Cultures of Use

Culture and its change are an important dynamic. An apparent rise in consumption of a psychoactive substance, or a connection between its use and groups seen as threats to social order, can make the practice appear as a social problem. In the eighteenth and early nineteenth centuries, drink was built into the fabric of English social life. It played a part in nearly every public and private ceremony, commercial bargain and craft ritual. Paying wages in pubs was common. But such practices were less welcome in the context of a maturing industrialised economy that required more disciplined and time-aware workers (Burnett, 1999). Likewise, the use of opiates, which was also commonplace for both medical and non-medical reasons (the distinctions we would draw were absent then) was seen as more problematic when associated with the industrial working class, or with the Chinese in the docklands area of London in the late nineteenth century.

Who is seen as using drugs and how threatening those groups appear to be in the context of the time are important in defining which drugs are a 'problem'. There can also be the opposite effect, a lack of perceived threat when the problematic aspects of legal substances are played down to the detriment of users and families. The worldwide use of Valium, mainly by women, was a case in point. Current discussions of the balance of concern, and allocation of policy time and resources between the problems of illicit drug use and problems associated with legal substances such as alcohol and tobacco, indicate the strength of the 'fear factor' and its importance in looking to the future.

Problem definitions themselves have an impact on cultures and help to frame a process of cultural destabilisation. Opiates in the nineteenth century provide one example of this. Today there is much discussion of the 'normalisation' of drug use, but it is important to remember that, in the nineteenth century, using opiates was far more normal for the vast majority of the population than it is today. In more recent times, during the last 50 years, the culture of smoking in the UK and other countries such as the US has changed. In the late 1950s the Cabinet Secretary of the day, Norman Brook, was horrified that it might one day be considered inappropriate for the Prime Minister to smoke in public. Nowadays it would be unthinkable that Tony Blair would do so, or indeed would smoke at all. Smoking has moved from being a cross-class activity in the 1950s to one associated in policy terms today with lower social classes and with teenage mothers in particular (Berridge, 2003). Such processes of cultural change contribute to the definition of a problem.

3.2 The Role of Technology

Technical change can also lead to sudden changes in patterns of use. For the opiates, the advent of the alkaloids (morphine and codeine in the early nineteenth century) and of hypodermic medication led initially to the restriction of the mass market and a more medicalised model (Berridge, 1999; Musto, 1999; Courtwright, 2001a). Initially, medical enthusiasm for the new mode of injection was great. Dr Francis Anstie's enthusiastic welcome for the hypodermic injection of morphia in 1868 (quoted in Berridge, 1999: 141) has contemporary echoes in the enthusiastic welcome for 'safer' drugs with no 'addiction potential' today:

> ... it is certainly the fact that there is far less tendency with hypodermic than with gastric medication to rapid and large increase of the dose, when morphia is used for a long time together.

But because hypodermic administration was more under medical control, the usage of this form of the drug was more visible and fears of an epidemic of morphine injection consequently greater. For its time, the hypodermic administration of medication was very near the leading edge of medical innovation. But medicine was not modernising in a vacuum. Medical changes such as the increasing refinement of opium and the invention of the syringe were embedded in a society that was experiencing a host of other technological 'revolutions' (Howard-Jones, 1947). The addiction concept thus came to embody not simply concerns over the risks attendant in the hypodermic injection of morphine, but also much broader fears that humans might somehow become the slaves of their own technological innovation (Hickman, 2004).

For alcohol, technological change meant an amplification of the mass market and the ability to produce and market a standardised product. The advent of flue-cured tobacco and the Bonsack machine for the mass-produced cigarette led to market expansion. The chewing of coca leaves in South America caused little comment because there the substance was used as an aid to work and to help contain social problems. The isolation of alkaloid cocaine in the late nineteenth century and its importation into western societies was initially also seen within the 'aid to work' model. But medical enthusiasm for the new drug again led inexorably to fears of epidemic usage (Berridge, 1999).

So technological development can have a dual impact. It can expand usage of a particular substance, or it can be met with an over-optimistic welcome followed by a subsequent over-reaction to an apparent epidemic spread, which contributes to our process of 'problem definition'. Technology impacts in other ways too, in the development of new techniques for the production and dissemination of knowledge, which is discussed below.

3.3 Professional Interests

Professional interests also play a significant role in the process. In the nineteenth century, opium use did present problems. A large number of infants and adults died from opium overdoses, and opium poisoning was frequent because of the uncertain standardisation of the drug. But those who led concern over the use of the drug, in particular the public health movement and the medical and pharmacy professions, the latter leading the initial move for legal restrictions on its sale, also had professional motivations in view. The 1868 Pharmacy Act, for example, aimed to place sale of the drug (until then available over the counter) under pharmaceutical control. But its main aim was not to restrict sales so much that the profits of pharmacists were reduced. Britain had a system of pharmaceutical regulation of what would later be called 'dangerous drugs' at least until the First World War. As we will see later in this chapter, that system changed to a medico-penal one in the 1920s, a reflection of the influence of the medical profession, which had been establishing its professional authority since the 1850s (Berridge, 1999). The role of the American medical profession was weaker in comparison, only establishing its professional status in the early twentieth century. This difference affected approaches to drug control in both countries (Musto, 1999).

A more recent example of this process of professional influence in defining the nature of a problem comes with the changes in drug policy in Britain in the 1960s. Until then, drug addiction had been dealt with by a range of professional medical personnel, including those who ran private nursing homes and practices, general practitioners and NHS consultants. Much drug addiction (as it was then called) was dealt with within general practice. Drug users were typically middle-aged and middle class, often with some medical connection themselves. The expansion of drug use in the 1960s and the use of drugs by a younger and more hedonistic group led to two committees of enquiry and to the ultimate replacement in the late 1960s of this earlier system by one based in hospital drug dependence units and run by consultant NHS psychiatrists. By the late 1970s and early 1980s these specialists, based primarily in London, had introduced abstinence-based regimes (Stimson and Oppenheimer, 1982). This period is still controversial, but it has

been cogently argued that such professional interests, in the context of other changes, led to an amplification of the problem and helped create a drug 'black market'.

3.4 Scientific Theories

Scientific theories can also be seen in this dual light – of helping to explain and helping to amplify a problem. It is important to note that the addiction concept is animated by the play of two diametrically opposed meanings embedded in the definition of the word 'addiction' itself. These two senses of the word differ in how they assign responsibility for the condition's origin. The word 'addict' first appeared in English around 1529 as a legal adjective derived from the Latin *addictus* which, according to the *Oxford English Dictionary* (OED), meant to be assigned by decree, made over, bound, or devoted. In this sense, the word described the state of someone who was formally bound (to another) by a court of law. This definition was set against a second, reflexive sense that emphasised the volition of the defendant, rather than the strict sense of judicial assignment pronounced in the legal term. It thus meant 'to bind, attach, or devote oneself as a servant, disciple, or adherent (to any person or cause)' and also 'to devote, give up, or apply habitually to a practice' (OED 'addict'). Both of these meanings of the word are at play in the noun '(drug) addict'.

'Modern' theories of addiction go back only into the nineteenth or late eighteenth century. Their emergence used to be seen simply as 'medical progress', medical science gradually explaining behaviour which had previously been inexplicable. But historians have developed a more complex understanding of such developments which in turn throws light on the use of such concepts in contemporary policy.

Until the mid- and late-nineteenth century, the belief was strong in the medical profession that drink was good for you, and many medical preparations contained alcohol. Pharmacists often held alcohol licences. Drink was often prescribed, as hospital and infirmary records tell us. Regular drinking and opium-taking were seen as 'habits', not as addictions.

But at the same time, medical opinion hostile to alcohol was emerging – dating back at least to 1804 when Thomas Trotter published his *Essay, medical, philosophical and chemical on drunkenness*. Trotter, like Benjamin Rush in America, called the habit of drunkenness a disease, which should be managed by the discerning physician (Lender and Martin, 1987: 36–40). The US sociologist Harry Levine has ascribed these developments within the context of a broader shift in notions of the relationship between will and desire at the turn of the nineteenth century. Perhaps more importantly, Levine's work shows that the disease concept of habitual alcohol use, which he identifies as synonymous with the addiction concept, relied on broader social and cultural beliefs that had little to do with the pharmacological or social effects of drug use (Levine, 1978).

In Britain, the historian Roy Porter pointed out that the components of what were later to be determined addiction were around in the eighteenth century. But it was only later that structural changes in society made them significant. He identifies the rise of Evangelism and philanthropic lobbies, alliances with the nascent temperance movement, and the medicalisation of drunkards into alcoholics. Porter's work rightly stresses the importance of structural factors in making habitual use a significant concept. This is often forgotten by commentators who seek to trace discussion of addiction back into the sixteenth century or before. It is not that people did not discuss these ideas then, but the issues failed to attain social and medical significance (Porter, 1985). Why people choose to use such categories at one point in time and not at another is a central concern for our present argument.

At the end of the nineteenth century, these beliefs coalesced into a scientific specialism. In England, the Society for the Study and Cure of Inebriety was established in 1884 (Berridge, 1990). Such medical societies were established in other countries as well, including the United States. Drinking was a disease, initially the disease of inebriety and later that of addiction. This was, by the time of the First World War according to Sir William Collins, president of the Society:

> a disease of the will – if one may couple terms derived from the opposite poles of the material and the volitional – and assuredly a disease in which the individual possessed has in many instances a most essential cooperative influence in his own worsement or betterment.

Collins and his supporters were both doctors and temperance supporters. They hoped that their work would put the temperance cause on more 'scientific', and therefore firmer, ground. It is important to remember that their theories applied to the opiates as well as to alcohol.

Ideas about addiction changed over time. In the late nineteenth century, under eugenic influence, inebriety and addiction were seen as a hereditary condition. The Lamarckian idea of the 'inheritance of acquired characteristics' underpinned much discussion. The focus at this time was on the role of women and the impact on children through the transmission of the characteristics of drinking. These debates are revived, unconsciously it seems, in scientists' contemporary discussions of the transmission of genetic characteristics.

The 'alcoholic family' was a matter of concern in the late nineteenth and early twentieth centuries. It is important to locate such ideas and concepts in the context of the time. They were of particular prominence because of concern about Britain's future as an imperial power in the wake of the failures of the Boer War and the lack of physical fitness of the working-class population which had been revealed. There was concern about the 'future of the race'. Such concepts are rooted in political imperatives and situations and often fulfil a political role. Such formative influences should also be considered in the present.

Such hereditary ideas were seen as outmoded after the First World War. 'Addict' became the dominant name for an habitual drug user, or, someone who suffered from an 'addiction', at around this time. Again this change reflected structural factors rather than 'medical progress'. The fear of technology was amplified by the horrors of the First World War. Psychological emphases grew more common after the wartime development of interest in the neuroses. Their popularity was also related to a change in positioning of the psychiatric profession, which was moving out of the asylum to seek a middle-class clientele. Such theories assumed their greatest importance after the Second World War.

In the 1960s the concept of dependence was used to bridge the categories of addiction (with physical connotations) and habituation (mind). Theories of the mind and body were also linked in the practice of giving up. Such categories were reinforced through their elaboration and dissemination at the international level through the authority of the World Health Organisation, established in 1948. Psychologists disputed individual and collective psychology at this period and wondered whether there was such a thing as an 'addictive personality'. Today concepts of mind and body are coming together in a different way through the discipline of psychopharmacology.

Addiction is thus not a timeless concept but has been the outgrowth of changing interest groups and structures within societies. Some commentators have seen the function of the definition as one of medical surveillance (Valverde, 1998). Such analyses are illustrated by the example of substances not initially categorised as addictive.

Tobacco, for example, is a latecomer in this respect and the concept of addiction has only been significant (in the sense that Porter discussed addiction to alcohol) since the 1980s or 1990s. This can be related to a number of factors quite external to 'scientific progress'. Among them are: the different historical route taken by the scientific investigation of tobacco, through public health epidemiology rather than psychiatry; the closer linkages with primary care and psychology in the 1970s; the distance of such networks

from psychopharmacology; the differing role of the law; and different relationships with the industry. Again, structural and professional rationales determine the nature and timing of concepts.

More recently, there have been moves to extend the concept of addiction to include other activities such as shopping and eating and to see it as a feature of social dislocation within free-market economies. The increasing elasticity and diversity of the concept may make it less useful in the future.

Increasingly in the last few decades, policy has been framed within what is termed an 'evidence-based' format. As well as considering the rise, acceptance and expansion of addiction as a concept, we should also consider the role and diffusion of 'new knowledge' more generally about the impact of psychoactive drugs. For example, the postwar rise of risk-factor epidemiology (initially significant in relation to smoking and lung cancer) saw this method become part of the 'toolkit' of public health (Berridge, 2003). Such methods have influenced the development of measures of harm (for example, units of alcohol consumption) and facilitated the categorisation of populations into categories for intervention (Thom, 1999; Berridge and Thom, 1996).

3.5 Economic Positioning

Economic positioning is an important variable in deciding what counts as a problem and what does not. The historian David Courtwright points out that, at the turn of the twentieth century, the economic embedding of alcohol was considerable (Courtwright, 2001b). The alcohol industry had a size and fiscal importance in western nations that dominated economic and diplomatic affairs. The French alcohol industry affected the livelihoods of 4.5–5 million people, or roughly 13 per cent of the French population. At the same time, alcohol taxes were a bedrock of western government finance. The same was true for many colonial governments in Africa and Asia. Industrial interests, from the early twentieth century at least, were allied with political ones – the drink trade's connection with the Conservatives in Britain began after the People's Budget of 1909.

There was an emergent difference with the opiates. By the end of the nineteenth century, the pharmaceutical industry was becoming established. But in general, production and trade in opium products and coca was more confined. Poor nations and colonies in southeast Asia grew most of the opium. Peru and Java accounted for most of the coca. A handful of industrial nations manufactured morphine and cocaine. Germany was the world's major producer of cocaine, and Britain the main manufacturer of morphine. Both resisted international regulation just before the First World War, but through the Board of Trade rather than any political alliance. The economic and political embedding of cocaine was weak in comparison with that of alcohol and it was an easier candidate for restriction.

Economics affects the ways in which the use of different drugs is perceived. It also affects the ways in which the usage of different drugs spreads globally. Courtwright again speculates on why some substances have attained global status as items of consumption and as 'problems', while others have not. He traces a continuum of spread from local to regional to hemispheric and to worldwide use. Tobacco has had the most dramatic historical movement along the continuum over a period of centuries. But other substances have not made the transition. A world of betel juice and kava bars is now unlikely (Courtwright, 2001b: 65).

Plant drugs now have to compete with chemicals. In fact the stories of morphine and cocaine provide some of the earliest examples of the transition of plant to manufactured medicine. The more recent history of khat illustrates how a lack of technological innovation can impede the wider diffusion of a substance. The drug has to be imported weekly into the UK as it quickly loses its potency.

The introduction of synthetic drugs by multinational pharmaceutical companies provides a major economic incentive in the market today and these are inevitably seen as 'clean' alternatives to plants. Some will also translate into underground usage. Some of the earlier drugs in turn are shifting their markets into the developing world. Tobacco, heroin and alcohol all provide examples of this reverse process.

3.6 Internationalism

As the above discussion suggests, the perception of any given psychoactive substance as a problem has also been affected by over 500 years of globalisation. Internationalism remains a key feature of anti-substance alliances. The first international alcoholism congress was held in Paris in 1878. In 1906 the first international association on the subject was set up and located in Lausanne, where it still sits, now called the International Council on Alcohol and Addiction (ICAA)

But alcohol was never a serious candidate for international regulation. The closest approximation to international effort was in the African-based regional control arrangement arrived at between the parties to the General Brussels Act of 1889–90 and included in the anti-slavery provisions of the Act (Bruun et al., 1975).

Paradoxically it was the opiates – with the focus of anti-opium effort being overseas – which ended up with an international control system that has dominated and helped to determine systems of domestic regulation. The story is one of those strange historical conjunctures whereby an earlier draft regional system (set up by the Shanghai Opium Commission in 1909) was transmuted through American efforts, in their turn prompted both by missionary concerns and strategic imperatives, into a nascent worldwide system before the First World War (Berridge, 1999; Musto, 1999). Germany and Britain resisted, defending their trade interests in the manufacture of cocaine and morphine. But the post-war settlement saw these export controls imported into the peace settlement under the supervision of the League of Nations. In the interwar years, the international system operated simply as a trading control mechanism and defined the boundaries between medical and non-medical use.

As historians such as William McAllister (1999) have recently shown, that system of control of trade changed after the Second World War, again under US influence, into a strongly prohibitory regime whose impact continues to be felt in smuggling, illicit trade and domestic drug-control legislation. Control, as it changed, helped to create and amplify the problem.

The attraction of the profits to be made in the illicit drug trade have distorted the agricultural economies of countries such as Mexico, Peru and Afghanistan, where growing crops that are restricted in the rich countries of the first world has advantages. US drug policy has increasingly been marked by a willingness to intervene in the affairs of other countries and to demand the support of other 'drug-consuming' nations in achieving its goals. The involvement of the CIA in drug running in Vietnam or, more recently, US support for the Taliban's ban on opium cultivation in Afghanistan, reflects a process of globalisation and international control that is now nearly a century old (McCoy, 1972; Berridge, 2002).

4 WHAT ARE THE EFFECTS OF USING PSYCHOACTIVE SUBSTANCES?

The American psychiatrist Norman Zinberg (1984) famously stated that the effect of a particular drug was dependent on 'set and setting', ie the situation in which the drug was taken, the expectations of the user and so on. There were no intrinsic effects of substances, but much depended on the social situation of the user. To this, we add the historical dimension. The effects of particular drugs and the ways in which those effects are talked about will vary according to positioning in time.

If we look at opium as an example, this becomes very clear. As we have seen, the concept of addiction was not an important part of discussions of drug use in the early nineteenth century. Opium had the same pharmacological properties then as now, and what we would now call its addictive properties were discussed in great detail by Thomas De Quincey in his *Confessions of an English opium eater* in 1821. But this was met with little concern and aroused relatively little comment at the time. The setting within which such comments were published was not one where the elements of 'problem definition' we have discussed above had yet coalesced. De Quincey's writings were more significant in this way later on in the century.

In the nineteenth century the concern was for balancing good and bad effects. The overuse of drugs was seen as a bad habit, rather like overeating, and long-term use was of little concern. Dean Isaac Milner told the reformer of the slave trade, William Wilberforce, who had originally started taking opium in 1788 to relieve a stomach ulcer:

> Be not afraid of the habit of such medicine, the habit of growling guts is infinitely worse. There is nothing injurious to the constitution in the medicines and if you use them all your life there is no great harm. But paroxysms of laxity and pain leave permanent evil.

The distinction between what we would now term medical and non-medical usage and effects was not established at this stage. De Quincey, who used opium for its power 'over the grander and more shadowy world of dreams' had initially taken it to relieve the curse of toothache. Such origins of use and for continuation became a matter of debate between De Quincey and Samuel Taylor Coleridge. De Quincey claimed after Coleridge's death that the poet had taken opium not for medical reasons but as a source of luxurious sensations.

That these arguments could take place indicates that the historical setting of particular effects and how they are defined is important. Overtly recreational use was, at that time, largely confined to a small circle of Romantic writers and poets and generally disapproved of by respectable society, although no more than overindulgence in alcohol. In the public discussions of opiate use that did take place, for example, in the public health movement and the public enquiries of the 1840s and 1850s, the effects of opiates were often compared with those of alcohol. The passivity induced by opium was, it was argued, preferable to the violence and lack of control of the drunkard. Such views were related to the fears of the industrial working class brought about by urbanisation and the separation of classes (Berridge, 1999).

But, as well as the public discussion of different effects and their political rationale, there is evidence of self-moderation of consumption, of lay knowledge of effects and how to moderate them. This emerges in some accounts of opiate use in the Fenland area, where usage was particularly high in the nineteenth century because of the marshy and malarial nature of the land. A Dr Hunter, reporting to Sir John Simon of the Privy Council Office in 1863, wrote:

> A man who is setting about a hard job takes his pill as a preliminary, and many never take their beer without dropping a piece of opium into it. To meet the popular taste, but to the extreme inconvenience of strangers, narcotic agents are put into the beer by the brewers or sellers (quoted in Berridge, 1999: 40).

The perceived effects of drugs also varied according to who was seen to be using them. We have already discussed the connection between the effects of drug use and the industrial working class. Beliefs about drug effects also expressed the racial fears of the late nineteenth century. In the turn-of-the-century US, discussions of cocaine fitted strongly with formulations of racial difference. The widespread belief that cocaine use was a distinctive element in many African-American communities has been challenged by historians (Musto, 1999;

Spillane, 2000; Helmer, 1975), but thinking about the figure of the black cocaine user within its wider cultural context helps us to understand Dr Christopher Koch's 1914 claim that 'most of the attacks upon white women of the south . . . are the direct result of a cocain-crazed Negro brain' (Koch, 1914). Writers such as Koch were alarmed by the perception of a threat borne by black emancipation. Writers found in cocaine use a powerful figure for what they believed was the threat held by the new social reality of black freedom – the emancipation of a predatory 'brute' into free, white society.

Such views were the expression of wider fears and tensions in American society of the period. In Britain, fears about race were expressed differently, through the image of the threatening Chinese opium smoker in dockland areas, most notably the fog-shrouded East End of London. Such views, like the American perceptions, have been critiqued by historians and others have seen in them an orientalist discourse which had its origins with De Quincey (Berridge, 1999; Hickman, 2000). They were part of the expression of contemporary fears of the 'residuum' that might overwhelm society and also of the potential domestic legacy of Britain's empire. The racial issue and its connection with drugs was formulated and expressed differently in different national situations.

As well as race, gender and childhood have also been important factors in perceptions of drug effect. In the late nineteenth century, it was women who, in Britain and the US, were seen as particularly prone to the non-medical hypodermic injection of morphia (Campbell, 2000; Courtwright, 2001a). Women as mothers were also of concern for the movement against alcohol. Juvenile smoking was associated with the menace of the lower-class 'hooligan' who threatened the future of the nation (Welshman, 1996). Such fears of drug effects have their contemporary echoes in the media condemnation of 'laddette' culture or the fears of public disorder by young people under the influence of alcohol.

The legal setting has also influenced the effects of using drugs. It has helped to produce the sense that drug use somehow equates with social rebellion, and this has proved to be attractive to many people who feel a need to challenge what they see as the conventional boundaries of 'normal' society. Ironically, the vehemence of the antidrug crusaders has fuelled the drug use which has typified various countercultural movements, particularly in the twentieth century.

Narcotics have played a similar countercultural role ever since De Quincey suggested that drugs might offer a pathway out of the accepted intellectual conventions of his day. This idea has gained wider appeal as drugs drew ever more negative publicity in the second half of the twentieth century. Put another way, when Nancy Reagan exhorted American youth to 'just say no' to drugs, there was a sizeable minority who were eager to say 'yes, please', simply because Nancy Reagan said do the opposite. Fashionable, countercultural drug use has flourished in the setting produced by anti-drug programmes that have demonised drug use as immoral or antisocial and it remains attractive to many people today, something most recently demonstrated in the so-called 'heroin chic' fashion photography of the 1990s (Hickman, 2002). In Britain, the anti-heroin campaign posters of the mid-1980s made their way onto the bedroom walls of teenagers in Liverpool – the model became an icon rather than a warning.

5 WHAT MECHANISMS DO WE HAVE TO MANAGE THE USE OF PSYCHOACTIVE SUBSTANCES?

History provides many examples of the mechanisms that have been used to manage psychoactive substances. Societies and governments have responded to drug use in different ways. In this section, we briefly survey a number of case studies in which use of substances has been responded to

by different mechanisms. We focus primarily on those used by western governments, although we are aware that non-western and colonial governments have often used different forms of regulation from those in place at home (Mills, 2003; Newman, 1995; Dikotter et al., 2004).

Our case studies are:

- alcohol controls during the First World War
- prohibition in the US
- drug policy in the US and UK in the 1920s
- US soldiers returning from the Vietnam War in the 1970s
- drink driving in the UK
- decline in tobacco consumption since the 1970s
- the rise, fall and rise of cocaine use in the twentieth century
- alcohol policy in Russia in the 1980s and 1990s.

5.1 Alcohol Controls During the First World War

Although the 19th-century temperance movement had long called for controls on the sale of alcohol, a comprehensive strategy was adopted only during the First World War under the impact of wartime conditions. Munitions-makers and shipbuilders had complained that drunkenness was a cause of low productivity. The government set up the Central Control Board and this imposed a wide range of restrictions in 1915. These included reducing the hours of sale of alcohol (the afternoon closure), lowering the alcohol strength of some drinks and outlawing the sale of alcohol on credit. In some areas, for example in Gretna, the trade was brought under state control.

Beer and spirit production was reduced by half during the last years of the war. This was at a time when a wartime spirit prevailed and greater restrictions on personal freedom proved acceptable (Turner, 1980; Rose, 1973).

The impact of these changes is measurable through the decline in deaths from cirrhosis of the liver (Smart, 1974). These dropped dramatically after the restrictions were introduced, as did overall alcohol consumption and convictions for drunkenness among civilians in areas affected by the Board's controls and, indeed, outside them.

Other factors could also have affected these outcomes. Levels of drinking had been falling slowly since 1900 and remained low until after the Second World War. The depression of the 1930s and expanding alternative leisure activities also had an impact. But the restrictions on production and increases in price were clearly important. The Central Control Board did not long survive the war but its restrictions remained in place into the 1960s and consumption remained low.

5.2 Prohibition in the US

The case study of US prohibition is often used to support an argument that stringent restriction of psychoactive substances doesn't work and leads inevitably to the creation of a criminal black market.

The historians' assessment of the 'prohibition experiment' makes a different case (Tyrell, 1997). The 1920 Volstead Act was the outgrowth of earlier localised experiments in individual 'dry' states. It represented the interests of the older rural Protestant interests in American society, supported by industry and by women's campaigns. Prohibition was never a total ban and a complicated licensing system provided many loopholes. Sources of illicit alcohol soon appeared in the industrialised cities where the culture of drinking was much more entrenched (Lender and Martin, 1987).

But the effects of prohibition were remarkable. In the early 1920s, consumption dropped to about 30 per cent of pre-prohibition levels. In areas where there was public support for the laws, they were effectively enforced and patterns and forms of drinking changed. The old culture of the saloon with its heavy drinking ended, and new groups of drinkers such as women emerged. Spirit drinking rose.

Certainly prohibition did see the growth of a criminal black market and illegal speakeasies, but, by 1927, drinking was still only at two-thirds the level it had reached before the war. Prohibition came to an end not because it failed, but because of the advent of the Great Depression in 1929. The prospect of taxable revenues from alcohol was too much for the government to resist, and restriction appeared also to be outmoded.

5.3 Drug Policy in the US and the UK in the 1920s

Prohibition also had its impact on the development of drug control policy in the US and the UK in the 1920s. Here, the contrasting policy routes taken by the two countries are often used to point to a 'lesson from history'. American-style prohibition of drugs led to an amplification of the black market, while the British liberal and medical control system resulted in a 40-year 'calm' when drug problems were minimal. Again, the work of historians doesn't completely support these interpretations.

Controls were introduced just before the First World War in the US and just after the war in the UK. The operative factor was the existence of a new system of international control of drugs, given force by its incorporation in the Versailles peace settlement after the war. This international system was the outgrowth of US missionary and strategic concern about opiate use in the Far East. Controls at national level in the US came through the Harrison Narcotics Act of 1914, interpreted through legal decisions to implement a policy where maintenance on opiate and other drugs through a medical practitioner was forbidden (Musto, 1999). A large-scale criminal black market was a result and drug users were confined, often against their will, in treatment centres which were like prisons. As Courtwright has commented (2001a: 147), by 1940, the US addict population had been transformed: 'The secretive, female, morphine addict had given way to the hustling, mainlining male junkie'. But, Courtwright argues, the policy changes of the post-war years can't be given sole responsibility for this change. The decline in medically induced addiction had been marked before the 1914–18 war and the pattern of addiction was shifting. Legal changes had not been solely, or even primarily, responsible for the transformation of the addict population, and government policy simply succeeded in making a bad situation worse.

In Britain, the opposite occurred, at least ostensibly. The British medical profession was more powerful earlier than that of the US and was far more entrenched in the treatment of addiction. It stood firm against Home Office moves to introduce a US-style system which could see addiction stamped out. Home Office officials were also uncertain about the medical rationale for control practices and had to turn to the profession for validation of their policy approach. The Rolleston Committee on morphine and heroin addiction (1924–26) is often seen as having introduced a 'British system' of medical maintenance prescribing, which prevented the development of a black market and was widely commended by US observers of drug policy in the 1960s as a suitable model to follow.

The reality, again, was rather different. The 'British system' was continued in the 1920s because addict numbers were low and were mainly middle class and iatrogenic. The system reflected and did not create this addict profile. The 'British system' was the result and not the cause of Britain's lack of an addict problem for the next 40 years. The system was less medical than it seemed. What had been established was a mixed criminal justice and medical system of control in which the balance of power could alter as the pattern of addiction itself shifted, as it did in the 1960s (Berridge, 1996, 1999).

These two examples show us that policy changes do not have the immediate impact on patterns of drug use which commentators often suppose. In both the US and the UK, policy changes fitted into already existing patterns of changing drug use, both reflecting and reinforcing them.

5.4 US Soldiers Returning from the Vietnam War in the 1970s

The story of the epidemic of drug use among US soldiers in Vietnam which disappeared, or was replaced by less harmful forms of drug use, on their return to the US, is widely known through the work of Lee Robins. Wartime availability of cheap heroin in smokable or 'snuff' form led to a huge demand for the drug in the war zone. But, of those who returned home, within a year, only 5 per cent of those who had been addicted to opiates in Vietnam were still addicted. Nearly half the men who considered themselves addicted in Vietnam tried opiates after their return, but only 6 per cent became addicted again, and few received any treatment for their drug use. Many changed to safer forms of drug use on returning home, most notably the widespread use of cannabis (Robins, 1974, 1993).

The story of the Vietnam veterans illustrates the importance of the 'set and setting' thesis which we discussed in section 4. It demonstrates the significance of environmental impacts on patterns of drug use and of cultural norms and shows that many drug users are able to moderate patterns of use without formal interventions.

5.5 Drink Driving in the UK

The arrival of restrictions on drinking and driving in Britain in the 1960s and 1970s provides an example of the complexity of interactions within policy and with culture. As Greenaway has pointed out (2003: 166–174), there was a background of clear and mounting scientific evidence, backed up by policy change in other countries.

Public and media opinion pressed for action, although politicians remained cautious for some while. Sections of the drink industry were supportive since they had much to gain from improved standards in this area. The policy area was defined as road safety, where the tendency was for greater regulation, rather than drink, where the trend was for liberalisation. Pressure group input was important.

Regulation (although not random testing) was accompanied by large expenditure on anti-drink-driving publicity and by a significant decline in road casualties as a result of drink. Drink driving shows how regulation and culture can interact, with one feeding off the other. It also shows the importance, for an intervention, of how the area of concern is defined. Its definition as road safety rather than drink was at a time when society favoured a liberal approach to drinking.

5.6 Decline in Tobacco Consumption Since the 1970s

There has been a substantial reduction in the proportion of smokers in the UK population, from 51 per cent of men and 41 per cent of women in 1974 to 28 per cent and 26 per cent respectively in 1998. The number declined steadily throughout the 1970s and 1980s, levelling out in the 1990s. However, figures for the second half of the 1990s showed smoking falling again among both men and women.

A clear class gradient in smoking has developed since the 1970s, when smoking was a cross-class activity. In 1998, men who lived in 'unskilled manual' households were nearly three times as likely to smoke as those who lived in professional households. The trend has been particularly marked for women, where smoking and lone teenage mothers have been closely associated (Graham, 1987; Berridge, 2003).

The reasons for this decline are various. Government policy throughout the 1970s and into the 1980s pursued a twin-track approach. It worked with the tobacco and pharmaceutical industries to modify the product (safer smoking and tobacco substitutes), and its marketing (packet labelling) and to produce cleaner, more medicalised, supplies (nicotine replacement). It also helped to fund anti-tobacco pressure-group

activity (for example, by Action on Smoking and Health (ASH)) which gained a high media profile, and by raising taxes and mounting health education campaigns. Government pursued a policy balancing act which was successful in reducing the consumption of tobacco (Berridge, 2003).

In more recent times, prohibition has come onto the policy agenda through the advertising ban and smoking bans in pubs and open spaces. Government has felt able to introduce more stringent regulation as the normality of smoking and its cultural embedding has declined. This in turn will contribute to further decline and to the confirmation of a hard core of users, now increasingly defined as 'addicts'. These developments have been paralleled by an interesting counter-process, the apparent liberalisation (although this has been disputed) of the law on cannabis and the rise of cannabis smoking as a more culturally acceptable activity.

5.7 The Rise, Fall and Rise of Cocaine Use in the Twentieth Century

For our last two examples, we turn from 'success stories' to those where drug use has not been contained. Cocaine proves one example. As Musto (1999) has pointed out (also Courtwright, 2001b) cheap cocaine fed a global epidemic which lasted from the 1890s to the mid-1920s, with peaks in different nations at different times (Spillane, 2000). Medical and semi-medical usage was common at first, followed by a spread to the underworld where opium smoking and drinking were already common. The first two decades of the twentieth century were full of reports of increased cocaine use in the 'demi-monde'. Then in the late 1920s the epidemic subsided and world exports began to decline. As was the case with the opiates, the drug was scarce in Europe and the US at the outbreak of the Second World War. This is partly attributable to a generational learning pattern amongst physicians, but the drying up of supplies was also important (Courtwright, 2001a).

The rise of cocaine use from the late 1960s was associated with more abundant supply but was initially a matter only for middle-class whites in the US. The arrival of crack cocaine in 1985 saw cocaine acquire a reputation as a dangerous and addictive substance. Patterns of usage were important in this perception. Crack contributed to the problems of poor inner-city areas. But its usage by those already feared – poor immigrant and ethnic groups – contributed to its image.

The subsequent 'War on Drugs' policy followed by the Reagan Government in the 1980s saw a move away from treatment towards criminal sanctions, law enforcement and international control efforts. The number of Americans using drugs continued to decline in the 1980s and 1990s but the harm experienced by those who did use and by the rest of society was amplified. The supply of drugs remained plentiful and producer countries expanded their crops, while problem drug use increased in the US, as did the violence associated with the crack trade.

5.8 Alcohol Policy in Russia in the 1980s and 1990s

Alcohol consumption increased in the then Soviet Union from the 1960s. Interventions had little effect. In 1984, Mikhail Gorbachev introduced restrictions to limit the availability of alcohol and launched a mass campaign against drink. The campaign failed but it achieved some striking early success between 1984 and 1987. Fewer people died from alcohol-related causes, and life expectancy increased sharply for both sexes during that period.

But these successes were only temporary, and drinking and drink-related harm soon began to rise. As with US prohibition, the restrictions underpinned new patterns of drinking, with a rise in spirit consumption. The already-existing Russian black market was capable of supply and the later stages of the campaign coincided with a freeing up of the economy which reduced the state's

ability to control supply. The price of alcohol relative to other products fell, and alcohol became an item of barter in the developing black economy (White, 1996).

6 CONCLUSIONS

The case study examples lead us to some general conclusions about the means by which substance use can be reduced or managed. Change can come about through policies and interventions specifically directed at the perceived problem, but these must be carefully timed and must attune with social, economic and cultural change.

The belief that policies can deal with problems is common, in particular with discussions of drug policy which use historical examples. But policy alone has relatively little impact.

The prevalence of drug use often converges over time in countries with widely differing policies. The cultural context is of vital importance in reinforcing, or legitimating, forms of regulation. No British politician would have considered introducing smoking bans in the 1950s because of the political implications of introducing such a culturally and electorally unpopular measure. The example of Russian alcohol policy shows what happens to a policy without social and economic support. The drug policies credited with bringing about diverse effects in the US and UK in the 1920s were, in fact, building on already existing patterns of use.

We may be dealing with cycles of drug use which relate to broader issues beyond the impact of formal policies. The recent decline in tobacco use and rise in the use of cannabis may be a local example of this. In more distant history, similar processes were at work. As opiate use declined in China at the end of the nineteenth century, tobacco use began to rise (Cox, 2000).

Prohibition or strict regulation can work, at least initially, as the examples of US prohibition and the short-term results of Russian alcohol policy show. How one defines success in these circumstances is, of course, important. A total ban may reduce overall numbers of users but increase harms for those persisting in use, as did US policy on cocaine and other drugs in the 1980s and 1990s. The balance between different forms of intervention, between health and criminal justice approaches and the differing emphasis over time on one or the other seems to be the most common form of policy choice.

Culture and its change is a vital component in the equation. Policy, of course, reinforces culture but there are other engines of change. The combination of science, the media and health activism has certainly been important in the British context for smoking, bringing a 'tipping point' in which smoking has been increasingly seen as a deviant rather than normal activity. Whether that is a desirable result should also be part of the discussion of 'success'. Destabilising and redefining use and the user brings its own harms and potential dangers. Such processes of cultural change have typically been initiated by the middle class and framed with working-class consumers in mind, of which smoking offers the most recent example. There is often little understanding of working-class cultural norms, or they are seen as unacceptable.

The timing of interventions in relation to culture is also important, as the examples of Vietnam, drink driving and smoking demonstrate. Interventions of different types can be made, either before drugs are well established with extensive marketing networks, or, alternatively, when the process of cultural destabilisation is underway and resistance is likely to be less. And such sanctions, as the example of alcohol control in the First World War shows, must have the support of economic interests.

One can also see a staging of different forms of intervention dependent on the stages of culture reached. Where a drug is regulated, demand can more easily be influenced through taxation and the control of distribution.

The case studies also underline the importance of industry partnerships in these forms of regulation. Although public health interests are now often hostile to involvement with industry in harm-reduction strategies (there are current examples from the tobacco and alcohol fields), such strategies have brought public health and industry interests together in the past and have been seen to have advantages.

The availability of substitute drugs also affects the impact of policy. Cannabis use by Vietnam soldiers in the 1970s and the current availability of nicotine replacement therapy for smokers have both provided alternatives for users.

References

Berridge, V. (1990) The Society for the Study of Addiction, 1884–1988. *Br J Addict* 85(8): 985–1087.

Berridge, V. (1996) 'Stamping Out Addiction': the work of the Rolleston Committee, 1924–1926. In: G.E. Berrios and H. Freeman (eds), *150 years of British psychiatry, 1841–1991, Vol. II: the aftermath*. London: Athlone Press.

Berridge, V. (1999) *Opium and the people: opiate use in nineteenth and early twentieth century England* (enlarged edition). London: Free Association Books.

Berridge, V. (2001) Altered states: opium and tobacco compared. *Soc Res* 68(3): 655–675.

Berridge, V. (2002) Re-review of McCoy's The Politics of Heroin in S.E. Asia *Addiction* 97: 1615–1616.

Berridge, V. (2003) Post-war smoking policy in the UK and the redefinition of public health. *Twentieth-Century British History* 14(1): 61–82.

Berridge, V. and Thom, B. (1996) Research and policy: what determines the relationship? *Policy Stud* 17(1): 23–24.

Bruun, K., Pan, L., and Rexed, I. (1975) *The gentlemen's club: international control of drugs and alcohol*. Chicago and London: University of Chicago Press.

Burnett, J. (1999) *Liquid pleasures. A social history of drinks in modern Britain*. London: Routledge.

Campbell, N.D. (2000) *Using women: gender, drug policy, and social justice*. New York: Routledge.

Courtwright, D.T. (2001a) *Dark paradise: opiate addiction in America* (enlarged edition). Cambridge, Mass.: Harvard University Press.

Courtwright, D.T. (2001b) *Forces of habit: drugs and the making of the modern world*. Cambridge, Mass.: Harvard University Press.

Cox, H. (2000) *The global cigarette. Origins and evolution of British American Tobacco, 1880–1945.* Oxford: Oxford University Press.

Dikotter, F., Laamann, L., and Xun, Z. (2004) *Narcotic culture: a history of drugs in China.* London: Hurst & Co.

Graham, H. (1987) Women's smoking and family health. *Soc Sci Med* 25: 47–56.

Greenaway, J. (2003) *Drink and British politics since 1830.* Basingstoke: Palgrave.

Helmer, J. (1975) *Drugs and minority oppression.* New York: Seabury Press.

Hickman, T.A. (2000) Drugs and race in American culture: orientalism in the turn-of-the-century discourse of narcotic addiction. *Am Stud* 41(1): 71–91.

Hickman, T.A. (2002) Heroin chic: the visual culture of narcotic addiction. *Third Text* 16(June): 119–136.

Hickman, T.A. (2004) 'Mania Americana': narcotic addiction and modernity in the United States, 1870–1920. *J Am Hist* 90(4): 1269–1294.

Howard-Jones, N. (1947) A critical study of the origins and early development of hypodermic medication. *J Hist Med Allied Sci* 2(2): 201–249.

Koch, C. (1914) Quoted in this drug-endangered nation. *The Literary Digest* 48(11): 687.

Lender, M.E. and Martin, J.K. (1987) *Drinking in America: a history.* New York: The Free Press.

Levine, H.G. (1978) The discovery of addiction: changing conceptions of habitual drunkenness in America. *J Stud Alc* 39(1): 143–174.

McAllister, W. (1999) *Drug diplomacy in the twentieth century: an international history.* New York: Routledge.

McCoy, A.W. (1972) *The politics of heroin in southeast Asia.* New York: Harper and Row.

Mills, J.H. (2003) *Cannabis Britannica. Empire, trade and prohibition.* Oxford: Oxford University Press.

Musto, D.F. (1999) *The American disease: origins of narcotic control* (3rd edition). New York: Oxford University Press.

Newman, R. (1995) Opium smoking in late imperial China: a reconsideration. *Mod Asian Stud* 29(4): 765–794.

Porter, R. (1985) The drinking man's disease: the 'pre-history' of alcoholism in georgian Britain. *Br J Addict* 80: 383–396.

Robins, L. (1974) Drug use by US army enlisted men in Vietnam: a follow-up on their return home. *Am J Epidemiol* 99: 235–249.

Robins, L. (1993) Vietnam veterans' rapid recovery from heroin addiction: a fluke or normal expectation? *Addiction* 88: 1041–1054.

Rose, M. (1973) The success of social reform? The Central Control Board (Liquor Traffic) 1915–1921. In: M.R.D. Foot (ed.), *War and society.* London: Joseph Elek.

Smart, R. (1974) The effect of licensing restrictions during 1914–1918 on drunkenness and liver cirrhosis deaths in Britain. *Br J Addict* 64: 109–121.

Spillane, J. (2000) *Cocaine: from medical marvel to modern menace in the United States, 1884–1920.* Baltimore: Johns Hopkins University Press.

Stimson, G. and Oppenheimer, E. (1982) *Heroin addiction: treatment and control in Britain.* London: Tavistock.

Thom, B. (1999) *Dealing with drink. Alcohol and social policy: from treatment to management.* London: Free Association Books.

Turner, J. (1980) State purchase of the liquor trade in the First World War. *Hist J* 23: 589–615.

Tyrell, I. (1997) The US prohibition experiment: myths, history and implications. *Addiction* 92: 1405–1409.

Valverde, M. (1998) *Diseases of the will: alcohol and the dilemmas of freedom.* Cambridge: Cambridge University Press.

Welshman, J. (1996) Images of youth: the issue of juvenile smoking, 1880–1914. *Addiction* 91(9): 1379–1386.

White, S. (1996) *Russia goes dry. Alcohol, state and society.* Cambridge: Cambridge University Press.

Zinberg, N. (1984) *Drug set and setting: the basis for controlled intoxicant use.* New Haven: Yale University Press.

Life Histories and Narratives of Addiction

Brian Hurwitz, Caroline Tapping and Neil Vickers

1 EXECUTIVE SUMMARY

Addiction has a generally low profile in literature, but addictive themes are apparent in modern biography and memoirs and sometimes assume an organising role in extended narratives. Such works we term 'addiction narratives'. This study examines:

- what addiction narratives can tell us about the effects of using psychoactive addictive substances
- whether addiction narratives can tell us anything about the psychoactive substances of the future

- whether such narratives indicate which kinds of intervention might be successful in preventing addiction.

Because modern addiction narratives sit on the shoulders of earlier nineteenth-century literary models, we also describe these in the report. However, we pay special attention to modern narratives chosen from a sample of such narratives with the following selective considerations in mind:

- the need to cover a range of addictive substances and behaviours
- the requirement that narratives considered should offer a breadth of description
- sufficient complexity of self-analysis and retrospection to allow an in-depth reading
- the need to include a mixture of narrative types.

1.1 Findings

Our analysis finds that addiction supports great narrative versatility. Many addiction narratives conform to one of the three basic types of illness narrative as set out by Arthur Frank. But they neither exactly mirror nor objectively describe the social or natural worlds. Addiction as related in narrative is not the same as addiction lived and lived with. These narratives cannot therefore be analysed for clues to questions seeking predictive replies.

1.1.1 What are the Effects of Using Psychoactive Addictive Substances?

For nearly 200 years, encounters with opium have been consistent preoccupations of addiction narratives. A multiplicity of other substances and behaviours have come to the fore in the past 50 years.

Concerning the effects of using psychoactive substances, the accounts we have read constitute a rich repository of narratively framed experiences occurring as a result of drug ingestion. A dominant contemporary addiction story is the confessional narrative

of a sick self, one that requires treatment. Achieving health is the quest of many such addiction narratives.

The quest narrative – frequently a story of recovery – indicates that becoming healthy is dependent on perceiving addiction as an illness requiring treatment. As a consequence, recollections of pleasurable experiences do not feature regularly in these narratives. Furthermore, attachment to an addictive substance or activity is perceived as wrong, even as a sign of weakness. The quest to undo the illness and the affliction of addiction is seen as a spiritual endeavour in which the 'true' identity of the addict needs to be recovered. This (self-)treatment narrative may have relevance for future treatments, the Foresight Project's third question.

Many addiction narratives move beyond a strictly scientific view of addiction. The addict's illness is perceived as a psychological and emotional journey in which the sickness of the physical body gathers less significance. Addiction narratives inherently tend to moralise the experience of addictive processes, diminishing in the process consideration of the physical or physiological aspects of addiction.

Addiction to heroin is reflected on in many narratives as a method of redesiring the first, exhilarating hit, whereas addictions to alcohol, food and sex are perceived as ways of comforting and steadying selfhood. In accordance with many illness narratives, the physical body is read as an emotional being, a belief that is borrowed from the culture of popular psychology.

1.1.2 What will be the Psychoactive Substances of the Future?

Addiction accounts are predominantly retrospective reconstructions confined to following and interpreting rather than to anticipating trends. They cannot predict what the psychoactive substances of the future will be.

1.1.3 What Kinds of Intervention might be Successful in Preventing Addiction?

One of the most striking features of addiction narratives from a clinical point of view is their lack of interest in the part played by environmental factors in the formation of the addiction. Heroin addicts in treatment often report that they find it easier to cut down on or even give up the drug altogether when they go away from their normal environment because they are not constantly faced with people offering to supply them with drugs. The narratives we looked at suggest that writers of addiction narratives tend to downplay this aspect of addictive experience. This is but one instance of what might be termed the narrowing of context that afflicts many addicts. Unless viable healthy alternatives are on offer, the attractions of addiction can be huge – the disaffected unemployed youth on run-down housing estates has far fewer options than those with good access to education, secure parental support, adequate financial means and a pleasant environment.

What separates the addiction narrative from other contemporary illness narratives is its tendency to understand addiction as a spiritual affliction. Here, the addictive substance or activity is of less relevance: only when addicts have realised the burden of addiction, when they are at rock bottom, may they return to a state of spiritual well-being. This reflects the ethos of Alcoholics Anonymous (AA) and similar organisations. This approach has the advantage that it counteracts the popular notion that addiction can be overcome by 'willpower' alone. Its disadvantage is that it tends to downplay the agency of the addict in aligning themselves with forces of recovery or degradation. We need to build on the AA narrative, but to find language and models that can appeal to a wider audience – especially for those without strong religious leanings.

Addiction narratives might usefully form part of the National Curriculum and Healthy Schools Initiative as part of the safety rubric which includes as one of its strands 'Police Liaison and Drug and Alcohol Awareness'. Such tales could be read and discussed in class at a stage before teenagers become involved in drugs.[1] Among the texts considered here that might serve this purpose, we would highlight those written by teenagers, such as *Go ask Alice* and Joan Donlan's *I never saw the sun rise*. Further research is required before we can take a view on whether narratives can 'inoculate' young people against addiction. But, given the well-established importance of the peer group in shaping pre-teenage and teenage behaviour, it may be an avenue worth pursuing.

2 INTRODUCTION

The place of addiction in literature is tiny compared with that of, say, emotion, misfortune or illness. Yet addiction and addictive processes are becoming increasingly prominent in modern biography and memoirs and they also feature in extended narratives. This developing literary profile may reflect both the twentieth-century medicalisation and destigmatisation of addictive behaviours (Neve, 2005: 21), and the widening purview of a concept that is now claimed to have some applicability to a dizzying array of substances and human behaviours, including: alcohol, drugs, food, gambling, tranquillisers, stimulants, nicotine, caffeine, sugar, chocolate, water, sex, masturbation, television and video games, haste, work, shoplifting, self-induced epilepsy, self-mutilation, spending money, religiosity and fasting, overcompetitiveness and many kinds of compulsions to repeat activities (Elster, 1999: 52; Elster and Skog, 1999: 4).

The Foresight Review Team asked us to consider three questions relating to addiction:

- what are the effects of using addictive substances?
- what will be the psychoactive substances of the future?
- what kinds of intervention might be successful in preventing addiction?

These questions are addressed in detail in sections 7 and 8 of this report. We should state at the outset that we had to change the terms of the second question as neither the narratives considered nor narrative theory can contribute to answering it directly, though they can make observations about the cultural widening of addictive identities.

In addition to tackling questions posed by the Foresight team, this study has two additional aims. First, it describes the contribution that narrative theory might make to the study of addiction narratives. In broad terms, we find that narrative theory suggests that readers of narrative should be wary of taking addiction narratives at face value. Second, it reads a number of modern addiction narratives (published after 1950; see Appendix) through the lens of this theory. Although it is fairly easy to demonstrate biases in addiction narratives – they follow conventional literary patterns very consistently and often ignore scientific knowledge – we think nevertheless that they retain an exemplary importance in shaping popular conceptions and popular attitudes to addiction. On that account alone they merit study.

Modern addiction narratives sit on the shoulders of earlier nineteenth-century models which we describe in the report. But, because we are concerned with the cultural power of addiction narratives today, we pay special attention to modern narratives (section 8). However, it is not our intention to provide an exhaustive or a comprehensive history of the genre of addiction narrative and we would not wish to claim to have considered a formal representative sample of modern works falling into this genre.

We conclude by suggesting a range of addiction narratives that might be presented to schoolchildren which could be read and discussed in class at a stage before teenagers become involved in drugs. The aim would be to see whether narrative can 'inoculate' young people against addiction.

3 NARRATIVE THEORY

There are at least two major bodies of scholarship interested in narrative, the literary and the psychological. For the literary theorist, narrative might be defined as 'the relation of a sequence of events in time'.

3.1 Relation

The fact that narrative always involves relation or telling immediately confers on it a double character. The listener, spectator or reader must imagine not only the events that 'actually happened', they must also bear in mind the ways in which these are arranged in the telling. Some literary critics call the former the 'story' and the latter the 'plot'. The plot construes the story in a certain way. We do not have to accept the plot's construal. Indeed, it is far more usual for the reader to experience the plot as another 'level' of the story, distinct from their experience of the whole. But plot always offers at least the beginnings of an interpretation by giving our experience a shape distinct from the original, embodied in the 'story'.

3.2 Sequence

One aspect of plot that is especially relevant to this work of proto-interpretation is the sequence. For, as Dr Johnson was fond of saying, the sequence in which events occur can often make as strong an impression on us as the events themselves. Sequence determines the psychological process the reader goes through in living with the plot. Two bad events followed by a good one will usually make a different final impression on us from a good event followed by two bad ones. It is widely held that if a narrative is to hold our attention, plot and story must always at some level be at odds with one another and this end is often achieved by manipulating the sequence. Narrators often lead us to expect one kind of sequence only to introduce events in the story that imperil such expectations. Just as often, they generate secrets that are withheld at least until the end of the work, as for example when we discover at the end of an Agatha Christie thriller that the narrator was the murderer. Studies by the literary scholar Frank Kermode (1968) elucidate this point at length.

3.3 Events in Time

The temporal dimension of narrative is undoubtedly the most complex and the hardest to do justice to in a short summary. The most striking and influential claim is that made by the French philosopher Paul Ricoeur that we do not experience time at all directly or consistently (Ricoeur, 1984). The temporal markers on which narrative relies are second-order constructions that impose order on something which, at the time it was lived, was experienced as uneven and often vague. Of course, this does not stop us from telling each other stories about what happened to us, say, yesterday. But that alters nothing. Because telling always involves altering the sense of time (usually by making time much more definite), telling is a transformative experience. For Ricoeur and most literary theorists of narrative, to confer temporal unity on a sequence of events is by definition to give them a new coherence.

These three characteristics of narrative – relation, by means of its introduction of a second point of view or perspective or mode; sequence, by its management of our psychological response to both; and temporal markers and the peculiar definition they bring in combination with the other two characteristics – are proto-interpretative. They result in a transformation of facts. In a literary narrative, their interaction (along with other kinds of interpretative 'prompts' such as those supplied by allusion) will often form a significant part of the work's design. This theoretical account of narrative has the cautionary virtue of deterring the unwary from equating narrative with 'data' or even 'experiences'. Narrative is a device that reflects on and transforms data or

experiences. It should not be conflated with data or experience *tout court*.

The psychological account of narrative, the account that dominates the social sciences, has no major disagreements with the literary theory just sketched, though it values narrative on different grounds. The literary theorist of narrative is interested in narrative as a means of investigating literary structure and literariness. The psychologist is interested in narrative because of the particular constellation of mental competences it calls upon. When we think in narrative terms we engage our cognitive processes, our memory and especially our moral sympathies. We open ourselves up to multiple ways of seeing events. In the medical world, the most influential account of narrative is probably that of the American psychologist Jerome Bruner. Bruner (1999) argues that we relate to our lives as narratives, with meaning, not as ongoing phenomenological trains of experiences.

> A life is a work of art, probably the greatest one we produce. It is not simply art in the *living*. For we do not live our lives in any naked sense, save when we are caught aback and leave our faces behind. Rather, the art is in the *telling* – the telling after the fact to ourselves and others. But it is *not* a fiction, life, nor is it, for that matter, the real thing. It is some amalgam of the two – both theater and what theater's about.

It is this prospect that has paved the way for physicians' interest in narrative. It is now commonly claimed that through the study of narrative, the physician can better understand patients' stories of sickness and his or her own personal stake in medical practice. It is often further claimed that 'narrative conveys far better than any purely clinical account both the concrete particularity and the metaphorical richness of the predicaments of sick people and the challenges and rewards offered to their physicians' (Charon et al., 1995).

Narrative studies are still at a fairly early stage in their evolution. They have probably been applied most successfully to the structural analysis of fiction. Because narrative is held to be a human universal ('Man is a story-telling animal'; MacIntyre, 1981) it has recently attracted the attentions of cognitive psychologists such as Bruner. Since the 1980s, it has also been employed by some philosophers as a means of thinking about, responding to and evaluating our lives and the actions that compose it (see, for example, *Philosophical papers*, 2003). The paradigm that will be used in this study is the literary paradigm.

4 CONCEPT OF ADDICTION

Today addiction signifies a relationship of enslavement to non-essential substances or activities, characterised, subjectively, by craving (strong desires and intense longings) and the clear wish and inability to quit and, objectively, by tolerance, withdrawal syndromes and harm to health (Elster and Skog, 1999: 1–29). The modern meaning of addiction derives from a theory that links overwhelming desire for a substance (or activity), escalating ingestion of it, unpleasant and potentially harmful effects of withdrawal (implying dependency), and loss of moral and physical self-determination by habitués (addicts) (Iversen, 2001).

This cluster of psychic and behavioural inter-relationships first began to be delineated in the eighteenth century, in relation to substances such as opium, although some important elements of what was later to become a theory of addiction were identified earlier. For example, the Italian anatomist and physician, Fallopius, described tolerance in Persian opium-eaters in the first half of the sixteenth century (credited by Sonnedecker (1963) as the first such description), whereas the phenomenon of withdrawal is credited to the Reverend Dr John Jones's 1701 description:

> The Effects of a Sudden Leaving Off of Opium after a Long and Lavish Use Thereof [include] Great and even Intolerable Distresses, Anxieties and Depressions of

Spirits, which in a few days commonly ends in a most miserable death.

In the eighteenth century, these and other elements, including the effects of high dosage on individuals, began to be considered to be related, as a result of medical attempts to explain the protean effects of opium and alcohol on health.

The word 'addiction' has lexical and semantic roots in Roman law, where *addictin-em* referred to a formal giving over or forced surrender of a person to a master by sentence of a court. The term therefore has its origins in legal processes binding a person subserviently to another. In early modern usage, it also denoted voluntary placement under the control of another, and devotion to a cause as a servant or disciple: 'He addicted him selfe to neyther of them: but now he semed to incline to the Emperour' (*Oxford English Dictionary* (OED) *Online*, 1560) and 'True bishops should addict themselves to a particular flocke' (*OED Online,* 1621) are examples of this usage.

In the seventeenth century, the meaning of addiction included voluntary commitment to something that was beneficial. Thus, in 1667, the Secretary of the Royal Society, Henry Oldenburg, pleaded the importance of developing new tastes to ensure safer drinking water: 'If these men would addict their palats to the pure fountains, and not wander after every poluted stream', he opined that there would be less illness (*OED Online,* 1667). In the eighteenth century, these semantic elements were occasionally stretched to include freely entered-into commercial relations, hence in the economic sphere, 'addiction of goods' referred to their consignment to a buyer (*OED Online,* 1751).

Today, the attachment of a person to a substance or activity denoted by addiction is that of enslavement, whether imposed by judicial sentence or by ownership. But in the modern theory of addiction, the enslavement is rooted in processes of attraction, which arise, on the one hand, from within an individual (the addict) as a result of potent experience involving euphoria and dysphoria and, on the other, from weakness of will in relation to a substance or activity that is thereby said to have an addictive power.[1]

5 ADDICTION – ITS LITERARY DEPICTION IN THE NINETEENTH CENTURY

Until the 19th century, literary depictions of addiction were dominated by attitudes to alcohol. When De Quincey published the first version of his *Confessions of an English opium-eater* in 1821, he claimed to be bringing to public notice facts which were known only to a small but growing circle of those who relied on opium under pain of death. These people, whom posterity would recognise as addicts, even if De Quincey's contemporaries would not, were deprived of public sympathy for two reasons. The first was racial: opium-eating might have been thought a serious moral failing in Turks, but it was not viewed as such in the British who regarded themselves – from the renaissance until the middle of the eighteenth century – as immune from such a sensuous pursuit. The implication was that anyone, of any race, could give up taking opium if they chose to. Turks chose not to because they had no moral fibre. The same would not apply to Englishmen, or so the prejudice held.

Following the Gin Craze of the 1730s and 1740s, English society became alert to the dangers of alcohol. Roy Porter has put forward a convincing case to suggest that, by the middle of the eighteenth century, as a direct consequence of the Gin Craze and its catastrophic social effects on the urban poor, habitual drunkenness was seen as a physiological condition characterised by physical dependence on the poison in alcohol (Porter, 1985). Paradoxically, this very recognition meant that eighteenth-century Britons were slow to see the dangers of opium. They tended to be masked by the more visible effects of alcohol, as most opium addicts of the late eighteenth and early nineteenth centuries took their opium in the form of laudanum, grains of raw opium dissolved in brandy. The English habitual drunkard was thus seen as sharing something with the Turkish opium addict – having surrendered their moral faculties to the pursuit of pleasure.

De Quincey, it should be noted, did not set the record straight from a modern scientific standpoint. Indeed, the standing of his book owes much to the fact that it traces the addictive process to physiological infirmity (in his case, a predisposition to stomach trouble and facial neuralgia) and imaginative greatness. De Quincey goes out of his way to contrast his own use of opiates with that of Turks ('I question whether any Turk, of all that ever entered the Paradise of Opium-eaters, can have had half the pleasure I had') as he found that they generally lacked these characteristics. (The same convention underpins Samuel Taylor Coleridge's *Kubla Khan* (1798) the published preface to which, in 1816, invites the reader to see the paradisal visions as the effects of opium on the poet's mind. The poem was then subtitled 'A poet's reverie'.) De Quincey's refusal to anchor addiction in physical phenomena alone is one of the things that has assured his book a long posterity.

De Quincey's book enjoyed a mild *succès de scandale* for the rest of the century. But attitudes to addiction continued to be dominated by alcohol (Berridge, 2004). Although opium addicts made more regular appearances in fiction as the century went on, they were depicted for the most part as vicious and their living conditions as sordid. Opium addiction was cowardly and was often caused by an inability to face the pains of life. George Eliot's description of Molly, the secret first wife of Godfrey Cass in *Silas Marner* (1863) brings this aspect out well:

Molly knew that the cause of her dingy rags was not her husband's neglect, but the demon Opium to whom she was enslaved, body and soul, except in the lingering mother's tenderness that refused to give him her hungry child. She knew this well; and yet, in the moments of wretched unbenumbed consciousness, the sense of her want and degradation transformed itself continually into bitterness toward Godfrey. *He* was well off; and if she had her rights she would be well off too. The belief that he repented his marriage, and suffered from it, only aggravated her vindictiveness. Just and self-reproving thoughts do not come to us too thickly, even in the purest air and with the best lessons of heaven and earth; how should those white-winged delicate messengers make their way to Molly's poisoned chamber, inhabited by no higher memories than those of a barmaid's paradise of pink ribbons and gentlemen's jokes? (Chapter 12)

The ribbons and the jokes are emblems of the false hopes opium is intended to sustain.

Wilkie Collins's *The Moonstone* (1868) begins the process of rehabilitating the opium addict's moral character by emphasising the difference between the drug's effects and those of alcohol. The moonstone of the title is an enormous diamond that was given to an English girl, Rachel Verrinder, on her eighteenth birthday, only to be stolen. The thief is revealed as the heroine's cousin, Frank Betteridge, whose consumption of opium had led him into sleepwalking (the stone is quickly stolen from him in turn). Betteridge is an honest man with desperate, confused and almost dishonest intentions. As he explains to the narrator:

> For ten years past I have suffered from an incurable internal complaint. I don't disguise from you that I should have let the agony of it kill me long since, but for one last interest in life, which makes my existence of some importance to me still. I want to provide for a person – very dear to me – whom I shall never see again. My own little patrimony is hardly sufficient to make her independent of the world. The hope, if I could only live long enough, of increasing it to a certain sum, has impelled me to resist the disease by such palliative means as I could devise. The one effectual palliative in my case, is – opium. To that all-potent and all-merciful drug I am indebted for a

respite of many years from my sentence of death. But even the virtues of opium have their limit. The progress of the disease has gradually forced me from the use of opium to the abuse of it. I am feeling the penalty at last. My nervous system is shattered; my nights are nights of horror. The end is not far off now.

Notice how the abuse of opium here is credited to the worsening of an underlying disease and not to an addictive process. Collins's friend and patron, Charles Dickens, gives us an opium addict in his unfinished novel, *The mystery of Edwin Drood* (1870). This time, however, the addict is portrayed as sinister. The precentor of Rochester Cathedral, John Jasper, is the uncle of the novel's eponymous hero who falls in love with his nephew's fiancée, Rosa. Though outwardly kind, he foments enmity between Edwin and Neville Landless, another of Rosa's admirers. Edwin and Rosa break off their engagement and Edwin disappears, never to return. As with Collins's Mr Betteridge, Jasper seems to be divided against himself and it is unclear whether he is aware of the fact.

6 ILLNESS NARRATIVES

Personal stories that recall the experience of illness have been analysed by anthropologists and social scientists, who argue that the relationship between illness and narrative, and the way in which illness may be reconstructed through autobiography, offer important insights into changes in subjectivity accompanying physical disease (Williams, 1984). On this view, narrative offers a mode of expression for the autobiography of illness. A personal story or an interview may unravel and unburden the individual's changing relationship to the surrounding world as a result of sickness. A narrative of this kind reveals the 'experience' of illness (Frank, 1995; see also Hyden, 1997), and is an alternative account to the medical account of disease. For Arthur Frank, 'a published narrative of an illness is not the illness itself, but it can become the experience of the illness' (Frank, 1995: 22).

Such illness or recovery narratives tend to fall into three types:

- short narratives recorded as a result of interviews (often for analysis by social scientists)
- personal stories that form substantial, published textual narratives
- Internet first-person accounts of illness found on self-help or recovery websites and websites for charities.

This report is concerned primarily with the second of these, published, textual narratives that recall varying experiences of addiction. Whether, on the grounds that addiction is itself an illness, addiction narratives should be treated as illness narratives, will be considered in section 10.

6.1 Illness and Recovery Narratives

The nature of the autobiographical narrative that reveals illness, with respect to the process of recovery, has been previously explored and five different story types outlined: the Alcoholics Anonymous (AA) story, the growth story, the codependence story, the love story, and the mastery story (Hanninen and Koski-Jannes, 1999). The recovery narrative has also been delineated and understood as a method of constructing 'a non-addict identity' (McIntosh, 2000). Furthermore, teenage girls' stories about cigarette addiction elaborate additional narrative types designated 'invincibility', 'giving in' and 'unanticipated addiction' (Moffat and Johnson, 2001).

Arthur Frank's investigation into illness narratives is auto-ethnographic, anthropological and sociological. He does not necessarily treat the illness narrative as a literary narrative, but his understanding of the illness narrative incorporates the notion of storytelling, the organisation of plot, the physical body, and the relationship between the text and the sociological context of illness and health. He suggests that people tell their own particular stories, but in doing so they

draw on the narrative types that cultures make available, and he proposes three such narrative types:

- the restitution narrative
- the chaos narrative
- the quest narrative.

The restitution narrative is learnt from institutional stories in which good health is considered the norm and which tell us that illness can be cured. In the restitution narrative, the storyteller yearns to find again the body's predictability. Such narratives tend not to show the reader the 'struggles of the self' but rather let them witness the 'expertise of others' (Frank, 1995: 92). According to Frank, the chaos narrative is the opposite of the restitution narrative because it never imagines change or improvement to the physical body. The chaos illness narrative drowns in suffering, and may offer little or no narrative sequence or any sense of past or future. Through it, arguably, no 'self' can be told.

Many contemporary illness narratives fit the quest schema, in which illness becomes a journey replayed through the act of narration, where the ill person acts as a witness. Notably, the quest narrative features a change in character as a result of suffering endured through sickness. Physical symptoms, such as pain, are often written about in some depth in this narrative. Frank suggests three facets to the quest narrative (often these will be combined): the memoir, the manifesto and automythology. Of particular importance to the quest narrative is the manner in which the storyteller connects with their reader. An ethic of solidarity and commitment is expressed, whereby the author 'offers his voice to others, not to speak for them, but to speak *with* them as a fellow-sufferer' (Frank, 1995: 132); equally, the storyteller displays an ethic of inspiration as they demonstrate what may be accomplished in difficult times. Of the narratives examined in this report, Caroline Knapp's *Drinking: a love story*, Joan Donlan's *I never saw the sun rise: the diary of a recovering chemically dependent teenager*, Alfonsi and Pesnot's *Satan's needle: a true story*, Sue William Silverman's *Love sick: one woman's journey through sexual addiction*, and Margaret Bullitt-Jonas's *Holy hunger: a woman's journey from food addiction to spiritual fulfillment* follow the schema of the quest narrative. Not all Frank's typologies precisely fit the addiction narratives considered below. However, his directives provide the beginning of a framework for this report.

6.2 Selection of Narratives

To select the works for consideration, we undertook a keyword search using the terms 'first-hand account' and 'addiction' in DrugScope's database, 'Drugdata', which comprises 85 000 records of its library's holdings about drug use and policy in the UK. This threw up some 300 records, including articles and secondary literature, from which 130 first- and third-person narratives were identified (many other narratives in the original list were not relevant or were not first-person accounts). Those published after 1950 were considered and discussed by the researchers (see Appendix).

Selection criteria included:

- the need to cover a range of addictive substances and behaviours
- the requirement that narratives considered should offer a breadth of description
- sufficient complexity of self-analysis and retrospection to allow an in-depth reading
- the need to include a mixture of narrative types.

The selection finally made is inevitably somewhat arbitrary but offers, we believe, sufficient experiential depth, organisation and content to withstand and benefit from analysis (including aspects of craving, guilt, personal fragmentation and attempted withdrawals and treatments; see Table 17.1).

TABLE 17.1 Narratives selected for analysis.

Type of text	Number	Works selected and read
First-person accounts	10	Aldous Huxley, *The doors of perception* (1953) Henri Michaux, *Miserable miracle* (1956) Joan Donlan, *I never saw the sun rise: the diary of a recovering chemically dependent teenager* (1977) Caroline Knapp, *Drinking: a love story* (1996) Ann Marlowe, *How to stop time: heroin from A to Z* (1999) Margaret Bullitt-Jonas, *Holy hunger: a woman's journey from food addiction to spiritual fulfillment* (2000) John Moriarty, *Liquid lover: a memoir* (2001) Sue William Silverman, *Love sick: one woman's journey through sexual addiction* (2001) E.L. Seidner, *Hit me: the true story of 60 years in the life of a compulsive gambler* (2004) Richard Craze, *The voice of tobacco: a dedicated smoker's diary of not smoking* (2003)
Narratives by family members or observers	2	Philippe Alfonsi and Patrick Pesnot, *Satan's needle: a true story of drug addiction and cure* (1972) Vicki D. Greenleaf, *Women and cocaine: personal stories of addiction and recovery* (1989)
Autobiographical accounts under the guise of a novel	1	William Burroughs, *Junkie* (1953)

6.3 Narrative Framing

In considering any narrative account of addiction, a number of factors must be taken into account before generalisations can be made.

The first question that a narrative theorist is likely to ask is: what kind of relationship is this narrative trying to establish with its readers? Is it an attempt to contribute to science? Is it an addict's *apologia pro vita sua*? And, though it might seem a strange question to the scientist, what is the function of addiction in the narrative? De Quincey wrote his *Confessions* in order to vindicate a particular view of the development of the creative mind. Revealing the evils of habitual opium-eating was at best a secondary aim. His life supplies an example of the peculiar kind of development he is interested in and his addiction, he suggests, helped to throw this process into sharper relief. Many writers since De Quincey have used addiction for a similar purpose.

Bluntly stated, addiction is well suited to a certain sort of literary game. We think of it as an experience of such an overwhelming kind that we readily understand everything that happens in addiction narratives as being about addiction. Hidden in the narrative detail, however, there may be the lineaments of a revelation relating to something that has nothing to do with addiction per se but which turns out to be the major subject of the narrative. Very often that something is God or the imagination or, in the case of William Burroughs, a different way of experiencing and relating to the social world. The conclusion that narrative theorists draw from this is that addiction is, among other things, a resource of great narrative versatility. This is not to deny its terrible and real consequences in the world. It is to insist that addiction as related in narrative is not the same as addiction lived and lived with. Addiction in narrative provides an organising framework through which individuals can communicate all manner of experiences of the world. The reader who approaches addiction narratives with an eye to their 'constructedness' will not see them as naïve communications. In particular, they will be careful not to treat them as repositories of raw data from which a narrative of addiction is to be reconstructed (Williams, 1984).

A question we have asked of our texts is whether they are illness narratives. Not all the narratives we looked at took the form of illness narratives. But illness narratives necessarily take up a certain stance in relation to the reader. They involve a sick role, a role within the story defined and dominated by the experience of sickness and by others' reaction to it. In a first-person narrative, the sick role will be taken up by the narrator. In a third-person narrative, the sick role will still act as a prism through which critical ideas can be refracted and perhaps deflected. The sick role is, of course, full of narrative flexibility: it can be that of victim and it can be defiant ('you probably pity me but actually I'm thriving in ways you couldn't begin to imagine'); it can be mawkish; it can and often does provide a platform for evangelism ('I thank God that He exposed me to the tribulations of my disease, for having come through it I am surer than ever of His higher power; addiction was part of His plan for me, a process of personal revelation'). The sick person may offer themselves as a hero for the (often-healthy) reader, going through experiences that the reader has not had to go through first-hand. In a recent essay on illness narrative, the social scientist, Alan Radley, argued that illness narratives as a genre 'problematise life as a work of freedom' (Radley, 1999). By bringing us face to face with constraints on freedom in the shape of illness, they make us appreciate the freedom of being able-bodied, and search for new kinds of freedom in disability. We find this argument persuasive and think it holds true of the narrative accounts of addiction that we have considered.

The question of the kind of relationship that the narration seeks to establish with the reader can often be tempered by narrative atmosphere. One of the most remarkable features of popular confessional alcoholism narratives is their ability to reproduce the ethos of an AA meeting. The reader is to imagine himself or herself not as one of hundreds or thousands of readers but as a member of a small group hearing a harrowing tale in an intimate setting.

The narrative theorist will also be interested in the extent to which addiction narratives reflect the time they were written in. Changing perceptions of addiction alter what is at stake in presenting oneself as an addict. When the great literary addicts of the 19th century presented themselves to the world, they embraced opprobrium with the relish of true innovators. The stakes are now much lower in terms of damage to one's public reputation.

This is, in part, the result of the collapse of the distinction between addiction and compulsion. The word 'addiction' is now used in everyday English to refer to almost any compulsive behaviour. This is a recent development, dating only from the 1980s. The half-ironic term 'shop-a-holic' has given place to the more earnest 'shopping addiction'. The concept of sex addiction no longer meets the scepticism that would once have greeted it. If it would be going too far to say that 'we are all addicts of some sort now', it might safely be suggested that with so many mass-market addiction narratives in bookshops concerning so many different kinds of addiction, the moral costs of describing oneself as an addict (in a narrative, at least) have never been lower. This destigmatisation is probably a function of changing cultural perceptions of addiction, informed, to an extent, by the need to reconceptualise behaviour so apparently common and 'normal' and which medicine is beginning to be understood as nothing but a form of chemical misuse. Recall that, in the 1950s, half the population smoked.

Historically, addiction and compulsion were seen as distinct. Addictions always involved compulsion but not all compulsions were seen as addictions. In the medical world, the distinction has lost significance because of the ascendancy of the neurobiological theory of addiction. All addictive activities, it is claimed, enhance dopamine neurotransmission. As a result of this biological process, the addictive activity becomes invested with 'incentive salience' (the urge to do the addictive thing takes up an ever bigger share of our minds that, before long, we cannot bear not to do it); but in time, the pleasure once associated with the addictive activity ceases to matter to us because we will go to extraordinary lengths to engage in it. For the neurobiologist, however much the addict may rationalise the processes involved, they are always in the end the slave of a biological impulse. It is the biological process that holds together the constellation of behaviours that constitutes the addiction. If that biochemical matrix could somehow be taken away, the addictive behaviours would cease.

In popular culture, the distinction between addiction and compulsion does not weigh very heavily for a different reason. All of the main modes of popular culture are driven by narrative, and narrative moralises. It moralises because it seeks to invest life with meaning. For this reason, it has little use for the physical except as something to be transcended. We see this especially in mass market addiction narratives. The more an addiction narrative relies on the conventions of mass entertainment – tabloid reportage of the kind that supplies the tone of most popular books on addiction, or soap opera – the less likely it is to be preoccupied with the physical basis of addiction. When a football star brought down by drink or drugs writes a book about his experiences, he will typically explain his recourse to these in terms of 'battling demons'. This may not mean that he subscribes to a purely psychological account of his addiction. But in mass-market narrative, it is not uncommon for the physical to be glossed over using psychological shorthand.

Precis of the selected works are summarised in the Appendix.

7 ADDICTIONS OF THE PAST, PRESENT AND FUTURE

7.1 Psychoactive Substances of the Future, the Past and the Present

Contemporary reflections on addiction in narrative are not dominated by one substance, although personal accounts of addictions to opium have been consistently published for nearly 200 years. After Thomas De Quincey, Charles Baudelaire, Jean Cocteau and William Burroughs, the physiological and psychological effects of taking heroin have been recalled from a personal perspective in, for example, Alexander Trocchi's *Cain's book* (1963), Philippe Alfonsi and Patrick Pesnot's *Satan's needle: a true story of drug addiction and cure*, Eric Detzer's *Monkey on my back: the autobiography of a modern opium eater* (1988) and Ann Marlowe's *How to stop time: heroin from A to Z*.

Jack London's *John Barleycorn: memoirs of an alcoholic* (1913) is an early personal account of alcoholism. However, it is not strictly autobiographical and the narrative is difficult to classify generically. (Crowley (1994) suggests the narrative sits somewhere between fictionalised autobiography and autobiographical fiction.) There have been many authors in the twentieth century who have experienced problems with alcohol (Eugene O'Neill, F. Scott Fitzgerald, Ernest Hemingway, Tennessee Williams and Jack Kerouac, to name but a sample), but few early narratives from a personal perspective exist. Early examples of shorter, personal narratives have been published in *The big book* for Alcoholics Anonymous, and Billie Holiday's ghost-written autobiography, *Lady sings the blues* (1956), which documents the performer's difficult relationships with alcohol and drugs. Perceiving alcohol addiction as an illness that requires unburdening and reflecting on in narrative form is a recent development, which arguably has been encouraged by the growth of AA. The publication of narratives such as Caroline Knapp's *Drinking: a love story*, John Moriarty's *Liquid lover: a memoir*, Nick Johnstone's *A head full of blue* (2002), John Sutherland's *Last drink to LA*, James Frey's *A million little pieces* (2003) and the earlier confessional narrative by Rosie Boycott, *A nice girl like me: a story of the seventies* (1985), suggests that addictions to alcohol desire the therapeutic act of narration.

Encounters with mescaline have been reflected on in the past by Huxley and Michaux. Personal experiences of cocaine addiction have been commented on in Vicki D. Greenleaf's *Women and cocaine: personal stories of addiction and recovery* and Katy Hendrick's *The party's over: diary of a recovering cocaine addict* (1992). Two early narratives, Joan Donlan's *I never saw the sun rise* and *Go ask Alice* (Anonymous, 1972) reorganise the personal experiences of taking LSD and speed. Olivia Gordon's *The agony of ecstasy* (2004) is a recent memoir considering ecstasy addiction and Elizabeth Wurtzel has reflected on her addiction to Ritalin in *More, now, again: a memoir* (2002).

7.2 Behavioural Addictions

Until recently, behavioural addictions were absent from narrative accounts and, even now, extended gambling and smoking narratives remain rare, despite many invitations for shorter confessionals on websites. The emergence of narratives recalling and reflecting on a persistent attachment to food or sex (Margaret Bullitt-Jonas's *Holy hunger: a woman's journey from food addiction to spiritual fulfillment* and Sue William Silverman's *Love sick: one woman's journey through sexual addiction*) marks a shift in the portrayal of the addict identity. The focus on the particular addictive behaviour is of less significance than the drug 'chosen' in the case of substance-misuse narratives, behavioural addiction being portrayed in these narratives as an overwhelming sickness that is not determined by the specific object of attachment. Personal experiences of behavioural addiction look set to continue to be reflected on in narrative in the future.

7.3 The Effects of Psychoactive Substances, the Motivations for Taking Psychoactive Substances and the Addict's Perception of Addiction

Confessional narrative is the most common form of narrative in which contemporary, personal experience of illness is reflected on. This narrative may take the form of the memoir, following the quest and recovery, chaos and/or restitution formats. These can encompass many forms of illness experience, including mental health problems, sexual abuse, physical disease and addiction. The narratorial or authorial motivation behind the publication of a confessional narrative is occasionally implied in the text and, when this occurs, the author frequently wishes to convey to readers an ethic of solidarity with fellow sufferers, with the aim of helping them to understand their own experiences.

For the confessional addiction narrative, realising one's identity as an addict (both during the illness and in recovery) is essential to the story. Through the publication of the self-story, the author inevitably 'comes out' as an addict, recalling the self-help ethic of AA. The confessional narrative is also influenced by popular psychology in which self-help seems to lead to peace and 'inner strength'.

Narrative accounts confirm that addiction expresses powerful attachment to a substance or activity. The addiction narrative tends also to reflect on and transform the experience of this attachment, reordering, in many cases, the complex relationship between addict and substance or activity. The subjective experience of addiction is frequently implied through the identity of the addict in the narrative, conveying how the self (both sober and addicted) negotiates its relationship to the outside world.

7.3.1 Self-medication and Self-therapy

The confessional self-story embarks on a quest to make sense of some parts of the addictive encounter, notably from a psychological perspective. Not all the recovery narratives will necessarily fulfil the quest, but attempts will often be made to understand both the immediate and long-term emotional effects of the substances. In the quest and recovery narrative, attachment to an addictive substance or activity may be viewed as a method of steadying and assuring selfhood. The addict's relationship to others is incomplete or without foundation, and they seek confirmation of identity from outside the self. At least this is how the narrator and addict understands addiction as a result of reflecting on their experience in narrative form. For Caroline Knapp, Margaret Bullitt-Jonas and John Moriarty, the failure to attain some sense of a coherent self begins in childhood. Attaching oneself to something outside the body is learnt at an early age.

When the recovered addict transforms the addictive encounter into narrative, the physiological aspects of addiction diminish in significance. Although addiction narratives occasionally offer descriptions of withdrawal or the unpleasant effects of the addictive substance on the body, these are overwhelmed by the quest to understand the psychological effects of the substance. Addiction is primarily understood as an emotional journey. Knapp notes the immediately therapeutic properties of alcohol ('Liquor soothes and protects, a psychic balm'; Knapp, 1996: 59) and she also implies that alcohol may be used to temporarily fill an emotional hollow or to fulfil an emotional state, thereby allowing a sense of completeness: 'Fill it up, fill it up, fill it up. Fill up the emptiness' (Knapp, 1996: 56).

Feelings of comfort and numbness postpone feelings of anxiety. Bullitt-Jonas recognises the sedative effects of binge eating: 'A binge often began with an angry mind, but by the end of the binge, the anger would be comfortably cloaked and soothed'

(Bullitt-Jonas, 2000: 63). Yvonne, one of the addicts interviewed by Greenleaf, believes that cocaine helped in the management of anxiety: 'I thought I wasn't worth anything, and the anxiety that brought had to be medicated' (Greenleaf, 1989: 57). Yet, attempting self-medication is conceived as pointless by the recovered addict, although achieving a temporary sense of well-being was once desperately important: 'Feed me until I feel better. Feed my hungry heart until I feel better' (Silverman, 2001). For the recovered addict, self-medication is wrong and it is an excessive, unnecessary desire. Perhaps the most misguided effort to assure selfhood is enacted by the narrator of Silverman's *Love sick* – her attachment to men defines her addict identity. She is able only to conceptualise her existence through having sex with others: 'I fuck therefore I am' (Silverman, 2001). The recovery narrative considers an attachment of this kind false. Recovering from such an addiction requires a heroic quest to discover and accept the identity that was once masked.

7.3.2 Re-desiring the First Hit

Mescaline has the power immediately to alter the sober, subjective experiences of time and space. Huxley's (1953) account of his psychological experiment is helpful here, since his encounter has not been refashioned through the recovery quest: 'Space was still; but it had lost its predominance. The mind was primarily concerned, not with measures and locations, but with being and meaning' (p. 9). As a result of ingesting mescaline, he is able to move beyond the construct of his own subjectivity:

> The other world to which mescaline admitted me was not the world of visions: it existed out there, in what I could see with my eyes open. The great change was in the realm of objective fact. What happened to my subjective universe was relatively unimportant to (p. 6).

His perceptions of colours also increase: 'lapis lazuli books whose colour was so

intense, so intrinsically meaningful, that they seemed to be on the point of leaving the shelves to thrust themselves more insistently on my attention'.

Such examples demonstrate the powers of mescaline to change the surrounding landscape, transforming the ordinary into a more appealing experience. Mescaline and heroin allow the addict to experience existence in a fresh way: 'Without hero, without opium', Pascale's senses are paralysed, 'I am a wall. I am doors. I am bars' (Alfonsi and Pesnot, 1972: 31). After injecting heroin, she recalls intense hallucinations:

> I lit a cigarette ... Swallowed the smoke, holding it deep in my lungs. Its taste increased tenfold, hundredfold! I was lying on the bed. No, in a field, grass all around me, soft, gentle grass. I stretched voluptuously. My legs and arms sank into the wild grass. And what flowers! (p. 58)

One way of appreciating addiction is to recognise the desire for escape: the addict continues to return to a place that appears more peaceful, more spiritual, or more intense.

Yet the effects produced by heroin contrast with the personal experiences of alcohol offered in the recovery narratives. Heroin may offer a 'new' euphoric experience – 'My whole body quivered with pleasure. Tiny needles danced on my skin' (Alfonsi and Pesnot, 1972: 58)[2] – and Marlowe (1999: 18) is not ashamed to express heroin-induced pleasurable experiences:

> There is this moment of exultation just when the dope hits your bloodstream, and you feel so good you have to share it, so you talk, you talk as you have never talked before ...

However, the 'first hit' of alcohol does not produce the same exhilaration, and neither does it necessarily offer access to a new sense of being. Alcoholism masks, displaces, or destroys feelings: 'I was drinking every night, drinking to get drunk, to obliterate' (Knapp, 1996: 49). Heroin is perceived by the addict as a substance that may block out or reduce sober experiences ('Heroin allows you to experience your feelings as feeble, remote and even pitiable little phenomena, rather than the frighteningly overwhelming experiences you may have known before'; Marlowe, 1999: 129), but it also achieves a new one in the process.

The repeated desire for heroin is, Marlowe suggests, an attempt at rediscovering the first 'hit'. Marlowe's narrative is not primarily a story of recovery in which Frank's quest is journeyed; in fact it works against such a form, both in its narrative content and structure. The narrative continues to return to one particular event, the first time the author took heroin:

> The initial highs did feel better than the drug will ever make you feel again (p. 9).
>
> The only problem is, the wonderful First Time becomes more and more difficult to recapture, even with a larger amount of dope (p. 59).

The narrative repeats and acknowledges the 'first time', recognising that its beauty is also its disappointment, and the first experience is lost for ever. Although Marlowe grapples with her own addict identity, heroin fascinates her and ultimately disappoints her: 'The chemistry of the drug is ruthless: it is designed to disappoint you' (p. 9). Desire for the initial 'hit' remains the basis for her addiction, as she understands it.[3]

7.4 Addiction as Illness

The addict is a sick identity in the quest recovery narratives (*I never saw the sun rise, drinking: a love story, holy hunger, hit me* and *love sick*). These narratives organise past experiences of addiction from the point of recovery. Caroline Knapp's *Drinking: a love story* desires the health of the author and her recovery from an addiction to alcohol. The narrative seeks to return to what culture conceives as normal, namely to be healthy and free of addiction. In this and other narratives, attachments to alcohol, food, gambling and sex are portrayed as unhealthy. The

physical symptoms of the addiction illness are rewritten by Bullit-Jonas:

> I'm plugged with food. My legs are swollen. They ache when I walk. My cheeks are fat. My stomach bulges. I hate my body. I'm ashamed of what I've done to it so quickly, so ruthlessly. There is such despair within the greed.

Bullitt-Jonas (2000: 60) is unequivocal in assessing her addiction to food – 'In fact I was dying from it' – and after meeting with Rick for sex, the narrator of Silverman's *Love sick* (2001: 20) complains 'My body feels sticky and smudged. It feels unhealthy'. Here the restitution narrative is clearly borrowed. Addiction is an illness and achieving sobriety is synonymous with being healthy.

The identity of the addict in narrative is not necessarily shaped by the substance of attachment. The sex-addict narrator of *Love sick* considers that many substances and activities have the same purpose. Her realisation (p. 157) is offered in hindsight, after a rehabilitation programme: 'We use sex, food, alcohol and money – external objects of false gratification – to try to fill inner emptiness, loss, need – in this emotionally purblind world'. The illness of addiction belongs inside the addict. Knapp expresses this in terms of hunger:

> Most alcoholics I know experience that hunger long before they pick up the first drink, that yearning for something, something outside the self that will provide relief and solace and well-being.[4]

This narrative framing is learnt from the Twelve-Step Program and the cultures of Alcoholics Anonymous, Overeaters Anonymous, Sex Addicts Anonymous (SAA), Gamblers Anonymous and Narcotics Anonymous.[5] The substance of attachment is not especially significant: the disease of addiction must be treated through the programme and the identity of the addict should be fully realised.

The quest recovery narrative demonstrates that becoming healthy is dependent on perceiving addiction as an illness requiring treatment. As a consequence, recollections of pleasurable experiences do not regularly feature in the narratives. Furthermore, attachment to an addictive substance or activity is perceived as wrong, even as a sign of weakness. The quest to undo the illness and the affliction of addiction is a spiritual endeavour, in which the 'true' identity of the addict needs to be recovered. Huxley rejoices in the spiritual experience mescaline provides for him in the early narrative, *The doors of perception*. Conversely, the quest narrative seeks elevation through sobriety. Donlan and Bullitt-Jonas's narratives in particular realise peace and spiritual fulfilment at their conclusions. Only when Donlan's (1977: 166) narrator is free of drugs can she have 'new' eyes: 'The sun is real again, and it's not temporary anymore'. Donlan is able to see the 'real' sun: she no longer requires artificial substances to appreciate natural beauty and she does not need to demand anything in excess of God's creation.

8 WHAT KINDS OF INTERVENTION MIGHT BE SUCCESSFUL IN PREVENTING ADDICTION?

What separates the addiction narrative from other contemporary illness narratives is its tendency to understand addiction as a spiritual affliction. Here the addictive substance or activity is of less relevance: only when addicts have realised the burden of addiction (when they are at rock bottom) may they return to a state of spiritual well-being (reflecting the ethos of AA and similar organisations). This approach has the advantage that it counteracts the popular notion that addiction can be overcome by 'willpower' alone. Its disadvantage is that it tends to downplay the agency of the addict in aligning himself or herself with forces of recovery or degradation. We need to build on the AA narrative, but to find language and models that can appeal to a wider

audience – especially for those without strong religious leanings.

Addiction narratives might usefully form part of the National Curriculum and Healthy Schools Initiative as part of the Safety rubric, which includes as one of its strands 'Police Liaison and Drug and Alcohol Awareness'. Such tales could be read and discussed in class at a stage before teenagers become involved in drugs. Among the texts considered here that might serve this purpose, we would highlight those written by teenagers, such as *Go ask Alice* and Joan Donlan's *I never saw the sun rise*. Further research is required before we can take a view on how best such texts could be used in the classroom or at which school stage they might be introduced. Whether introduction to certain narratives can 'inoculate' young people against addiction is an eminently researchable question amenable to trial design.

9 CONCLUSIONS

Addiction is highly amenable to narrative representation. With regard to what will be the psychoactive substances of the future, we have shown that narratives of addiction exemplify types of illness narrative that neither exactly mirror nor objectively describe the social or natural worlds. So they cannot be analysed for clues – let alone for answers – to a question that seeks predictive replies.

Although addiction narratives have hitherto not confined their focus to any one substance, for nearly 200 years encounters with opium have been consistent preoccupations of such narratives, a multiplicity of other substances and behaviours gaining their focus in the past 50 years. Addiction accounts are predominantly retrospective reconstructions confined to following and interpreting rather than to anticipating trends in availability of psychoactive substances.

Concerning the effects of using psychoactive substances, the accounts we have read constitute a rich repository of narratively framed experiences and consequences in later lifetime. The contemporary addiction story is the confessional narrative of a sick self, one that requires treatment; and achieving health is the quest of many such addiction narratives.

But the contemporary narrative often moves beyond the strictly scientific view of addiction. The addict's illness is perceived as a psychological and emotional journey in which the sickness of the physical body gathers less significance. Addiction narratives inherently tend to moralise experience of addictive processes, diminishing in the process consideration of physical or physiological aspects of addiction.

Addiction to heroin is reflected upon in many narratives as a method of redesiring the first, exhilarating hit; whereas addictions to alcohol, food and sex are perceived as ways of comforting and steadying selfhood. In accordance with many illness narratives, the physical body is read as an emotional being, a belief that is borrowed from the culture of popular psychology.

One of the most striking features of addiction narratives from a clinical point of view is their lack of interest in the part played by environmental factors in the formation of the addiction. Heroin addicts in treatment often report that they find it easier to cut down on or even give up the drug altogether when they go away from their normal environment because they are not constantly faced with people offering to supply them with drugs. The narratives we looked at suggest that writers of addiction narratives tend to downplay this aspect of addictive experience. We can only speculate as to the reasons. It may be that the AA narrative with its emphasis on the addict's helplessness necessarily downplays the addict's agency in the recovery process.

But what separates the addiction narrative from other contemporary illness narratives is its tendency to understand addiction as a spiritual affliction. Here the addictive substance or activity is of less relevance: only when the addict has realised the burden of addiction may he or she return

to a state of spiritual well-being, reflecting the ethos of Alcoholics Anonymous and similar organisations. In such a way, addiction narratives demonstrate that addiction is not specific to personality, gender or class. Rather, addiction has the power to afflict many of us. The substance of addiction may in the end be only a contingent means to an end.

Acknowledgements

The authors are grateful for comments from Professor Sir Kenneth Calman and Dr Jeremy Holmes on an earlier draft of this report. Although not all of their points could be fully addressed, we have endeavoured to take account of most and have incorporated many into the final report.

NOTES

1. See for example King (2005; review of Cohen, J. (2004) *The new primary school drugs education pack*, Healthwise.
2. Cocaine seems to have the power to induce euphoria but for Sandie (in Greenleaf, 1989: 86), this also coincided with offering her a new identity: 'Sandie loved cocaine for its ability to mask her emotions as much as for the euphoric high it provided'.
3. In Greenleaf (1989: 154), Cathy's perception of her addiction to cocaine is similar: 'Personally I believe the first time an addict gets high, we spend the rest of our lives trying to recapture that feeling'.
4. Not all addicts adopt this philosophy. For example, a letter is included in Mary Kenny's *Death by heroin* (1999: 43) in which 'Paul' speaks about his experience: 'I must say that you do choose to be an addict, you are not a victim of a disease as some would say'.
5. Indeed, the recovery narratives of Knapp (1996) and Seidner (2004) include a list of questions designed to determine the extent of one's addiction. In the epilogue,

Seidner encourages the reader to attend a Gamblers Anonymous meeting.

References

Alfonsi, P. and Pesnot, P. (1972) *Satan's needle: a true story of drug addiction and cure.* Translated by J. Wilson. London: Hodder and Stoughton.

Berridge, V. (2004) Punishment or treatment? Inebriety, drink, and drugs, 1860–2004. *Lancet* 364: S2–3.

Bruner, J. (1999) Narratives of aging. *J Aging Stud* 13(1): 7–9.

Bullitt-Jonas, M. (2000) *Holy hunger: a woman's journey from food addiction to spiritual fulfillment.* New York: Vintage.

Burroughs, W.S. Junkie (1953) Confessions of an unredeemed drug addict. New York: Ace.

Charon, R., Trautmann, J., Banks, J., Connelly, E., Hunsaker Hawkins, A., Montgomery Hunter, K., Hudson Jones, A., Montello, M., and Poirier, S. (1995) Literature and medicine: contributions to clinical practice. *Ann Intern Med* 122 (April): 599–606.

Crowley, J. W. (1994) *The white logic: alcoholism and gender in American modernist fiction.* Amherst: University of Massachusetts Press.

Craze, R. (2003) *The voice of tobacco: a dedicated smoker's diary of not smoking.* Devon: White Ladder Press.

Donlan, J. (1977) *I never saw the sun rise: the diary of a recovering chemically dependent teenager.* Minnesota: Compcare Publications.

Elster, J. and Skog, O.-J. (1999) Introduction. In: J. Elster and O.-J. Skog (eds), *Getting hooked.* Cambridge: Cambridge University Press.

Elster, J. (1999) *Strong feelings.* Cambridge Mass: MITP.

Frank, A.W. (1995) *The wounded storyteller: body, illness and ethics.* Chicago: The University of Chicago Press.

Greenleaf, V. (1989) *Women and cocaine: personal stories of addiction and recovery.* Los Angeles: RGA.

Hanninen, V. and Koski-Jannes, A. (1999) Narratives of recovery from addictive behaviours. *Addiction* 94(12): 1837–1848.

Huxley, A. (2004) *The doors of perception.* London: Vintage (1953).

Hyden, L. (1997) Illness and narrative. *Sociol Health Illness* 19(1): 48–69.

Iversen, L.L. (2001) Addiction. In: C. Blakemore and S. Jennett (eds), *The Oxford companion to the body.* Oxford: Oxford University Press: 8.

Jones, J. (1701) *The mysteries of opium reveal'd.* London: Cruttenden and Cox: 89.

Kenny, M. (1999) *Death by heroin.* Dublin: New Island: 43.

Kermode, F. (1968) *The sense of ending.* Oxford: OUP.

King, A. (2005) The principles of drug education. *Drug Linn* 20: 28.

Knapp, C. (1996) *Drinking: a love story.* London: Quartet Books.

London, J. (1913) *John Barleycorn: memoirs of an alcoholic.* In: J. Barleycorn, '*Alcoholic memoirs*' edited with an introduction by John Sutherland. Oxford: Oxford University Press, (1989).

MacIntyre, A. (1981) *After virtue: a study in moral theory.* London: Duckworth and Co: 29.

Marlowe, A. (1999) *How to stop time: heroin from A to Z.* London: Virago: 18.

McIntosh, J. (2000) Addicts' narratives of recovery from drug use: constructing a non-addict identity. *Soc Sci Med* 50: 1501–1510.

Michaux, H. (1956) *Miserable miracle. Mescaline.* (Translated by Louise Varese. San Francisco and London 1963).

Moffat, M. and Johnson, J. (2001) Through the haze of cigarettes: teenage girls' stories about cigarette addiction. *Qual Health Res* 11(5): 668–681.

Moriarty, J. (2001) *Liquid lover: a memoir.* Los Angeles: Alyson Publications.

Neve, M. (2005) Historical keywords: addiction. *Lancet* 365: 21.

OED OnLine **1560** *J. Daus Sleidane's Comm.* 138a http://dictionary.oed.com/

OED OnLine **1621** *1st & 2nd Bk. of Discipline* 86 http://dictionary.oed.com/

OED OnLine **1667** II. 413 http://dictionary.oed.com/

OED OnLine **1751** *Chambers Cycl.* http://dictionary.oed.com/

Philosophical Papers (2003) Special edition devoted entirely to philosophical explorations of narrative). 32(3) November.

Porter, R. (1985) The drinking man's disease: the 'pre-history' of alcoholism in Georgian Britain. *Br J Addict* 80: 385–396.

Radley, A. (1999) The aesthetics of illness: narrative, horror and the sublime. *Sociol Health Illness* 21(6): 778–796.

Ricoeur, P. (1984) *Time and narrative.* Chicago: Chicago University Press.

Seidner, E. (2004) *Hit me: the true story of 60 years in the life of a compulsive gambler.* Indiana: Author House.

Silverman, S.W. (2001) *Love sick: one woman's journey through sexual addiction.* London: W.W. Norton.

Sonnedecker, G. (1962) The emergence of the concept of opiate addiction. *J Mondial de Pharmacie* 3: 273–5.

Sonnedecker, G. (1963) The emergence of the concept of opiate addiction. *J Mondial de Pharmacie* 1: 27–34.

Williams G.H. (1984) The genesis of chronic illness: narrative reconstruction. *Sociol Health Illness* 6(2): 175–200.

10 APPENDIX: SUMMARIES OF POST-1950s ADDICTION NARRATIVES CONSIDERED

Appendix: Summaries of post-1950S addiction narratives considered

1. *The doors of perception* (1953) recalls Aldous Huxley's psychological experiment with mescaline. A first-person account, part auto/ethnographic, part manifesto, it is unrestricted by the restitution narrative.

2. William Burroughs' *Junkie: Confessions of an unredeemed drug addict* (1953) is a novel that is widely thought to be autobiographical. It tells the story of William Lee (Lee was Burroughs' mother's maiden name), a young man from a family of real social eminence in the Midwest – they are listed in the Social Register – who finds himself selling drugs to feed his habit in New York City. By turns, he sells and uses morphine, marijuana and cocaine before finally settling on heroin, the ultimate junk. The narrator is portrayed as a rootless, unfeeling homosexual (though we discover he is married to a woman on page 61, about a third of the way through the book). Most of the story is concerned with describing how drug addicts obtain their drugs, how they avoid the police, how they use the drugs, as well as the criminal activities they engage in in order to go on using them. Heroin addicts become prostitutes and rent boys. If they are from respectable, moneyed families (as they very often are in this book), they pawn heirlooms. Heroin addiction, says Burroughs, is not 'a kick, or a means to increased enjoyment of life. It is a way of life'. When not in prison and not on junk, the narrator presents himself as a drunkard in pursuit of oblivion. The novel ends with the protagonist fleeing to Mexico, having served a sentence in jail and with many of his peers dead from the effects of 'junk'. Though officially 'clean', he remains an amoralist, on the margins of society. The moral lesson of *Junkie* seems to be that the heroin addict, with his strange argot and difficult lifestyle – though a poor disciplinarian of himself – is an excellent witness of the ills of industrial society.

3. Henri Michaux's *Miserable miracle* (1967) is an example of first-person ethnography within a chaos narrative. Much of the narrative was written while Michaux was feeling the effects of mescaline. Where Huxley's narrative is written retrospectively, Michaux narrates the sensations arising from his mescaline trips as they occur, using the acts of writing and drawing as methods of illustrating the drug-taking experience.

4. Philippe Alfonsi and Patrick Pesnot's *Satan's needle: a true story of drug addiction and cure* (1972) is an illness/quest narrative, offering a mixture of first- and third-person perspectives from the two women addicts and also the two journalists who observe them. Much of the narrative, especially the first half, is told in the first person, as a result of taped sessions with Pascale and Mireille. The narrative quests for recovery but fails.

5. Joan Donlan's *I never saw the sun rise: the diary of a recovering chemically dependent teenager* (1977) is an illness/quest narrative from a first-person perspective.

Addiction is treated as a disease which demands to be cured. The lived experience of her addiction has been reflected on in the narrative from the point of recovery, offering a construed diary. In accordance with *Go ask Alice* (first published in 1972), which also reflects on similar substance dependencies, the identity of the author has been withheld: the author of Go a*sk Alice* is anonymous; Joan Donlan is a pseudonym.

6. Each person who has experienced addiction in Vicki D. Greenleaf's *Women and cocaine: personal stories of addiction and recovery* (1989) has achieved recovery. In this way, all the narratives gathered here are illness/recovery narratives. Addiction is presented here as an illness that requires healing, reflecting the restitution narrative. Both first- and third-person accounts help to construct each recovery story.

7. Caroline Knapp's *Drinking: a love story* (1996) is a first-person illness/quest narrative that reflects aspects of the restitution narrative. This is the 'AA story' in which Alcoholics Anonymous is of overwhelming importance. Her 'disease', as she refers to it, demands reordering and healing in the process of storytelling.

8. Ann Marlowe's *How to stop time: heroin from A to Z* (1999) is a first-person illness narrative considering heroin addiction. *How to stop time* also features aspects of the chaos narrative and the text allows for an experimental narrative style. Although the author is a recovering addict, the narrative does not search for redemption.

9. Margaret Bullitt-Jonas's *Holy hunger: a woman's journey from food addiction to spiritual fulfilment* (2000) is an illness/quest narrative: the narrative is confessional and is written from the perspective of recovery. The narrator reorders the lived addictive encounter and with retrospective analysis seeks to understand why the author has suffered from an addiction to food. The narrative also provides an insight into Overeaters

Anonymous. Finding resolution in 'spiritual fulfilment', the author *of Holy hunger* finds inner peace which suggests that her suffering has changed her irrevocably.

10. Sue William Silverman's *Love sick: one woman's journey through sexual addiction* (2001) is an illness/quest narrative from a first-person perspective. The text features aspects of both the restitution narrative and the quest narrative. The narrative yearns for a full recovery, or for normalcy, and the reader is offered insights into the author's time in rehab, her therapy sessions and Sex Addicts Anonymous meetings. The narrative fails to reach fulfilment, either through the narrator's sexual exploits or as a result of therapy for her addiction to sex.

11. John Moriarty's *Liquid lover* (2001) is a memoir written by an alcoholic gay man in his forties. The author grew up in Chicago in the 1960s to Irish parents. Drinking was an important part of family life, especially among his male relatives. When he was twelve, Moriarty began drinking beer. One day, he stole into an empty house in order to drink alcohol with the brother of one of his friends. The other boy raped him. Moriarty told his friend (the rapist's brother) and was badly beaten up for his pains; he also lost his friend. During adolescence he decided he was homosexual. In his twenties he feared alcoholism and, though he did not give up alcohol altogether, he was careful not to drink too much. He was successful in his chosen career as a journalist and freelance writer. He also had a series of unhappy relationships with men, which usually ended with him getting drunk and beating his lovers up. By the time he was in his mid-thirties, his drunkenness had become part and parcel of his everyday life. He took himself to AA meetings, expressed remorse, but always held back the fact that he was homosexual. AA meetings never restrained him for very long. Finally, as a result of a four-day

binge, he nearly died and realised that either he would have to give up alcohol for good or he would die. This time, when he went to AA meetings he told his fellow alcoholics that he was gay and about everything that had happened to him as a child and adolescent. Moriarty claims that his inability to give up alcohol was related to his shame at having been raped, which ruined his homosexuality. The key to his giving it up was proclaiming his homosexuality in spite of the rape.

Moriarty's memoir takes the form of a series of fragments in which the reader is asked to believe that they are in Moriarty's presence as he shows them a series of mementoes. The author frequently adopts a hieratic stance, presenting himself in the guise of the Buddha of countless self-help books: 'Find me. I will wait. Capture my heart. I will capture yours. Take this moment to tell me one secret. Breathe this life into your soul. Angels come when we are ready. Find me'. It is profoundly religious in tone though perhaps not in imaginative reach.

12. Richard Craze's *The voice of tobacco: a dedicated smoker's diary of not smoking* (2003) is not a typical illness narrative although the narrative quests for a full recovery. The author has committed himself to quitting and the diary provides a construed account of the experience of withdrawal over a period of three months. Craze does not analyse why he chose to smoke and instead focuses on the desire to choose not to smoke.

13. Ed Seidner's *Hit me: the true story of 60 years in the life of a compulsive gambler* (2004) is an illness narrative reflecting on the author's experience of gambling addiction. Seidner's narrative is uncomplicated in its structure, failing to offer much retrospective analysis of the experience of this addiction. Rather, his past experiences are reclaimed in the narrative and the consequences of his gambling addiction are offered through the story, rather than through authorial intervention. He provides an ethic of solidarity to his fellow gamblers, pleading with others to reconsider their motives and actions when attending casinos.

CHAPTER

18

Drugs Futures 2025? Perspective of the Pharmaceutical Industry

Ian Ragan

1 EXECUTIVE SUMMARY

The Foresight project on Brain Science, Addiction and Drugs asked Dr Ian Ragan of CIR Consulting Ltd to find out the views of the pharmaceutical industry on the use of psychoactive substances in the future.

A questionnaire was sent to 16 pharmaceutical and biotechnology companies soliciting their views on the types of psychoactive substance that could be discovered within

the next 20 years, and the changes to societal attitudes and business practices that would be needed to make these drugs available to patients and the general public. Of the 16 companies approached, nine responded.

The industry is cautious about the commercial viability of treatments specifically aimed at addiction, and has mixed views on the role that vaccines could play in its prevention. The industry is also much concerned about the ethics of preventative treatments.

Nevertheless, there is optimism that drugs to enhance executive function, decrease impulsivity, and reduce stress and craving will be discovered anyway, whether specifically aimed at addiction or not. These could form part of a treatment regimen that combines the identification of at-risk groups, pharmacological and psychological treatments to reduce craving and prevent relapse, while simultaneously addressing comorbid conditions.

Optimism about new treatments for neuropathic, inflammatory and functional pain is being driven by a better understanding of central sensitisation mechanisms and the role of inflammatory factors, as well as by confidence in drugs now in their early stages of development. However, the barrier to success is high because of concerns about safety, the poor predictive value of animal models, the lack of surrogate markers and abuse potential. In particular, there was no consensus among the industry respondents as to whether new treatments would be free from potential abuse.

In the area of mental health, the industry is optimistic that new treatments for depression and anxiety will be available in 5–10 years' time, showing that companies are already researching in these areas. Drugs for cognitive enhancement are seen as more challenging, because of difficulties with predictive animal models and with clinical trials. In schizophrenia, advances in the near future will be in new adjunct therapies to support the atypical antipsychotic drugs by enhancing efficacy and reducing side-effects. The prevention of schizophrenia is not inconceivable from the scientific point of view but will be very difficult and ethically challenging. Other areas where new treatments may become available are sleep disorder, attention-deficit hyperactivity disorder, mood stabilisation and autism.

The industry believes that new diagnostic descriptions, definitions and subdivisions of mental illnesses will arrive within 10 years, based perhaps on a better understanding of the pathophysiology and genetic basis of the disease, but more likely on treatment responsiveness. Lack of progress in this area could impede the proper understanding and use of genomic information in disease treatment. New drugs based on new definitions will follow with a 5–10-year lag.

In the area of treatments for specific age groups, the industry believes that paediatric medicine is especially difficult. Extrapolating from the adult what will happen in the child or adolescent is problematic, and therefore giving psychoactive substances to the developing brain brings real concerns about efficacy and long-term safety. The recent publicity over the use of antidepressants in adolescents will cast a shadow over the field for a long time to come. In geriatric medicine, there is more optimism and more investment. There is huge unmet medical need in Alzheimer's disease, Parkinson's disease, depression and sleep disorder among the elderly.

The industry is united in believing that greater transparency is essential over the societal changes needed to allow some of these scientific possibilities to reach the public. The industry will have a major role in providing information on how drugs will be used in the next few years and will make efforts to restore its tarnished image through early and open publication of clinical trial data. The industry hopes that its efforts will be reciprocated by increased understanding from the public and greater appreciation of risk and benefit from the regulators. The dangers are the trend towards increased post-launch monitoring and of greater risk-averseness stifling innovation.

The industry is unanimous in its lack of enthusiasm for developing drugs for non-medical purposes. Most found the idea ethically indefensible in the current climate. Even if society changed to make it more acceptable, the industry's concerns about the risk and benefit of medicines where the benefit is medically marginal and where there is potential abuse or misuse remain a considerable obstacle. Therefore, the view is that non-medical uses will only arise off-label from drugs developed for real medical conditions, although the boundary between medical and non-medical is likely to change over the coming years. The areas in which this could happen are sleep, mood, stress, anxiety, impulsivity and vigilance.

The industry regrets what it perceives as the inadequacy of the national strategy for mental health, which it feels puts the UK at a disadvantage compared with the US. Many respondents reiterated that the proper treatment of mental illness could never be purely pharmacological. The future lies in better prevention, diagnosis and screening, the identification of at-risk groups, tailored pharmacological intervention, and counselling and psychological support. The industry no longer believes in magic bullets for mental illnesses.

2 INTRODUCTION

2.1 The Current State of the Industry

In considering future developments in psychoactive substances, there is a great disparity between what is theoretically possible and what the pharmaceutical industry would consider pursuing. This involves more than estimating the probability that theoretical ideas might be realised or that there would be appropriate reimbursement for new substances. The industry is concerned about the ethical issues that have to be addressed when considering the future for the pharmacological manipulation of mood and cognition. An appreciation of the complexity of the question requires an understanding of the current state of the industry and the internal debate about the future shape of the business.

The current woes of the pharmaceutical industry are the subject of much attention these days (*Innovation in the pharmaceutical sector*, 2004; Boston Consulting Group, 2004; PharmaFutures, 2004; IBM Business Consulting Services). It is apparent that the optimistic view of the 1980s and 1990s that new technology would transform the business has not yet been realised. The reasons include long lead times, higher-than-predicted levels of attrition in development of medicines

and the lack of use of surrogates as regulatory endpoints for licensing. It is true that the way in which drug discovery is carried out has changed utterly, especially in the early phases where molecular biology has been astonishingly powerful in redefining the business. In addition, medicinal chemistry has been transformed by the development of automated synthesis and library generation, even if the initial enthusiasm for creating massive combinatorial libraries has waned. Armed with genome information, thousands of new drug targets and high-throughput methods, it is not surprising that the industry was bullish about the future. What has happened to dampen this enthusiasm?

Many internal and external influences have led to the sector's present lack of confidence. The basic fact is that the rate of launch of new products has not matched the increased investment. Some analysts foresee a continuing decline in the number of new chemical entities receiving approval, (Lehman Brothers, 2003) while others view the present state as a temporary blip which is already changing as the refocused efforts of the industry put new molecules into early clinical development (*Innovation in the pharmaceutical sector*, 2004). However, there is no doubt that costs have increased dramatically, while attrition rates have not reduced significantly along the value chain. Estimates put the cost of bringing a new molecule to the market at around \$1 billion (Tufts Center for the Study of Drug Development, 2003). The cost is spread across the entire chain from early screening to clinical trials because the lower costs per molecule at the early stage are cancelled out by their high failure rate. Drug discovery may be a complex and highly technical process but it still relies heavily on trial and error. The effect of increasing costs is obvious. A greater return per launched product will be required. Even now, only one-third of launched drugs recoup their costs and are profitable for their discoverers. Small wonder, then, that the industry markets its successful products so aggressively and defends their patent exclusivity with such determination. This analysis therefore leads to another question. Why has all this new science not led to a reduced attrition rate?

There are many possible answers of varying plausibility. The human genome has provided us with many thousands of potential drug targets, but not as many as we hoped for when we thought that the genome contained up to 100 000 genes. Estimates of the size of the subset of these that could be targets for effective small-molecule therapies are obviously imprecise, but it is not likely to be more than a few per cent. The prospect of increasing the number of druggable targets by including biologicals (peptides, proteins and antibodies) will continue to be a rare or remote possibility for central nervous system (CNS) disorders. Therefore, the discovery that there may not be virtually limitless numbers of undiscovered drug targets has led to increased speculation that we may already have picked all the easy targets by traditional methods of discovery. If so, the remaining targets are going to be more challenging at the scientific level and the treatments are going to be less effective in the clinic. This could explain why attrition rates continue to be so high and why increased investment has not brought a corresponding return. The problem could be circumvented if methods of predicting drug efficacy at an early stage were more advanced. This applies especially in psychiatry and neurology, with higher attrition rates currently than in other therapeutic areas (Tufts Center for the Study of Drug Development, 2004) despite the possibility of better predictive tools such as PET and fMRI.

The failure of many plausible ideas to translate into effective therapies in the clinic, even with encouraging animal data, has already led to signs that some companies are beginning to re-assess the emphasis they put on CNS research, despite growing clinical need. The industry has to invest most heavily where it can succeed, and it does not have the luxury of responding only to medical need if the challenge of creating an effective medicine is too great.

The preceding argument has focused on factors that increase the cost of basic research. But the costs of clinical research have also risen dramatically. The number and complexity of the studies required has grown, as has the individual cost per patient in the developed world. The number of trials and the number of patients enrolled into them have risen in response to the need for more data on both efficacy and safety. Competition between companies is much greater than it was, even 10 years ago, and differentiating a new drug from competitor products is becoming more difficult. Thus, the need to have comparative studies to support marketing, formulary negotiations and reimbursement decisions has increased. The recent spate of high-profile withdrawals, such as that of the painkiller Vioxx (www.vioxx.com/rofecoxib/vioxx/consumer/index.jsp) continues to fuel the demand for more reassurance about safety in the context of the benefit that the medicine brings. The regulatory authorities increasingly mandate commitments to post-marketing studies as a condition for approval. Temporary pauses in clinical trials to address safety issues have trebled in the past few years compared with the late 1990s (Boston Consulting Group, 2004).

At a time when the industry struggles with its ability to innovate, there is increasing downward pressure on the returns for innovation. Price regulation and cost containment measures are common throughout Europe (*Innovation in the pharmaceutical sector*, 2004) and it is likely that the same trends will occur in the US. The squeeze on the profits from existing drugs causes the industry to reflect on its portfolios and adopt a more conservative approach to its future investments in research and development. Already companies are investing very much less in blue-sky research than they were 15 years ago. This is not necessarily a bad thing if companies focus their minds on drug discovery and the academic sector is able to provide the basic science.

The collapse of the sales of the antidepressant, Prozac, after its patent life expired was a spectacular example of the power of the generics industry. The industry has to accept that the patent life of a product is the only period in which it can make money for its discoverers. Generic substitution also forces the realisation that in the future, mere incremental innovation will not lead to large sales, even if approval is gained. However, there is reason to hope that real innovation will continue to be rewarded, if the extension of data protection and market exclusivity for new indications remains. This will act as real encouragement.

One of the most obvious industry responses to these challenges has been merger and acquisition. The concept of merging two complementary entities, getting rid of the overlap and slimming the combined workforce is attractive from the business perspective and especially so for those who act as brokers in the process. In reality, the short-term effect is a loss of productivity and adverse effects on morale and the reputation of the industry (*Innovation in the pharmaceutical sector*, 2004). In the long term, the loss of total research and development (R&D) is potentially damaging. But reducing the competition may improve the chances that the survivors will succeed (*Innovation in the pharmaceutical sector*, 2004). However, as a strategy, it has no long-term future because eventually the world will run out of companies to merge. When mergers do occur, assets are divested. Smaller companies can develop these with lower needs for a return. Such firms provide equity to the market themselves and build market capital, as well as collaborating with mainstream pharmaceutical companies. However, bigger companies are needed to develop these assets through to the market and make R&D affordable and sustainable in the long term. Likewise, the move of R&D to Asia, where costs are much lower, is helpful, but does not in itself address the underlying malaise of the industry.

Other responses such as focusing efforts on the core business, creating flexibility through outsourcing, and working in partnership with other stakeholders, hold out promise for a radical re-engineering of the way drug discovery and development are done, with the end goals of lower costs, faster development times and reduced attrition rates. Much of this depends on the success of new ideas in translational research and experimental medicine, and the promise of personalised treatment arising from the application of pharmacogenetics and pharmacogenomics (Little, 2004; Evan and Relling, 2004). Even then, the industry is nervous about the return on investment from such a radically changed business model. Success therefore depends as much on changes to the regulatory process as on basic science. The low esteem of the industry in the eyes of the world is a real impediment to a constructive dialogue on solutions to the industry's problems and on how to provide effective and much-needed medicines. The industry, battered by public opinion, is at risk of retreating into its shell at a time when working with other stakeholders is vital for medical progress.

In the context of possible future psychoactive substances, it is clear that the industry does not relish taking on all the scientific possibilities that might present themselves. Our survey reveals that the industry is very aware of the ethical, legal and societal impacts of this kind of work and, while its reputation languishes at the same level as the tobacco industry, it is not surprising that there are areas into which the industry would not wish to stray when there are so many diseases for which treatments are genuinely needed.

2.2 Psychoactive Substances for Medical Use: Drivers and Influences

In the light of present concerns about the stability and future prospects of the business, this section looks at the positive drivers, influences and potential impediments to the development of new psychoactive substances for purely medical conditions. It concerns itself less with the scientific possibilities, which need to be considered case by case, and more with general considerations of the pros and cons of investing in this field and the way in which medical treatments are likely to evolve as a result of societal changes.

First and foremost, the driver for continued industry interest in this field is the huge unmet clinical need. This provides unlimited opportunities for novel breakthrough therapies and enormous market potential. The disease burden of CNS disorders is extraordinarily high (Olesen and Leonardi, 2003) and even in areas of past success, such as depression, anxiety and schizophrenia, the proportion of patients receiving effective therapy is low, either because the treatment is ineffective, or because their problems have been undiagnosed or misdiagnosed, or because they have not received or taken effective treatment. Western society at least expects to have effective treatments for mental health conditions that are increasingly accepted as real illnesses (but see below). However, there will be increasing pressure for drugs that affect the course of a disease rather than just relieving its symptoms. Other influences will be those already identified as necessary to transform the business model. For example, the heavily marketed blockbuster will give way to personalised medicine, while the belief in magic bullets for complex CNS disorders is already seen, in retrospect, as naive. Effective treatments will require combination therapies, polypharmacy and an individualised approach based on screening, early detection and monitoring.

The impediments to progress are formidable. The problem of attrition rates and increasing clinical trial burden is higher for CNS drugs than for others (Tufts Center for the Study of Drug Development, 2004) creating tension between unmet need and huge market potential on the one hand, and high risk of failure on the other. Companies may become risk-averse over both their science and their reputations. There is already suspicion that the industry invents diseases in order to sell cures, and that it actively promotes the medicalisation of

normal life. An example that has attracted much publicity is attention-deficit hyperactivity disorder (ADHD), regarded by some as society's failure to deal properly with the unusual behaviour of certain children. According to this viewpoint, drug companies have developed and marketed drugs for a condition that does not really exist, and the availability of behaviour-modifying drugs masks the real need to address the underlying cause of the behaviour (see discussion in *Connecting brains and society*, 2004). The truth is that ADHD is a real condition that can be controlled with drugs, but that pharmacology should be seen as part of a treatment regimen that must include appropriate attention to understanding the child's problems. To dismiss ADHD as a marketing department ploy is demeaning to all those who suffer from this condition. However, this example illustrates the extreme vulnerability of the industry to reputational damage if it is perceived to be taking advantage of societal ills to promote drug sales.

The issue is exacerbated by the inability to control the off-label use of a drug. At present, companies only develop drugs for bona fide medical conditions for which they conduct clinical trials. These conditions are those for which the drug is approved and which appear on the drug label. However, off-label use is both widespread and legal and can lead to a drug finding therapeutic and commercial success for conditions for which it was never designed (eg gabapentin (Mack, 2003) and modafinil (www.modafinal.com/article/off-label.html)). This is beneficial under the right circumstances as it maximises the medical utility of the drug and recognises the fact that predicting therapeutic utility is still an imprecise science. In the absence of clinical trials of the new indication, however, the evidence for safety and efficacy can be said to be anecdotal, or at best uncontrolled. In the absence of robust evidence to confirm the efficacy and safety profile, there is a potential increased risk to patients and prescribers. Furthermore, there are other off-label uses ranging from the benign to the criminal that point up the dangers inherent in mood-altering drugs. At one end of this spectrum are the media stories about selective serotonin reuptake inhibitor (SSRI) antidepressants being used inappropriately by non-depressed people as pick-me-ups. They are unlikely to be effective as these drugs are not mood-altering per se. At the other end, there is the abuse of IV temazepam (Ralston and Taylor, 1993) and even worse, the date-rape drugs, Rohypnol, gamma-hydroxybutyrate (GHB), ecstasy and ketamine (see eg www.4woman.gov/faq/rohypnol.htm). It is inevitable that non-medical off-label use is going to occur with the kinds of new drugs envisaged in this survey, particularly if they are in general safer than earlier generations of medicines, as one would predict. There will be nervousness about the abuse potential of new mood-altering drugs, a problem that just does not arise in any other therapeutic area. It is an unfortunate fact that non-medical use of mood-altering drugs not only undermines the credibility of the companies which develop and market them, but also affects the patients who really need them.

Finally, there is the very complex and emotive issue of the safety of mood-altering drugs. New forms of substitute prescribing inevitably carry a risk of abuse. Perhaps the most widely debated issue among the public has been whether SSRI use is associated with increased risk of suicide. The debate continues, although there is no evidence that an increased risk exists in adults, despite the drugs' use in many millions of patients over many years. Recent regulatory reviews have confirmed that the risk–benefit ratio remains positive in all the licensed indications for SSRIs (BMJ, 2005). The future may provide the tools to screen out at-risk patients if rare but serious consequences turn out to have a genetic basis, but this is unknown. At present it seems logical to assume that any drug that alters brain chemistry will have the potential for causing thought disturbance in vulnerable people such as one might expect to find in a psychiatric population. The more

successful the industry is in producing drugs with a more favourable risk–benefit ratio, the more likely it is that they will be used off-label for non-medical conditions.

2.3 Psychoactive Substances for Non-medical Use: Drivers and Influences

This section considers whether the industry would, or could undertake the de novo discovery and development of drugs purely for non-medical purposes. This is quite distinct from the off-label use referred to above. The issues that face the industry in providing a new generation of psychoactive substances for medical use are exaggerated manyfold when non-medical use is considered. Some of these are scientific but many depend critically on public attitudes. It would be foolish to assume that these will remain fixed for the next 20 years.

Non-medical use should not be equated with recreational use. It is hard to imagine that the industry would set out to create a drug purely for mood alteration, with all the dangers of abuse that would come with it. More plausible is the idea that the boundary between medical and non-medical use will shift as a result of greater societal acceptance of pharmacological intervention. According to a recent conference on the future of brain science (*Connecting brains and society*, 2004), voluntary use of drugs for non-medical purposes (including recreational use) does not seem to be a major societal issue. What concerns people more is the 'medicalisation of normalcy', with the implicit fear that redefinition of what is normal will bring with it some form of compulsion to treat perceived deviations from the norm.

What are the non-medical non-recreational uses to which new psychoactive substances might be put? First, the control of 'abnormal' behaviour in normal settings, for example, aggression in schools, is already a topic of much current debate and concern. For those who do not accept that ADHD is a true disease, the custom in the US that children so diagnosed must be medicated in order to enter the school system is an example of what the future might hold.[1] Second, the enhancement of cognition to improve intellectual performance goes far beyond mere recreational use. Third, there is the use of drugs to normalise, or cope with responses to, abnormal situations. Sleep deprivation and abnormal sleep patterns are a major cause of distress to the elderly, in which context it is a medical issue. However, large numbers of people enter professions voluntarily where sleep disturbance is an unavoidable consequence of the work, e.g. shift-workers and airline crews. Such uses encourage fears of future civil control by pharmacological intervention, however unlikely this may be.

The driver for the industry actively to seek the development of such drugs is linked to what society finds acceptable. The market potential is obviously enormous. Who among us would not be tempted to use a safe, effective cognition enhancer if one were available? The trend to greater acceptability is already clear. Tinkering with Mother Nature, whether via botox, liposuction or drugs, is no longer veiled in secrecy. When the idea of designing drugs for weight loss was first discussed, there were many voices in the industry who claimed that obesity was a lifestyle issue and that it was not the proper business of pharmaceutical companies. However, the view prevailed that pharmaceutical companies had no right to make moral judgements over a major cause of premature death. Furthermore, there is a lifestyle element to most major illnesses such as cardiovascular disease, cancer, arthritis and metabolic disorders. It is a much smaller step these days to the treatment of lifestyle alone than it was 15 years ago.

The impediments, though, are daunting and in essence are the same as for medical uses (section 2.2) but more so. The safety aspects assume much greater importance for non-medical use. Although personalised medicine may help mitigate previously unforeseen and perhaps mechanistically unrelated side-effects, there is little doubt that the desired action of the drug will carry some risk for the user. When there is no disease to be treated, side-effects are clearly not tolerable, either from marketing or ethical perspectives. The financial and reputational risks are off-putting. There are also difficulties in the discovery and development of such drugs. Under the UK's 1986 Animal (Scientific Procedures) Act (www.archive.official-documents.co.uk/document/hoc/321/321-xa.htm) regulated procedures on protected animal species are only permitted where there are no scientifically suitable alternatives. In addition, the likely benefits (to man, other animals, or the environment) must be weighed against the likely welfare costs to the animals involved. Clearly, for non-medical uses, the benefit is harder to demonstrate. While the expansion of knowledge is also a legitimate justification for the use of animals in scientific procedures under UK law, it is difficult to see what reason there would be for causing pain, suffering or distress to animals in order to develop cognition enhancers for normal people, or to alleviate the stresses of modern lifestyle habits such as erratic working hours. In addition, regardless of the legal position, the sensitivity of the industry to its current poor image is likely to weigh heavily in any decisions. And from a purely scientific perspective, it is unclear what kind of animal models could be used to demonstrate efficacy for non-medical uses, and how clinical trials would be conducted.

3 SURVEY RESULTS

3.1 The Questions

The intention was to ask the respondents what developments they thought possible over the next 20 years, but also to indicate the probability that these might occur within this timeframe and to add comments on their reasons. Section 1 of the survey focused on putative psychoactive substances for the treatment of addiction, pain, mental health and paediatric and geriatric care, topics that emerged as important from the

Brain Science, Addiction and Drugs Project's scoping workshops. Section 2 asked questions about the ethical and regulatory aspects of drug development in the future and how these might help or hinder medical advances. Section 3 considered whether it would be possible to develop drugs specifically for non-medical purposes and, if so, in which areas. Finally, Section 4 asked for thoughts on topics not considered elsewhere, within the scope of the survey, where scientific advances could be used or stimulated to provide therapeutic advances. Nine companies listed in the acknowledgements contributed their ideas to the survey questions, which can be found in the online version of the report (www.foresight.gov.uk). A copy of the letter sent to companies inviting them to participate and a copy of the questionnaire used to collect data is in the Appendix.

3.2 What New Prevention/Treatments for Addiction and Problem Use May be Developed?

Addiction is now increasingly accepted as a complex disorder of the brain that has environmental, drug-related and genetic components. (Kreek *et al.*, 2004; Volkow and Li, 2004). It is defined as an intense compulsion to take a drug, over which the individual has impaired control, despite serious adverse consequences. The development of addiction requires chronic exposure to the drug whose initial acute effects typically activate brain pathways associated with positive reinforcement. The volitional phase of early drug use weakens as drug exposure leads to remodelling of brain pathways. This results in a complex set of behaviours that characterise addiction in which negative reinforcement plays an important part (tolerance, sensitisation, dependence, withdrawal, relapse sensitivity). This evolving pattern of addiction has led to distinction being drawn between drug addiction (associated with reward) and drug dependence (associated with withdrawal symptoms) as the adaptive

changes and triggers are different. This separation has practical applications as it provides treatment options aimed at reducing craving, ameliorating withdrawal, normalising behaviours and preventing relapse that involve many aspects of human brain function such as reward, motivation, learning, inhibitory control and executive function. This means that strategies need to address more than one aspect of addiction to be successful; pharmacology, psychology and social support need to work in partnership, and comorbid conditions such as depression or schizophrenia need to be treated in parallel. As with all mental illnesses, complex disorders require complex and thoughtful intervention strategies. There are no magic bullets for addiction and never will be.

A further important aspect of drug addiction is the evidence that it is a developmental disorder. Normal adolescent characteristics, such as increased risk-taking and sensitivity to peer pressure that make experimentation with drugs more likely, may reflect incomplete development of brain regions involved with executive function. But, in addition, it seems plausible that drugs taken at this developmental stage may have much greater propensity to remodel the brain than in adults. Certainly, exposure to alcohol and nicotine at an early stage results in greater vulnerability to addiction than later, adult exposure. This vulnerability is compounded by genetic factors, some of which have already been identified. However, polymorphisms in genes involved in the metabolism of drugs do not offer themselves as plausible targets for pharmacological intervention and, as yet, while there are interesting hints that polymorphisms in receptors in key reward pathways alter addiction vulnerability, translating such findings into effective therapies is not trivial. Finally, environmental factors play a major part in the development of addiction. Stress increases vulnerability to addiction and to relapse, while drugs of abuse cause abnormal responsivity to stress. It is hardly surprising therefore that low socioeconomic class, low self-esteem and poor parenting go hand in hand with drug availability and abuse. Even in non-human primates, cocaine self-administration is linked to group status, with dominant animals showing less desire than those lower down the pecking order.

In their comments, the pharmaceutical company respondents covered a wide range of scientific and business issues that could have an impact on the development of new treatments. Improved identification of the genetic contribution to addiction could help through pharmacogenomics to identify treatment groups, even if such work did not lead easily to new molecular targets for therapy. On the other hand, progress with understanding the genes involved in alcohol addiction has identified some putative targets (eg gamma-aminobutyric acid type A (GABA-A) receptor subtypes) that are already under investigation for other CNS disorders. In this way, pharmacogenomic studies could provide the impetus to test novel drugs in addiction. Furthermore, since addictions resulting from various drugs of abuse (eg opiates, cocaine, nicotine, alcohol) share some key features in common, it is likely that therapies aimed more downstream of the original site of action will generalise. An example is the use of opiate receptor antagonists such as naltrexone, for the treatment of both opiate addiction and alcoholism.

There are considerable difficulties that could impede progress to more effective therapy for addiction. The small size of the existing market, caused by the poor efficacy of current drugs, is a disincentive to entering the field as it would require an innovative approach to sales, marketing and distribution in order to create therapeutic and commercial success. Addicts frequently do not seek pharmacological treatment, and compliance is poor. One respondent proposed depot injections of drugs, as used in the treatment of schizophrenia, as a possible solution to this. Indeed, depot naltrexone is under evaluation at the current time. Physicians are often not proactive in making therapy available, and treatment centres, staffed largely by non-physicians, have the reputation of being anti-medication.

Many countries do not provide reimbursement for the evaluation or treatment of drug abuse and addiction, which has discouraged the involvement of both the medical profession and the industry. There are also difficulties in conducting clinical trials. So it is not surprising that mainstream pharmaceutical companies have not shown a great appetite for this field in the past. However, effective partnership between the industry and government bodies concerned with health, the law and education could change the landscape greatly if society decided that this was a pressing enough need. There are already encouraging examples of success with Zyban (bupropion) and Subutex (buprenorphine; Lingford-Hughes et al., 2004).

On specific treatments, the respondents were divided on the likelihood of vaccines for treatment and prevention. Opinion ranged from placing the possibility as quite high within 5 years to low even in 10 years. Doubts were also expressed about the commercial viability of such products and the ethics of their use. A changed paradigm for drug development in this field could alter the financial picture, but some respondents found it difficult to imagine the circumstances in which a vaccine could be used preventatively. Addiction is not a communicable disease, although its propagation may have aspects of one. Therefore, concepts of social responsibility and herd immunity used to justify mass vaccination do not strictly apply. Furthermore, if the effect of the vaccine is to blunt or negate the rewarding properties of a drug, the risk is that the addict will simply self-administer higher doses. Such a strategy would only be successful where addicts are highly motivated to stop anyway, as in smoking. This group will inevitably have a choice whether or not to take the vaccine. However, there could be some instances where the imposition of a vaccine might be considered, as with cocaine addicts who have been incarcerated because of drug-related crime, and for whom vaccination might be made a condition for early release from prison.

The ethical question of removing the choice of the addict to be treated is one that will have to be faced if and when such treatments become available. For nicotine and cocaine, this could be in 5 years.

Vaccination technology could also be used to help prevent the initiation of the drug-taking habit. The most obvious target here is the adolescent. The ethical implications of giving a vaccine when it may neither be necessary, nor the choice of the recipient, again would need to be fully considered. There may be ways to help identify those most vulnerable, using a combination of environmental (eg lower socioeconomic group) and genetic factors. The former would no doubt bring accusations of class bias and stigmatisation, unless cocaine vaccination was imposed on the young urban professional class as well. The leading addiction vaccines in development at the moment are for nicotine and cocaine, but this list could be extended to other drugs of abuse, including heroin and phencyclidine (PCP) in the 10-year timeframe.

Drugs to enhance executive function were perceived as important and likely treatments. Different respondents expected them to become available in 5–20 years but added that they were unlikely to be specifically developed for the treatment of addiction.

Opinion on drugs to unlearn addiction was very mixed, ranging from never, to low probability even in 15 years, to moderate probability within 5.

Better agreement was reached on the importance of anti-stress drugs, not only for relapse but also for drug seeking. Given the importance of this area for a wider variety of CNS disorders, all respondents predicted moderate to high probability of success in the 10–15-year timeframe or even less. One respondent foresaw a future in which the addict received inpatient treatment to become 'clean' and subsequently was put on a relapse prevention programme comprising both social aspects and the use of anti-craving drugs.

On one area, all correspondents were in accord. Combinations with psychological approaches were seen as absolutely inevitable in the next 5 years. Addiction will always need a combined approach. One respondent looking further ahead described the ideal future preventative treatment as one involving pharmacogenomics to identify the at-risk group, and then counselling and drug treatments to enhance executive function and decrease impulsivity.

Looking even further out, one respondent speculated about the use of imaging to identify brain regions associated with craving, with the patient able to use electrical stimulation of those regions to control desire. The success of deep brain stimulation in Parkinson's disease and pain control clearly has potential in other conditions.

Some specific treatments were mentioned by a number of correspondents as being feasible in this 20-year timeframe. These included anti-craving drugs, drugs to improve compliance, drugs to ease withdrawal, specific treatments for alcoholism and the need for simultaneous treatment of psychiatric comorbidities such as depression and schizophrenia. The list illustrates the wide range of options available for intervention in this complex area and the continuing need to consider multiple simultaneous approaches for effective therapy.

3.3 What is the Likelihood of New Treatments for the Management of Pain?

To answer this question, it is important to define the kind of pain under consideration. There are four main categories of pain: nociceptive, inflammatory, neuropathic and functional (Woolf, 2004). The sensation of pain has strong cognitive and emotional components and is linked to autonomic function. All of these components contribute to the actual experience of pain. The perception of a painful stimulus relies on a specialised subset of nerves called nociceptors that relay signals to the brain via the spinal cord. As people are aware from those rare individuals who are genetically incapable of experiencing noci-ception, this form of pain is a very valuable warning and defensive system whose com-plete suppression by drugs is not desirable. If the nociceptive system fails to prevent tissue damage, the healing phase is pro-moted by inflammatory pain in the affected area, whose increased intensity serves to remind the individual to protect the tissue. Inflammatory pain should resolve as heal-ing progresses. While this is a normal and positively beneficial process (so-called adap-tive pain), it sometimes needs managing, for example, following surgery or traumatic injury or in abnormal states such as chronic inflammatory disease. The aim is to nor-malise pain responses, not to remove them entirely.

Other forms of pain are called maladaptive because they arise from abnormal sensory processing and are persistent or recurrent. The unmet need here is huge as treatment options are limited and understanding of the causes is at an early stage. Neuropathic pain arises from lesions of the peripheral nervous system caused by diseases such as diabetes, AIDS and post-herpetic neuralgia and from lesions of the central nervous sys-tem in such conditions as spinal cord injury, multiple sclerosis and stroke. Functional pain remains the least understood, as it is not associated with any deficit, lesion or abnor-mality. Functional pain conditions include fibromyalgia, irritable bowel syndrome and tension-type headache. Inflammatory, neu-ropathic and functional pain share the com-mon feature of hypersensitivity in which normal innocuous stimuli become painful or mildly painful sensations become more severe. This sensitisation process has contri-butions from both the peripheral and central nervous systems and occurs at the level of the nociceptor terminals, the central ascend-ing pathways to the brain and the descend-ing inhibitory pathways, which offer a wide selection of plausible drug targets. Finally, not all forms of pain fit neatly into these categories. Migraine, for example, has both neurologic and inflammatory components. Cancer pain can be caused by inflammatory

responses in affected tissues, and by nerve damage.

The prospects for future developments depend on the availability of plausible tar-gets and the effectiveness of current treat-ments. In the treatment of nociceptive, inflammatory and neuropathic pain, there are efficacious treatment options currently available such as the opiates. Attention has focused on reducing side-effects, of which abuse potential is the most serious. Recent concerns about the safety and future prospects of the cyclo-oxygenase 2 (COX-2) inhibitors, Vioxx and Celebrex, have cre-ated a huge hole in treatment provision for inflammatory pain that will no doubt spur further efforts by the industry.

The respondents were in good agree-ment that new treatments would be available within 5 years, and 10 at the most. This pre-sumably reflects the fact that most major companies have active pain programmes that are in some stage of clinical develop-ment and would be expected to reach the market in this time. Most effort is directed to chronic neuropathic and inflammatory pain, as opiates are hard to beat in terms of effi-cacy in acute pain. The prospect of replac-ing them for non-scheduled treatments was considered unlikely.

This optimism was illustrated by one respondent who went into some detail about the increasing understanding of neuronal pathways and the influence of inflammatory signals. Insight into the central sensitisation mechanisms thought to be responsible for chronic spontaneous pain has provided sev-eral new molecular targets for drug discov-ery and development. Drug candidates for some of these that are already in early clinical trials could provide new treatments as early as 2010–2015. Other respondents supported the view that many new targets were also being pursued for neuropathic pain. This optimism has to be tempered by concerns voiced by the same respondent and others that drugs for pain have to be very safe, as most conditions to be treated are not life-threatening. This is a serious hurdle to be overcome. In addition, the pain area has an unenviable record for the poor predictive value of animal models. Clinical development is hampered by the unavailability of surrogate markers of pain and therefore it is necessary to go to patients for the first indications of efficacy, something that the industry would prefer not to do. This can lead to competition for patients, which means delays in enrolment and completion of trials, and greater up-front costs before efficacy can be established.

Perhaps the most interesting disagreements were to be found in answer to the question about the development of drugs without abuse potential. The optimistic view was that most new targets have no theoretical abuse liability, presumably because they do not invoke opioid pathways, and therefore that the new drugs emerging in the 10–15 year timeframe would be free from this taint. Cymbalta (duloxetine) and Neurontin (gabapentin) were cited as examples of treatments already in use for neuropathic pain that apparently avoid this problem. However, the conservative view was that all drugs carry some risk of abuse, especially where reward is involved. In the case of pain, the reward is the removal of something unpleasant rather than the receipt of something pleasurable, but this means that any analgesic carries risk of abuse in patients, though not in the normal population.

3.4 What is the Likelihood for the Development of New Drugs for Mental Health?

It is difficult to generalise across so broad a field. The detailed subquestions covered depression, anxiety, cognitive enhancement in schizophrenia, cognitive enhancement in neurodegenerative conditions, and prevention of schizophrenia. The field has been waiting a long time for a truly innovative breakthrough.

In depression, current treatments can trace their history back to the early fortuitous discoveries of iproniazid and imipramine that led to the formulation of the monoamine hypothesis of depression (Wong and Licina, 2004). Since then, this has been the mainstay of efforts to develop new antidepressants. To search outside this zone of comfort is necessary but carries risk of failure. Excitement around neuropeptide targets has not abated totally, despite the disappointing failure of the neurokinin-1 (NK-1) antagonist, aprepitant (Ranga and Krishnan, 2002), and this and other targets (eg corticotrophin releasing factor (CRF-1) receptor) continue to be proposed and developed as our knowledge of the pathophysiology of depression accumulates. The field was given an enormous jolt by the discovery that the previously noted promotion of neurogenesis by antidepressants was necessary for their behavioural effects (Santarelli et al., 2003). This together with the evidence of stress-induced neuronal loss and its blocking by antidepressants has provided a whole new slant on depression and its treatment. Much work is going on in pharmacogenomics to trace common pathways, uncover new targets and determine disease and treatment susceptibility, but its impact on drug discovery is low at present. The field continues to debate the appropriateness of animal models of depression as opposed to behaviours responding to existing therapies, and this debate will continue until radically new ideas are tested in the clinic.

In anxiety, the story is much the same. Several companies have tried and are trying to develop second-generation anxiolytics based on subtypes of the GABA-A receptor that avoid the well-known side-effects of benzodiazepines. However, no new targets have yet provided anxiolytics that have been proven in the clinic.

The modest therapeutic success of the acetylcholinesterase inhibitors, donazepil, rivastigmine and galantamine, has certainly encouraged the search for new and better cognition enhancers. The thinking behind such drugs was simply to replace a known deficiency, that is, to boost acetylcholine levels that had declined because of the loss of cholinergic neurones. There is probably a feeling that the acetylcholine deficiency in Alzheimer's disease has already been dealt with as well as possible and the applicability of the concept to other cognitive disorders is limited. Therefore the field has moved on to consider other neurotransmitters such as glutamate (Lynch, 2002), or the downstream cyclic AMP response element binding protein (CREB) pathway (Tully *et al.*, 2003). Here the emphasis is less perhaps on restoring a simple neurochemical deficit and more on boosting existing systems and ultimately stimulating plasticity and brain repair. The latter thinking is behind the study of 'non-specific' cognitive enhancement in such conditions as stroke, hydrocephalus and acute brain injury. As in other areas of brain disease, the biological validation of new targets in animal models or tests remains problematical until these new ideas have been tested in the clinic. The appropriateness, or even feasibility, of testing cognition enhancers in animals presents problems on two fronts. The first is how to choose a suitable deficit model in which to test drugs, particularly if the aim of the drug is not neurotransmitter replacement. The second bears on a later question in the survey over whether it is possible to develop cognition enhancers to augment normal function in man, and therefore whether it would be necessary to demonstrate efficacy in normal animals to justify development.

In the field of schizophrenia, the success of the atypical antipsychotics in providing some alleviation of most of the core symptoms of the disease has to be set against the fact that no one knows exactly why these drugs are effective (Roth *et al.*, 2004). The reason is simply that the most successful have very complex pharmacology and act at many different CNS receptors. The field has moved from believing that one of these receptors was responsible for all the positive benefits to the understanding that it is the mix of effects that brings therapeutic utility. Theories abound on which aspects of the pharmacology are related to the efficacy of these drugs and which to the side-effects. It is by no means clear that the two will separate cleanly anyway. Consequently, the industry struggles to identify

plausible new approaches, and it recognises the extreme difficulty of reproducing or improving the mix of pharmacology present in successful drugs such as Zyprexa (olanzapine) and Clozaril (clozapine). Experience in this area has led to an increasing belief in the industry that magic bullets based on single mechanisms of action do not exist for CNS disorders. Furthermore the call for 'magic shotguns' (Roth *et al.*, 2004), ie selectively non-selective drugs, underestimates the enormous challenge that this creates for medicinal chemistry.

The respondents gave a wide range of views on the future. There is a degree of optimism that new treatments will be coming forward, but not imminently. Some felt that the lack of a national strategy on CNS disorders to bring together pharmaceutical companies, academia and government was a hindrance to the successful development of new drugs for mental health in general. However, the creation of UK Clinical Research Collaboration (UKCRC) may provide a framework for such a development in the future. It is interesting that, at a European level, through the European Federation of Pharmaceutical Industries and Associations (EFPIA) and organisations such as the European Brain Council, the industry is promoting brain disease as an area for co-ordination of effort and investment. Many felt that new technologies would be important for future success. Pharmacogenomics and pharmacogenetics were frequently cited, although there was less agreement on when these techniques would really feed into the development of new treatments, with projections ranging from 10 to 20 years ('a long march' as one described it). Certainly these techniques will be needed if we are to move from symptomatic treatment to early identification and prevention of disease. The genetic basis of depression may be understood within 10 years, leading to greater patient segregation on the basis of prognosis and treatment modalities, as well as providing potential new targets and biomarkers to aid the drug discovery process. Some companies were optimistic that new understanding of neurotransmitter systems in cognition would bear fruit in providing cognition enhancers for a broader range of conditions, but probably in 10 years rather than 5. Others considered more radical approaches to therapy, such as implants and electrical stimulation of key brain areas, manipulation of gene expression through targeted activation of systemically delivered drugs, stem cell therapy (more than 20 years) and the use of small molecules to activate brain repair mechanisms.

Most respondents were highly optimistic that new antidepressants would be available in 10 years and perhaps earlier. As before, this confidence reflects the fact that many major companies have active research programmes in this area that should deliver in this timeframe.

There was somewhat less confidence about new anti-anxiety drugs in the 5-year horizon, despite the overlap between anxiety and depression and the new emphasis on stress disorders. But there was a degree of accord that in 10 years new treatments should be available.

Cognition enhancement, whether for schizophrenia or for neurodegenerative disease, is clearly perceived as more challenging, for the reasons given above. There are many druggable targets implicated in processes of learning and memory, but the demonstration of robust clinical efficacy is neither fast, easy nor cheap. Mention was made of the importance of rehabilitation plus pharmacological intervention in effective therapy for neurological conditions. This applies equally for traumatic injury (eg stroke) and for degenerative diseases such as Alzheimer's. Concern was expressed that treatments intended to arrest cognitive decline, such as the promising anti-amyloid strategies being used in Alzheimer's disease, could lead to the problem of long-term stabilisation of the impairment with no prospect of improvement. Obviously early and accurate diagnosis would be a key advantage.

The notion of preventative antipsychotic drugs caused concern about how these would be developed and ethically tested in people. It would be necessary to be able to diagnose prodromal schizophrenia with great accuracy to justify the administration of drugs to those who are ostensibly well. The genetic basis of schizophrenia could be unravelled in 3–8 years and might provide the required diagnostic tools. There was a feeling that blocking the transition of the prodromal state to full-blown disease was challenging but not outside the bounds of possibility. Several respondents commented that advances in schizophrenia treatment are going to be difficult and that the more immediate future (5–10 years) lay in adjunct therapy in combination with atypical antipsychotics to broaden efficacy and reduce side-effects.

Many respondents listed other areas of mental health not covered by the main questions. Foremost among these was sleep disorder and the likelihood of new drugs within five years to treat lack of sleep, as well as addressing the need for increased wakefulness. Insomnia has been regarded as secondary to other conditions such as depression, but this picture is changing as it becomes increasingly recognised that insomnia is at the core of many CNS disorders and that treatment of insomnia will have a major impact on mental health. Successful treatments for stress disorders are likely in the 5–10-year timeframe as stress pathways are increasingly targeted for novel therapies. New treatments for ADHD, Parkinson's disease (symptomatic), mood stabilisation and even, surprisingly, autism, were all mentioned by one or more respondents as likely within 5–10 years.

3.5 What is the Likelihood of the Development of New Descriptions or Definitions of Mood Disorders?

There was a remarkable consistency in the responses to this question. New descriptions and definitions are expected with high probability in 5–10 years. One respondent felt that the development of new diagnostic criteria was critical but not being given adequate priority for funding. The failure to improve outdated rating scales based on behavioural descriptors will impede our ability to incorporate genomic information arising in the next 5–10 years, which might then take as long as 20 years to become useful. For example, entirely different symptom clusters might add up to the same Hamilton Depression Rating Scale score, but it is unlikely that the underlying genetic factors are identical. More likely is that new descriptions and definitions will be based on treatment responsiveness and will thereby redefine the disease itself. For example, drugs reducing stress responses will probably be effective in a subset of so-called depressed patients whose exaggerated stress is responsible for their depression. These patients could therefore be rediagnosed as suffering from a stress disorder rather than major depression.

Respondents were also in agreement that the development of new mood-altering drugs based on new definitions would eventually occur but would lag behind, with 15 years as the most likely timeframe. Subclassification of symptoms associated with a core disease (e.g. cognitive impairment associated with schizophrenia) could lead to a clearer framework for polypharmacological approaches. Several warnings, though, were raised, such as the risk of blurring the boundary between therapeutics and 'cosmetics' a common concern with mood-altering drugs. Effective new medicines will inevitably be abused, in the sense that people will take them if they provide a pleasurable sensation, leading to psychological, if not physical, dependence. In an ideal world, such drugs would be used to help individuals susceptible to mood disorder and they would be provided with a proper mix of pharmacological and psychological support.

3.6 What is the Likelihood of the Development of Specific Drugs that are Targeted to Paediatric or Geriatric Care?

Paediatric medicine is a difficult area for the industry and there was little consistency in the answers received. Some saw new drugs arising within 5 years, while others thought that 20 years was the minimum time needed to address all the questions. The safety issue is clearly uppermost in people's minds and is in marked contrast with the development of drugs for geriatric care where very long-term use and developmental toxicology do not require attention. One respondent commented that recent publicity over the use of antidepressants in children would overshadow the development of drugs for paediatric mental health for some time to come. ADHD has been more or less successfully tackled so the obstacles are not insurmountable, and new ideas about autism could bear fruit within 10 years. The view was expressed that a focus on severe genetic or developmental illnesses would be ethically more acceptable than a focus on conditions for which behavioural therapy offers an alternative. However, developmental disorders such as autism have a poor prognosis and, even if treatments were available, toxicity issues would impede development, however efficacious the drug. As in many topics of this survey, the use of pharmacogenomic and pharmacogenetic tools to identify individuals at risk could change the balance in favour of new paediatric drugs.

There is more optimism in geriatric medicine. Current market opportunities are perceived as greater in today's climate, the hurdles are less severe (e.g. toxicological) and both of these are reflected in the emphasis that the industry is placing on mental diseases of old age, primarily Alzheimer's, Parkinson's, depression and sleep disorder. The last of these should definitely be regarded as a primary medical problem in the elderly that remains largely unmet and contributes greatly to the tribulations of old age. In the care setting, one respondent expressed a wish for drugs to improve the quality of life of the elderly rather than just to sedate and manage them, a process that causes impaired rather than the improved cognitive performance that is needed.

One respondent pointed out that, despite the understanding that drug metabolism, efficacy and side-effects of drugs are age-dependent, clinical trials tend to be run in the 60–75 year age group, which is not geriatric by present-day standards.

3.7 Cultural, Ethical, Legal, Societal, Business or Regulatory Changes Required to Allow Development of New Drugs for Medical Purposes

Every respondent thought that the industry would have a major role in providing information on the way to use drugs in the near future, the majority predicting within 5 years. Patients have progressed rapidly in recent years from being mere consumers of healthcare decisions made by the medical profession, through a stage of being better informed, to the present state in which they are involved in making decisions about their own care (the 'expert' patient). This change is desirable and inevitable, but does not necessarily make life easier for the physician or the patient. The access of patients via the Internet to various levels of information, from the traditional, academia-driven and peer-reviewed to the anecdotal, ill-informed and wildly illogical means that the industry should be in the forefront of initiatives to disclose data in order to protect themselves and their products. However, the industry has not moved fast enough in the eyes of the external world and the recent scramble to publish clinical trial data has been motivated more by external legal proceedings than by a genuine desire for openness. As one respondent put it, accusations of lack of transparency over the effects of Vioxx (rofecoxib), Seroxat (paroxetine) and Prozac (fluoxetine) have increased the public's suspicion of the industry, forcing greater openness on the one hand and a demand for more drug monitoring on the other. Nevertheless, more openness is a good move and nearly all respondents were of the opinion that complete reporting of all clinical trial data will be the norm within five years, whether this is voluntary or legislated. A separate issue is how the information that individual companies hold on their products can be conveyed to the patient. National policies on direct-to-consumer advertising differ widely, but patient groups do not want gatekeepers controlling the information they are allowed to receive.

Changes in the way drug discovery is done and delivered to the patient will also have an impact on the transparency issue. The expected development of personalised medicine will lead to the industry offering both diagnostic tools and treatments, bringing them much closer to the patient and requiring more data disclosure and a greater involvement of the patient in decision making.

The industry would like its increased openness to be accompanied by improved understanding on the part of external stakeholders. Public education will be needed and the industry will have to make efforts to provide information in a way that the public can understand. Regulatory agencies have a major role to play in interpreting data in a rigorous and dispassionate manner that strikes a fair balance between the pros and cons of a treatment option. Knee-jerk responses to setbacks may be an inevitable response to the threat of litigation but do little to benefit the patient. Several voices from outside Merck commented that the Merck's defensive withdrawal of Vioxx from the market made no medical and scientific sense and severely limits treatment options for patients in need. Significantly, since these comments were received, the US Food and Drug Administration has given its cautious blessing for Merck to allow Vioxx back onto the market, but only under severely restrictive conditions.

The need for public debate and understanding is most necessary in the areas of greatest sensitivity, for example, where treatment could be imposed for perceived individual or societal gain. With regard to vaccines for the treatment of addiction, the role of the pharmaceutical industry in providing information on the way to use such drugs in the future will be very important but possibly quite restricted. The clinical studies that will be needed to understand the limits to the use of these vaccines as a therapy and as a preventative will be strongly influenced by the regulatory authorities. While the latter are very keen to support the development of new, effective therapies to help current addicts, they may have a strict view about running studies in adolescents to establish the impact these vaccines have on preventing the initiation of drug taking. This aspect of vaccine use in addiction has not yet been discussed in any detail, but will likely involve a number of different social, ethical, government, and regulatory and pharmaceutical groups.

Most respondents believed that regulatory and societal changes will therefore serve to both help and hinder new developments in mental health. On the positive side, greater transparency and a better-informed public debate on risk and benefit could lead to an appreciation that drugs can never be absolutely safe. This appreciation could help counter the present negative image of the industry, restoring confidence in and within the sector and removing the dead hand of risk-averseness from initiatives to develop innovative treatments. Nevertheless, many respondents felt that the inevitable price of recent events would be more post-launch monitoring for side-effects, and more regulation to protect patients, even at the cost of creating barriers to drug discovery. An interesting alternative view was put forward by one respondent who believed that a combination of patient demand and funding problems would eventually reverse the trend towards greater safety as soon as the baby boomers really reached old age. The choice could be either to lower the regulatory hurdle for approval of new treatments in order to lower the costs of care, or to legalise euthanasia.

3.8 What Psychoactive Substances Could be Developed Specifically for Non-medical Purposes?

The attitude conveyed by the responses from the industry ranged from 'impossible' to 'why not?'. The essential issue which all recognised was that scientifically there is no

reason why not, but the question is whether society is prepared to accept this development. As described in section 2.3, this question was not about the off-label use of drugs developed for medical purposes (section 2.2), although several respondents chose to focus on the ethical, legal and social acceptability of mental performance-enhancing drugs rather than the route by which they were developed. Consequently the timelines vary enormously. Several respondents felt that cognition and attention enhancers might be available in 10 years, but this implies that the industry is currently working on drugs for strictly non-medical purposes, which is certainly not the case. However, there are shades of grey between the all-white of purely medical and the black of totally non-medical. Drugs might be developed for particular medical conditions that drive clinical trials and allow the regulators to approve the drugs, when in fact no one is fooled into thinking that they will be restricted to that use. The obvious example that several respondents quoted is that of modafinil (Provigil), approved for the rare condition of narcolepsy, but widely used and prescribed for dealing with various conditions of sleep deprivation, few of which would be considered medical. The regulatory path to create a purely non-medical drug for sleep-deprived, overworked Western man and woman is now clear and will no doubt be taken again in the future.

In their comments, many respondents tackled the general ethical issues around this topic. Taking the question in its intended literal sense, most thought that the answer was that it would never be possible to develop drugs in the foreseeable future purely for non-medical uses, even if those uses were acceptable to society. Major social change would be required to permit this to happen. As one correspondent put it, we are already in the era of non-medical drugs, it is just that we prefer not to admit it yet. What percentage of Viagra (sildenafil) sales is for genuine male erectile dysfunction? Is the enormous effort devoted by the industry to obesity just intended for those whose weight poses them a serious medical problem?

We are already beginning to treat deviation from the norm rather than a specific medical condition. Perhaps normalising blood pressure in patients with hypertension was an early example of this. The societal change needed is greater honesty about what we really want, but this could take many years. The industry is reluctant to push the issue because of the impossibly high standards of safety that would be demanded of a drug developed exclusively for non-medical use. However, greater societal acceptance (or honesty) in this regard would deflect current criticism of the industry, based on the view that it creates diseases in order to sell its products (such as ADHD). The link between what the industry produces and medical need would be severed and replaced by what society wants. The debate about whether industry is trying to move the defining line of normality would become irrelevant.

However, in the current climate, the industry is very sensitive to these issues and, not surprisingly, cautious. Defining the border of normal is difficult, as one respondent said. Another described the issue in terms of public attitudes to increasing performance, providing pleasure and decreasing the stress and strains of daily living. If athletes provide themselves with the best of nutrition to optimise their physical performance, what is to stop the public demanding chemical nourishment for their brain processes? If it really works and is safe, acceptance would be inevitable, although demonstrating efficacy and safety is not trivial.

The safety question may be the greatest impediment to the industry, which is why many respondents thought that the only route to non-medical use was via the demonstration of safety and efficacy in a medical condition. Screening for potential abuse in both animal and human studies is a regulatory requirement and the industry would consider this as part of the entire risk–benefit profile before deciding to continue development of a medicine. A positive screen or abuse test is seen as a major issue, with implications for storage, distribution and ease of writing prescriptions. So such a compound would only be pursued as a medicine if the

medical benefit was considerable. Furthermore, the risk to those taking part in clinical trials is counterbalanced by the potential therapeutic benefits. Regardless of society's acceptance or desires, the industry seems likely to adopt this lower-risk approach and, even then, there would need to be increased public awareness that drugs for non-medical uses still carry risk. It would be easy for the general public to assume that such products were inherently safer than drugs for medical conditions, in the way that many people already take drugs such as ecstasy on a regular basis with little concern for the consequences. As one respondent put it, 'just because you can buy it, doesn't mean it is safe'. A 'happy pill' will always be open to abuse and there will always be the suspicion that industry is putting people at risk for profit, and that government permits this in order to avoid dealing with the root causes of drug-seeking behaviour.

The types of non-medical use that the respondents identified included mood enhancers, anxiolytics, sleep promoters, wakefulness promoters, impulsivity controllers, reaction time modulators and vigilance enhancers. All of these could have bona-fide medical uses as well. The most likely in the 10–20-year timeframe were cognition enhancers, drugs to improve attention (a better caffeine) and drugs to deal with sleep disturbance. There was no agreement on whether it was likely that substances such as nicotine could be delivered in drinks. The response was probably 'yes, but why bother?'.

3.9 Are There Any Other Key Broad Issues Not Covered Elsewhere?

There were few responses in this section and of these, several had already been considered by others in their responses to previous questions. Here two themes are picked out which resonated with many of the comments received. The first is that the successful development of new drugs for mental health would be greatly aided by better national co-ordination of research efforts as already occurs in the US, and that there should be better collaboration between government, the industry and academia to focus resources on critical areas of need. The now defunct UK National Neuroscience Research Institute was an attempt to do this, and it is to be hoped that the UKCRC will help to bring together a national strategy for mental health. Failing this, the European initiatives mentioned earlier may provide a suitable framework. The second is that the treatment of mental illness will change. Better diagnosis and risk-factor assessment, the use of imaging and other technologies will aid appropriate pharmacological intervention. But proper treatment will need to integrate this with behavioural and psychological approaches. As has already been said, there are no magic bullets for mental illness.

3.10 Acknowledgements

The author would like to thank all those companies who participated in this survey and gave so freely of their time and opinions. They were: Amgen, GSK, Lilly, Merck, Neurocrine, Pharmidex, Pfizer, Roche, Xenova.

NOTE

1. Website of the US Center for Cognitive Liberty, which campaigns on this issue: www.cognitiveliberty.org/makingchoices/index.htm.

References

BMJ, (2005) Editorial: Suicide, depression, and antidepressants. *BMJ* 330: 373–374.

Boston Consulting Group. (2004) *A comprehensive assessment of the declining drug development performance of the US pharmaceutical industry.*

Connecting Brains and Society. (2004) The King Baudouin Foundation and the Rathenau Institute.

Evan, W.E. and Relling, M.V. (2004) Moving towards individualized medicine with pharmacogenomics *Nature* 429: 464–468.

IBM Business Consulting Services. (2002) *Pharma 2010: The threshold of innovation.*

Innovation in the pharmaceutical sector. (2004) A study undertaken for the European Commission by Charles River Associates. November.

Kreek, M.J., LaForge, K.S., and Butelman, E. (2002) Pharmacotherapy of addictions. *Nature Rev Drug Disc* 1: 710–725.

Lehman Brothers. (2003) *PharmaPipelines.*

Lingford-Hughes, A.R., Welch, S., and Nutt, D.J. (2004) Evidence-based guidelines for the pharmacological management of substance misuse, addiction and comorbidity: recommendations from the British Association for Psychopharmacology. *Psychopharmacol* 18(3): 293–335.

Little, S. (2004) *Curr Drug Disc* October 2004: 25–27.

Lynch, G. (2002) Memory enhancement: the search for mechanism-based drugs. *Nature Neurosci* 5(Suppl): 1035–1038.

Mack, A. (2003) Examination of the evidence for off-label use of gabapentin. *J Manag Care Pharm* 9(6): 559–568.

Olesen, J. and Leonardi, M. (2003) The burden of brain diseases in Europe. *Eur J Neurology* 10: 471–477.

PharmaFutures. (2004) *The pharmaceutical sector. A long-term value outlook.* December.

Ralston, G.E. and Taylor, J.A. (1993) Temazepam abuse. *Addiction* 88(3): 423.

Ranga, K. and Krishnan, R. (2002) Clinical experience with substance P receptor (NK1) antagonists in depression. *J Clin Psych* 63(Suppl 11): 25–29.

Roth, L.R., Sheffler, D.J, and Kroeze, W.K. (2004) Magic shotguns versus magic bullets: selectively non-selective drugs for mood disorders and schizophrenia. *Nature Rev Drug Disc* 3: 353–358.

Santarelli, L., Saxe, M., Gross, C., Surget, A., Battaglia, F., Dulawa, S., Weisstaub, N., Lee, J., Duman, R., Arancio, O., Belzung, C., and Hen, R. (2003). Substance P antagonists: meet the new drugs, same as the old drugs? Insights from transgenic animal models. *Science* 301: 805–809.

Tufts Center for the Study of Drug Development. (2003) *Impact Report* 5(3).

Tufts Center for the Study of Drug Development. (2004) *News release* 29 April.

Tully, T., Bourtchouladze, R., Scott, R., and Tallman, J. (2003) Targeting the CREB pathway for memory enhancers. *Nature Rev Drug Disc* 2: 267–277.

Volkow, N.D. and Li, T.K. (2004) Drug addiction: the neurobiology of behaviour gone away. *Nature Rev Neurosci* 5: 963–970.

Wong, M.-L. and Licino, J. (2004) From monoamines to generic targets: a paradigm shift for drug discovery in depression. *Nature Rev Drug Disc* 3: 136–151.

Woolf, C.J. (2004) Pain: moving from symptoms control toward mechanism-specific pharmacologic management. *Ann Inter Med* 140(6): 441–451.

4 APPENDIX: SURVEY MATERIAL

This appendix contains a copy of the letter sent to companies inviting them to participate in the study and also a copy of the questionnaire used to collect data.

4.1 Copy of the Letter

The aim of the Foresight on Brain Science, Addiction and Drugs project is to look to the future situation in 2025 and beyond, to consider various ways in which psychoactive substances might be produced, used and regulated. Psychoactive substances are those that are for mental health, pleasure, to enhance cognition or to modify mood.

The key question that the project is addressing is: How can we manage the use of psychoactive substances in the future to best advantage for the individual, the community and society?

Foresight has commissioned 15 state-of-science reviews to provide a scientific basis to explore the key question. The project is looking at a 20-year timeframe, so we are thinking about 2025. This review was commissioned to ensure there was input to the project from an industry perspective. The attached questionnaire is to help you formulate your responses and to enable the writing of a consensus industry view of 2025. The survey is based around three main questions, with a fourth section to cover anything that you consider important which is not covered elsewhere in the survey.

These three questions are: What will be the psychoactive substances of the future (for medical purposes)? What regulatory and societal changes would be required to allow these drugs (for medical purposes) to be developed and marketed? What psychoactive substances could be developed specifically for nonmedical purposes? Obviously any information you can provide should be non-confidential and will be non-attributable. The companies that participate in this survey will be listed and thanked for their input but comments from individual companies will not be identified. I hope that this will encourage the free flow of creative and imaginative juices and therefore please do not feel constrained by the size of the comments boxes. Put down everything that occurs to you. It is likely that the report that is written will eventually be made available publicly through publication in a report in hard copy or downloadable from a website.

The timescale of this exercise is unfortunately very short and, therefore, if you are unable to participate because of lack of time, please delegate the job to those who have, or preferably get a small group to brainstorm the questions. I would appreciate your response by 4 February 2005 at the latest.

Thank you for your time and assistance.

C. Ian Ragan

4.2 Copy of the Questionnaire

Section 1 of the Questionnaire

We would like you to speculate about what types of psychoactive substances there might be in the future. We would like you to consider the role that advances in pharmacogenetics and pharmacogenomics and other technologies will play in realising these developments and the extent that the field could move from symptomatic treatment to cure, prevention or disease modification.

Where possible, please indicate the probability of such developments in the times shown. A separate box is available for you to comment on these or other developments of these types and to expand on your responses.

1. What new preventions/treatments for addiction and problem use may be developed in the following areas?	5 years	10 years	15 years	20 years	Never
Vaccines (for prevention and treatment)					
Drugs to enhance executive function					
Drugs to unlearn addiction					
Anti-stress drugs (as stress has been associated with relapse)					
Combinations with psychological approaches					
Other preventions/treatments not listed that you think the project should consider and when they might be developed					
Comments (eg scientific constraints, impact of technology, genomics etc.)					

2. What is the likelihood of new treatments for the management of pain?	5 years	10 years	15 years	20 years	Never
What is the likelihood of there being effective drugs that do not carry the risk of abuse?					
Comments (eg scientific constraints, impact of technology, genomics, other management of pain issues not listed that you think the project should consider)					

3. What is the likelihood for the development of new drugs for mental health in the following areas?	5 years	10 years	15 years	20 years	Never
New antidepressant drugs					
New anti-anxiety drugs					
Cognition enhancement for those with schizophrenia					
Cognition enhancement for those with neurodegenerative conditions, eg Parkinson's disease, stroke, brain injury					
Preventative antipsychosis drugs					
Other drugs for mental health not listed that you think the project should consider and when they might be developed					
Comments (eg scientific constraints, impact of technology, genomics, opportunities for disease modification, etc.)					

4. What is the likelihood of the development of new descriptions/definitions of mood disorders?	5 years	10 years	15 years	20 years	Never
If so, is it likely that this will lead to the development of new treatments?					
Other issues to do with the development of mood-altering drugs not listed that you think the project should consider and when these might arise					
Comments (eg impact of genetics, pharmacogenetics, pharmacogenomics, etc., possible new or redefined mood disorders)					

	5 years	10 years	15 years	20 years	Never
5a. What is the likelihood of the development of specific drugs that are targeted for paediatric care?					
5b. What is the likelihood of the development of specific drugs that are targeted for geriatric care?					
Other issues to do with the development of mood-altering drugs not listed that you think the project should consider and when these might arise					
Comments (eg impact of genetics, pharmacogenetics, pharmacogenomics, etc., possible new or redefined mood disorders)					

Section 2 of the Quextionnaire

For this section we would like you to consider what cultural/ethical/legal/societal/business/regulatory changes may be required to allow drugs (for medical purposes) to be developed and marketed. Where possible, please give some indication of the importance or likelihood of such developments in the times shown (eg little, a lot, etc.). A separate box is available for you to comment on these or other developments of these types and to expand on your responses.

	5 years	10 years	15 years	20 years	Never
6. How important a role will the pharmaceutical industry have in providing information on the way to use drugs in the future?					
7. How open will be the disclosure of research results?					
8. Will changes in context, whether regulatory or social, occur which will help or hinder advances in these developments or their deployment?					
9. Will there need to be greater safeguards in drug use, for example through drug monitoring?					
Other – any issues not covered by questions 6–9 that you think the project should consider and when these might arise					
Comments (eg communication of information, disclosure of research results, nature of societal changes)					

Section 3 of the Questionnaire

In Section 3 we would like you to speculate on what psychoactive substances could be developed specifically for non-medical purposes. Where possible, please indicate the likelihood of such developments in the times shown. A separate box is available for you to comment on these or other developments of these types and to expand on your responses.

	5 years	10 years	15 years	20 years	Never
10. What is the likelihood of the development of drugs specifically for non-medical use?					
11. What would these drugs be? Please make suggestions with probabilities and times					
12. What changes would be needed in society, in the development and regulatory processes and in the market to allow this? Please list, with likelihood.					
13. What is the likelihood of delivering products such as nicotine in drinks?					
14. What is the likelihood of delivering cognition enhancers that could be used for non-medical purposes?					
Other – any issues not covered by questions 10–14 that you think the project should consider					
Comments					

Section 4 of the Questionnaire

Are there any other key broad issues that are not covered elsewhere in this survey that are being driven by advances in science capability that you think the project should consider? If so, please would you comment?

19

The Scenarios

Office of Science and Innovation

1 INTRODUCTION

1.1 The Brain Science, Addiction and Drugs Project

The UK Government's Foresight programme is managed by the Office of Science and Technology and exists to produce challenging visions of the future to ensure effective strategies now.

The aim of the Brain Science, Addiction and Drugs Project, announced in July 2003, is to provide a vision of how scientific and technological advances may impact on our understanding of addiction and the use of psychoactive substances[1] over the next 20 years by answering the following key question: How can we manage the use of psychoactive substances in the future to best advantage for the individual, the community and society?

As part of the suite of tools designed to answer this question, the project team commissioned Waverley Management Consultants and Henley Centre to develop a set of scenarios which describe four alternative views of the future socioeconomic context in which psychoactive substances will be used.

Foresight has defined a psychoactive substance as 'any substance or surrogate intervention that affects brain function through its chemical neurotransmitters. The term includes recreational, psychiatric, cognitive enhancing or mood-altering drugs and also future technology such as transcranial magnetic stimulation or neural prosthetics'.

2 SCENARIO PLANNING

2.1 Introduction

Scenarios help people imagine and manage the future more effectively. The scenario process highlights the main drivers and uncertainties surrounding a given policy area or activity and explores how they might play out in the future. The result is a set of stories that offer alternative views of what might happen if certain trends – most of which are observable today – continue to a logical conclusion.

There are four broad stages in developing scenarios:

- Stage 1: Identification and analysis of change drivers
- Stage 2: Identification of predetermined elements and critical uncertainties
- Stage 3: Construction of the scenario matrix
- Stage 4: Construction of the scenario narratives.

Sections 2.2–2.5 provide an overview of each of these stages. The specific methodology used in this project can be found in the Appendix.

2.2 Stage 1: Identification and Analysis of Change Drivers

Change drivers are factors which shape the future environment. Some are highly visible now, but others are less so. While it may be possible to determine the effects of change drivers on the present and the near future, it can be less easy to determine their effects in the medium to long term.

It is therefore important during this stage of the scenario process to identify a broad range of drivers and to consider which will be most important in the future – rather than to focus solely on those which are most important today.

Typically at this stage, therefore, drivers are prioritised according to their future policy importance.

2.3 Stage 2: Identification of Predetermined Elements and Critical Uncertainties

Once drivers have been prioritised, the next step is to consider how the important ones might play out in the future. In some cases, drivers will be predetermined elements and their outcome will be quite clear. Other drivers will have uncertain outcomes.

It is important during this stage of the scenario process to identify and characterise both types of outcome. For uncertain drivers, it is essential at this stage to identify the nature of the uncertainty and the range of possible outcomes. It is also important to explore the dynamic interplay between drivers over time.

The critical output from this stage is a number of 'axes of uncertainty' which describe the range of uncertainties for the future, together with the range of possible outcomes. These uncertainties are used to define the scenario space and to shape narrative production. Predetermined elements define strategic issues that need to be addressed across all the scenarios.

2.4 Stage 3: Construction of the Scenario Matrix

The scenario matrix is a 2 × 2 schematic that defines the main parameters of the scenarios. It is constructed by juxtaposing the two axes of uncertainty that reflect the most important uncertainties, offer the most insight, or provide the most intriguing glimpse of the future.

Matrix construction is an art rather than a science and the final 2 × 2 is often decided through negotiation, intuition and testing.

2.5 Stage 4: Construction of the Scenario Narratives

The scenario narratives are constructed within the logical framework provided by the scenario matrix. The narratives draw on all the material in stages 1 and 2 and also on wider research, such as the state-of-science reviews commissioned as part of the Brain Science, Addiction and Drugs project. The narratives can either describe 'end states' – what the world looks like in the future, without any sense of how that future evolved – or 'timelines' – a description of how the future has evolved from the present day. The narratives should present the perspectives of different stakeholders in order to provide a

sense of the different priorities and issues that exist in each future.

Wherever possible, stakeholders should be involved in testing and exploring the emerging scenario narratives.

2.6 Working with the Completed Scenarios

Once the scenarios are completed, they can be used by policy-makers and their organisations to explore how they would act in the different futures. These users can evaluate different policy options, identify success criteria and determine the effect of different policy instruments. Generally, these differ in each scenario and the discussion can help participants build a shared understanding of how the increasingly complex changes taking place in the world are likely to affect their activities.

Policy makers can also use the scenarios to explore the issues and choices facing them today. All scenarios contain elements of today extrapolated to a logical future conclusion. Exploring them allows policy makers to see the consequences of making – or not making – certain policy decisions that might be facing them in the near future.

3 OVERVIEW OF THE SCENARIOS

3.1 Introduction

This section presents the scenario matrix and provides an overview of the scenarios. The detailed methodology employed in the project (including prioritised drivers, predetermined elements and critical uncertainties) is presented in the Appendix.

3.2 The Matrix

The scenario matrix juxtaposes two axes of uncertainty.

Life enhancement–life preservation describes the basis for psychoactive substance use. The axis relates to the views of the individual, community or society. At one extreme, life enhancement involves continuous modification of mood and behaviour. It may also include faster transition to medicalisation and more regulatory, market, or cultural adaptation to non-medical uses. At the other extreme, life preservation includes all psychoactive substance use for therapeutic conditions. The axis provides a certain degree of flexibility about what is classed as a disease, which may change over time.

Evidence-based regulation and view-based regulation describes the basis for regulation. This axis relates to factors which underlie the regulation and control of drug use by government. Evidence-based regulation is informed by current scientific knowledge and is considered in light of the harms and benefits to the individual, community and society that are attached to the use of different psychoactive substances. View-based regulation describes an apparently arbitrary, historic, moralistic and non-science-based policy approach to psychoactive substance control. It involves the control of psychoactive substances purely on the basis of their psychoactive properties, rather than taking into account their other effects, whether beneficial, harmful or pleasurable.

The axes combine to create a scenario space with four scenarios (Figure 19.1).

3.3 High Performance

High Performance is a competitive world where people work and play hard. Cognition enhancers have become highly popular and, following a period of unregulated use, are now used openly to enhance most

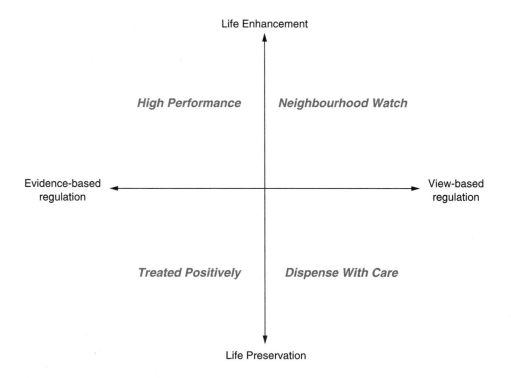

Source: Henley Centre/Waverley Management Consultants

FIGURE 19.1   The scenario matrix.

types of work, under strictly controlled conditions that minimise harm. After some initial concerns, UK society is now ready to accept the use of some recreational drugs, but only under equally strict and regulated conditions. People are able to identify their personal vulnerability profile and take responsibility for choosing substances likely to cause least harm. Addiction is seen solely as an illness to be treated, not a behaviour to be punished, and the number of problem drug users in society is falling. There is still, however, a level of hardcore supply and street use that needs to be tackled, both nationally and internationally.

3.4 Neighbourhood Watch

Neighbourhood Watch describes a world where policy decisions are made according to the prevailing social view and where the approach to drug policy changes regularly. Following a period of tolerance, particularly among the professional classes, drug use is now seen as a social ill that must be stamped out. Locally-based community partnerships implement policy on drug testing in schools and the workplace. Their approach is punitive, with offenders subject to a 'one strike and you're out' policy. Research into the causes and mechanisms of addiction is not valued and there is little interest or investment in treatment. There are concerns over the sustainability of this approach; some regions are relaxing the rules and the UK's strong focus on domestic policy has resulted in continued failure to tackle the international supply chain.

3.5 Dispense With Care

In Dispense With Care, the UK's ageing and demanding population places the NHS under severe strain. The number of conditions that can be treated has increased dramatically and the new generation of 'consumer patients' wants access to all treatments, irrespective of cost. But demand is not matched by a willingness to invest in

the public sector and the NHS is forced to cut back on the number of drugs available to patients. This has led to an increase in private sector healthcare. In general, people are well educated about their health, and drug use has declined. Vaccinations against diseases such as Alzheimer's disease (and against certain forms of addiction) have increased but these are generally only available through the private sector. The NHS has been forced to exclude those requiring treatment due to self-harm.

3.6 Treated Positively

In Treated Positively, advances in our understanding of the molecular mechanisms of disease have transformed the nature of treatment and of the pharmaceutical industry. New, smaller, manufacturers use open-source technology to quickly create customised precision treatments that match individual disease profiles and the large pharmaceutical companies' dominance of the market is threatened. Greater understanding of genetic susceptibility to addiction means that individuals are able to select which psychoactive substances to avoid and even manipulate their own vulnerability profile. Cannabis is used therapeutically by the terminally and chronically ill and psychedelic drugs are being considered as therapeutic agents. Illicit drug manufacture – which has also benefited from advances in science – is cheap and sophisticated.

3.7 Comparison Chart

Table 19.1 describes key differences between the scenarios according to:

- the basis of decision making by policy makers, individuals and society
- how psychoactive substances are used and viewed by society
- what is happening to manufacturers
- how society views addiction
- the ethical issues to be addressed.

TABLE 19.1 Comparison of the scenarios.

	High Performance	Neighbourhood Watch	Dispense With Care	Treated Positively
Decision making	Based on scientific knowledge	Based on the prevailing social view	Based on the prevailing social view	Based on scientific knowledge
How psychoactive substances are used	Widespread, sophisticated use to optimise performance. Harm is minimised	Used according to personal cultural context and peer behaviour	General intolerance of psychoactive substances other than for treatment	Widespread acceptance for treatment, but use for recreation or performance enhancement is less readily accepted
Manufacturers	UK firms are strong suppliers; and move into manufacture and supply of cognition enhancers	UK firms are strong suppliers. Generics are plentiful	UK firms have withdrawn from the development of new medicines for mental health	China and India are key suppliers to private sector. Big companies under threat from open-source niche players
	Generics are plentiful. The black market thrives	Illicit manufacture moves along the international supply chain		Illicit production is cheap and sophisticated
Addiction	Not stigmatised	Not tolerated	Not tolerated	Not stigmatised
	Viewed as an illness to be treated	Punitive and criminalising regime	Addicts not criminalised, but excluded from support frameworks.	Society is increasingly using preventative treatment for those at risk
Ethical issues	Whether to broaden controlled use	Whether the punitive approach is suitable and sustainable	How to deal with the legacy of the socially excluded	Whether to allow widespread interventions to prevent those at risk falling into harm

4 HIGH PERFORMANCE

4.1 Context

It is 21 August 2025. The UK is enjoying a period of high economic growth fuelled by innovation, long-term investment in technology and the sustained acquisition of knowledge, which is now pursued as the key source of value for companies and the key source of wealth creation for nations.

The UK is a strong global player in goods, services and (particularly) talent. Many commentators attribute the UK's current prosperity to the constant churn of 'knowledge nomads' – the newly emerged class of elite knowledge workers who roam the globe constantly in search of new challenges and interests and who regard the UK as one of the most progressive societies in which to live and work. The UK remains confident in a world where trade and production are increasingly concentrated in a small number of large multinationals, but it is also aware that its continued success depends on remaining attractive to nomads.

People work and play hard. There is plenty of opportunity for those who want it – most do – and plenty of reward for those who are successful. Consumption is high and conspicuous; the service sector is thriving and the switch to full electronic service delivery (ESD) means that public services are rightly regarded as among the best in the world.

There is, of course, no such thing as a free lunch and the UK's prosperity has a price tag attached. Continuous innovation and the adoption of technology have created many new jobs and industries, but have also destroyed old ones; growth in the service sector has mopped up a lot of unemployment, but the jobs are not always the ones people want; wealth and opportunity have become concentrated in the cities, while rural areas are under threat; and people are ultimately more concerned with their own interests than with those of the wider community.

Responsible use of psychoactive substances – whether for recreation or performance enhancement – is allowed under regulated conditions and these products are sold in licensed premises. Recreational drugs are expensive and the cost is normally borne by consumers directly. Some employers are willing to subsidise cognition and performance enhancers.

There are no global regulatory standards and the UK is flooded with cheap generics and bootleg drugs from countries with less rigorous quality assurance and testing. Some are sold legitimately, but most are imported over the Internet and sold on the street. Many people are still using black-market drugs.

4.2 Historical Development: the Perspective from 2025

In all the excitement over last week's publication of the UK's latest productivity figures, most people missed the announcement that the number of problem drug users in the UK is continuing to fall steadily (Figure 19.2). While it was perhaps less newsworthy than the economy's improved performance, it is nevertheless a major achievement and one that should not pass unnoticed. Perhaps the fact that it almost did is a mark of how far the UK has come in the last 25 years.

Even back then, the UK was bucking trends. It continued to enjoy steady economic growth during the first years of the new millennium despite the global recession that affected its neighbours, allies and competitors. In 2003, the average couple was twice as well off as their parents had been a generation before. House prices, home ownership and consumer spending all rose strongly and even the least well-off had access to what appeared to be limitless amounts of credit to fuel their demand for consumption.

It was something of a hard-won battle, however. Many employees were struggling to achieve a work-life balance and had little time or energy for leisure pursuits, community participation or self-improvement; and the rising cost of living led to significant numbers of low-paid workers – many of them in the emergency services and other public sector jobs – moving out of the major towns and cities. There was a prevailing mood of short-termism that left many feeling anxious and dissatisfied. The divorce rate rose as the stress of trying to keep afloat took its toll on families and relationships.

The social divide that had plagued the UK since the post-war period was still a problem at that time. Until the end of the twentieth century, the incidence of 'problematic drug use' (as heroin use was defined then) was highest among low-income individuals and the socially deprived. However, alcohol and drug use increased dramatically in the middle classes and among the young as social and economic pressures rose.

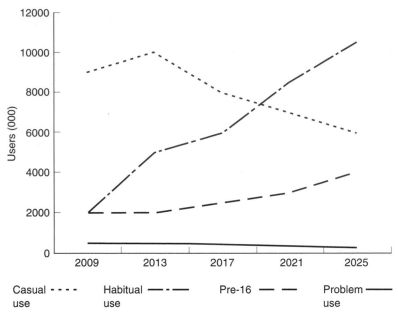

Source: Journal of Addictive Behaviour. Volume 25: August 2025

FIGURE 19.2   Use of Psychoactive Substances 2009–2025.

The majority of middle-class users stuck to cannabis and ecstasy, but growing numbers turned to more powerful drugs like cocaine and even heroin. By 2009, 8 per cent of the adult population – 2.5 million individuals – were estimated to be habitual drug users; 30 per cent (9 million) admitted to occasional use and the number of problematic drug users was continuing to rise.

While these levels of use seem low by comparison with today's standards, drug taking in 2009 was still non-certificated and indiscriminate, and users had no way of knowing what long-term harm they were doing to themselves. Moreover, deterrence – the principal basis of public policy at that time – was unable to contain the social harms caused by increasing numbers of problematic users and the aggressive sales techniques of those who were seeking continued growth of a black market worth £7 billion.

Somewhat perversely, perhaps, the UK's journey out of this tangled web of ethical and social issues began as a result of economic rather than social pressures. By 2010,

the UK's future prosperity was looking less assured and although UK output continued to grow (even if, at 1.5 per cent per annum, it remained significantly below the global and European averages) unrestrained consumer credit, declining productivity and unstable IT were creating mounting concern about the long-term health of the economy.

The UK's concerns were not helped by the continuing growth of the Chinese economy, which had confounded those who thought that it would have to mark time while fiscal reform and infrastructure development caught up. Its continuing – and mutually beneficial – relationship with India and the renaissance of Japan's economy after a decade of painful economic reform meant that suddenly Asia appeared to be right back in the race and the US in particular was looking over its shoulder with rather less amusement than before.

A key factor in the growth of the Asian economies was the level of foreign direct investment in the region. Growing numbers of UK employees found themselves spending time in Beijing and elsewhere and assimilating the distinctive work culture – which included extensive use of drugs designed to enhance wakefulness and intellectual performance. Use of these substances – locally manufactured modifications of second-generation performance enhancers – seemed logical to a workforce made up of sports fanatics who had watched their athletes participate in the drugs 'arms race' of the last three decades and who now believed themselves to be engaged in a similar battle for global economic supremacy.

Performance enhancers began to appear in the UK around 2011. Most employers were aware of their presence, but none would admit it – the prospect of increased wealth and productivity from an enhanced labour force was too much to resist. The UK pharmaceutical companies spotted the potential and quietly began to look at the science underpinning the new psychoactive enhancers. Equally quietly, they began to share their findings. In 2014, PharmUK (the industry representative body) hosted a series of informal private dinners for business and political leaders to discuss the UK's response to cognition enhancement in the labour force.

These were landmark events. By concentrating on the economic and scientific arguments – demonstrable improvement in individual, commercial and regional performance and the potential to develop third-generation drugs that offered little or no risk of harm – the drug companies built a compelling case for the controlled and monitored use of cognition enhancers ('cogs') in the workplace. Their commercial scenarios were compelling too, showing (conservatively as it turned out) a £100 billion market with projected annual growth rates of 5 per cent.

The politicians were willing to listen. All sides of the spectrum recognised the need for a fundamental shift away from the increasingly untenable view-based policies that had dominated successive governments' approaches to drug use. Cog users – motivated by ambition and the desire for greater personal performance rather than the pleasures of intoxication – were different from other drug users. The politicians recognised that the introduction of controlled cog use might offer a route to longer-term acceptance of drugs in society.

And, of course, it was clear that the Asian economies were ready to legalise cogs.

Things began to happen following the landslide victory in the 2015 election, fought on the 'five pledges for prosperity' manifesto which included the promise to 'maximise the benefits from safe use of cognition enhancers and minimise the harms from unsafe use of other psychoactive substances.'

Having won this mandate, the government's first step was to set up the Office of Drug Policy and Testing (ODPT) to oversee the development and delivery of its promise. Its second was to launch an extensive campaign of public engagement designed to inform and stimulate debate and to address the (still considerable) concerns among some parts of the community that the UK was heading down the road to perdition. Getting the media on board was key but, while they were broadly supportive of controlled use, they were sceptical of the government's commitment to drive through the reforms and concerned that a half-hearted approach would do more harm than good. Their scepticism was instrumental in the Government securing all-party support and, once this was in place, the media came on side.

The business community – and particularly the drug manufacturers – also got involved, supporting a series of town hall meetings across the UK and hosting discussion groups on the Internet. They were passionate advocates of enhancers, arguing that regulated use within a controlled environment was considerably safer than unregulated and unsupervised clandestine use.

This was a vigorous debate which helped shape the legislation and, when the bill allowing controlled use of performance enhancers in safe working environments was passed in 2017, the government had no concerns over the political viability of its approach. It was, anyway, a gentle introduction. The Act did not allow enhancement in workers with responsibilities for others (drivers, pilots, teachers or doctors, for example) or in vulnerable groups (the young, the old, those genetically predisposed to addiction, for example). By emphasising that customer safety and product liability rested with employers, the Act ensured that safe use in the workplace was a shared responsibility.

Following the successful pilot of the cannabis blood-level tests and the impact study on cognitive enhancement, two key pieces of legislation were announced in the 2021 King's speech: the amendment to the 2017 Safety at Work Act, extending the category of workers allowed to use performance enhancers; and the Licensed Premises (Cannabis) Act which finally became law last year.

Both initiatives are currently being evaluated by the ODPT and we won't know the policy impacts for another couple of years, but the early indications are positive. The biggest concern about licensing cannabis – that certificated users would resist the random blood tests – has not been an issue so far; and efforts to produce a non-invasive test continue. And far from 'staying away from the airlines in droves', passengers profess to feel safer with cog-enhanced crews. The airlines' investment in smart cockpits which won't let pilots fly until they have passed the functional tests has helped and we can expect to see this technology rolled out to other services and consumer products in the next decade – probably with substance testing as well as performance testing.

It is not surprising that consumers accept these developments. The civil liberties lobby may still regard predictive screening as an intrusion, but most people regard it as a sophisticated way to identify personal vulnerabilities and to take control of their own behaviour. Although some dangers remain – the misconception that it provides a safe way of choosing cocktails, for instance – its benefit in helping people understand addiction and harm is undisputed. Society has benefited too. It is unlikely that the demise of alcohol would have happened without people having access to clear personalised evidence about the harm it causes.

No one can predict who will win the forthcoming election, but it will make little difference to this agenda at least. All four of the main parties have pledged to continue the reform programme and it is likely that the new government's legislative programme will widen the range of substances available in licensed premises. It is also likely that calls to lower the legal age for performance enhancers will be resisted. All parties agree that the evidence on potential harm to young plastic brains still supports the current limit.

Most importantly, the treatment programme launched this year will remain secure. Perhaps this government's greatest triumph is that addiction is now seen solely as an illness to be treated, not a behaviour to be punished. Increased understanding of the neurological mechanisms that cause addictive behaviour and the development of combination therapies are proving as effective

TABLE 19.2   Summary of historical events.

Year	Event
2007	Many struggling with work-life balance
2007	Dramatic increase in drug use among middle classes
2009	2.5 million habitual users
2009	Public policy unable to contain social harm
2009	The UK's future prosperity looking less assured
2010	Extensive use of cognitive enhancers throughout emerging economies
2011	Performance enhancers begin to appear in the UK
2013	Pharmaceutical companies host round-table discussions on future of cognitive enhancers
2015	Office of Drug Policy and Testing set up
2015	Widespread public debate
2017	Safety at Work Act introduced
2019	First cannabis blood-level tests piloted
2021	Licensed Premises (Cannabis) Act passed by Parliament
2021	Safety At Work Act amended to broaden categories of employment
2024	Addiction seen solely as an illness to be cured
2025	Problematic drug use continues to fall

15 June 2025

Party leaders hail decline in problem drug use

Leaders of all the main political parties last night welcomed the news that problem drug use is continuing to fall. Announcing the results, Donal Moore, chair of the cross-party working group on drug use, praised the Office of Drug Policy and Testing.

22 May 2015

Office of Drug Policy and Testing launches Citizens' Forum

The UK government is launching a nationwide forum to build public understanding of the benefits of controlled use of cognition enhancing drugs.

Thursday, 21 August 2025

Come along, now!
It's time to clean up our streets

The lives of thousands of residents across Britain are still blighted by drug dealers – despite the rise in licensed premises nationwide.
It may be true that on-street dealing is falling, but the statistics provide little comfort to those on the front line of Britain's war against the dealers.
"They don't even try to be discreet anymore" said one resident. "they just hang about, waiting for

Tuesday, 6 September 2011

Beaten by a head?

Li Quon Shing is a charming and affable young man who is saving hard to travel to Europe for the Olympics next year.
Quon, a keen amateur sprinter, has an encyclopaedic knowledge of past medal winners, their times and their race histories. It is a remarkable feat of memory which becomes rather more disconcerting when he demonstrates his equally detailed knowledge – and insightful analysis – of the financial services sector in South

May 29 2017

The cogs of industry

Social policy in the early years of this century was dominated by concerns over illicit drug use. Some of those concerns remain today, but things may be about to change now that performance enhancement is an acceptable part of the knowledge professional's tool kit.

as the early promise suggested – and the patients themselves have pointed out that making addiction a health issue rather than a criminal one also makes it easier for them to avoid the social situations and peer pressures that has kept them ill. There is every reason to suppose that the number of problem drugs used on our streets will stay low – and perhaps even reduce further.

There is another benefit of removing drug use from the criminal justice system. The police can now concentrate on the social harms caused by the black market. There is still a level of hardcore supply and use that needs to be tackled, both nationally and internationally. Now that we have chosen to put more of our wealth into healthcare, this must be the next priority.

5 NEIGHBOURHOOD WATCH

5.1 Context

It is 5 May 2025. The UK is suffering something of an identity crisis and is struggling to find its place in the world (prompting some cynics and foreign observers to point out that, actually, it has . . .). Large parts of the UK's administration have been devolved and, while some regions have a greater sense of identity and self-determination, there is growing unease about the consequent loss of social cohesion and the absence of a shared political purpose.

The UK is performing less well economically. Some regions perform better than others. Productivity and profitability generally remain below the European average. Companies are highly cost-conscious. Consumer confidence is low. Economic migration within the UK – towards the more successful regions – is on the increase.

Central government is faced with the challenging task of leading the national response to key strategic issues while continuing to allow local decision making to flourish. This can seem an impossible task – particularly since there is not much money available to fix systemic problems – and it is perhaps no

surprise that government's main priority at the moment is to be seen as a safe pair of hands.

While the decline in political engagement that began at the end of the twentieth century has not yet been reversed, there are some signs that the effort to focus people on their own communities is bearing fruit. It is an important issue and community regeneration is a key challenge for the UK.

People across all strata of society still use psychoactive substances. Consumption of alcohol and tobacco has fallen, but illicit substance use – while in slow decline – is more widespread than it used to be. There has been a strong moral backlash to drug use, however, and communities are working together to tackle the problem. Concerns remain over the effectiveness of the approach in certain regions.

5.2 Historical Development: the Perspective from 2025

It is rumoured that the UK's 'drugs tsar' – chief executive of the Government's current anti-drugs initiative, Be Safe: Getting it right? Avoid Drugs (BSAD) – will plead for more time when she presents her annual review to the Regional Government Summit later this month. Delegates are, of course, used to a succession of tsars, advocates and champions explaining that 'we're not quite there yet, but it's definitely going to be much better soon.' This year, however, they are expecting a celebration and are going to be surprised if the rumour mill is right.

The trouble is that we have begun to believe our own hype. While it is undeniably true that the regional business community partnerships (RBCPs) have made a real difference in tackling drug use over the last six years, their punitive approach does not look economically, morally or socially sustainable. This is not a popular message and the tsar's efforts to stimulate the debate do her credit; as does her insistence that the UK must regain its trust in science and bring it back into the policy process.

May 2–9 2025

Getting it right?

Britain's approach to drug use over the last five years has transformed social attitudes and had a major effect on criminal behaviour. There is much to be pleased about – but there is a lot to be done yet if the country is to maintain the moral high ground and not fall back into a depressing cycle of

---

2 November 2017

Drug taking is 'normal behaviour' in society today

Frederick Brooke, Chief Executive of Safe Society, has warned that drug use in Britain has become normalised, and many people are now resigned to its constant presence as a social ill.

Tuesday, 17 February 2009

Break the habit!

British scientists learn how to control bad behaviour

A team of top British scientists has figured out how to treat addictive behaviour, holding out the possibility that addiction to drink, drugs, chocolate – and even shopping – could soon be a thing of the past. The brainy boffins have discovered why some of us are more likely than others to slip into bad habits and are now working on ways to treat those of us who do. They have identified

---

28 April 2019

New partnerships to tackle drugs

The Government has announced that it will fund a number of Regional Business Community Partnerships (RBCPs) to tackle drugs in their own areas. The Partnerships will represent all parts of the community and will have the powers needed to make and implement local policy. They will be encouraged to focus on school and workplace policing initially, but will have the freedom to move into any aspect of control that their Boards

---

26 June 2025

The Drugs Issue

- Regaining the moral ground.
- Treating addicts: Who cares?
- Controlling the control centre.
- Cause and effect.

The tsar is a determined advocate for legislative development – but is she right?

Part of the answer to that question lies in the long-run consequences of the constantly changing policy framework – sometimes liberal, sometimes punitive, sometimes both together – caused by the coming and going of successive governments. But to fully understand the tsar's unease about the future, we must look at the shifting cultural context of drug use in the UK over the past 40 years.

The emergence of AIDS in the 1980s resulted in an unprecedented campaign to raise awareness of the public health issues, and focused society on the dangers of injecting drugs. As fears that tens of thousands of injecting users would become HIV positive receded, a countercultural movement that saw the campaign images as icons – rather than warnings – took off. The emergence of 'heroin chic' in the 1990s lifted problematic drug use out of deprived housing estates and established it as a rebellious counterculture for the well-heeled. The growth of individualism and self-fulfilment combined with increasing consumption and declining moral authority to make illicit substance use a regular feature of everyday life for a whole new group in society who were anything but economically and politically marginalised.

The number of middle-class users remained relatively low at first – due as much to the high costs and unreliability of supply as to any questions of legality or personal risk – but grew steadily as prices fell. By 2007, the view that illicit psychoactives were a rather more glamorous alternative to the legal ones had firmly taken hold among the professional classes. 'Money, phone, keys, cocaine' was a common checklist before going to meet friends for a night out.

The growth in middle-class users through the mid- to late-noughties was facilitated partly by confusion arising from conflicting policy messages and partly by the new sensibility – reflected in the hit pop song of 2008 and promoted fairly unsubtly through the media – that it was 'trendy (to be tolerant)'. Psychoactive drug use was looked on indulgently as a rite of passage and any

attempt at prohibition was considered to be political suicide. Moreover, the growing publicity given to treatments based on the manipulation of the M-CRM model of addiction (Memory-Control, Reward, Motivation) was (wilfully?) misinterpreted to mean that addiction was under control. By the time of the 2010 election, society – or the better-off parts of it at least – took the view that the drugs issue had been contained, if not eradicated. The election campaign focused on more urgent matters and parents who were hard pressed to pay school fees encouraged their children to use enhancers to help them pass their exams.

While their middle-class cousins were racking up a couple of lines between the tiramisu and double espresso, residents of less well-off communities were facing a rather different reality.

Despite continued efforts to improve living standards across the UK, poverty remained entrenched in certain social groups and geographical areas. Despite regional governments' efforts to use education and entrepreneurialism as ways to raise individuals' aspirations and to empower them to make their way out of poverty, crime – with its low start-up costs, high potential returns and no minimum age requirement – offered a quicker and more exciting route. On-street crime rose sharply as groups of teenagers headed off to the wealthier neighbourhoods nearby.

Drug culture flourished against this background of perceived and often real – loss of opportunity. The 2014 Safe Society Survey (Figure 19.3) showed that teenage drinking and smoking were on the increase (bucking the national trend); that the number of young people taking recreational drugs had increased significantly, with one in ten preteen children admitting using recreational drugs without parental approval; that the prevalence of strokes, psychosis and other illnesses among long-term cannabis users had increased; and that 'cocktailing' (combining drugs in novel ways to get a new high or to stay awake and functioning following consumption) was on the increase. Worst of all

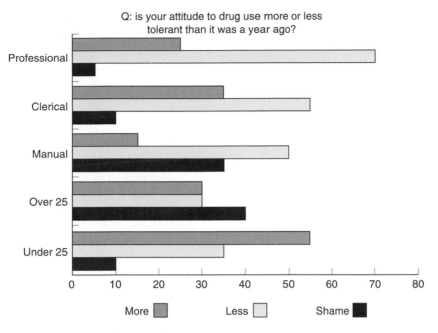

FIGURE 19.3 Safe society survey 2005.

was the level of problematic drug use. It had doubled over the decade, with concomitant and dramatic increases in drug-related crime, infection and death.

In these communities, then, illicit drug taking had become part of everyday life – but unselfconsciously so. Getting together for a drink, a smoke, a toke or a hit was simply what people did when they weren't working. There were no distinctions between 'legal' and 'illegal' substances, since these definitions originated in and related to a world that these particular consumers cared little for and which seemed to care even less for them. Any brushes with authority – and they were rare – were easily shrugged off.

Given these facts, it is shocking to recall the furore that greeted the chair of Safe Society when he suggested, in his 2015 report to the select committee, that drug use had become normalised across society.

While the Safe Society Survey was a pivotal moment in the UK's fight against drugs, it might be described as the warm-up. The main act – which hit the stage in 2017 – was the Spiritual Alliance Against Drugs' seminal book, *The Canute effect: losing the fight against drugs*. The book's use of personal

stories and family histories to illuminate the statistics was revelation enough. But it was the introduction of the Alliance's socioeconomic harm model – and, in particular, the interactive version that allowed readers to input their own postcode and see the impact of drug use on their own community – that really shocked people.

The Canute effect provided a wake-up call for society. Its central thesis was that the responsibility for the growth in the abuse of illicit substances – which was destroying lives, families and communities throughout the UK – was a collective one. The book was particularly dismissive of science, ranking its 'failure' to contain drug abuse alongside its 'failure' in GM, global warming, cyber crime and intelligent road safety. But it also lambasted civic society for effectively sticking its head in the sand, local governments for failing to work together across regional boundaries, providing suppliers with the oxygen for growth, and the pharmaceutical companies which were continuing to produce psychoactive substances, albeit legally.

The book reserved its greatest contempt, though, for what it scathingly called 'the immoral minority' – those members of the middle classes who should (the book argued) know better than to put their own health at risk and to ignore the real price of consumption: misery on the streets in the UK and funds for the regimes and organisations supporting production in Colombia, Afghanistan and elsewhere. In the final chapter, *A learnt habit*, the authors used the harm model to show the impact of parental and sibling drug use on children and, horrifically, what would happen to the UK if just one in ten of the children being encouraged to use cognition enhancers moved on to other drugs.

The Canute effect provided a voice for non-users, pointing out that they were neither intolerant nor abnormal for being against drugs. On the contrary, it argued, non-users were the moral custodians of the future. The Alliance called on them to stand up and be counted.

They did – in droves – and the tide began to turn. Community leaders across the UK began to mobilise citizens and make representations to the regional authorities. The most successful regions were those that involved locally based business in their plans. Engagement was an obvious choice for many businesses increasingly concerned about the consequences of drug use in their current and future labour forces, but especially for the drug companies, which saw involvement as an essential part of their corporate responsibility and a way to strengthen their reputation.

When central government set up the Regional Business Community Partnership Fund in 2019, it received bids for matched funding from all regions. The first RBCPs – with boards comprising community leaders, business leaders, law enforcement officers and health professionals, were incorporated in 2020. They immediately began to build acceptance for the new legislation on mandatory testing in the will workplace and in schools and to oversee its implementation.

The RCBPs have moved from strength to strength over the past five years. Their biggest impact has been keeping communities informed about and involved in new developments and approaches. The best of them have been highly successful in securing consensus to pilot new zero-tolerance programmes such as 'one strike and you're out' – by involving citizen panels in the evaluation process. There is real evidence from the 2024 Safe Society Survey that drug use has dropped significantly among the professional classes and is slowing elsewhere.

It does all feel rather good at the moment – but the tsar is right to be concerned about the sustainability of the UK's current regulatory framework. Moral approaches work best when they are in tune with the morality of the day, and there have been some other – and more disturbing – rumours circulating that some regions might once again be prepared to turn a blind eye to certain types of recreational drug use, as the price for attracting and retaining certain types of wealth creators. If that happens, the whole pack of cards will fall.

The Canute effect's greatest legacy is that it did, indeed, turn the tide but by playing the morality card and castigating science for its 'failures', it unwittingly contributed to the continuing erosion of trust in science. As a result, much of the existing research into the causes and treatment of drug use has been sidelined; and very little new work has been funded in the last decade. The tsar is right to want to bring science back into the policy and regulatory process. If she fails to do so, there is a real danger that the UK's policy approach will return to the liberal/punitive cycle.

There is another factor as well. The UK's continuing struggle to get its own house in order means that we have made little or no effort to tackle the international supply chain that continues to operate effectively, delivering huge quantities of drugs here and elsewhere. We need to pay more attention to finding effective ways of working with our international partners to shut the supply chain down.

There is still, therefore, a lot for the tsar to do. Let's hope delegates at the Summit recognise that.

TABLE 19.3   Summary of historical events

Year	Event
2007	Illicit psychoactive use firmly taken hold of the professional classes
2008	Prevailing sensibility of tolerance to drug use
2010	Better-off parts of society perceive that drug use has been contained
2010	Drug culture is flourishing in poorer communities
2014	Increasing prevalence of drug use in preteens
2014	Increase in problematic drug use
2015	Drug use has become normalised across society
2017	Spiritual Alliance Against Drugs publish *The Canute effect: losing the fight against drugs*
2020	First Regional Community Business Partnerships incorporated
2020	Introduction of mandatory testing in the workplace and schools
2024	Safe Society Survey shows a drop in casual drug use
2025	Drugs tsar pleads for more time

6 DISPENSE WITH CARE

6.1 Context

It is 20 July 2025. While the UK economy can hardly be described as being in difficulty, there is no room for complacency. The UK, in common with most regions of Europe, is trying to simultaneously ride out and correct the 'demographic imbalance' (Figure 19.4) which has seen the worker:pensioner ratio fall dramatically over the last decade: 30 per cent of the population now is over 60; 10 per cent is over 70.

The government has few options. Its efforts to attract young overseas workers and their families to the UK with the offer of jobs, housing, quality of life and opportunity has had limited success due to the highly competitive nature of the marketplace – and the UK's reputation for not welcoming migrants. Another plank of its strategy, investing in UK plc's human resources by encouraging people to stay fit and healthy, has been more successful, but is not itself enough to rectify the situation. Consequently, the UK is a country stretched to capacity. Labour and skills shortages, coupled with inadequate pension arrangements, mean that many people work past the statutory retirement age (now set at 67), but not in sufficient numbers to meet the increasing costs of healthcare and other public services. Personal taxation is higher now than at any time in the last 30 years.

The state remains the main provider of healthcare, but spiralling costs – caused by the ageing population and the growing number of treatments available – have meant a decline in service in recent years. Those who can afford to are moving to the private sector, but the majority don't have the luxury of this option. Grey campaigners – a motivated, skilled and powerful lobby – have brought care for the elderly to the forefront of the political agenda.

Government has acknowledged the need to provide better healthcare, and the cost of treating 'self-inflicted' illness has been shifted to the individual. Those who suffer problems as a direct result of misusing psychoactive substances (including legally produced mood enhancers and cognition enhancers) have to pay for their own healthcare. Some take out specialist medical insurance.

6.2 Historical Development: the Perspective from 2025

ELZ's share price rose today following the CEO's announcement that the company is to begin full-scale production of ADVantage, the vaccine for preventing Alzheimer's disease. 'Vaccines have long been a key public health tool for preventing bacterial infections,' he told delegates and press at the launch event in Beijing this week, 'but this will be the first product that prevents the onset of a non-infectious disease'. ADVantage is good news for ELZ and for millions of patients around the world, and also for

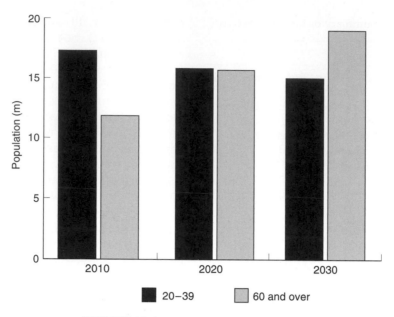

FIGURE 19.4   Population trends, 2010–2030.

the pharmaceutical sector at large, which has been needing a bit of a boost. But unfortunately for those in the UK who suffer from or are predisposed to Alzheimer's, cost considerations mean that ADVantage won't be available to everyone until after the statutory probationary period required to test value for money. Given that there is little doubt it will pass and that the funding problem will have to be addressed anyway, there is a strong argument for probation to be relaxed, allowing ADVantage to be introduced more quickly.

ADVantage has once again focused public attention on the difficulties of choosing between competing needs and treatments in healthcare. The usual explanation for these difficulties is that the UK is a victim of its own – and others' – success in medical advancement. The real story is rather more complicated, and is dominated by increasing patient expectations and the demographic shift that has taken place in the UK over the past 20 years.

When the National Health Service was established in 1948, it offered to provide citizens with 'all medical, dental and nursing care. Everyone – rich or poor, man, woman or child – can use it, or any part of it. There are no charges, except for a few special items'. It was a wonderful, heroic and reckless promise that people took up with such enthusiasm that spending in the first nine months – expected to be £198 million – actually hit £276 million.

Over the following 50 years, any notions that this initial overspend was the legacy of war, rationing and a backlog of untreated cases were quickly dispelled. The funding required to fulfil that initial promise rose in step with medical advancement and by the time the NHS reached its 50th birthday, people were so used to having health services on tap that they took it for granted. In fact, people were so used to having everything on tap that consumption had reached astonishing levels. Two decades of (more or less) sustained world economic growth had created a materialistic and demanding society full of consumers seeking instant fulfilment. The market satisfied their every need and they expected public services to do the same.

Consumer patients, as they were dubbed, were certainly a force for change over the first decade of the twenty-first century – though whether for good or ill remains hotly contested, even today. Consumer patients were very focused on getting what they wanted and constantly sought improvements in care, either for themselves at the point of service, or for society as a whole through political debate in the media. The view that came to dominate public opinion was that the individual's right to health, like his or her right to goods and services, should be met at all costs.

'All costs' rose considerably throughout the decade. While expert commentators argued that a public health system needs sophisticated and principled consumers if it is to develop and provide high-quality services, the 'consumer patient' revolution was blighted by the fact that consumers were not as sophisticated as they thought they were. Although generally well informed about health matters and the latest medical developments, they had a poor understanding of risk, public health issues and how to evaluate the choices needed to run a public health service. They were also particularly susceptible to every latest health scare and, for a while, resource allocation in the NHS began to look dangerously like a ping pong ball policy bouncing here, there and everywhere in response to demand.

Demand grew fastest in the steadily growing elderly population. The over-65s were pretty healthy mechanically, but by 2010, one million of them – one in twenty – suffered from dementia. The number rose to one in five in those over 80. Alzheimer's, the most common dementia, accounted for nearly 500 000 sufferers. Treatments were available, but their efficacy was disputed and the cost was high – over £500 million a year for Alzheimer's alone. The NHS tried to withdraw some of the most expensive and disputed drugs from the market, but found itself at the centre of a huge political storm. This, remember, was the SKIer generation ('spending the kids' inheritance'), having fun after a lifetime of toil. They redefined 'senior' citizens as a moral and political force, using their considerable energy, wealth and time to demand that the state look after them and

their parents. The treatments remained in place for the time being.

The younger generation, meanwhile, were pursuing their own agenda. For a variety of reasons – which ranged from the view that money can buy anything to the view that the state should provide for everybody – it wanted treatment for an increasing number of conditions which had once been considered 'social' or 'psychological'. As consumers used to getting what they wanted, they found it intolerable that they should feel stress, have cravings for chocolate, cigarettes or cannabis, or that their children should not be vaccinated against the threat of behavioural or substance addiction. The number of prescriptions for behaviour-controlling drugs increased fivefold between 2007 and 2012, without patients properly understanding the possible harms they were being exposed to and before the medical profession could establish appropriate levels of prescribing.

If these rising demands had been backed up by concomitant levels of investment, the 'consumer patient' phenomenon might have created a virtuous spiral of improvement. But instead, focused as always on their own interests rather than the collective good, the NHS's 'shareholders' constantly voted for the parties of low taxation. This was not a sustainable position. By 2014, many commentators were concerned that the NHS was on the brink of terminal decline. The electorate took the view that the media was crying wolf – and kept up the pressure.

The surge in demand caused by the 2015 flu pandemic nearly did push the NHS over the brink. Simultaneously its finest hour and its worst, the pandemic served to remind society that you get what you pay for. It also, sadly, reminded them what was truly important. All the previously warring communities were affected to some degree.

Once the pandemic was over, society began to take a hard look at its priorities. The soul-searching and breast-beating which filled the media long afterwards marked a shift away from the culture of consumption and towards a more balanced, ecological

21 July 2025

ELZ gains ADVantage as shares soar

Share prices rose steeply overnight as ELZ, the Chinese pharmaceutical giant, launched its long-awaited vaccine against Alzheimer's Disease yesterday. ADVantage is the latest product to appear from ELZ's highly innovative research laboratories. ELZ has defended the cost of ADVantage and it appears unlikely that it will have significant

Wednesday 19 January 2011

How dare they?

Patients denied 'expensive' drugs

Five patients suffering from Alzheimer's Disease have been told they will not receive their medication any longer because it is too expensive. Sarah Andrews, who cares full time for her father, Jack, 75, was told by her local health authority that he can no longer have the drugs that helped him and that he must take an alternative, cheaper drug. "He used to have this drug and it was hopeless," Sarah told us

June 21-27 2012

Welfare in a state

It has always been true that you get what you pay for. Most of us recognise this fact, which is why we generally tend to spend as much as we can possibly afford when buying anything new – whether it be a tennis racquet or a house. The rule holds for just about anything – except healthcare, where we are most certainly not

30 June 2025

NHS 'no longer able to help those who don't help themselves'

The Minister for Health announces that, due to rising healthcare costs, certain illnesses resulting from 'self-harm' can no longer be treated on the NHS.

approach to living. People accepted the need to invest more in society and in the public infrastructure needed to maintain and care for it.

They also recognised the need to take more direct responsibility for their own health. They called for – and paid attention to – better information on diet, exercise and general health. There was a renewal of interest in simple, freshly prepared food. The UK lost its crown as the fast-food king of Europe and the nation got off the couch and began to swim, cycle and play football again.

The use of illicit drugs declined in the young and middle-aged middle classes. While this was partly caused by abstinence – the shift towards a healthier culture meant that some people were persuaded to 'go for a run instead of popping a pill' – much of it was due to consumers switching substance. Continued ambiguity about the link between depression, psychosis and the long-term use of drugs such as cannabis and ecstasy persuaded floating users to switch to alcohol which they perceived to be less harmful in light of its legal status. There was a consequent increase in antisocial behaviour due to drinking but any concerns were overridden by a decline in drug-related crime. Tobacco consumption also increased slightly, most significantly among the young.

The shift towards greater personal responsibility for healthcare was not just restricted to behaviour. By 2020, over one-third of the UK population – and one in four of those over 60 – had taken out supplementary private medical insurance. Patients mainly used the private sector for health 'events' such as birth, operations or long-term care, and stayed within the NHS for day-to-day treatment.

These improvements were not enough to offset the legacy of years (some said decades) of under-investment in the health sector, so no one was surprised when COPE – the Centre of Practice Excellence – introduced stringent probationary procedures in 2021 to reduce the cost and number of new drugs made available through the NHS. UK manufacturers, already under pressure to reduce costs, were forced to consolidate product ranges and concentrate on lower-risk, higher-value drugs. Development of new medicines for mental health stopped entirely, leaving the market for new treatment of central nervous system disease open to less regulated producers in China and India. Some consumers chose to access producers directly through unregulated routes, such as the Internet.

COPE's reduction programme has clear consequences for the treatment of dementia and a vast array of medicalised disorders, but the most significant impact is likely to be on the new generation of drugs being developed to treat addiction and tackle vulnerability. Not only are they unlikely to get onto COPE's register, but the prevailing view now is that addiction is a self-imposed illness that individuals should deal with through the private rather than public sector. The fact that this consigns a large swathe of users to a future they prefer not to contemplate is a regrettable but unavoidable consequence.

The private sector providers are certainly appraising their options. They have already picked up on concerns about addiction and vulnerability and have cleverly (cynically?) targeted worried parents by offering vaccinations against the common drugs of addiction (cocaine, heroine, nicotine and cannabis – but not as yet, alcohol) in children's formulations. The government's view that there is no evidence to suggest long-term harm will be good enough to offset any lingering doubts.

As for the over-65s, they are philosophical – mellow, even – about the changes of the last decade. They have been able to make alternative arrangements for many of the ailments of old age, but dementia is one condition that still relies on big pharma. Big pharma perhaps relies on it too, knowing that the private healthcare market is not going to be sufficient to sustain them. There may be no precedent for COPE to relax its probation protocols for ADVantage, but it doesn't really need one. We could all be winners.

7 TREATED POSITIVELY

7.1 Context

It is 17 March 2025. The UK is facing a number of challenging social and political issues including global warming, terrorism and global equity, and the government is as concerned with foreign policy as it is with domestic matters.

The UK's citizens are concerned about these issues too and have adopted the values and principles that underpin the need to tackle them. Society places greater importance on lifestyle, on taking care of one's self and one's family and on developing community. Consumerism has become less important and people are willing to make the investment necessary to fund a higher, more equitable quality of life.

Economic growth is still market-driven, but it has been slower than in the past. There have been higher levels of taxation and investment. The regulatory regime

TABLE 19.4 Summary of historical events.

Year	Event
2005	Emergence of 'consumer patient' phenomenon
2008	Poor public understanding of choices in health policy
2010	Dementia sufferers approach 1 million in the UK
2011	SKIer generation become a strong political force
2012	Five-fold increase in prescription of behaviour-controlling drugs
2014	NHS on brink of terminal decline
2015	Flu pandemic
2016	Shift away from the culture of consumption towards a more balanced, ecological approach to living
2017	Decline in illicit substance use with associated rise in alcohol and tobacco use
2020	One-third of UK population has private medical insurance
2021	COPE introduces new probationary procedures to help with prescription drug reduction
2023	UK pharmaceutical sector stops development of new medicines for mental health
2024	Private health providers diversify
2025	Full-scale production of ADVantage, a vaccine for Alzheimer's disease

encourages wealth distribution through fair trade. Tariffs are negotiated through a constant and dynamic process.

There is a general shift towards smaller businesses. This reflects the benefits of smaller, nimbler structures rather than any particular view that big capitalism is bad.

Increased understanding of the harm that drug users inflict on themselves, their families, their communities and society drives policy. The approach has been particularly successful in well-educated and middle-class families (Figure 19.5). It is, however, regarded with suspicion by the less well-educated and they are less willing to seek help. Consequently, there is concern that they are in danger of excluding themselves from treatment.

The UK is an acknowledged leader in addiction treatment, but is still frustrated by its own (and the international community's) failure to tackle supply – a failure which continues to cause tension between nation states.

7.2 Historical Development: the Perspective from 2025

The Medicines Review Commissioner today launched a robust defence of his decision that psychedelic drugs should not be used in the treatment of conditions such as alcoholism, depression and post-traumatic stress disorder. 'The latest research on the efficacy of psychedelics on these conditions is inconclusive,' he said, adding, 'I am not, however, closing the door on their use in the future'.

The ruling has disappointed a number of pharmaceutical companies which were hoping for a more favourable outcome, but they have taken his remarks to mean that the next review will allow psychedelics to be used, at least for treating depression. This will probably be enough to keep them happy in the meantime – alcoholism is a shrinking market anyway and using psychedelics to treat stress disorders is still fraught with ethical difficulties.

The Commissioner was also at pains to emphasise that his ruling is for the immediate future and that rehabilitation of psychedelics is not being blocked. He simply wishes to ensure that the evidence is in place before making his recommendation one way or another.

Science was somewhat in the doldrums in the early noughties, poorly perceived, poorly valued and mistrusted by large parts of society. People laboured under two general misapprehensions about scientific endeavour: first, that it was founded on the discovery of absolute and incontrovertible truths and, second, that it could fix anything. This led to unrealistic expectations, and whenever a crisis or health scare arose, people wanted to know what was going to be done

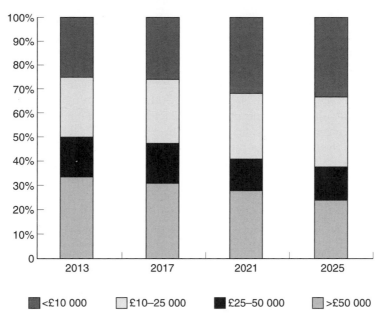

Source: Medicines Review Commission, 2025

FIGURE 19.5 Number of occasional drug users by income.

about it, by when, why the situation had been allowed to arise in the first place and who was to blame. Any delays, or attempts to explain why something couldn't be done immediately, were interpreted as procrastination or evasion.

Scientists' efforts to make science more accessible – by engaging in public debate about the interpretation of data and the ethics and impact of new discoveries – were generally misrepresented by a media which sought 'the answers' and which tended towards sensationalist rather than measured reporting. Wilfully or otherwise, they presented differences of opinion as being politically motivated, or as proof of some vested interest. It didn't help that politicians were quick to pick up the data and arguments that suited their purposes and quick to discard those that didn't.

Life scientists had a particularly trying time, caught up in ethical issues such as cloning, GM food and extended longevity, and decried for playing God or for putting profit before people. It is a happy irony, therefore, that they were mainly responsible

for the sea change in society's attitude that began in 2007 with the unravelling of the basic molecular biology of cancer and continued with the subsequent development of today's array of genetically based precision treatments.

The cultural and political reverberations of these developments were profound. This was still the era of so-called 'blockbuster' drugs that were handed out to all patients, but which offered different levels of efficacy and variable, sometimes extreme, side-effects. The government's first challenge, therefore, was to understand the regulatory and economic implications for the drugs industry of precision treatments for cancer. The second was to work out the cost implications to the health service.

The Medicines Review Commission, set up in 2010, was charged with identifying the issues and making policy recommendations to the Prime Minister. The Commission was encouraged to interpret its brief widely and it quickly began to examine the feasibility of extending the range of illnesses understood at the molecular and genetic level. One of its first recommendations was that the government increase funding in a number of areas, including addiction.

The Commission also began to look at some wider issues of patient care and, particularly, the use of cannabinoids to treat distress in terminally ill patients. Cannabis had been used by cancer sufferers and other seriously ill patients to alleviate pain and distress for many years. Patients were resigned to being classed as criminals and, while not happy about the situation, generally had more pressing issues to worry about. Many of them, however, became reluctant causes célèbres (some said pawns) as they were drawn into highly politicised debates on legalisation that did little to advance society's understanding of the moral, sociological or scientific issues involved. The Commission sought to move the debate on by introducing some rational analysis and exploding some of the myths put forward by both sides.

The UK was not alone in wrestling with this dilemma and the debate certainly moved on when the US decided to legalise cannabis treatment for the terminally ill. America's hard-line stance on cannabis had been weakening for some time, due in part to the growing number of states allowing medical marijuana use in defiance of federal law. More significantly, though, its longstanding position that abstinence should be promoted at all costs and that initiatives such as needle exchange promoted drug use and blood-borne disease became increasingly untenable in light of growing evidence to the contrary. When Europe finally lost patience with US intransigence, it used the United Nations to negotiate a shift in position as its price for joining the global coalition. The rest, as they say, is history. The US legislation was passed in 2013 and the UK followed a year later with the Cannabinoid Act.

As in the US, cannabis-based treatment was initially limited to the terminally ill. Although the 2018 review of the act widened use to all cancer patients in chemotherapy and to patients with long-term degenerative illnesses such as multiple sclerosis, it resisted calls for more general release, noting that prescription for more general ailments relied on subjective judgements by GPs that were open to abuse by unscrupulous patients. Aside from the moral issues involved, the Commission remained concerned to protect the vulnerable, particularly young users and those with depression, from the as yet unproven effects of long-term cannabis use.

These concerns prompted the Commission to recommend that UK research concentrate on the molecular mechanisms of addiction. The Brain Imaging Institute, a joint venture between government, academia and industry, was set up in 2012 to build this understanding and to test new approaches to treatment. The Institute used new fluorescent markers to identify which areas of the brain were involved in addiction by observing where and how certain molecules acted. The collaborative approach was powerful and quickly led to advances in the understanding of addiction and the effects of psychoactive substances. Working together through the Institute, academia and industry were able to rapidly develop and test the efficacy of new agents designed for precision treatment.

One unintended spin-off from the Institute's work was the development of a vulnerability test which combined genetic and imaging data to suggest susceptibility to addiction. The test was trialled in 2017 with some success and, although it remains a costly and low-volume option, research is continuing into the benefits of making it more widely available. There are hopes, too, that mass screening will allow the prediction of sensitivity to drugs and quantify the risks of dangerous drug interactions. There remains, though, a question about how acceptable this will be to a society of individuals who still retain the right to their own genetic information. By 2020, the shape of the new pharmaceutical sector was beginning to emerge. Although big drug companies still dominated the market, there was a growing number of low-cost specialist manufacturers using 'open source' – collaborative knowledge-based systems that use pharmacogenetics and other research data to create new precision treatments. Open source remains an exciting development in the industry today, increasingly allowing small and micromanufacturers to quickly create customised treatments to match individual disease profiles. Many of the incumbents dismiss it, but no one really believes that there is any future in the fortress approach to in-house development that sustained blockbuster drugs.

Open source is also an exciting development for illicit drug manufacturers. There are signs that the next generation of illicit substances will also be precision drugs, targeted at the individual's brain's reward system. The sudden appearance of 'brainbursts' in 2022 shows how sophisticated illicit manufacturing processes have become. Precision illicits offer high returns – more intense effects, cheaper to make, easier to cut – and users appear to be willing to try anything once.

17 March 2025

Psychedelics: Case Not Proven

The Medicines Review Commission's decision to refuse a licence for psychedelic drug use in treating depression and other illnesses is a disappointment. It means that a great many users will need to stay outside the law for the present time.

1 October 2010

End of the blockbuster?

- Targeted Treatments.
- Mass Profiling?

Friday 21 September 2018

Government denies drug testing plans

New government-funded research means that doctors will soon be able to test everyone for drug addiction. The test – which has already been trialled – uses DNA data and brain imaging to work out whether someone is likely to take drugs or not. Sarah Smith, Director of Privacy, claimed that government plans to test everyone are illegal – but a spokesman for the Department of Information said that there were no such plans and that the tests

Indeed, the past decade's efforts to understand addiction and identify precision treatments have not been matched by investment in tackling the problem on the street. Education, and increased awareness of the health (rather than moral) dangers of taking psychoactive substances, mean that some people think carefully about consuming recreational or performance-enhancing drugs. But the evidence suggests that the less well-off and the most vulnerable are still generally unaware of the potential risks.

The combination of new research with significant advances in clinical and experimental psychology, particularly in the management of behavioural addiction and the neuropsychological processes involved in relapse, has created a multidisciplinary approach to treatment that is highly effective. The simple fact remains, however, that the supply of patients is showing no sign of drying up.

Society may have resolved some of the ethical dilemmas of 20 years ago, but new ones have emerged to take their place. Open source, with all its potential benefits, requires regulation. The development of new pharmacogenetic and pharmacogenomic tools offers the possibility of genetic modification to treat or reduce the risk of addiction, whether voluntarily or not. Children, too, could be vaccinated against addiction. Society will have to address these issues sooner rather than later and it is likely that the Commission will launch the debate soon.

Meanwhile, the Commission needs to look more closely at the research on psychedelics. The scientific evidence for psychedelics' efficacy as therapeutic agents is compelling, but there remains the wider concern that they are still too closely associated with leisure use. The 2023 review of the Cannabinoid Act concluded that cannabis remains open to the dangers of abuse and did not widen use. The same argument applies to psychedelics and, at a time when society needs to revisit the balance between treatment, research and the fight against illicit use, their introduction might just be a step too far.

TABLE 19.5 Summary of historical events.

Year	Event
2007	Molecular biology of cancer is unravelled
2010	Medicines Review Commission set up
2012	Brain Imaging Institute set up
2013	US legalises cannabis treatment for the terminally ill
2014	UK legalises cannabis treatment for the terminally ill
2017	First trial of vulnerability testing
2018	Review of Cannabinoid Act widens use to treatment of chemotherapy and the seriously ill
2020	Open source begins to change the structure of the pharmaceutical industry
2022	Illicit manufacturers move towards precision drugs
2023	Illicit drug use remains a problem
2023	Review of Cannabinoid Act maintains use but doesn't widen it
2024	Ethical dilemmas emerge around regulation and treatment and control of addiction
2025	Medical Review Commissioner announces that the evidence for introducing psychedelics is not conclusive

8 WORKING WITH THE SCENARIOS

8.1 Introduction

This section of the report offers some suggestions for how to work with the scenarios. The approaches described here are based on those used in other Foresight projects (principally the Cyber Trust and Crime Prevention project) and in other public sector scenario projects.

The list is not comprehensive, but does offer some insights into how to use the scenarios to inform strategy. The approaches described here work best in facilitated workshop sessions with upwards of 12 participants. Typically, they require one full day, although it is possible to hold productive conversations with fewer people and, if required, in less time.

Three approaches are described here. None of them suggest that those involved identify the scenario they want to happen and then identify what to do to ensure that it does. Mainly that is because the scenarios describe possibilities rather than predict outcomes. The reality is that the future will contain elements of all four scenarios. The uncertainty is which elements – and, consequently, which challenges – will dominate.

8.2 Gaming

The basic approach to gaming involves exploring the scenarios from the perspective of a number of different stakeholders and then using the futures perspective to devise recommendations for the present.

A typical gaming workshop can be structured in six steps:

- Step 1: Carry out a SWOT (strengths, weaknesses, opportunities, threats) analysis of the first scenario from the perspective of one of (say) three stakeholders (government, citizens, industry, law enforcers, illegal manufacturers and users are all suitable candidates in the present case).
- Step 2: Use the SWOT discussion to determine the extent to which each stakeholder likes living and working in the scenario and identify what they want government to do to maintain or improve their level of satisfaction.
- Step 3: Step out of role – and, imagining that the scenario is an accurate representation of the future – make a number of recommendations for current policy. These recommendations should reinforce the elements of the scenario which participants believe to be beneficial to the UK and should address those elements which are likely to be less beneficial.
- Step 4: Consider the risks to government (or other key actors) in pursuing the policy recommendations made in Step 3. Develop a strategy for managing risk.
- Step 5: Repeat steps 1–4 for the other three scenarios. An alternative approach is to work in parallel across the scenarios.

- Step 6: Compare the results of the different scenario discussions to identify robust policy challenges, those which appear in all or most of the scenarios, and scenario-specific challenges. Gaming workshops offer a rich perspective on the policy challenges facing government and other actors. The outputs from gaming workshops generally highlights a number of significant policy challenges and risk issues that need to be addressed in the near future.

8.3 Windtunnelling

'Windtunnelling' describes the process where the scenarios are used to test the robustness of a particular policy or strategy under development.

A typical windtunnelling workshop can be structured in six steps:

- Step 1: Agree the wording, purpose and desired outcomes of the policy or strategy.
- Step 2: Carry out a SWOT analysis of each scenario from the perspective of one of (say) three stakeholders (government, citizens, industry, law enforcers, illegal manufacturers, or users are all suitable candidates in the present case).
- Step 3: Identify the factors supporting – and barriers holding back – successful implementation of the policy or strategy in each scenario.
- Step 4: Clarify whether the policy or strategy is robust, redundant, or in need of modification in each scenario.
- Step 5: Agree the main steps required to deliver the policy or strategy in each scenario.
- Step 6: Discuss which scenario is closest to current reality and which scenario is closest to the 'official' future – and use this discussion to draw together the discussion from the earlier steps in order to identify what can be done to deliver the policy or strategy now, what needs further analysis and testing, and what – if any – further research needs to be carried out.

8.4 Reverse Engineering

Reverse engineering is a process of deconstructing the scenarios, using similar techniques to the ones used to develop them, to identify future events which require a policy or strategic response.

A typical reverse engineering workshop can be structured in five steps:

- Step 1: Discuss the benefits and disbenefits of a given scenario.
- Step 2: Identify trends and events which need to happen for the scenario to occur (some of these events are embedded in the narrative, but the group should identify more).
- Step 3: Map trends and events on a 2 × 2 matrix, according to whether they are certain or uncertain and whether they will have a high or low impact on a given policy area or actor.
- Step 4: For high-impact events that are certain to occur, ask the group to identify whether:

  o the events will occur in the short, medium or long term

  o whether the impact is positive or negative

  o what the response should be.

- Step 5: Repeat across all scenarios.

Reverse engineering exercises use the scenarios to identify opportunities and threats facing the organisation in the short, medium or long term. They are a powerful and productive way of setting a forward agenda for action.

9 APPENDIX: METHODOLOGY

9.1 Introduction

Henley Centre used a three-stage process for this project, consisting of driver assessment, scenario development and scenario testing. This approach is based on current thinking about how organisations learn. Stakeholders are involved from the first stage of the process – reviewing the drivers – through to the development of the scenarios and their implications (see Figure 19.6).

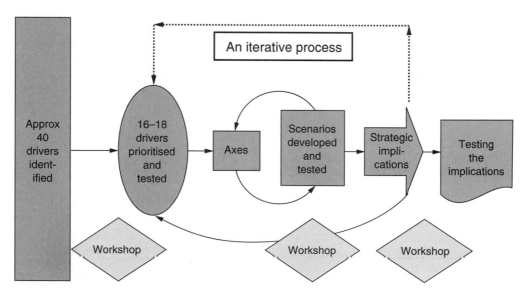

Source: Henley Centre

FIGURE 19.6 Project process.

9.2 Stage 1: Driver Assessment

In preparation for the first workshop, Henley Centre assembled approximately 40 drivers of change, broadly speaking across the so-called 'STEEPO' categories: Social, Technological, Economic, Environment, Political and Organisational (see Figure 19.7). A significant proportion of these drivers were specific to the area of brain science, addiction and drugs, although some captured wider social trends such as attitudes to leisure. They included technology and regulatory drivers. Sources included:

- analysis of the Brain Science Addiction and Drugs project output to date
- the Henley Centre's Knowledge Bank of drivers and trends, both qualitative and quantitative, including changes in consumer attitudes and behaviour as well as major shifts in society
- the initial scoping work conducted by Henley Centre for the project.

This stage concluded with a structured workshop which enabled participants to test the drivers in a number of ways including individual assessment, group review and plenary response, offering a valuable triangulation process to test the data. Techniques used included a proprietary Henley Centre technique based on 'Futures Wheels'. Importantly, the porous workshop process provided an opportunity for participants to add drivers they felt were missing.

The output of this first stage was a prioritised set of drivers, tested for both importance and uncertainty. There was a significant degree of consensus about those drivers which seemed most important in determining the future of brain science, addiction and drugs. The final prioritised set of drivers, in no particular order, is listed below:

- increasing social cost of drug use
- increasing drive to a performance culture
- increasing healthcare costs
- ageing population
- technological surveillance and control
- increasing knowledge about drug effects among professionals and users
- widening gap between rich and poor
- increasing individualism
- new markets for psychoactive drugs and treatments

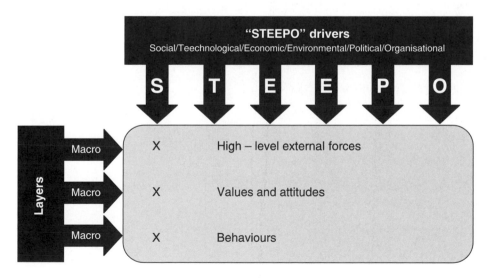

Source: Henley Centre

FIGURE 19.7   STEEPO process.

- increasing geopolitical instability
- increasing market for lifestyle drugs
- several generations having grown up with drug use
- convergence of food and drug industries
- shift towards harm-based view of regulation.

9.3 Stage 2: Scenario Development

In consultation with the core Foresight team and Waverley Management Consultants, Henley synthesised the output from stage 1 to generate a proposed set of scenario axes and, subsequently, a short set of initial scenarios drafted by Alister Wilson of Waverley Management Consultants.

In order to develop the axes, the priority drivers listed above were assessed in terms of their relative impact on the other shortlisted drivers. This 'dependency analysis' identified:

- those drivers which are dominant and therefore have a major impact in terms

of affecting change ('predetermined elements')
- those drivers which are dependent and are therefore relatively uncertain in their impact, as they tend to follow change ('critical uncertainties').

The drivers, which are both dominant and uncertain, give the greatest scope for creating divergent possible futures and are consequently the key focus. The dependency matrix resulting from this analysis is in Figure 19.8.

The drivers that emerged as being both relatively dominant and relatively dependent were then clustered and synthesised to generate two axes or dimensions, which in turn create a framework on which the scenarios could be developed.

The prioritised drivers were:

- increasing social cost of drug use
- increasing healthcare costs
- increasing knowledge about drug effects (by both professionals and users)
- widening gap between rich and poor

Dominance			
H	- Increasing drive to a performance culture - Ageing population - Increasing individualism		- Increasing healthcare costs - New markets for psychoactive drugs and treatments
M	- Several generations have grown up with drug use	- Widening gap between rich and poor	- Shift towards harm based view of regulation - Increasing market for lifestyle drugs - Increasing social cost of drug use - Increasing knowledge of effects of drugs (professionals and users)
L	- Increasing geopolitical instability	- Convergence of food and drug industries	- Technological surveillance and control
	L	M	H　　Dependency

Source: Henley Centre

FIGURE 19.8 Dependency matrix.

- new markets for psychoactive drugs and treatments
- increasing market for lifestyle drugs
- shift towards harm-based view of regulation.

The two emerging clusters and the drivers which they captured were:

- Regulation

  - shift towards harm-based view of regulation
  - increasing social cost of drug use
  - increasing knowledge of effects of drugs (by both professionals and users)
  - increasing healthcare costs.

- Psychoactive substances use and supply

  - new markets for psychoactive drugs and treatments
  - widening gap between rich and poor
  - increasing market for lifestyle drugs.

When building the scenario axes, consideration of three factors is important:

- there should be a degree of uncertainty about each axis
- there should be a degree of complexity about each axis
- axes should be different in nature (ie not collapse on top of each other).

Various iterations of axes were considered. The final combination was regarded as being the set which most rigorously reflected the output of the dependency matrix, and which created strategically useful and interesting scenarios for Foresight.

9.3.1 The Vertical Axis: Basis for Psychoactive Substance Use (Life Enhancement ↔ Life Preservation)

This is a versatile axis which may relate to the views of the individual, community or society. The communities may be ethnic, geographical or demographic in their nature. At one extreme, life enhancement involves continuous modification of mood

and behaviour. It may also include faster transition to medicalisation and more regulatory, market, and cultural adaptation to nonmedical uses. At the other extreme, life preservation includes all psychoactive substance use for therapeutic conditions. As an axis, it provides a certain degree of flexibility. For example, history shows us that what is classed as a disease may change over time. This axis allows for such changes to be reflected in the scenario narratives.

9.3.2 The Horizontal Axis: Basis for Regulation (Evidence-based Regulation ↔ View-based Regulation)

This axis relates to factors that underlie regulation and control of drug use by government. Evidence-based regulation is informed by current scientific knowledge and is considered in light of the harms and benefits to the individual, community and society that are attached to the use of different psychoactive substances. At the other extreme, view-based regulation describes an apparently arbitrary, historical, moralistic or non-science-based policy approach to psychoactive substance control. It incorporates the control of psychoactive substances purely on the basis of their psychoactive properties, rather than taking into account their other effects, whether beneficial, harmful or pleasurable.

Based on these two axes, short scenarios or potential futures were developed for each of the four possibilities using combinations of the extremes of each scenario axis (see Figure 19.1). It was recognised that parts of each of these scenarios could play out at different times in different cities, or indeed different households. The 'real' future probably lies in some combination of these wide-ranging possibilities.

The subsequent workshop allowed these scenarios to be tested and developed in a series of facilitated groups and plenary review sessions by the attendees.

The narratives were then written up as a fuller set of contextual scenarios by Alister Wilson.

9.4 Stage 3: Scenario Testing and Assessment

The third phase tested the scenarios for robustness and credibility and included two key strands. The first involved validating questions about the scenarios which emerged from the development phase. This was done via a combination of group discussion and plenary review and response.

The second involved constructing plausible journeys across the timeframe of the scenarios, focusing on the key turning points in each narrative. This is a critical element of scenario planning. The literature points out that good scenarios 'explain how the change unfolded'. Finally, a 'plausibility and favourability' exercise was carried out in order to test, explore and validate the assumptions of participants relating to the scenario narratives.

This final workshop provided the remaining input to the full-length scenarios which can be seen in sections 4–7.

Acknowledgements

To all those participants who contributed so constructively and enthusiastically to the workshops, which ran between November 2004 and March 2005.

NOTE

1. The term 'drug' is used to signify a psychoactive substance.

Author Index

Subject Index

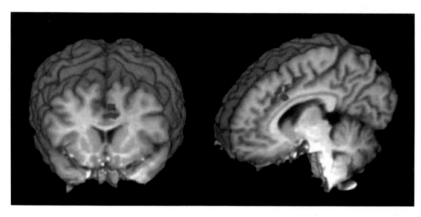

FIGURE 9.2   Reduced anterior cingulate activation observed in cocaine users relative to controls in response to commission errors on a GO/NOGO task.